# ALLERGY AND IMMUNOLOGY

## AN OTOLARYNGIC APPROACH

# ALLERGY AND IMMUNOLOGY

## AN OTOLARYNGIC APPROACH

*Editors*

### JOHN H. KROUSE, M.D., Ph.D., F.A.C.S., F.A.A.O.A.

*Professor of Otolaryngology*
*Department of Otolaryngology*
*Wayne State University*
*Detroit, Michigan*

### STEPHEN J. CHADWICK, M.D., F.A.C.S., F.A.A.O.A.

*Associate Professor of Surgery*
*Section of Otolaryngology*
*Southern Illinois University School of Medicine*
*Past President, American Academy of Otolaryngic Allergy*
*Springfield, Illinois*

### BRUCE R. GORDON, M.D., F.A.C.S., F.A.A.O.A.

*Instructor, Department of Otology and Laryngology*
*Harvard University*
*Cambridge, Massachusetts*
*Associate Surgeon, Associate Staff*
*Massachusetts Eye and Ear Infirmary*
*Boston, Massachusetts*
*Chief of Otolaryngology*
*Cape Cod Hospital*
*Hyannis, Massachusetts*

### M. JENNIFER DEREBERY, M.D., F.A.C.S., F.A.A.O.A.

*Associate*
*House Ear Clinic and House Ear Institute*
*Los Angeles, California*

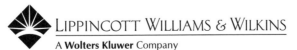

LIPPINCOTT WILLIAMS & WILKINS
A **Wolters Kluwer** Company
Philadelphia · Baltimore · New York · London
Buenos Aires · Hong Kong · Sydney · Tokyo

*Acquisitions Editor:* Jim Merritt
*Developmental Editor:* Michael Standen
*Production Editor:* Thomas Boyce
*Manufacturing Manager:* Christopher Rice
*Cover Designer:* David Levy
*Compositor:* Maryland Composition
*Printer:* Edwards Brothers

© 2002 by LIPPINCOTT WILLIAMS & WILKINS
530 Walnut Street
Philadelphia, PA 19106 USA
LWW.com

**Library of Congress Cataloging-in-Publication Data**

---

Allergy and immunology : an otolaryngic approach / editors, John H. Krouse ... [et al.].
    p. ; cm.
  Includes bibliographical references and index.
  ISBN 0-7817-2628-X
  1. Respiratory allergy. 2. Otolaryngology. 3. Otolaryngology—Immunological aspects.
I. Krouse, John H.
  [DNLM: 1. Hypersensitivity. 2. Otorhinolaryngologic Diseases. WD 300 A43285
    2001]
  RC589 .A45 2001
  616.97—dc21

                                                                    2001033873

---

Care has been taken to confirm the accuracy of the information presented and to describe generally accepted practices. However, the authors, editors, and publisher are not responsible for errors or omissions or for any consequences from application of the information in this book and make no warranty, expressed or implied, with respect to the currency, completeness, or accuracy of the contents of the publication. Application of this information in a particular situation remains the professional responsibility of the practitioner.

The authors, editors, and publisher have exerted every effort to ensure that drug selection and dosage set forth in this text are in accordance with current recommendations and practice at the time of publication. However, in view of ongoing research, changes in government regulations, and the constant flow of information relating to drug therapy and drug reactions, the reader is urged to check the package insert for each drug for any change in indications and dosage and for added warnings and precautions. This is particularly important when the recommended agent is a new or infrequently employed drug.

Some drugs and medical devices presented in this publication have Food and Drug Administration (FDA) clearance for limited use in restricted research settings. It is the responsibility of healthcare providers to ascertain the FDA status of each drug or device planned for use in their clinical practice.

10 9 8 7 6 5 4 3 2 1

# CONTENTS

# CONTRIBUTING AUTHORS

**Mark B. Abelson, M.D.** Associate Clinical Professor of Ophthalmology, Harvard Medical School, Boston; Senior Scientist, Schepens Eye Research Institute, Boston, Massachusetts

**Steven S. Ball, M.D.** Resident, Division of Otolaryngology–Head and Neck Surgery, University of North Carolina, Chapel Hill, North Carolina

**Karen I. Berliner, Ph.D.** Consultant, Clinical Studies Department, House Ear Institute, Los Angeles, California

**Joel M. Bernstein, M.D., Ph.D.** Professor of Clinical Otolaryngology and Pediatrics, Department of Otolaryngology, State University of New York at Buffalo, Buffalo, New York

**Edwyn L. Boyd, M.D., F.A.A.O.A.** Private Practice, Hoover Ear, Nose, and Throat Associates, Hoover, Alabama

**Stephen J. Chadwick, M.D., F.A.C.S., F.A.A.O.A.** Associate Professor of Surgery, Section of Otolaryngology, Southern Illinois University School of Medicine, Past President, American Academy of Otolaryngic Allergy, Springfield, Illinois

**Matthew J. Chapin, B.S.** Ophthalmic Research Associates, Inc., North Andover, Massachusetts

**M. Jennifer Derebery, M.D., F.A.C.S., F.A.A.O.A.** Associate, House Ear Clinic and House Ear Institute, Los Angeles, California

**Ivor Emanuel, M.D., F.A.A.O.A.** Affiliate, University of California Teaching Hospitals and California Pacific Medical Center, San Francisco, California

**Berrylin J. Ferguson, M.D.** Associate Professor, Department of Otolaryngology, University of Pittsburgh School of Medicine, Pittsburgh, Pennsylvania

**John A. Fornadley, M.D.** Department of Surgery, Division of Otolaryngology, Pennsylvania State University, Hershey, Pennsylvania

**W. Whitney Gabhart, N.D.** Ohio Valley Integrated Medicine, New Albany, Indiana

**Bruce R. Gordon, M.D., F.A.C.S., F.A.A.O.A.** Instructor, Department of Otology & Laryngology, Harvard University, Cambridge; Associate Surgeon, Associate Staff, Massachusetts Eye & Ear Infirmary, Boston; Chief of Otolaryngology, Cape Cod Hospital, Hyannis, Massachusetts

**Anil Gungor, M.D.** Assistant Professor of Otolaryngology, Department of Pediatric Otolaryngology, Children's Hospital of Pittsburgh, Pittsburgh, Pennsylvania

**James A. Hadley, M.D., F.A.C.S.** Department of Surgery, Division of Otolaryngology, Clinical Associate Professor of Surgery (Otolaryngology), University of Rochester Medical Center, Rochester, New York

**Richard C. Haydon III, M.D., F.A.C.S., F.A.A.O.A.** Associate Professor of Surgery, Division of Otolaryngology, Department of Surgery, University of Kentucky College of Medicine, Lexington, Kentucky

**Hueston C. King, M.D., F.A.C.S., F.A.C.A.A.I., F.A.A.O.A.** Clinical Professor, Department of Otorhinolaryngology, University of Texas Southwestern Medical Center, Dallas, Texas; Clinical Professor, Department of Otolaryngology, University of Florida College of Medicine, Gainesville, Florida

**Helen Fox Krause, M.D., F.A.C.S., F.A.A.O.A.** Department of Otolaryngology, University of Pittsburgh, Pittsburgh, Pennsylvania

**Helene J. Krouse, Ph.D., A.R.N.P., C.O.R.L.N.** Professor of Nursing, College of Nursing, Wayne State University, Detroit, Michigan

**John H. Krouse, M.D., Ph.D., F.A.C.S., F.A.A.O.A.** Professor of Otolaryngology, Department of Otolaryngology, Wayne State University, Detroit, Michigan

**Richard L. Mabry, M.D.** Clinical Professor of Otolaryngology, Department of Otolaryngology–Head and Neck Surgery, University of Texas Southwestern Medical Center, Dallas, Texas

**Alan B. McDaniel, M.D.** Ohio Valley Integrated Medicine, New Albany, Indiana

**Bradley F. Marple, M.D.**   Associate Professor of Otolaryngology, Department of Otolaryngology–Head and Neck Surgery, University of Texas Southwestern Medical Center, Dallas; Chief of Otolaryngology, Dallas Veterans Administration Hospital, Dallas, Texas

**Jeffrey J. Miller, M.D.**   Resident, Department of Otolaryngology and Communicative Sciences, Medical University of South Carolina, Charleston, South Carolina

**John David Osguthorpe, M.D.**   Professor, Department of Otolaryngology and Communicative Sciences, Medical University of South Carolina, Charleston, South Carolina

**Michael J. Parker, M.D.**   Department of Ear, Nose, and Throat, Community General Hospital, Syracuse, New York

**Kim E. Pershall, M.D., F.A.A.O.A.**   Private Practice, Lubbock, Texas

**Harold C. Pillsbury III, M.D., F.A.C.S.**   Professor and Chief, Thomas J. Dark Distinguished Professor of Surgery, Division of Otolaryngology–Head and Neck Surgery, University of North Carolina, Chapel Hill, North Carolina

**Karen Rhew, M.D.**   Assistant Professor, Department of Otolaryngology–Head and Neck Surgery, University of Colorado School of Medicine, Denver, Colorado

**Renee Z. Rinaldi, M.D.**   Associate Clinical Professor of Medicine, UCLA School of Medicine, Los Angeles, California

**Elizabeth R. Sandman, B.S.**   Clinical Research Associate, Ophthalmic Research Associates, Inc., North Andover, Massachusetts

**Richard J. Trevino, M.D.**   Private Practice, Ear, Nose, and Throat Allergy, San Jose, California

**Maria C. Veling, M.D., F.A.A.O.A.**   Assistant Professor, Division of Otolaryngology, Department of Surgery, University of Louisville School of Medicine, Louisville, Kentucky

**Michael H. Weisman, M.D.**   Professor of Medicine, Division of Rheumatology, Department of Medicine, University of California at San Diego, La Jolla; Director, Division of Rheumatology, Cedars–Sinai Medical Center, Los Angeles, California

# ACKNOWLEDGMENTS

We dedicate this book to our many teachers, colleagues, and friends who have guided our journey in the quest for knowledge. Through their support and encouragement we have worked to advance the science and practice of otolaryngic allergy and immunology. In specific, we acknowledge three of our predecessors who have exemplified the spirit of otolaryngic allergy in their research, teaching, and clinical care of patients. This text is therefore published with honor and respect to Drs. French Hansel, George Shambaugh, and James Willoughby. It is through their unwavering commitment to excellence and their compassion for those whose lives they crossed that we are able to author this book, bringing their lives and their knowledge to present and future generations of physicians. It is our hope that we have captured their spirit with both fervor and humility.

*John H. Krouse*
*Stephen J. Chadwick*
*Bruce R. Gordon*
*M. Jennifer Derebery*

I acknowledge with love my wife and partner, Helene, and my two children Beth and Daniel. They have been inspirations to me, and I share this text with them.

*John H. Krouse*

I thank Mrs. Karen Stoner, Chief Librarian of the Decatur Memorial Foundation Library, for her untiring energy and invaluable assistance with research. I thank my transcriptionists, Julie Causey and Susan Dunham, for their patience and good nature. I thank my wife Melinda and my son Nicholson for their patience and understanding. Lastly, I dedicate these words to the memory of my parents, Bernice and Charles, and my father-in-law, Gale Hedrick, all of whom departed during the writing of this textbook. They will be missed.

*Stephen J. Chadwick*

I acknowledge my teachers, Drs. Hueston King, William King, Walter Ward, Hamilton Dixon, James Willoughby, Frank Waickman, and Helen Krause. They sparked my interest in otolaryngic allergy, and helped me to learn about it. I also acknowledge my wife, Shirley Beth Gordon, and my adult children, Andrea Ellen Gordon and William Michael Gordon, who encouraged my attending meetings and conferences because they knew how important teaching was to me. Finally, I express my thanks to my co-editors and contributing authors, since they have all traveled the same road with me as students and teachers of otolaryngic allergy.

*Bruce R. Gordon*

To my husband Gregory Spahr, and daughters Alexandra and Madison, for the soccer games I missed. I also thank my friend and professional mentor, Dr. Howard P. House.

*M. Jennifer Derebery*

# PREFACE

By all indications, the interest in allergy and immunology among otolaryngologists has been steadily increasing over the past decade. There is a wide range of factors that has fueled this rapid growth: the failure of surgical interventions to cure common problems, such as rhinosinusitis and otitis media with effusion; a population that has been searching for alternatives to pharmacotherapy and surgery; a changing pattern of reimbursement among insurers; and the recognition that allergy plays a central role in the pathogenesis and treatment of many common otolaryngological disorders. As otolaryngologists have included allergy management in the routine care of their patients with otitis, laryngitis, pharyngitis, and rhinosinusitis, they have seen improved patient outcomes and increased patient satisfaction. Success breeds success, and allergy practice among otolaryngologists continues to grow and flourish.

When the authors first met to discuss this textbook in the fall of 1998, this growth was clearly evident. The American Academy of Otolaryngic Allergy had noted a steady increase in the number of members as well as an accelerating attendance at instructional courses. The number of billed procedures related to allergy testing and management was growing. Interest among residents as well as the recruitment by practices of otolaryngologists trained in allergy and immunology was rising. Not only have these trends continued in the new millennium, they have continued to escalate. One tangible measure of the impact of allergy in the current practice of otolaryngology is the fact that the American Academy of Otolaryngic Allergy has grown to be the largest of the otolaryngology subsocieties.

With a keen awareness of this accelerating interest, it was clear that there was no current, comprehensive, research-based textbook in the field of otolaryngic allergy and immunology. In 1998 we therefore set out to draft such a text, inviting the major thought leaders, teachers, researchers, and clinicians in the field to participate in writing a comprehensive volume on this growing subject. The authors were charged with two important tasks—to thoroughly review the current literature related to their topic, and to prepare a chapter that was comprehensive and grounded in research. We have been pleased at the outcome of this process, and hope that the reader will find each discussion to be pertinent, accurate, thorough, and evidence-based.

It is the purpose of this textbook to review the field of otolaryngic allergy and immunology historically, to present the science that underlies our practice, and then to discuss, in detail, those disorders that the practicing otolaryngologist will encounter on a daily basis. In addition, this book reviews related allergic disorders and their treatments, the impact of allergies on society, and alternative and complementary approaches to allergic diseases. It concludes with a discussion of future areas for investigation and research.

It was our privilege and pleasure to prepare this textbook for the use of practicing otolaryngologists and other physicians, residents, students, nurses, and other allied health personnel. We hope that the reader will find it to be a practical reference for the daily practice of allergy and immunology, as well as a thorough guide for the scientist interested in clinical and basic research. We look forward to the future evolution of this fascinating field, and to sharing with and learning from our partners in this journey.

*John H. Krouse*
*Stephen J. Chadwick*
*Bruce R. Gordon*
*M. Jennifer Derebery*

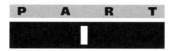

# BACKGROUND AND BASIC SCIENCES

# 1

# A HISTORY OF OTOLARYNGIC ALLERGY

## HUESTON C. KING

A chapter in history can be presented as a series of dates, most of which no one will remember, interspersed with an itemization of scientific occurrences, many of which will have little meaning outside their immediate context. The same history, on the other hand, can be a portrait of the people involved in producing the history, both as individuals and as a group, and of the ongoing events occurring at the time in the medical world, and in the world in general, which influence the progress of medicine, and otolaryngic allergy in particular. This is the story behind the history, and often makes for more interesting reading. Scientific developments are essential in providing the impetus for the evolution of a medical specialty or subspecialty, but it is the manner in which such events are perceived and applied by the people involved that channels and directs the overall tide of the specific historical course. It has been said that much of history is just gossip that has grown old gracefully. This may well be true. Documentation of the history of otolaryngic allergy is in woefully short supply. The author was present and involved in much of the history presented here, and received considerable information from others who had experienced personally or heard discussed previous aspects, but memory is fragile and, to be placed in perspective, much of the material presented is subject to the author's observation and interpretation. No apology is made for this. The goal is to place events occurring over the better part of a century in such a form that not only the events themselves, but the cause and results of these events as well as the concerns of the people involved will provide a better picture of whole evolution. If we do not learn from history, we are destined to repeat it.

## EVOLUTION OF OTOLARYNGOLOGY

Otolaryngology as a whole is a relatively small specialty, although immensely diversified. Allergy, or hypersensitivity,

although one of the most extensive influences on overall health, has occupied a relatively small nook in the practice of otolaryngology until recent years. This is to be regretted, because with today's understanding of the ramifications of allergy, a conservative estimate of 50% of otolaryngic problems can be attributed fairly directly to allergy. There can be no placing of blame for this failure on otolaryngology, however. The same laxity reigned for decades in essentially all specialties. To understand this, it must be remembered that it was not unusual as recently as the 1970s to have competent physicians describe allergy as probably "largely in the mind." (The existence of allergy was known, of course, but was largely associated with anaphylaxis and asthma.)

The medical community, then and now, has been addicted to the findings of the laboratory. Anything that cannot be produced, and reproduced, in numerical parameters is subject to question. Like most concepts, this one has its upside and its downside. The upside is that random anecdotal material, not subjected to controlled study, usually is discarded as of no value. The downside is that that same material is often the start of a study, which will never occur if the original limited observations are discarded before they can be evaluated. Demonstrations of allergic reactions on an in vivo basis, such as the Prausnitz-Kustner test reported in 1921 (1), were well established, but not of a laboratory type. Not until the identification of immunoglobulin E in the late 1960s (2) did allergy emerge as a source of interest to a wide range of different specialties, and become a political and scientific football.

All of the preceding philosophical overview is designed to set the stage for a better understanding of the actual evolution of otolaryngic allergy. Although some acceptance of allergy has its roots in ancient history, and various discoveries since have updated the acknowledgment of the condition by the medical community, specialization is largely a 20th century phenomenon. If the development of otolaryngic allergy is to be properly understood, the evolution of the specialty of otolaryngology itself needs to be reviewed.

Otolaryngology is one of the oldest recognized special-

**H. C. King:** Department of Otorhinolaryngology, University of Texas Southwestern Medical Center, Dallas, Texas.

ties, its certifying board having been founded in 1924. All this is well documented. Its parameters were limited at its inception, as they were in essentially all specialty fields, because of the limitations of medical knowledge and technology at the time. Nonetheless, it provided fine services to the community within these limitations for nearly two decades. Much less well recognized is the situation in the immediate post-World War II years. As often occurs in wartime, medicine advanced at an unprecedentedly rapid pace. There simply was not time enough to perform the extended studies on promising drugs and procedures usual in a time of peace. In addition, immediate lifesaving procedures took a prominent position in the medical hierarchy. Rarely does otolaryngology find itself involved in such procedures. (To be sure, there are exceptions, but in the overall cosmos, the exceptions are not large.) Otolaryngic allergy, and allergy in general, occupies an even smaller part of the overall picture. Allergies can certainly kill, as has been well demonstrated by anaphylaxis from drug reactions, but the vast majority are discomfort problems. Such problems the prognosticators of medicine during the war and immediate postwar period felt could wait for better times, a decision that could not be criticized, but inevitably influenced long-term medical practice.

Bearing in mind the situation of medicine in the nation in general during the immediate postwar era, the place of otolaryngology in general in the frame of things requires consideration before the place of otolaryngic allergy can be considered. At this time, subspecialization in otolaryngology was minimal, largely limited to a few groups of hardy individuals who pursued postgraduate training through courses presented by individual professors scattered over the country. Most residency programs concentrated on tonsils, adenoids, septa, mastoids, and head and neck cancer. When the author decided to go into the field, the advice from several sources was that it would be best to plan something else because the probability was that the entire specialty would be dead within a few years. Antibiotics, only recently available to the public on an adequate basis, would eliminate the problems of tonsillitis, sinusitis, and middle ear disease. General surgeons would take over the cancer surgery niche until such time as research finally eliminated the need for such procedures. Facial plastic surgery was in its infancy, with the few otolaryngologists involved in it facing a head-to-head turf battle with the general plastic surgeons, and finding themselves vastly outnumbered. The entire specialty had shrunk to the point that at a time when universal military training was required for all physicians, a full deferment was permitted to anyone accepted into a recognized otolaryngology residency anywhere in the country. The still fully active military was desperate for otolaryngologists to care for the troops and their dependents, a service needed currently, and was not finding nearly enough available. Some assistance was obtained by developing a 3-month intense specialty program in otolaryngology and making it available

to drafted family physicians (the "90-day wonders"), who were then able to handle routine problems, usually but not always serving in isolated bases. The supply of fully trained specialists and those entering training, however, was progressively shrinking. In about 1957, the Army closed all of its residencies except Walter Reed and Letterman. Various reasons were given, but the understanding of those involved at the time was that there simply were not enough residents coming into the program to keep the residencies open. As already described, the field was felt to be dying a slow death, and probably not appropriate for young men preparing for a lifetime medical career.

Then the situation abruptly changed. In 1957, the World Congress of Otolaryngology was held in Washington, DC. The magic words were "middle ear surgery." The operating microscope had arrived from Germany, reconstructive tympanoplasty was presented, stapedectomy was introduced, a variety of variations on the recently developed stapes mobilization procedure were presented, and overnight it appeared that otolaryngologists could perform ear surgery the rest of their lives without ever catching up. The response was immediate and overwhelming. From not enough residents to fill the programs, the Army suddenly found itself with a 4-year waiting list to enter a residency, and a similar situation occurred in the civilian sector. Otolaryngology, and especially otology, was to be the field of the young.

Today it seems surprising that the long-term result of this relatively massive influx of aspiring specialists of similar age could not have been foreseen. The population was growing, but not at anywhere near the same speed as the otolaryngology population. Antibiotics did, in fact, reduce the prevalence of tonsillitis and adenoiditis, and concurrently with this reduction in the disease load, tonsillectomy was considered for several years to be contraindicated, especially in the asthmatic patient, because anecdotal reports linked tonsillectomy with precipitation of asthma in the allergic patient. This was subsequently disproved, but the reduction in the surgery pool was quite real. Infectious ear disease also was reduced, although surgery was by no means eliminated. In many cases, otosclerosis was the condition that brought the new wave into otolaryngology. In the mid-1960s I heard a colleague discuss the rapidly shrinking pool of stapedectomy candidates, and wonder if the disease was being significantly reduced by universal fluoridation of water. I brought to his attention that although the population of Miami, our home city, had grown 20%, the otolaryngologist population had grown 800%. At a certain point, when drained rapidly, the surgery pool simply dries up.

Now an economic situation enters the picture. It was during this period that the incumbent President decided that supporting the development, and therefore the number, of physicians in the United States would overload the market, and market pressures would then drive down the cost of medical care. It may be said in favor of medicine that technology developed at a sufficiently rapid rate to occupy the needs of most new physicians. Nevertheless, a large mass of young physicians entered the medical workforce, especially the field of otolaryngology, over a very short period, overloading a workforce previously minimally supplied.

Otology quickly succumbed. Although a large percentage of the new arrivals expected to practice only otology, only a limited number succeeded, and most of those confined their practice to tertiary care centers. The others quickly expanded their range to general otolaryngology. Even this frequently did not meet their needs. The families of these young physicians were growing, their children needed education, and a living wage at a professional level became an item of importance. For most, it was too late to consider changing fields to enter a specialty more in its infancy. The solution was the same as that for any business in which the future appears to be limited: diversify!

Fortunately, otolaryngology offered excellent opportunities for diversification. By necessity, otolaryngologists had long been forced to care for a wide range of conditions, and to apply a variety of solutions. Most were quite competent surgeons, and fully familiar with the nose. Expansion of septal surgery into rhinoplasty was a natural step. Once cosmetic nasal surgery became a part of the otolaryngologist's armamentarium, further cosmetic surgery followed rapidly. Otolaryngologists began to perform otoplasties, face lifts, and multiple cosmetic procedures in the head and neck area. Thyroid surgery and cleft palate surgery had for a time been included in some, but by no means all, accredited residency programs. The new wave of otolaryngologists rapidly embraced these additions to the surgical menu. Endoscopy expanded from foreign body to diagnostic. The otolaryngologist had accepted diversification.

Such changes were not obtained without difficulty. As already noted, this was the period in which an attempt was being made under federal mandate to flood the country with physicians to bring costs down by market pressure. Before this action, the country's supply of physicians tended to be somewhat less than ideal, except in certain areas, and physicians were more likely to find themselves overworked than in search of patients. The shift in policy changed that situation rapidly. The physician supply outstripped the need. Supply and demand problems ensued.

Other fields than otolaryngology also were being overloaded, and facing the same competition for patients. Such specialties as plastic surgery and general surgery also were diversifying and expanding their procedure base, and did not welcome the otolaryngologist offering the same procedures. A turf battle was inevitable, and developed, especially with plastic surgery. Much of this battle continues today. Now the government is attempting to reduce the number of physicians, especially specialists. The market rarely responds well in the long run to manipulation.

Back to the otolaryngology expansion program. It has already been noted that the specialty of otolaryngology has always been one of the smaller ones, and had shrunk still further in the immediate postwar era. When the need for expansion was seen, there were few programs well enough diversified to train properly the new group of otolaryngologists in all of the now needed procedures. The solution, and the only viable solution at the time, was to take advantage of the expertise of the few experts in various aspects of the field by means of intensive courses. These were available, and often were expanded as the need arose. Although the specialty has always been small, the field has always been highly diverse, and until the overall expansion in numbers most otolaryngologists contented themselves with general otolaryngology, or developed certain aspects of expertise by means of special programs. With the expansion in numbers, a wider range of expertise was needed by a wider number of otolaryngologists, but in many cases there were not enough professors with this range of expertise to provide full training at the resident level. Again, the answer was the postgraduate course, now usually open to the resident. Because the entire field of medicine continues to expand at an exponential rate, such courses are essential to keep up with new developments, so the pattern, adopted to supply special training to physicians with special interests, and then expanded to provide needed training to all, has proved in the long run to be the most viable means of continuing to update needed knowledge.

All of this background in the changes in the field of otolaryngology in general are of importance in placing the history of otolaryngic allergy in perspective. Allergy has always been an essential part of otolaryngology. As noted, it is estimated that 50% of the problems an otolaryngologist faces are directly related to allergy. Joseph Goodale (1868–1957) provided allergy care to his patients as an otolaryngologist well before the specialty was established as such (3). As has already been mentioned, however, it was not unusual as recently as the 1960s to have the public, and much of the medical community, describe allergy as "probably mostly in the mind." It is not surprising, therefore, that most otolaryngologists, while paying lip service to the importance of allergy in the practice, paid little attention to the actual condition in patients. The field was surgical, and surgery was the answer. If the problem could not be surgically corrected, it should be in someone else's province. There were always a few physicians who recognized the importance of allergy in otolaryngology and both practiced and taught it to those concerned enough to ask. In the early days, these were accepted as valuable, if somewhat eccentric, experts in a field that certainly was not oversupplied with physicians, and who could provide the needed expertise to those who, for one reason or another, chose to include this aspect of otolaryngology in their patient care program. The evolution of this group, and the expansion to the current state of otolaryngic allergy, is to be seen in the context of the changes in otolaryngology in general.

## The Specialty Dilemma

First, as already noted, otolaryngologists are by training surgeons. Allergy is not a surgical specialty. In spite of this basic bias in training, it does not usually take the otolaryngologist long to find out that in most cases he will be expected to act as a primary care physician for all that falls within his physical area. This includes medicine, surgery, allergy, and the multitude of special conditions peculiar to the ear, nose, and throat. A dichotomy already is present. The surgeon is trained to act on results (the "Surgical Personality"). If it seems to work, or if someone has reported good results from using the procedure, try it. The internist, also by training, needs to know the underlying mechanisms (the "Medical Personality"). The surgeon, therefore, is prone to forge ahead while the internist studies the ramifications of an approach. The two personalities are not by nature interchangeable. Whether the training produces the personality or the personality leads to the training is a moot question. The difference is there, and is at the heart of most of the divisiveness seen in the field of allergy over the succeeding decades, and is still present in the field today. The otolaryngic allergist, with the surgical personality, simply does not think along the same lines as the medically trained general allergist.

## EVOLUTION OF OTOLARYNGIC ALLERGY

Over most of the 19th century, and much of the early part of the 20th century, most medicine was practiced by observation, implications, and extrapolation. Laboratory confirmation was limited in most fields. The finest professors were those whose acute powers of observation and proper application of the findings were supported by astute history taking and detailed physical examination. Time was not of the essence, and much information could be derived by allowing the patient to go into detail in describing the presenting problem. (This, of course, could seriously strain the patience of the physician, but if allowed to proceed often resulted in providing the answer without extensive laboratory testing.) Nowhere more than in allergy is such a situation of greater importance. The critical aspect of allergy is individuality, which in essence means that statistics are of little value. Lucretius put it succinctly in "One man's meat is another man's poison." Establishing the percentage of patients sensitive to peanuts may be of general value, but it does not assist the physician caring for the peanut-sensitive patient in any way. The same can be said for the investigation of inhalant allergies, although to a lesser degree. The value of knowing blooming seasons can be of help, but in the final evaluation it is the specific exposure of the individual patient that must be determined to provide the necessary information properly to test and treat. Generalized statistics do not do this. Only a detailed patient history, coupled with appropriate tests or challenges, can elicit this information.

Inevitably, this leads to considerable experimentation, and experimentation was the byword for much of the first half of the 20th century. This was particularly true in allergy. Although immunotherapy had been introduced by Leonard Noon in 1911 (4), his concept, as a disciple of Jenner, was that allergy was produced by toxins, which could be neutralized by antitoxins as in smallpox. The concept was wrong, but the treatment worked. This philosophy of concept and clinical trial was particularly appealing to the surgically trained physician becoming interested in allergy, and resulted in a wide range of approaches to the allergy field, as well as other conditions that might be considered allergy related. (It must be remembered that medicine in general, and allergy in particular, was of necessity practiced more on an empirical than a controlled scientific basis.)

The general allergy field was not overcrowded at that time, and the otolaryngic allergy group was extremely small, allowing divergent growth with few close comparisons of care procedures, and minimal competition. Observation of patient results led to experimentation in ways to improve these results, and this was particularly true of the relatively impatient otolaryngic allergist. (The precursor of the "outcome results" studies in vogue today.) Because the mechanism behind the allergic reaction still was not understood, clinical results were the only realistic way to proceed, either for the general allergist or the otolaryngic allergist. The difference was that the otolaryngic allergist was quite ready and motivated to try applying any procedure that seemed effective, even in a limited number of cases, to other difficult problems the solution to which was unsatisfactory when approaches currently in general use were applied.

Many of the approaches used were well outside the range of "community standards," as considered today. Many worked, some regularly, some on occasion. Until the late 1960s and early 1970s, this had little effect on the progression of the field. To be sure, the general allergists frequently referred to the otolaryngic group as "cultists," and decried their procedures, but patients impatient with the results of conventional care continued to migrate to the otolaryngic allergist. The otolaryngic allergy group remained small, but dedicated. Their results were encouraging enough to produce a steady flow of patients. Although locally threatening to the establishment on occasion when success was achieved in the face of previous failures, the total effect was not great enough to be a problem, and therefore was largely ignored. The situation nationally, however, was about to change.

## The Personalities Involved

To follow the development of otolaryngic allergy from this point on, it is necessary to depart from the overall picture of otolaryngic allergy in the medical community, to backtrack a bit, and to focus on the specific development of the field from its inception. Any small field, and especially one divergent from its specialty, is a distillate of personalities and their viewpoints. A variety of personalities has produced the field of otolaryngic allergy, and all have had their influences. Not all, of course, can be recorded here. Seeing how the field evolved, however, allows one to have a better picture of the way that the field has achieved its current niche in the medical community.

Allergy, as previously noted, has been recognized since ancient times. Medicine in general has the same background in ancient history. Specialization, however, is a newer phenomenon. At what point the specialist began to emerge from the ranks of general medicine is not clear. Otolaryngology as a specialty, however, is over a century old. Even in the early days it must have been recognized that some influence (today recognized as allergy) was having a major effect on treatment results. As already mentioned, Joseph Goodale, an otolaryngologist of the last century, was aware of the effects of allergy and commented on them in his writings. No attempt to identify allergy as a major cause of otolaryngic problems occurred until appreciably later, however.

In 1921, French Hansel, the otolaryngologist generally recognized as the father of otolaryngic allergy, became interested in allergy when, in 1921, as a Fellow under H. I. Lillie at Mayo Clinic, he became involved in preparing a thesis on vasomotor rhinitis, a condition well recognized as within the province of the otolaryngologist. After studying 100 cases, he concluded that these were actually examples of allergy because skin tests for allergy were positive. After his fellowship, Dr. Hansel joined the Department of Otolaryngology at Washington University of St. Louis in 1923, and, influenced by the results of his previous study, began analyzing tissue specimens from sinus surgery cases. He noted marked infiltration of eosinophils and plasma cells, strongly suggesting allergy. This further propelled his interest, and in the absence of the strong turf battle later to develop, he was given a position as a consultant to the general Allergy Department at Washington University of St. Louis. As noted earlier, this was a period in which otolaryngology, although well established, provided most of its diversification through short-term courses or arranged visits to one of the few recognized experts in a limited aspect of the field. Allergy was no exception, and during his stay at Washington University of St. Louis, Dr. Hansel was visited by several practitioners, one of whom was Howard House, destined to become one of the country's finest otologists. Dr. House immediately recognized the importance of allergy in the field, and today the House Clinic provides extensive investigation and care in allergy.

During his stay at Washington University in St. Louis, Dr. Hansel produced many contributions to the literature, including definitive textbooks on allergy for the otolaryngologist (5). The incoming Dean of the Department of Otolaryngology allowed Dr. Hansel to establish an allergy clinic as a part of the department, providing access to information on allergy to a much wider range of otolaryngologists. Although on a small scale compared with the overall field of medicine, this access provided the first inroad to establishing otolaryngic allergy as a true medical field.

Over the years, a large group of students had studied with Dr. Hansel, and in 1941 members of this group felt that a recognized society should be established to provide a regular meeting ground and allow interchange of information on a regular basis. This society was chartered in 1941, with 40 members, as the American Society of Ophthalmological and Otolaryngological Allergy (ASOOA), and the first meeting was held in St. Louis in 1942. World War II then interfered with further meetings, and the next meeting was held in 1947. By this time the membership had increased to 78, not a large group in proportion to other medical societies. The membership roster, however, contained such universally recognized names in otolaryngology as Victor Goodhill, Howard House, George Shambaugh, Eugene Derlacki, Russell Williams, and Sam Sanders.

It was fortunate that the national society had been established independently, because in 1944 L. W. Dean retired from Washington University and his successor, Theo Walsh, had little interest in allergy and closed the otolaryngic allergy clinic. Dr. Hansel, as a result, retired from the department, and encouraged by Dr. W. E. Owen, established the Hansel Foundation to provide for a continuation of the courses he had directed while in the university. Sixty students attended the first course, presented in St. Louis in 1948. The enrollment represented a far cry from today's course attendance, but demonstrated interest even at a time when the field of otolaryngology as a whole was undergoing a distinct decline.

French Hansel made certain unique advances in the field of allergy, which first separated otolaryngic allergy from general allergy. The first and most definitive of these was the concept of titration, or quantitative evaluation of allergic sensitivity in both testing and treatment. Although the established concept of scratch and prick testing presented by Dr. Leonard Noon had already been modified to some degree to provide some quantification by conjunctival sac testing (the "Noon Unit"), and further quantified by Dr. R. Cook, the quantified approach was not in general use even by a group. It remained for Dr. Hansel to note that high doses of antigen tended to produce adverse reactions, that smaller doses relieved symptoms without as great a risk, and that such variation could be made antigen by antigen. This resulted in the development of "serial endpoint titration," today known as *skin endpoint titration*. Dr. Hansel used a 1:10 dilution of extract both for testing and treatment, individually testing each appropriate antigen, and treating to a level of symptom relief. This format was in use by Dr. Hansel's students until modified by Dr. Herbert Rinkel some years later.

If French Hansel was the father of otolaryngic allergy, surely the title of the sustaining force in the field belongs to a student of Hansel's, Herbert Rinkel. Dr. Rinkel was trained in internal medicine rather than in otolaryngology, but became more identified with the format of otolaryngic allergy than any other practitioner, including French Hansel. Only 3 years younger than Hansel, Dr. Rinkel became affiliated with Balyeat's Clinic in Oklahoma City after his training, and while there developed a pronounced interest in allergy, especially in the concept of cyclic food allergy, which he developed largely through astute observation. He helped many patients through dietary manipulation alone, but never revealed his results to Balyeat because of a developing professional conflict that eventually led to a dissolution of the relationship, with a clause preventing Dr. Rinkel from practicing in any state contiguous to Oklahoma In many aspects of medicine, territorialism was strong during this period. Financial issues cannot have been a major concern in producing a clause involving not one but a group of states—only prestige.

Banned from Oklahoma, and with some financial problems, Dr. Rinkel went into practice in Kansas City with an old medical school colleague, Dr. Ben Withers. Dr. Zeller from Chicago was studying with Dr. Withers at the time, and he and Dr. Rinkel worked out an agreement whereby Dr. Rinkel would teach Dr. Zeller allergy for the sum of $500. This aided Dr. Rinkel's situation, and became the start of a lifelong friendship. Although Dr. Rinkel started his own practice in 1936, he and Dr. Zeller remained in close contact. In developing his practice, Dr. Rinkel expanded his studies on the benefits of quantification in the diagnosis and treatment of allergy, and revised his previous concepts borrowed from Dr. Hansel on using a 1:10 dilution format in testing and treating, noting difficulty in providing reliable repetition of tests and a tendency toward adverse reactions at higher dilutions. After several trials, he settled on a 1:5 dilution format for testing and treatment, which provided better reliability while retaining most of the decimal format familiar to all physicians (6).

Dr. Theron Randolph from Chicago visited Dr. Rinkel in 1942 and 1943, and became interested not only in the titration format but in the concepts of cyclic food allergy that Dr. Rinkel had developed while working with Balyeat. Working in conjunction, largely with regular correspondence, Rinkel, Randolph, and Zeller produced a landmark book on food allergy, published in 1951 (7). Rinkel's work was becoming known, both through publications and courses. A series of visits to Texas resulted in the formation of another group, later to become the Pan American Allergy Society. With this group and the ASOOA, organization of otolaryngic allergy was on its way.

It has been noted that personalities figure strongly in the development of any new, and especially a limited field. Both of the primary figures in the development of otolaryngic allergy to this point were described as unique personalities.

French Hansel was a strong individual with an inquiring mind, unwilling to abandon a project in which he believed even when pursuing such a project might compromise his position in his chosen field. Determination and persistence were bywords. He loved to teach, as evidenced by the courses he gave and his writings; however, he often had difficulty expressing himself, especially in public. His writings were erudite, but tended to be extremely detailed and convoluted. It was said of him that his best material was presented in the local bar after hours. Herbert Rinkel has been described as a brilliant and exciting teacher. In addition to his highly organized programs, he was a remarkably astute observer, and everyone fortunate enough to study under him has a wealth of stories about his observations and interpretations. Although he had minimal scientific equipment with which to substantiate his observations, little of what he discovered has since been disproved. On the personal side, he had his foibles. He is reported never to have been willing to drive an automobile, but used taxis until essentially every taxi driver in Kansas City knew him. While a clear and well organized teacher, he related better to his students on a one-on-one basis than when lecturing. It was frequently said of Herbert Rinkel that more was learned from him in the men's room than in the lecture hall. (Parenthetically, much the same may be said regarding the coffee breaks scheduled in today's teaching courses. Individual questions are clarified at those times on a one-on-one basis. May they never be eliminated!)

From the earliest part of this discussion, it has been noted that otolaryngic allergy grew apart from conventional allergy very early in the development of each field. It has been said by those unfamiliar with the principles involved that there are two different schools of thought on allergy. This is not, and has never been the case. The same principles are espoused by both approaches without exception. What has differed is the way in which such approaches are handled. The conventional allergy group approached diagnosis and treatment as a scientific study, whereas the otolaryngic allergy group approached the same problem as a challenge to produce a response. As a result, most of the early practices in otolaryngic allergy have no laboratory-based scientific support, but have been practiced and taught on the basis of clinical response only. This approach has been the basis of the charge of "cultism" in otolaryngic allergy. Before considering this, it should be remembered that only in the last three decades has laboratory evidence been available to support conventional allergy treatment, and that the otolaryngic allergists were far more ready to take advantage of the newly available material than were the competition. Over the years, much of medicine has been pioneered by physicians willing to take a leap of faith before the underlying mechanisms had been confirmed, and had such a leap not been taken, confirmation would never have been made because the incentive would not have been present.

## OTOLARYNGIC ALLERGY 50 YEARS AGO

### Inhalant Allergy

Let us take a look at the otolaryngic allergy procedures being taught, and therefore presumably in reasonably wide use, during the late 1960s. Inhalant allergy was fairly well defined, with full botanical evaluation of various parts of the country identified, although it was discovered in short order that many published botanical maps were decades out of date, not having been checked by botanists over a prolonged period. Still, the allergist had something with which to work, and allowing for cross-reactivity, a reasonably good result could be expected. Using the material available, and supplementing this information by personal observation, that is, visually checking the allergenic inhalants actually found in the area (strongly encouraged but rarely applied), the treating allergist could hope to select appropriate allergens with which to test the patient. The testing would then be performed using intradermal injections, 1:5 serial dilutions from a 1:20 concentrate, of the antigens suspected. Testing would be started with a very weak solution, usually a #10 strength by serial dilution (which amounts to roughly 1:2 billion.) and advanced progressively until a positive response was seen. A positive progressive reaction identified in this manner would be used to determine most of the offending pollens and molds, as well as the degree of sensitivity. A treatment mix could then be made, adjusting the concentrations on the basis of the test findings, and progressive injections could be administered to a level of symptomatic relief. Treatment was then to be held at that level for an indefinite time.

This approach, although successful in providing relief of symptoms for a large percentage of patients, had several disadvantages. First, a 1:2 billion dilution represented an allergen strength little better than that of water. This should not have been a problem because the testing was carried out with progressively stronger dilutions until a positive response was seen. However, a problem surfaced in this testing format that was not immediately recognized. Certain patients demonstrated a positive skin reaction at the #10 dilution level. Various bizarre whealing responses were seen and recognized, which are discussed elsewhere, but the critical aberrant response was the positive reaction at impossibly weak dilutions. This response led to the application of progressively weaker dilutions, until there were patients identified as frequently having positive responses at the #14 dilution level, a ratio of better than 1:1 trillion (8). Immunotherapy at this level could not be reasonably expected to alter the immune response in any way. Treatment at this level was used on occasion, however, and opened the way for a major political battle at a later date. This is discussed later.

The second problem had to do with misinterpretation of certain of Dr. Rinkel's teaching tenets. Rinkel clearly stated in his published work that the testing format he taught should be used only to determine a degree of sensitivity and a safe point at which to introduce immunotherapy. He never stated that the testing format could be used to determine the point at which treatment advancement should be terminated. However, for some reason, between the formation of the skin endpoint titration approach and the later courses presented in the early 1960s, the concept developed that treatment should be fixed at a 0.5-mL dose of the endpoint dilution unless subsequent testing determined a change in endpoint. How this misconception arose is a matter of conjecture. The only explanation currently suspected is that although Dr. Rinkel specifically stated that the testing determined only a safe starting point, and thereafter treatment should be carried out on a clinical basis, concurrently with this advice (and apparently as an aside), he commented that most of his patients in the Kansas City area endpointed at approximately a #2 to #3 dilution. This evidently was taken by some of those studying with him, and later undertaking to continue his programs, as indicating that this dose should be considered an arbitrary maintenance dose. No one seems to know how the misconception developed. This concept, however, contributed to the developing confusion that was seriously to hamper the quantitative approach during later years.

### Food Allergy

Food sensitivity had never been seriously approached by the general allergist. Anaphylactic responses were well recognized, and lip service was paid to the fact that there were many other aspects of food sensitivity, but because there was no objective means of identifying offending foods other than skin testing, which could reliably identify only type I reactions, much of the rest of food sensitivity was either ignored or relegated to the realm of "probably psychosomatic." The otolaryngic allergist, on the other hand, had been seriously interested in the effects of food on the body since the earliest stage of allergy evaluation. Dr. Rinkel began investigation into food sensitivity in the late 1930s. His book with Randolph and Zeller has already been noted. It was evident to the early observers, alerted to the ramifications of allergy, that food sensitivity was capable of producing a far wider range of reactions than was inhalant allergy. Although recognized as a major culprit, identifying offending foods proved to be a major problem. The only available test was elimination and challenge, which raised the immediate question of how long to eliminate and how to challenge. An immediate type of sensitivity caused no difficulty; even the patient was easily able to provide the information as to what food had been eaten minutes or hours before the allergic event took place. Keen observers, however, quickly noted that this type of reaction was relatively rare in proportion to the number of patients with chronic complaints difficult to attribute to obvious causes. (It must be remembered that this was a period in the evolution of medicine in which observation and history taking far outstripped laboratory studies in providing the information necessary to form a diagnosis.) It became evident to the allergist that the inhalant allergic patient had a basically compromised immune system, and was more likely than the immunologically normal patient to demonstrate food allergies. This was by no means a clear-cut division, but the concern alerted the physician already concerned with inhalant allergy to pay closer attention to the possibility of accompanying food problems.

Once recognized, it became incumbent on the treating physician to make every effort to identify the offending food and either treat of eliminate the problem. Little was known of immunology at this time, and patterns of sensitization depended more on clinical observation than upon laboratory diagnosis. Both the general allergists and the otolaryngic allergists were quick to divide food allergy into "fixed" and "cyclic" types. The "fixed" type (now known to be IgE mediated) was easy to identify owing to its predictable occurrence whenever the food was eaten, even in extremely small quantities, and even when the exposures were years apart. The "cyclic" type presented the greater problem. This type of sensitivity was obviously an entity, but one quite difficult to identify. Most general allergists chose to avoid dealing with this problem. The otolaryngic allergist, on the other hand, viewed cyclic food allergy as a challenge and immediately began to seek means of isolating the offenders. With no laboratory help, and an almost infinite range of symptoms attributable to foods, this was not an easy undertaking.

The gold standard of cyclic food testing, then and now, has been elimination and challenge. The difficulty with this format has always been logistics; an incumbent head of the American College of Allergy, Asthma, and Immunology (ACAAI) Committee on Food and Chemical Sensitivity commented in an introductory address to a seminar that "elimination and challenge was the gold standard of food testing, and was logistically impossible to perform accurately" (9).

Before the 1960s, the otolaryngic allergists had determined by trial and error that a 4-day elimination of a suspect food followed by a vigorous challenge on the fifth day was capable of producing the strongest and most definitive reaction, causing both strong symptoms and producing the specific symptoms due to the food in question. Today, the antigen–antibody ratio induced by this elimination and challenge explains the results, but in the 1960s this was not a known or even considered explanation. The test was the result of observation, and the results confirmed the test's validity.

Unfortunately, then as now, the described elimination and challenge, or oral challenge food test, was prohibitively time consuming if a number of foods were to be tested. Once a positive reaction appeared, no more challenges could

be performed until the symptoms produced by the positive challenge had cleared. This would be at least a matter of days, making one challenge a week a likely pattern. An attempt always was made to control the pattern by challenging foods less likely to be positive first, but the fact of the matter was that the patient was more concerned with the probably positive foods. A better form of screening was needed. Although Dr. Rinkel discussed other forms of food testing, it appears that Dr. Carleton Lee was truly the founder of the provocative food test (10). (Since Drs. Rinkel, Lee, Willoughby, Williams, and several other primary investigators taught and studied together, it often is difficult to identify one as the sole originator of a procedure.) At any rate, by the mid-1960s, the provocative-neutralization test was taught in all otolaryngic allergy courses. The test was the end result of various experiments, and never was fully established as a single entity. It appears that the initial approach was an attempt to apply the serial dilution inhalant pattern to food testing. This was not successful, in all probability because of the fact that all inhalant allergies use one immunologic pathway, whereas food sensitivity uses a variety of pathways. During the experiments, however, it was noted that a reasonably strong injection of a food extract, delivered either intradermally or subcutaneously, usually would induce the reactions attributable to consuming the food. It also was noted that a less concentrated injection of the food extract would eliminate the reactions induced by the stronger extract. No explanation was available for this phenomenon. Many corollaries to this pattern were later described, but these were less clear-cut. The format taught in the 1960s, however, included the ability to identify a cyclic food sensitivity by provocation-neutralization testing, and if the patient was unable to eliminate the food because of its widespread use, the regular use of a neutralization injection of the food extract would allow the patient to eat the food within limits without experiencing adverse reactions.

Provocation and neutralization was taught as a standard in all otolaryngic allergy courses. Certain difficulties were experienced, however. First, there was widespread disagreement over a proper way in which to provoke and to neutralize. Because the test had evolved from the oral challenge, this is perhaps not surprising. Some practitioners felt that the only correct way to apply the test was by subcutaneous injection of the stronger (provoking) dose of the food extract, and that the production of symptoms was the only reliable indication of sensitivity. Other practitioners used intradermal injections of the extract and depended on reading the whealing reaction on the skin. Some performed both provocation and neutralization by presenting the extract sublingually. Some investigators started at the highest dilution of the antigen prepared by the 1:5 format, a #1 dilution, and progressed to weaker dilutions if a positive response occurred. Others started with a #2 or #3 dilution, and if there was no response, tried the next higher dose as a "kicker," thereafter progressing serially to weaker doses seeking a neutralizing dose. Some based the neutralizing dose purely on symptom relief, whereas others looked for a loss of the whealing response. Some depended almost entirely on the production of the symptoms being investigated, whereas others described a wide variety of symptoms presumed to indicate an overdose or underdose of extract in performing the test. Dr. Lee strongly believed that an underdose produced more symptoms than an overdose, and that if the serial doses were continued past the point of neutralization, severe reactions might ensue. Other investigators disagreed.

As one with extensive personal experience in the use of provocation and neutralization over a number of years, the author noted approximately a 65% to 70% success ratio by using this approach, and most others agreed. The most surprising aspect of the procedure was that there did not appear to be any cumulative effect in the total amount of extract used in testing. Provoking doses followed by neutralizing doses could be alternated repeatedly, and the same results occurred each time the procedure was performed.

## Extrapolation of Provocation and Neutralization

Although the biologic mechanisms underlying the provocative test and treatment were unknown at the time, and still remain unsatisfactorily explained, the degree of success in the face of no other practical approach to food sensitivity inspired the aggressive "surgical" nature of the otolaryngic allergist to try applying the approach to other problems. Dr. Dor Brown in Texas began using the same method with viral vaccines to combat the symptoms of flu, and Dr. Joe Miller of Mobile used similar viral vaccines to combat the effects of herpes zoster. Again, there was a significant degree of success, although somewhat less than that seen in food sensitivity. It was not a great leap from this to using hormonal extracts to influence menstrual problems from irregularity to premenstrual syndrome. Again, there was a significant degree of success, and the approach gained converts. The teaching and practice of provocation and neutralization were universal in the otolaryngic allergy community during the 1960s and 1970s.

Other procedures were relatively unique to the otolaryngic allergy community at this time. Black's cytotoxic test for food allergy had been modified by William and Marian Bryan (11), and was accepted although not in wide use. It was generally agreed that the principle had utility, but the test had too many variables and too much subjectivity to become a standard of practice. Those who did use the test in practice primarily used it as a screening procedure from which to select foods to be tested by whatever procedure they preferred. Cytotoxic testing required the services of a good clinical pathologist. It was generally agreed that someone familiar with sperm counts was the best cytotoxic interpreter.

On the inhalant side, one of the greatest and frequently least appreciated advantages of skin endpoint titration was that the patient involved served as a standard for determining sensitivity. The titration format seen on the patient's arm provided a measurement of antigen strength and patient sensitivity independent of the antigen strength reported by the source of supply. This could be of major value because the variability between different suppliers at this time often was quite significant. It also allowed for the office preparation of extracts not available commercially. Although few practitioners would voluntarily prepare many of the extracts they used, there were times when a critical allergen simply was not commercially available. This usually represented a lack of demand. The otolaryngic allergy field was small, and if the region was somewhat isolated, there were times when the demand was not enough for the commercial laboratories to produce the vaccine needed. Kits were available to sterilize and prepare the vaccine, and were used effectively, even by the author, when needed.

There also were innovators in the field of inhalant allergy testing. It was known, for example, that pine pollen was minimally sensitizing, but that the pine turpene released by the pine needles in the country's extensive pine forests was quite capable of producing pronounced respiratory symptoms. One innovator, Dr. Ed Binkley, took his van into the forest, reversed his air conditioner fan to draw air into the van, passed the turpene laden air through a solution of cocoglycerine and thereby produced a turpene antigen supply. This was filtered and used in titration in the same manner as a commercial antigen, with satisfactory results. Although no laboratory measurement of the vaccine strength was available, the arm titration provided the measurement needed and a safe starting point for therapy.

It is easy to see that during the late 1950s and 1960s, the field of medicine was far different from that of today. Malpractice suits were practically unheard of, third-party payment was limited to a few insurance companies, Medicare had come into existence only in the early 1960s, and those patients unable to afford medical care were treated through charity clinics and, if hospitalized, placed on charity wards. Here, they usually received the same medical care as the paying patient, although with less personal contact. (As an aside, the author has yet to recall a single patient refused medical care during this era because of lack of funds.) With the lack of outside pressure, innovation was common. The procedures described demonstrate this clearly. Before the reader becomes aghast at the variety of treatment protocols in use at the time, and cannot understand the lack of serious side reactions, it should be remembered that extremely small amounts of antigen were used in all of these procedures. Serial dilution titration, used in the format described, used appreciably less antigen than is in general use today. Even the innovative procedures such as viral treatment and hormonal treatment used far less material in a total treatment format than would have been used in a single therapeutic injection for conventional purposes. The goal of these procedures was to stimulate the patient's immune system in some way to combat the problem. Although the method by which the patient's immune system reacted was not understood, this was not considered to be a deterrent. The goal was results, and if these seemed to be forthcoming, the treatment was pursued with enthusiasm.

## Early Education in Otolaryngic Allergy

During this period, an aspect of fiefdom was prevalent in much of the medical community. Unlike today, when discoveries are enthusiastically shared with the world (partially at least to have them credited to the original discoverer), during this period there was a tendency on the part of a successful physician who had developed a technique to capitalize on it by establishing himself as the guru of the procedure. To be sure, courses were taught to students interested in the procedures, but these students were largely expected to use the procedure as taught, and in most cases truly to become a disciple of the guru doing the teaching. Few of these professors accepted the findings of others as worthy, and possibly superior in some ways to the procedure they espoused. This was true not only of allergy, but of otology, facial plastic surgery, and much of otolaryngology. This was not truly surprising, because otolaryngology was just emerging from its leanest years and the exploding group of new physicians had not had time to develop enough expertise to compete with the few established experts in specific parts of the field. These scattered sources of true expertise forced the young physician determined to become proficient in many or all aspects of otolaryngology to pursue the available intensive specialty courses with vigor. The field had expanded faster than the supply of professors, and the average residency was not equipped to cope with all of the advances. This was to change.

Although certain other aspects of otolaryngology were taught in a variety of venues, otolaryngic allergy truly evolved from a single source. This field was the offspring of French Hansel, and subsequently Herbert Rinkel. While Dr. Rinkel was alive, his teaching provided the basic material needed by the aspiring young otolaryngic allergist to practice the field successfully. Unlike many of his counterparts in the surgical field, Dr. Rinkel was constantly inquiring, constantly observing, and making every attempt to improve and refine the techniques in use. Had Dr. Rinkel lived, most of the procedures probably would have greatly changed with time and medical progress, but unfortunately his life was cut short by cancer in 1963, at the age of 67. His courses lived on, but a strong tendency grew to revere Dr. Rinkel as almost a prophet, and maintain his teaching virtually unchanged, which is highly unlikely to have been the case in Dr. Rinkel's own hands.

Three major teaching courses evolved from Rinkel's own course. It has been reported that Dr. Rinkel charged the new course directors with using provocation and neutralization in different ways to see whether one was superior, but this has not been confirmed. That the courses would have left Dr. Rinkel's supervision had Rinkel lived is unlikely, but with his death three separate courses came into being.

One course, which superficially appeared to be two separate courses, for all intents and purposes was a single course presented by two directors in different locales but with the same faculty. This course was presented in Kansas City by Dr. James Willoughby, who had inherited Dr. Rinkel's practice, every other year, and on the alternate year essentially the same course was presented by Dr. Russell Williams, either at Jackson Hole, Wyoming, or at his base in Cheyenne, Wyoming. The faculty was the same, and the directors shared much of the load in both locations. There was no significant difference in subjects, and those taught were essentially pure Rinkel. The second course was presented in Memphis, Tennessee by Dr. Sam Sanders. This course was an annual one, and taught essentially the same material but with a slightly different approach. The third course was given by Dr. Dor Brown in Dallas, Texas.

As was the case among many professors of the day, much ego was involved. Dr. Willoughby was not an otolaryngologist, and Dr. Sanders would not allow a nonotolaryngologist at his courses, despite the fact that Dr. Willoughby had succeeded to Dr. Rinkel's practice. As would be expected, little interchange between the courses occurred. Dr. Brown's course was independent, and evidenced little contact with the other teaching programs, although much of the same material was covered. Throughout the 1960s these programs were the source of training for all aspiring otolaryngic allergists.

With such limited sources of training, it may well be asked why the aspiring otolaryngic allergist did not study with the general allergists. This has been a source of contention since the early days of allergy care in this century. As described early in the chapter, there is a basic difference in personality between surgeons and internists, and this difference led from the first recognition of allergy and Dr. Noon's immunotherapy to different approaches to the problem. It takes only a brief look at the procedures in use in the 1950s and 1960s by the otolaryngic allergist to realize that few internists, geared to investigating underlying principles, would accept such a trial-and-error approach. Actually, over the years before the formation of the American Board of Allergy and Immunology, a Conjoint Board of Internal Medicine and Pediatrics in 1971, four attempts were made to form a primary board of allergy, using the prescribed format of the American Board of Medical Specialties. This effort started in1943. All four attempts failed, and finally, in frustration, the American Board of Allergy and Immunology was formed. This organization was accepted by the American Medical Association (AMA), but instructed never to represent itself as a primary board. This mandate, however, was largely ignored. Regardless of the cause, the two disciplines steadily grew farther and farther apart, and at times became quite rancorous. This was of little concern to the otolaryngic allergist during the early decades because there was little external pressure and the patients were happy. Although the otolaryngic allergist was frequently criticized by the general allergist during this period, and often referred to as a cultist, there was little serious concern because the field of otolaryngic allergy was not large enough to be a threat. Although the general allergy group was not large, it was far larger than the small group of otolaryngologists practicing their approach to care.

The situation began to change when the rapidly growing group of young otolaryngologists entering the field under the stimulation of ear surgery found themselves short on patients and in need of diversification. Facial plastic surgery had already become a burgeoning field, and turf battles were raging between the otolaryngic facial plastic surgeon and the general plastic surgeon. To add to the problem, Medicare had come into existence, and other major medical insurance companies were expanding exponentially to cover those not under Medicare. Much of the plastic surgery battle was being waged over what procedures were eligible for insurance coverage. This could be solved by a delineation of procedures considered essential and subject to coverage, but a fine point was raised by proper definition of procedures. These could be varied to accomplish some degree of coverage.

About this time, the author was serving as a claims representative for the major insurance carrier in the state of Florida. Certain procedures were brought up for claims consideration, specifically some of the procedures practiced by the otolaryngic allergist. The procedures were explained satisfactorily on a local level, but decision on payment was referred to the home office, and in turn to the precursor of the Health Care Financing Administration (HCFA). Without any real investigation or literature search, the person in charge, an orthopedist, telephoned some of the local allergists and was told that the physicians practicing these procedures were "a bunch of cultists, and shouldn't be paid." (This was all confirmed in person.) The ramifications of this decision extended beyond simple payment, because during this time malpractice claims were appearing, and the basis of most of these claims was that the procedures in question were "not within the standard of the community." If claims were to be denied under these terms, it would almost predictably follow that suits would appear.

At this time, 1976, I also was serving as a relatively new member of the Council of the American Academy of Otolaryngic Allergy (AAOA). I received my first assignment: find out why these procedures were challenged in the first place, and get it taken care of. Based on the factors described previously, the importance of this decision should be evident.

What first appeared to be a designed attack in the devel-

oping turf battle between the general and otolaryngic allergists turned out actually to represent only the appearance on insurance claims of procedures of which the company, and HCFA, had never heard. Investigation quickly produced the fact that the key difficulty was that these procedures did not appear in Current Procedural Terminology-4 (CPT-4). As far as the insurance companies were concerned, anything not in CPT-4 did not exist. When I brought this information to the AAOA president, he asked, "What's CPT-4?" This gives an idea of the isolation of an entire school of practice at the time.

## Otolaryngic Allergy and Politics

My position in this situation quickly became apparent. I was one of those in the earliest ranks of the explosion into the otolaryngology field, and had taken and taught facial plastic surgery courses before enough otolaryngologists were practicing the procedures to present a serious threat to the general plastic surgeons. To be sure, the general plastic surgeons resented any intrusion into what they considered their field, but no significant concern existed. Then the ranks of the facial plastic surgeon began to expand rapidly, for reasons already discussed. The general plastic surgeons used a variety of approaches to limit the advances of the facial plastic surgeon, including resistance to any form of insurance coverage, protests that the facial plastic surgeons were not Board certified, attempts to limit hospital privileges, and other avenues if locally available. When the same group of neophyte otolaryngologists began to enter the allergy field, partly because of interest (allergy directly affects 50% of otolaryngology problems), and partly because of the necessity to diversify for economic reasons, much the same tactics were undertaken by the general allergist. Your author, previously exposed to the plastic surgery battles, was able to anticipate many of the approaches in advance. The two largest concerns, however, were (a) the procedures were not listed in CPT-4, and (b) the practitioners were not certified by the American Board of Allergy and Immunology. (Never mind that this board was not a primary board, but a conjoint board of other specialties, in much the same category as gastroenterology or nephrology. Nonphysicians do not understand these things.)

The first battle had to be the CPT-4 problem. On submitting our standard procedures for inclusion in the next edition, I was informed that these were "unproven and controversial." A careful examination of CPT-4 revealed any number of procedures, including coronary bypass surgery, which had never been proven by any form of scientific study. The next step was finding who determined the allergy procedures to be included in the volume, and to no one's surprise it was a general allergist. Two or three additional attempts at inclusion met the same fate, after which it became necessary to contact the editors of CPT-4 and find out what the actual criteria for inclusion were. These did not include scientifically proven or noncontroversial techniques, but only procedures in wide use in the medical community. Adding up the students who had taken any of the various courses in otolaryngic allergy and, having invested registration fees and expenses, were presumably using at least some of the procedures that they had learned, produced a large enough group of practitioners to have the procedures included in the next edition, but it took 5 years of lobbying to accomplish this goal.

This point in history is included in detail because of some subsequent reservations expressed by younger practitioners not involved in that battle. Inclusion in CPT-4 is important enough that over a decade after the original battle a major attempt was made by a group of general allergists to have these procedures removed from the volume. Only a lawsuit by a dedicated member of our organization forestalled this removal. The stronger managed care becomes, and the more restrictive insurance coverage becomes, the more important it is that our procedures be included in a resource base that is used by the managers. There may well be times when payment is denied for these procedures. It is reasonable to change the phraseology of the procedures reported when necessary, but if the procedure designations are removed, it is highly unlikely that they will ever again gain access to the resource volume. Payment may vary from year to year, but inclusion will not. If we do not learn from history, we may expect to repeat it.

## HISTORY OF THE AMERICAN ACADEMY OF OTOLARYNGIC ALLERGY

Under the earliest history of otolaryngic allergy it was noted that during French Hansel's teaching years, it was suggested that a formal organization be established to ensure the continuing viability of the teaching programs initiated by Dr. Hansel. The original organization, the ASOOA, was formed in 1941, the oldest allergy organization in the country. Although possibly prestigious, the organization was small, and primarily dedicated to an annual meeting at which ideas and suggestions were exchanged, sociability was encouraged, and a few papers were presented. These were published starting in 1960 in the *Transactions* of the society, a small journal, but registered with the Smithsonian Institute. When the turf battles became significant in the mid-1970s, it became evident that a powerful central organization was needed. It was only reasonable to use the already well established organization, the ASOOA, and expand it into a politically effective force. This was well under way within a few years. Representatives of the ASOOA were able to influence Washington on the widespread use of their procedures and on the fact that the organization was well established and represented a definite factor in providing medical care.

In 1977 and 1978, a change occurred in the mother academy, the American Academy of Otolaryngology. The goal was to gather all of the satellite societies under the umbrella of the mother, thereby gaining major support for the satellites and better cohesiveness for the mother society. This was accomplished, although in so doing the allergy society agreed to give up its *Transactions* and to publish through a journal established through the mother academy. The *Transactions,* therefore, was terminated in 1981, and potential publications were initially sent by agreement to the *Archives of Otolaryngology.* This affiliation, however, was transferred in 1984 to *Otolaryngology/Head and Neck Surgery* as a primary publishing source for articles on otolaryngic allergy. In maintaining visibility, is quite important for a relatively small organization to have a journal specifically interested in publishing articles related to that field. Random distribution of medical articles frequently results in important articles pertaining to limited areas of interest being lost. This had become painfully evident in the lack of literature available in 1976, when our procedures were challenged, and it was found that more articles had been published in the journals of the Society for Clinical Ecology than in otolaryngology journals.

To place this situation in perspective, it is necessary to take a somewhat broader look at the various organizations practicing allergy care and its various ramifications at this time. It should be evident from the otolaryngic procedures described that the otolaryngic allergy group was well to the left of the traditional allergy organizations. As far to the left of the otolaryngic allergy group as this group was to the left of the traditional allergists were the clinical ecologists. This group, organized as the Society for Clinical Ecology (now the Academy of Environmental Medicine), treated straightforward allergy in essentially the same manner as did the otolaryngic allergists, but were in addition deeply involved in claims of chemical sensitivity, environmental influences, and a great variety of things never subjected to any real attempts at scientific investigation or objective substantiation of treatment results. The otolaryngic allergist occupied a position somewhere between the two extremes. All three organizations deprecated the others, but the political and scientific acceptance cascade tended to run from right to left. Today, the traditional allergists have become more flexible, the otolaryngic allergists have accepted many of the tenets of the traditional allergists, and many of the procedures pursued by the clinical ecologists are now under study by national committees. Over the years, some of the lines dividing the approaches blur. However, there were three clear-cut camps in the 1970s, and it was a blow to the otolaryngic allergists to be required to turn to the clinical ecologist for support in published literature.

It has long been an axiom in academic circles that one must publish or die. The same does not apply to clinicians. Persuading a clinician to take time to prepare an article is a major endeavor, as editors of clinical journals are well aware. At that time, few otolaryngic allergists were in active academia, and, as was to be expected, the articles were few. This has improved to a degree over the years. Today, articles from otolaryngic allergists are readily available and generally well prepared and written, but the supply still is less than could be desired.

The otolaryngic allergy organization continued to grow. The courses, previously very closely circumscribed, became larger and in more demand. In 1973, the author arranged with Dr. Willoughby to give his course on a trial basis in Miami, Florida, because a request had been made to provide more postgraduate courses in the area. This course turned out to be the largest then on record, with 325 attendees. With this encouragement, a second course was held the following year, and courses using much of the same established faculty proliferated in New Orleans, St. Petersburg, Pittsburgh, and elsewhere. Evaluating the requests of attendees, more advanced courses were arranged in Williamsburg, San Diego, Orlando, Corpus Christi, and Baltimore. The basic courses continued, often expanded to twice a year, and the venue was moved to various locations to accommodate the regional attendees. The membership of the organization continued to grow, and in 1981 became the AAOA.

Although still small in numbers compared with the general allergy contingent, the AAOA and its teaching course graduates had grown large enough to draw the attention of the general allergy societies. There is a joint council of the general allergy societies, the JCAAI, that allows the group to act cooperatively when deemed necessary. The group had come to the conclusion that the otolaryngic allergists were teaching unacceptable techniques, and were therefore duping the American public. This opinion was apparently based on word-of-mouth information. None of the members of the three major allergy societies seemed to read any of the literature of the otolaryngic allergists, or this opinion might have differed. It is to the discredit of the otolaryngic allergists that, as noted, they were woefully lax in producing written material at this time, but such material did exist, and was available in established journals. Despite the availability of this literature, the author, a Fellow of the American College of Allergy, Asthma and Immunology (ACAAI), noted repeatedly at meetings of the College that when questions were raised about articles that had been so published, the answer inevitably seemed to be "I wasn't aware of that," or "I hadn't seen that article."

For whatever reason, the general allergy group became convinced that serial endpoint titration was still being performed as in French Hansel's original teachings, using homeopathic doses of antigen. Actually, this approach had been abandoned as a philosophy at the time of Dr. Rinkel's publications. Rinkel commented that after the endpoint had been determined, thereby establishing a safe point at which to initiate therapy, the treatment plan should be removed from the laboratory and escalated from the clinical point of view up to a symptom-relieving maintenance level. He then gave escalation formats covering three successive five-times-stronger dilutions. It is unfortunate that he also commented that the vast majority of his patients in Kansas City endpointed at the #2 of #3 level, and that maintenance was usually reached before the first upward conversion was needed. On Dr. Rinkel's part, this was an observation apparently designed to show his students how much closer to a maintenance dose titration was able to provide, but a large number of his followers took this to mean that 0.50 mL of the endpoint should be considered a maintenance dose, regardless of symptoms. This teaching crept into many of the otolaryngic allergy courses through the 1960s and 1970s. Fortuitously, a corollary of the plan was that if relief had not been obtained, the patient should be retested. This usually resulted in finding a higher endpoint, as which time a new escalation could be performed. The end result was usually continued progression, but without any real understanding of the pattern and with less than optimal results. A peculiarity of the original format, and possibly the factor that motivated Dr. Hansel throughout his teaching career, is that relief of symptoms often is obtained at extremely small doses of antigen, often even while testing. This relief, however, is not sustained.

Based on the conviction that Dr. Hansel's original homeopathic treatment was that practiced by the otolaryngic allergist in the late 1970s, the general allergy groups prepared a study specifically designed to discredit their concept of the otolaryngic allergist's teaching format. The study was carried out in 1978 and 1979. The goal of the study was commendable, if in fact the American public was truly being mistreated by an increasingly large and successful group of physicians. A group of several hundred allergy sufferers was recruited from the Washington, DC area, who skin tested positive to ragweed at dilutions of #9 and above. These patients were then given immunotherapy to a level of 0.50 mL of the endpoint, usually #9, and therapy was discontinued. Because a #9 dilution represents a dilution factor of 1:39,062,500, and even when carried out to the next dilution level in treating the dilution was 1:7,812,500, it came as no surprise to the participants in the study that the results were no better than placebo. Those participating in the study prepared for their role in testing by engaging in a brief visit to one of the otolaryngic allergist's offices, and no input to the study by the physicians familiar with the techniques was allowed. Much of the technique used was flawed, and no otolaryngic allergist would have terminated escalation at the level described, but the papers were published and used as a basis for advising third-party payers not to pay for treatment based on this format. The papers, known thereafter as the Hirsch-Van Meter papers, did extensive damage to the progress of otolaryngic allergy. Rebuttals were immediately written and published, but the general allergists again did not read the otolaryngic literature and hence continued to claim positive results from the study.

It is true that otolaryngic allergy at this time was taught in a rather haphazard manner, the various courses having little contact with one another and much of the material presented showing the bias of the presenter, although the overall pattern remained that of Herbert Rinkel. A major degree of relief from the disorganization was obtained by the development of the radioallergosorbent test (RAST). The original Phadebas RAST, presented in 1975, was hailed as a milestone in identifying allergy, but it was felt by the general allergy world that it probably would be of little clinical use because of the sacrifice of sensitivity for specificity. This test was modified in subsequent years to the Fadal-Nalebuff RAST, which used a more clinically realistic formulation that in turn closely paralleled skin endpoint titration. This provided a laboratory-based test to which the public could relate, and was quickly adopted by the otolaryngic allergist. One immediate benefit from the RAST was the proof that endpoints below #6 (1:312,500) represented only skin hyperreactivity and did not indicate immunologic activity. These factors aided immensely in bringing the heterogeneous teaching formats into line.

This event and recovery was not the end of the otolaryngic allergist's problems. The AAOA's position as the vehicle of otolaryngic allergy suffered what may have been its most serious educational challenge when its certification as a provider of continuing medical education (CME) credits was reviewed in 1982. Before that time, the AMA performed its own credentialing, sending a representative to the applicant organization's national meeting, who reviewed the organization's activities and then presented a report to the AMA. Between the successful credentialing in 1979 and the next review in 1982, credentialing was passed from the AMA to the Accreditation Committee for Continuing Medical Education (ACCME), a joint body composed of members of a variety of specialties and charged with demanding that programs of organizations providing CME credits be structured on an educational level comparable with that of university programs. The probation imposed on the AAOA was not on the basis of material taught, however, but on the lack of organization in how the programs were presented and portrayed to the potential attendee. It was quite a blow, however, to find the oldest allergy organization in the country on probation. The probation affected primarily the annual meeting because the courses actually were sponsored by individual universities or already-accredited societies, but the affiliation with the AAOA was essential if the field was to continue to progress. The AAOA was obviously the overall vehicle for an organization meeting increasing educational demand and increasing pressure from competition and third-party payers.

The dubious honor of restoring accreditation to the AAOA fell to your author. After the initial shock of perusing an application that ultimately required 148 pages of data, course and meeting reorganization, and program restructuring, it became evident that in the long run this would probably be the best thing that could have happened to the organization. To comply with the regulations, the errors that had crept into some of the programs would have to be eliminated and the courses structured in such a manner that uniformity would be established and current knowledge updated for each course. The lecturers would have to stay abreast of developments and maintain good presentational ability, or be eliminated from the field. This program was instituted. From the successful recovery from probation in 1988, the teaching courses all took on a much higher quality.

It may have been the probation that motivated Dr. John Boyles, president of the AAOA in 1985 to 1986, to institute a movement to have all of the otolaryngic allergy teaching courses brought directly under the umbrella of the AAOA. The courses at this point were still taught by their original directors, those who had established independent teaching courses after Dr. Rinkel's death. The faculty for these courses was selected by the course director, who also outlined the program. As noted, sponsorship to this date had been obtained from organizations already accredited for providing postgraduate CME credits. These were usually universities, such as the University of Tennessee and the University of Miami, but such organizations as the Missouri Allergy Society also were used. The AAOA also was an accredited teaching organization and provided CME credit for its national meeting. The course attendance was becoming steadily larger, however, bolstered by increasing national interest in allergy and the expansion and diversification of otolaryngology as a field. CME credits, formerly desirable but largely used to give a course prestige, had become essential for maintaining licenses to practice and continuing hospital privileges. A course not providing CME credits would be poorly attended, and arranging CME credits through a variety of sources could be difficult and expensive.

Change continued. Courses previously held in one location for years were moved around the country to take advantage of attractive and diverse locations (which encouraged the bringing of families and staff to the program), better facilities for teaching, and the practicality of including commercial exhibitors, which proved to be highly beneficial both financially and educationally. The necessity of establishing a uniform format in teaching was becoming evident, and it was becoming more difficult to obtain university sponsorship without giving up control of the course.

In 1986, all of the courses were placed under the direction of the AAOA, which was now able to provide full CME accreditation. Course directors were rotated to provide variety and maintain continuity. The course programs were reviewed and approved by the AAOA Education Committee, and a regular program for selecting and, if necessary, removing faculty was instituted.

## Fellowship Certification

The professional disagreement between the otolaryngic allergists and the general allergists continued. Much of the controversy, and at times vilification, was carried out with more heat than light. As has already been alluded to, the general allergists rarely read otolaryngic allergy literature, and hence were largely unaware of the changes in the otolaryngic allergy teaching programs. With their surgical personalities, otolaryngologists have always been eager to explore new events (as exemplified in taking immediate advantage of RAST at a time when the general allergists claimed that the minimal difference in sensitivity made RAST of little use, but confirming a high percentage of their studies with RAST). With the benefits of laboratory support, it quickly became evident that using extremely low doses of antigen in immunotherapy provided no prolonged relief. Progressing sequentially up to symptom-relief levels provided satisfactory results with minimal side effects, but if prolonged relief was to be obtained without regular injections, higher doses of antigen would be required. In other words, maximally tolerated doses of antigen, just below the level of adverse reactions, were the best course, as had been the policy of the general allergist. The skin endpoint titration format, however, allowed the desired level to be reached more rapidly and with better control. This approach, therefore, continued to be the standard of otolaryngic allergists, most of whom also made use of in vitro testing techniques because these were popular with patients and closely paralleled skin endpoint titration. All of these advances were freely taught and reported in the literature, but because few attempts were made to recognize these changes, many general allergists still believed that the techniques originally described by French Hansel and Herbert Rinkel several decades previously were in use, and denigrated the otolaryngic allergist as untrained.

It has already been noted that in 1971, after nearly 30 years of trying to establish a primary board of allergy, the American Board of Allergy and Immunology was formed as a conjoint board of internal medicine and pediatrics. An immediate attempt was made to exclude the otolaryngologist from the practice of allergy care on the basis of the lack of certification by that board. The American Board of Allergy and Immunology was considered by many to be basically a subspecialty board, much like that of cardiology or gastroenterology. The nonphysician, however, especially those involved in medical management, did not always think so. It would have seemed the most expeditious move on the part of the American Board of Otolaryngology to provide subcertification in such fields as facial plastic surgery and allergy, among other things. The American Board of Otolaryngology, however, has a reputation of being quite paternalistic, and has always felt that subcertification would tend to dilute the image of the otolaryngologist as a regional expert in all aspects of otolaryngology care. Such subcertification was not granted, therefore, in spite of recommendations from the American Academy of Otolaryngology. The otolaryngic allergist continued to have to battle for acceptance. Although he was boarded in otolaryngology, and one of the requirements of the American Board of Otolaryngology is a "knowledge, skill and understanding" in allergy and immunology relevant to the head and neck (11), the challenge of the American Board of Allergy and Immunology continued. It required intervention by the AMA Board of Trustees, who in 1976 issued Report W (12), a formal statement recognizing that the treatment of patients with allergic conditions is a regular part of the practice of otolaryngologists, that residency training in otolaryngology includes experience in the care of allergic patients, that both the profession and the public should recognize this as a part of their function, and that third-party payers should pay them for this function. The report also specifically forbade board certification as a means of restricting access to practice. The general allergy societies later endorsed this report, which gave the otolaryngic allergist a formal, if not always recognized, entry into the field of allergy care.

Not content with this legal form of access and anxious to raise its standards and achieve the best form or recognition, the ASOOA (soon to become the AAOA) in 1977 established its own Fellowship examination. This was patterned on the American Board of Otolaryngology examination, and required an extensive written examination. It also required the assembly of several case reports to be reviewed and examined by members of the Council, who would use these as the basis of an oral examination. Before applying for the examination, the candidate was required to attend several courses and annual meetings to become and remain upgraded in the current practice of otolaryngic allergy. This examination was felt to offer the clinician recognizable expertise in the field of otolaryngic allergy. Fellowship in this organization was not easy to obtain, and was not to be taken lightly.

## The More Recent Years

Most of the major crises described took place before 1985 or so. By then, the organization was well recognized, its presence felt even by the general allergists. By the 1990s, even some interaction between the otolaryngic allergy and general allergy organizations was beginning to occur. The name of the otolaryngic allergy organization, the ASOOA, was shortened to the AAOA. Membership in the AAOA enlarged, today exceeding 2,200, and a seat on the AMA House of Delegates was achieved. Research and fellowship training became available to those in or completing residency. The AAOA had become a fixture in the field of medicine. Current activities are ever expanding, and will differ by the publication date of this book. There appears no likelihood that, despite the constraints of managed care, the field of otolaryngic allergy will diminish in the foreseeable future.

## A FINAL VIEW

It is impossible to present a summation of a historical chapter because history never provides an end. By the time this book reaches publication, many changes will have occurred in the field of otolaryngic allergy, both scientific and political. No one can predict these changes, but an overview of the changes that have already occurred may aid those preparing to cope with future changes to plan for them in some sort of logical way.

It may have been noticed by those following this presentation that successive events have been presented more in the order of various aspects of the developing situation than in a simple chronologic order. As your author, I have been closely involved in much of the course of events, and have felt that these situations, told from the point of view of one involved, may present a more intimate picture than that provided by chronologic documentation. Such documentation is available, and presents the evolution of the specialty from a different aspect (13,14). Many of the situations discussed in this chapter have not been formally documented and could be subject to a different interpretation by other observers, but for those in which the author was present, every effort has been made to put the events in perspective. It is my hope this will provide an "up close and personal" look at much of the history of otolaryngic allergy, and perhaps give some guidelines for those pursuing the field in the future.

## REFERENCES

1. Gell PGH, Coombs RRA. *Clinical aspects of immunology.* Oxford: Blackwell Scientific, 1962:808–816.
2. Ishizaka K, Ishizaka T, Hornbrook MM. Physicochemical properties of reaginic antibody: V. correlation of reaginic activity with E-globulin antibody. *J Immunol* 1966;97:840–853.
3. Goodale JL. Pollen therapy in hay fever. *Bost Med Surg J* 1915; 2:42–48.
4. Noon L. Prophylactic inoculation against hay fever. *Lancet* 1911; 1:1572–1573.
5. Hansel F. *Allergy and immunity in otolaryngology,* 3rd ed. Rochester, MN: American Academy of Ophthalmology and Otolaryngology, 1975.
6. Rinkel HJ. The whealing response of the skin to serial dilution testing. *Ann Allergy* 1949;7:120–126.
7. Rinkel HJ, Randolph TG, Zeller M. *Food allergy.* Springfield, IL: Charles C Thomas, 1951.
8. Cowan DE. Serial dilution titration: technique and application. In: King HC, ed. *Otolaryngological allergy.* Miami: Symposia Specialists, 1981:56–75.
9. Kniker WT. *Introductory lecture: adverse reactions to foods and chemicals.* Toronto: International Food Allergy Symposium, American College of Allergists, 1989.
10. Lee CH, Williams RT, Binkley EL. Provocative testing and treatment to foods. *Arch Otolaryngol* 1969;90:173–177.
11. Bryan MD, Bryan WTK. Cytologic diagnosis in allergic disorders. *Otolaryngol Clin North Am* 1974;7:637–666.
12. American Medical Association. Proceedings of the House of Delegates, 125th Annual Convention, Dallas, Texas, June 27–July 1, 1976. Reference Committee C, (2) Report W, Allergy and Immunology.
13. Anon JB. Otolaryngic allergy: the last half century. *Otolaryngol Clin North Am* 1992;25:1–12.
14. Osguthorpe JD. Evolution of otolaryngic allergy and the American Academy of Otolaryngic Allergy. *Otolaryngol Head Neck Surg* 1996;114:4.

# 2

# IMMUNOLOGY OF ALLERGIC UPPER RESPIRATORY DISORDERS

## JAMES A. HADLEY

Comprehension of the structure and function of the immune system is a prerequisite to the study of allergic upper respiratory disorders. Rhinitis, both allergic and nonallergic, as well as chronic upper respiratory tract disorders represent a breakdown of the homeostatic immune state.

The immune system is a complex group of cells, organs, and chemicals that work to eradicate the body of infectious invasion.

The primary function of the immune system is to distinguish self from nonself and to protect the organism from invasion of foreign substances, or pathogens. It is made up of an elaborate system of cells and molecules that has effector and regulatory functions in addition to nonspecific functions. This system is a requirement for humans to prevent attack by microorganisms, toxins, tumors, and autoimmune disorders. If there is a breakdown of the immune system, a wide range of diseases or disorders may occur, ranging from allergic rhinitis to rheumatoid arthritis or combined immunodeficiency.

The immune system is the body's second line of defense. The first line consists of barriers to invasion such as skin, mucous membranes, acidity of the stomach, and cells that are nonspecific. The specific actions of the immune system are dependent on prior recognition of self-cells and destruction of nonself cells.

The immune system is extremely adaptive and is able to adjust to specific attack with a specific response. It responds to changes in environment and alters responses by remembering what stimuli had been encountered in the past.

The characteristics of the immune system include a genetically determined system with features of memory, specificity, self-recognition, amplification, feedback control, and recruitment of secondary defenses. The immune system remembers a prior infection such that resistance develops to subsequent reinfection by the same organism. Memory persists in T lymphocytes and circulating immunoglobulins.

The body is able to discriminate exceedingly minute molecular details, and closely related microbes elicit independent responses. The immune cells capable of reacting with self are selectively deactivated during development, thus reducing the possibility of self-destruction by development of autoimmune disorders. The immune system has the capability to produce on demand massive amounts of immune products and immune cells to amplify the response, but also has a regulatory system of feedback control to control the response, and it can call in a secondary line of defense.

## HISTORICAL VIGNETTES

The term *immunity* stems from the Latin term *immunitas* and refers to the exemption that was granted to Roman senators from legal prosecution. Exemption from disease states and infectious diseases generally is the meaning of the development of immunity. The immune system was designed to protect against invasion by other organisms and infectious or allergic agents, but some responses of the system can in themselves cause inflammation in the body and disease.

Seasonal catarrh, or hay fever, was first described in 1819 by John Bostock of London, but its cause, ragweed pollen, was not recognized until 1872 by Morill Wyman.

Ehrlich first described the mast cell in 1879. This set the stage for future investigations of the allergic reaction by this cell.

Edward Jenner noted that milkmaids who had recovered from cowpox infections never contracted smallpox. Transferring this knowledge, he developed the principle of vaccination, inoculating a young boy with cowpox to prevent the more serious related infection. He induced immunity to smallpox, and this early work led to our current knowledge of immunity.

Richet and Portier in 1902 coined the term *anaphylaxis* after they showed the development of anaphylaxis in dogs. Von Pirquet predicted that immunity and hypersensitivity would depend on interaction of a foreign substance and the

**J. A. Hadley:** Department of Surgery, Division of Otolaryngology, University of Rochester Medical Center, Rochester, New York.

immune system, and he used the term *allergy* to denote this reaction.

In 1921, Prausnitz and Kustner described the transfer of immediate hypersensitivity (to fish protein) by serum to the skin of a normal individual. Variations of this test remained the standard for measuring skin-sensitizing antibody for 50 years.

Coca and Grove in 1925 studied skin-sensitizing factor (termed *atopic reagin*) in sera of patients with ragweed hay fever. However, this antibody could not be measured at that time.

In 1967, Ishizaka and Ishizaka discovered that this antibody was immunoglobulin E (IgE) while they were studying IgA. Independently, Johansson also discovered this same relationship. IgE was thought to be the reaginic antibody responsible for allergic reactions.

Cellular and molecular immunology has been elucidated since the late 1970s with proper laboratory methodologies. Cytokines and chemical mediators are well known and serve as a basis for our current comprehension of immunology. It is an intricate system with many cells and molecules providing support for the defense of the organism.

## INNATE AND ADAPTIVE IMMUNITY

There are two main types of immunity: innate and adaptive. Innate immunity is the generalized response to an invasion by microbes or allergens: the body's protection by its epithelial barriers, first line of defense by phagocytosis, or a nonspecific response or activation of the complement system. These are relatively nonspecific responses that are classified as "innate." Adaptive immunity refers to the body's capability to mount specific responses to the invading microbe or allergen. These antigen-specific responses depend on the action of T cells and B cells. The initiation of adaptive immunologic responses requires antigen processing, recognition of the antigen by the cells, and subsequent expansion of the cell lines by cloning to enhance the number of effector cells. Adaptive immunity also involves memory, primarily residing in the T cells, which allows the body to develop a more rapid response to the next invasion of the same antigen. Both the innate and adaptive types of immunity enhance each other, providing a more general overall defense of the organism. Phylogeny has developed a much greater degree of adaptive immunity in higher organisms, whereas lower organisms depend largely on innate immunity.

## Features of Adaptive Immunity

Humans have a genetically determined immune system, which has the following features: specificity, memory, self-limitation, nonreactivity to self, amplification, feedback control, and recruitment of secondary defense mechanisms.

### Specificity

The immune system develops specific actions against specific antigens, and can recognize structural properties of macromolecules called *epitopes*. This specificity is mediated through antigen receptors on the cell surface or through the formation of specific antibodies.

### Memory

A second introduction of an antigen entices the immune system to develop a rapid response to that antigen. The second response is more rapid and quantitatively larger than at the first exposure, allowing a more efficient killing or targeting of the antigen. Clones of cells are produced on the second or subsequent exposures to the same antigen, or large amounts of antibody are produced.

### Self-limitation

The activity induced by an immune response eventually wanes and dies out. The immune response returns to its resting state. This is the process of homeostasis, a kind of feedback inhibition to downregulate the immune response.

### Nonreactivity to Self (Self-recognition)

The immune system is designed to eliminate nonself antigens while preserving self-cells. *Tolerance* is the term used for nonreactivity to self-antigens. The immune system eliminates those cells capable of reacting to itself. If there is a breakdown of tolerance, autoimmune disease may develop.

### Amplification

The ability to produce on demand a large quantity of immune products and immune cells is a critical feature. The booster or amnestic response is characteristic of amplification of the immune system. A second introduction of a foreign substance generates a much larger immune response than the first. Activation of the complement cascade may generate thousands of more active complexes for reduction of the foreign object.

### Feedback Control

Once upregulated, the immune system must have in place a system to begin to turn off the complex series of reactions that initiate the responses. Controls to downregulate the immune responses may be both cellular and molecular. Without feedback mechanisms, the immune system goes unchecked and altered immune states may be the result.

## *Recruitment of Secondary Defense Mechanisms*

Both cellular and chemical mediator responses are elicited by the initial reactions. Secondary defenses may result in the direct attack on pathogens, or phagocytosis. Not only is there a primary defense mechanism, but other methods are called into action such as complement and natural killer (NK) cells.

## COMPONENTS OF THE IMMUNE SYSTEM

## Cells of the Immune System

All the cells involved in the blood and immune system originate from pluripotent stem cells in the bone marrow. During hematopoiesis, these pluripotent cells give rise to two lineages: the lymphoid cells and the myeloid cells. The myeloid lineage of cells differentiates into all other cells, including red blood cells, platelets, basophils. eosinophils, neutrophils, and monocytes. The lymphoid lineage differentiates into the three different types of lymphocytes: T lymphocytes, B lymphocytes, and natural killer cells (Fig. 2.1).

## *Lymphocytes*

### General

Lymphocytes are derived from stem cells residing in the bone marrow. The bone marrow and the thymus are the primary lymphoid organs of the immune system. Once the pluripotent cells differentiate into a cell lineage, they become functional by passage through the thymus or the bone marrow. The spleen and the lymph nodes are secondary organs of the immune system. The role of the thymus gland is to produce mature T lymphocytes that distinguish self antigens from nonself. Primitive T lymphocytes migrate through the blood to the thymus gland, where they enter the peripheral cortex. After stimulation, they migrate to germinal centers, where they undergo rapid cell division and receive the imprinting that allows them to distinguish self from nonself. T lymphocytes that are beneficial to the immune system are spared, whereas those that may produce an autoimmune reaction are destroyed (Fig. 2.2).

Lymphocytes are the only cells that are capable of recognizing specific antigenic determinants, or epitopes, and thus

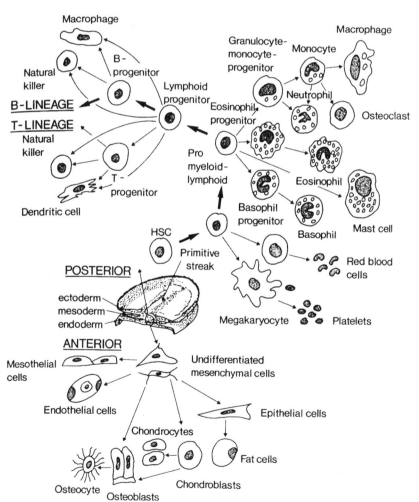

**FIG. 2.1.** Differentiation of cells from stem cell. (From Paul WE. *Fundamental immunology,* 4th ed. Philadelphia: Lippincott Williams & Wilkins, 1999:185, with permission.)

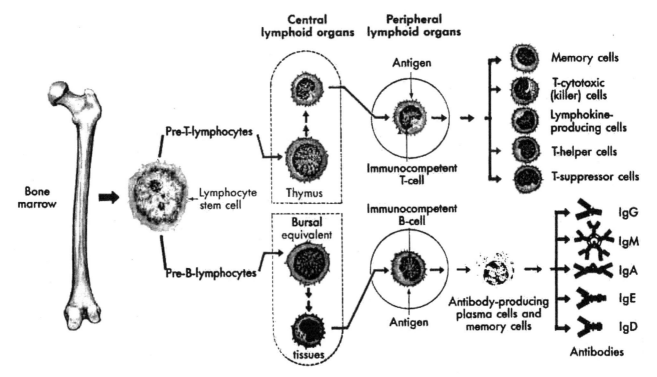

**FIG. 2.2.** Maturation, differentiation, and activation of lymphocytes. (From Grimes D. *Infectious diseases.* St. Louis: Mosby Year Book, 1991, with permission.)

are responsible for the adaptive immunologic responses of memory and specificity. Each lymphocyte is able to identify only one epitope or determinant. Each cell during development encodes its receptors by rearranging DNA to fabricate a unique antigen receptor. That cell and all of its clones therefore express receptors that are specific to that antigen. These memory T cells remain quiescent until an amnestic response occurs.

### Classes of Lymphocytes

Lymphocytes are divided into two subsets: B cells and T cells. They have the same morphology, but differ in function and their secretory products.

*T Cells.* T cells are distinguished from B cells by their cell surface receptors, designated α, β, γ, and δ. These receptors are complexed with other molecules and are described as a *cluster of differentiation.* These clusters of differentiation (CD3, CD4, CD8, and others) also provide other functions to differentiate the cells into functional units. CD3 is found on all T cells, CD4 is found on helper T cells, whereas CD8 is found on suppressor and cytotoxic T cells. The CD4/CD8 ratio is helpful in determining the status of the immune response in patients with acquired immunodeficiency syndrome (AIDS). A decline in the number of CD4 cells is seen in the later stages of the disease.

*T Helper Cells.* T helper cells may initiate responses and as well as provide help to other cells, specifically the B cells and cytotoxic T cells, in participating in the inflammatory response. Cytokines elaborated specifically by these T helper cells are responsible for the activation, proliferation, and differentiation of cells involved in the immune response. T lymphocytes can be classified according to their cytokine production into Th1 cells or Th2 cells.

The Th1 cells are characterized by elaboration of interleukin (IL)-2, IL-3, tumor necrosis factor-α, and interferon (IFN)-γ. They mediate cytotoxicity and local inflammatory reactions and thus are important for combating intracellular pathogens such as viruses, bacteria, and parasites.

The Th2 cells are characterized by elaboration of IL-3, IL-4, IL-5, IL-6, and IL-10. These interleukins perform helper functions in the immune response, especially with regard to B-cell production and elaboration of immunoglobulins. Th2 cells are in general more involved in humoral immunity. IL-4 and IL-10 may diminish activity of Th1 cells, which is useful in turning off the formation of antibody (Fig. 2.3).

*T Cytotoxic Cells.* These cells can have a direct cytotoxic effect on other cells, but require help from Th1 cells to proliferate and differentiate. They have the CD8 surface clusters and are suppressive in function.

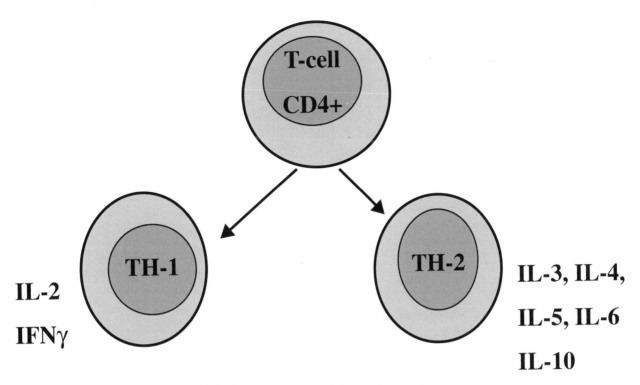

**FIG. 2.3.** Functional subsets of CD4$^+$ helper T cells.

*T Suppressor Cells.* These T cells have a negative regulatory function. They have CD8 clusters of differentiation and are involved with regulation of the intensity of a reaction, keeping it in check.

*B Cells.* B lymphocytes, so called because of their maturation in birds in the bursa of Fabricius, are the cells that produce antibodies. In humans, it is presumed that the B cells mature in the bone marrow.

The major function of B cells is to produce antibodies in response to foreign proteins of bacteria, viruses, and tumors. B cells are stimulated into differentiation by a specific antigen with the assistance of Th1 cells. They elaborate an immunoglobulin antibody specific to the antigen that stimulated their differentiation. The immunoglobulin produced is either bound to the surface of the B cells, ready to induce the B cell to proliferate and mature into a plasma cell to produce large amounts of the immunoglobulin, or then it is secreted by the plasma cells to target and complex with the antigen for eventual destruction by the organism (Fig. 2.4).

*Null Cells.* These lymphocytes are distinct because they carry neither a surface receptor nor an immunoglobulin. They consist of subsets of cells that include the natural killer (NK) cells, as well as lymphokine-activated killer cells and large granular lymphocytes. NK lymphocytes are able selectively to determine which cells have been altered (either by

malignant transformation or viral infection) and compare these altered cells with normal cells. Their activity is increased by IFN-$\gamma$ and IL-2, which leads to cell lysis.

Natural killer cells function as effector cells that directly kill certain tumors such as melanomas, lymphomas, and virus-infected cells.

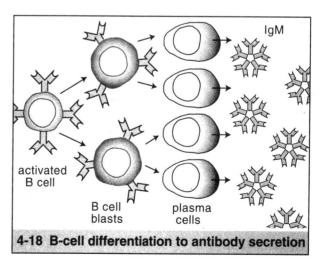

**4-18 B-cell differentiation to antibody secretion**

**FIG. 2.4.** B-cell differentiation into plasma cells and formation of antibodies. (From Sharon J. *Basic immunology.* Philadelphia: Lippincott Williams & Wilkins, 1998:44, with permission.)

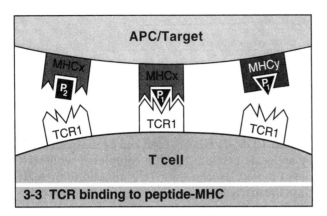

**FIG. 2.5.** Antigen-presenting cell presenting antigen to T cell. (From Sharon J. *Basic immunology.* Philadelphia: Lippincott Williams & Wilkins, 1998:27, with permission.)

## Mononuclear Phagocytes and Macrophages

The mononuclear phagocyte system has two functions: removal of particulate antigens by the phagocytes and the processing and presentation of antigens to T cells by antigen-presenting cells (APCs).

### Antigen-presenting Cells

These heterogeneous populations of leukocytes have an essential role in the activity of the immune system. They are immunostimulatory and induce the functional activity of T cells. APCs are specialized macrophages that recognize foreign substances as antigen and process the antigen by enzymatic degradation. They then put the fragments back on their surface in conjunction with major histocompatibility complexes I and II and "present" the antigen for recognition by a T helper cell. These cells are found primarily in the skin, mucosa, lymph nodes, spleen, and thymus (Fig. 2.5).

### Granulocytes

***Mast Cells and Basophils.*** Basophils represent only 0.2% of circulating granulocytes, and mast cells remain fixed in tissues but are indistinguishable from the basophil. Mast cells and basophils both contain granules that harbor histamine and other chemical mediators, and they have thousands of receptors for the Fc portion of IgE.

The stimulus for mast cell or basophil degranulation is the presence of an antigen cross-linking IgE molecules bound to the surface of the cell. When an antigen "binds" two adjacent IgE molecules on the surface of the mast cell, a signal occurs that leads to degranulation of the mast cell with the release of the chemical mediators, which are involved in the immediate hypersensitivity reaction (Fig. 2.6).

***Eosinophils.*** Human eosinophils are bilobed and usually comprise approximately 2% to 5% of granulocytes in a nonallergic person, but they may increase in numbers in the allergic state.

The eosinophil plays a role in the immune system in the late phase of the hypersensitivity response. Chemically attracted to the site of inflammation by chemotactic factors [e.g., eosinophilic chemotactic factor (ECF-A), granulocyte–macrophage colony-stimulating factor (GM-CSF)], the eosinophil releases its granules, which contain powerful enzymes and proteolytic agents such as major basic protein, eosinophil cationic protein, eosinophil-derived neurotoxin, and eosinophil peroxidase. The recruitment and activation of eosinophils in sites of inflammation is regulated by T-cell–dependent cytokines, especially IL-5 and IL-3, as well as GM-CSF and RANTES (regulated on activation, normal T-cell expressed and secreted).

***Neutrophils.*** These multilobed granulocytes comprise over 95% of the circulating granulocytes. Drawn to sites of inflammation by cytokines, the neutrophil uses its phagocytic activity to engulf and destroy pathogens. They have antibi-

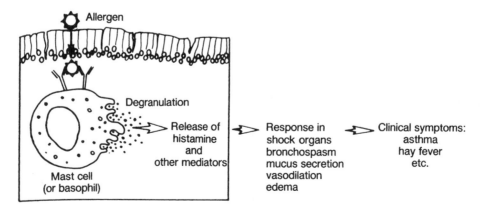

**FIG. 2.6.** Mast cell or basophil degranulation. (From Sheehan C. *Clinical immunology: principles and laboratory diagnosis,* 2nd ed. Philadelphia: Lippincott Williams & Wilkins, 1997:67, with permission.)

otic proteins stored in two types of granules. Lysosomes in the granules contain the acid hydrolases, myeloperoxidase and muramidase, as well as lactoferrin and other antibiotic defense proteins. The granules are released after stimulation by immune complexes.

### Platelets

Platelets are derived from megakaryocytes; the adult human produces $10^{11}$ platelets each day, 30% of which are sequestered in the spleen. In addition to their role in blood clotting, platelets contain granules that release serotonin and fibrinogen, which can activate complement and stimulate the inflammatory response.

## Molecules of the Immune System: Antibodies and Antigens

Antibodies (immunoglobulins) are proteins produced primarily after a response elicited by the immune system. They circulate in serum and specifically bind to antigens in both the recognition phase and the effector phase of humoral immunity.

Antigens are substances capable of eliciting an immune response. They react with lymphocytes to induce the formation of antibodies or sensitized cells.

### Immunoglobulins

There are five classes of immunoglobulins, which are distinguished by their antigenic and structural characteristics. The basic molecule of an immunoglobulin consists of four protein chains linked together by disulfide bonds in a "Y"-shape. The two arms of the "Y" form antigen-binding sites, and the base forms the cell-binding site. The use of enzymatic cleavage of the immunoglobulin molecule helps to define functions: papain cleavage produces the Fab portions and one Fc fragment.

**Production**
Immunoglobulins are produced by B cells after their transformation into plasma cells, which secrete only a specific type of immunoglobulin for the specific antigen. Immunoglobulins are glycoproteins consisting of two identical light chains of polypeptides (κ or λ) and two identical heavy chains, which confer immunoglobulin type (A, D, E, G, or M). Light chains may be produced in abnormal quantities in multiple myeloma and are detected as Bence-Jones proteins in the urine. The heavy chains, because of their structure, confer antibody class. Normal individuals secrete all the types of immunoglobulins (Fig. 2.7).

**Antibody Classes**
Characteristics of immunoglobulins are listed in Table 2.1.

***IgG.*** The major immunoglobulin in human serum is IgG, accounting for 70% to 75% of the immunoglobulin pool.

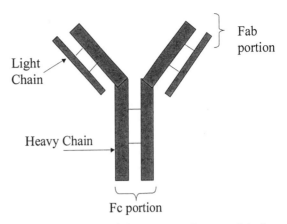

**FIG. 2.7.** Structure of the prototype immunoglobulin.

It is the major antibody of the secondary immune response. Maternal IgG confers immunity to neonates for the first few months of life because it readily crosses the placenta. The primary activity of IgG is to neutralize viruses, bacteria, and their toxins. There are four subclasses of IgG: IgG1, IgG2, IgG3, and IgG4 (Fig. 2.8).

***IgM.*** This pentameric antibody is the largest of the immunoglobulins and is largely confined to the intravascular space. It is the predominant early antibody after initiation of the immune response. Its structure allows highly effective antibody activity and it is the major defense against bacterial invasion (Fig. 2.9).

***IgA.*** This is the major immunoglobulin of body secretions and mucosal surfaces. It is found in saliva, colostrum, breast milk, tracheobronchial secretions, and genitourinary secretions. Two secretory subclasses are recognized: sIgA1 and sIgA2 (Fig. 2.10).

***IgD.*** Accounting for less than 1% of the total immunoglobulin pool, IgD is still poorly understood. It may have a role in antigen-triggered lymphocyte differentiation (Fig. 2.11).

***IgE*** Originally known as *reagin,* IgE is found only in trace amounts in serum. It is primarily membrane bound to effector cells (i.e., mast cells and basophils). It has a role in protection against parasitic infections, as well as in allergic diseases (Fig. 2.12; Table 2.1).

### Antibody Response to Antigen Challenge

The primary function of antibody is to bind antigen. Antibody can have a direct effect in neutralizing antigen, but in most cases antibody binding to antigen stimulates the complement cascade to eradicate the antigen.

**TABLE 2.1. PROPERTIES OF IMMUNOGLOBULINS**

| Isotype | Molecular Weight | Additional Components | Percentage of Serum Ig | Functions |
|---|---|---|---|---|
| IgA (dimer) | 385,000 | J chain Secretory piece | 0.3 | Provides antibodies for external body fluids |
| IgD | 180,000 | | <1 | Membrane bound; function unknown |
| IgE | 190,000 | | <0.001 | Bound to mast cells; role in immediate hypersensitivity |
| IgG | 145,000–170,000 | Subclasses IgG1, IgG2, IgG3, IgG4 | 75–85 | Found in secondary Ig responses |
| IgM (pentamer) | 970,000 | J chain | 6–8 | Prevalent in primary response; effective for agglutination and activation of complement |

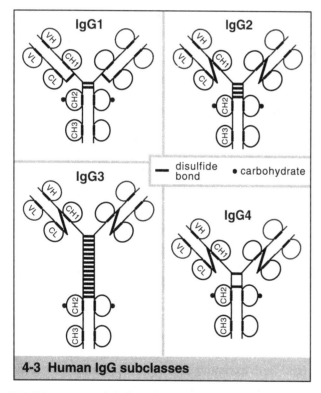

**4-3  Human IgG subclasses**

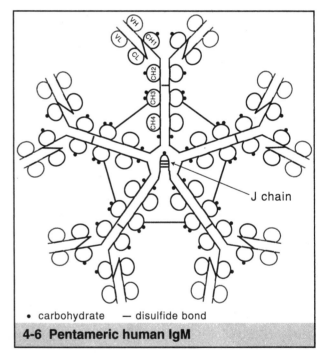

**4-6  Pentameric human IgM**

**FIG. 2.8.** Immunoglobulin G. (From Sharon J. *Basic immunology.* Philadelphia: Lippincott Williams & Wilkins, 1998:39, with permission.)

**FIG. 2.9.** Immunoglobulin M. (From Sharon J. *Basic immunology.* Philadelphia: Lippincott Williams & Wilkins, 1998:39, with permission.)

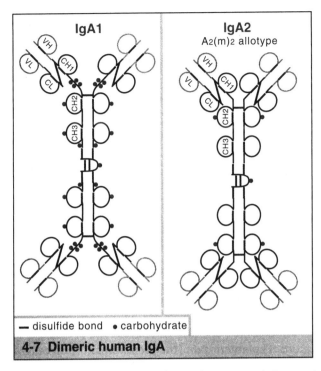

FIG. 2.10. Immunoglobulin A. (From Sharon J. *Basic immunology.* Philadelphia: Lippincott Williams & Wilkins, 1998:40, with permission.)

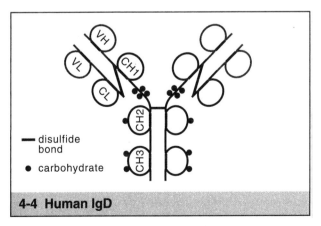

FIG. 2.11. Immunoglobulin D. (From Sharon J. *Basic immunology.* Philadelphia: Lippincott Williams & Wilkins, 1998:39, with permission.)

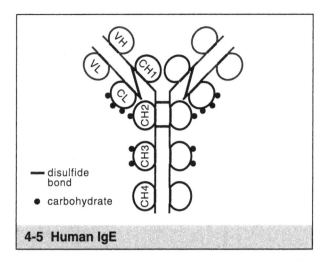

FIG. 2.12. Immunoglobulin E. (From Sharon J. *Basic immunology.* Philadelphia: Lippincott Williams & Wilkins, 1998:39, with permission.)

Antibody production is influenced by the primary and secondary immune responses. Initial contact with an antigen stimulates production of specific antibody to that antigen. Subsequent contact with the same antigen stimulates plasma cells to produce a massive response with production of large quantities of specific antibody to neutralize the antigen (Fig. 2.13).

## *Control of Antibody Synthesis*

Mechanisms to turn off antibody production include negative feedback inhibition and a shift in the balance of helper T cells and suppressor T cells in favor of suppression as the immune reaction nears completion.

## Nonspecific Mediators: Cytokines and Lymphokines

Cooperation in the immune system depends on an orderly group of molecules that send signals to the immune system to turn on some reactions and inhibit others. Communications between the T cells, B cells, and potent chemical messengers called *cytokines* enhance macrophage activity. Those cytokines produced specifically by lymphocytes are called *lymphokines,* and the mediators that act between leukocytes are called *interleukins.* Cytokines play a major role in immunoregulation because they enhance cell growth, direct the activation of cells, stimulate macrophages, and even destroy antigens.

Interferon is the prototypical lymphokine that was found in the supernatant of virally infected cultured cells. Its action was found to interfere with another virus infecting the same cells, hence the term *interferon.* Three types of IFNs have been identified: alpha-IFN (IFN-$\alpha$), beta-IFN (IFN-$\beta$), and gamma-IFN (IFN-$\gamma$). IFN-$\alpha$ and IFN-$\beta$ decrease viral replication and reduce proliferation of several different cell types. IFN-$\gamma$ is produced by activated T cells and macrophages and inhibits neoplastic cell proliferation.

Other cytokines act as growth factors for certain cell lineages; these colony-stimulating factors are produced by T

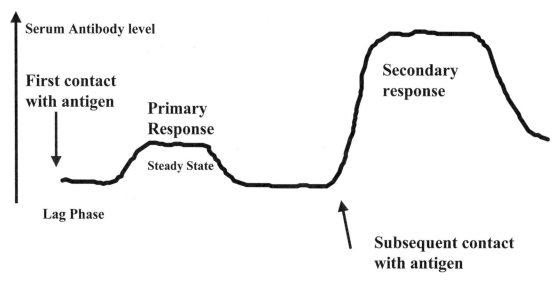

**FIG. 2.13.** Primary and secondary immune responses.

cells and provide a link between the lymphoid and myeloid hematopoietic systems (Table 2.2).

The interleukins are a group of chemical mediators produced primarily by lymphocytes and some macrophages that serve as directors of immune reactions. Structurally different, they function individually either to turn on the immune response or inhibit some reactions (Table 2.3).

## Complement

Complement is an essential component of the immune system. It has a role in both specific and nonspecific immune responses to infection. Complement is a series of protein molecules that act in a cascade, and each enzyme acts as a catalyst for the next. The end result is lysis of target cells or enhancement of other antibody responses. Ehrlich originally applied the term *complement* to describe the activity in serum that "complemented" the ability of specific antibody to cause lysis of bacteria. Various components of the complement reaction were discovered over a period of years, resulting in an illogical system of nomenclature. The proteins are numbered C1q, C1r, C1s, C4, C2, C3, C5, C6, C7, C8, and C9 (Fig. 2.14).

There are two main pathways for activation of complement; the classic pathway (adaptive pathway) and the alternative pathway (innate pathway). A third pathway (lectin pathway) also exists. All three pathways lead to the formation of an enzyme that cleaves C3 into C3a and C3b, which is the stimulus to activation of C5, followed by the components C6, C7, C8, and C9. This is the essential process of complement activation. The classic pathway is the main mechanism, and is activated by the formation of immune complexes containing IgM or IgG. C1 is the first enzyme in this cascade. The alternative pathway is activated by many bacteria, viruses, or parasites, as well as immune complexes containing IgA, IgE, or IgG, but it is less efficient. The lectin pathway is activated by many gram-positive and gram-negative organisms (Fig. 2.15).

The mechanisms of the complement system include op-

## TABLE 2.2. LIST OF CYTOKINES

| Cytokine | Source | Function |
|---|---|---|
| IFN-α | Leukocytes | Antiviral protection, inhibits cell proliferation |
| IFN-β | Fibroblasts, macrophages | Antiviral protection |
| IFN-γ | T cells, natural killer cells | Kills tumor cells, promotes inflammatory responses |
| Granulocyte-CSF | Monocytes, fibroblasts | Myeloid growth factor |
| Granulocyte–macrophage-CSF | T cells, fibroblasts, monocytes | Myelocytic growth factor |
| Monocyte-CSF | Monocytes, lymphocytes, fibroblasts | Macrophage growth factor |
| Transforming growth factor-β | T cells | Tumor defense, cell growth |
| TNF-α | T cells | Inflammation, tumor defense, wound healing |
| TNF-β | T cells | Inflammation, tumor defense, wound healing |

CSF, colony-stimulating factor; IFN, interferon; TNF, tumor necrosis factor.

**TABLE 2.3. LIST OF INTERLEUKINS**

| Interleukin | Origin | Function |
|---|---|---|
| IL-1 | Macrophages | Proinflammatory, augments immune response, activates T cells, endogenous pyrogen |
| IL-2 | T cells | Promotes growth and proliferation of T, B, and NK cells |
| IL-3 | T cells | Proliferation of early hematopoietic cells |
| IL-4 | T cells, mast cells | Growth factor for T cells, and activated B cells<br>Governs B-cell isotype switching to IgG and IgE |
| IL-5 | Macrophages, T cells, fibroblasts | Proinflammatory<br>Promotes growth and proliferation of activated B cells |
| IL-6 | Macrophages, T and B cells, fibroblasts | Promotes B-cell differentiation and growth<br>Proinflammatory |
| IL-7 | Bone marrow, thymus | Promotes growth of B cells |
| IL-8 | Macrophages, monocytes | Triggers neutrophil chemotaxis and activation |
| IL-9 | T helper cells | T-cell and mast cell growth factor |
| IL-10 | T cells, macrophages | Inhibition of cytokine synthesis<br>Inhibits proliferation of T helper cells |
| IL-12 | Mononuclear phagocytes | Mediator of immune response to intracellular microbes<br>Activates NK cells, promotes interferon-$\gamma$ production |
| IL-15 | Mononuclear phagocytes | Stimulates NK cells in response to viral infections |
| IL-18 | Macrophages | Induces cell-mediated immunity<br>Augments IL-12 reaction with NK cells to produce IFN-$\gamma$ |

IFN, interferon; NK, natural killer.

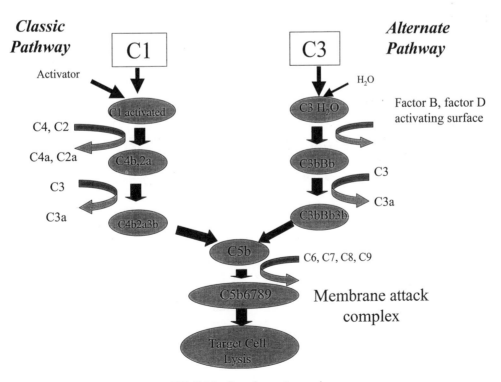

**FIG. 2.14.** Complement cascade.

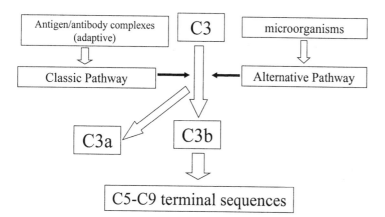

**FIG. 2.15.** Comparison of classic and alternative complement pathways.

sonization of microorganisms for phagocytosis, direct lysis of microorganisms, chemotactic attraction to sites of inflammation and activation of immune cells, processing of immune complexes, and induction of specific antibody responses. Opsonization occurs when complement proteins coat the surface of the target cell. Phagocytes that carry receptors for these complement components are able to bind to the target cell, which leads to phagocytosis of the target cell. Complement can distinguish self from nonself. C3b binds to nonself cells (e.g., microorganisms) or immune complexes, whereas self-cells are protected by surface molecules that limit C3b deposition and attachment.

## INTERACTIONS OF THE IMMUNE RESPONSE: HYPERSENSITIVITY REACTIONS

Hypersensitivity reactions occur when an exaggerated adaptive immune response occurs. They are the result of normally beneficial immune responses that act inappropriately and cause inflammatory reactions and subsequent tissue damage. Hypersensitivity reactions do not occur on first contact with antigens, but usually appear on subsequent contact. Gell and Coombs classically divided hypersensitivity reactions into four types (types I through IV); Shearer and Huston added other types of reactions. Types I through III are antibody mediated, whereas type IV is a T-cell–mediated reaction (Table 2.4).

### Type I: Immediate (Anaphylactic) Hypersensitivity

Mast cells bind IgE by their Fc receptors. When antigen is encountered, IgE becomes cross-linked, which then induces degranulation and release of chemical mediators that produce inflammatory reactions. This is the classic allergic reaction. Type I hypersensitivity is a rapid reaction occurring in minutes. The mediators released from the mast cells or basophils cause an increase in local permeability, resulting in edema, as well as vasodilatation, smooth muscle contraction, and stimulation of nerve endings, resulting in pruritus. These manifestations produce the classic allergic symptoms of swelling, itching, congestion, hypotension, and bronchospasm (Fig. 2.16).

### Early and Late Reactions

Type I reactions produce a dual-phase response. Liberation of chemical mediators from the mast cell, which include histamine, and other preformed chemical mediators, results in a cascade of events that initiate the allergic response. With degranulation, lysis of the cell wall generates the production of newly formed chemical mediators, which include leukotrienes and prostaglandins. These secondary chemical mediators are responsible for the influx into the site of reaction of multiple cells, particularly eosinophils and neutrophils, that induce the effects characteristic of the late phase of the allergic reaction. Toxic enzymes liberated by the eosinophils and the neutrophils result in further inflammation (Fig. 2.17).

### Type II: Antibody-dependent Cytotoxicity

Type II hypersensitivity reactions are mediated by IgG and IgM antibodies binding to specific cells or tissues (Fig. 2.18).

Type II antibody-dependent reactions are directed against antigen on an individual's own cells (target cells), which then leads to cytotoxic action by NK cells or complement-mediated cell lysis. Complement fragments (C3a and C5a) attract macrophages to the site and stimulate the activation of the classic pathway of complement action, with production of the C5b-9 membrane attack complex.

Hemolytic disease of the newborn is characteristic of this type of hypersensitivity reaction. Red blood cells leak into the mother's circulation during birth and stimulate production of anti-Rh antibody. Subsequent pregnancies involve transfer of these IgG antibodies across the placenta into the

**TABLE 2.4. GELL AND COOMBS HYPERSENSITIVITY REACTIONS**

| Type | Target Organs | Clinical Manifestations | Mechanisms |
|---|---|---|---|
| I. Anaphylactic | Nasal mucosa, GI tract, skin, lungs, conjunctiva | Allergic rhinitis, urticaria, atopic dermatitis, GI sensitivity, asthma | IgE |
| II. Cytotoxic | Circulating | Hemolytic anemia, hemolytic disease of newborn | IgG, IgM, phagocytes |
| III. Immune complex reactions (Arthus reaction) | Blood vessels of skin, joints, kidneys, lungs | Serum sickness, systemic lupus erythematosus, chronic glomerulonephritis | Antigen–antibody complexes (IgG) |
| IV. Cell-mediated reactions (delayed-type hypersensitivity reactions) | Skin, lungs, central nervous system, thyroid | Contact dermatitis, tuberculosis, thyroiditis | Sensitized T lymphocytes |

GI, gastrointestinal.

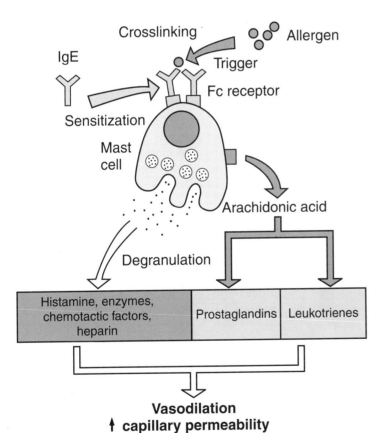

**FIG. 2.16.** Type I hypersensitivity reaction. (From Mudge-Grout C. *Immunologic disorders.* St. Louis: Mosby Year Book, 1993:26, with permission.)

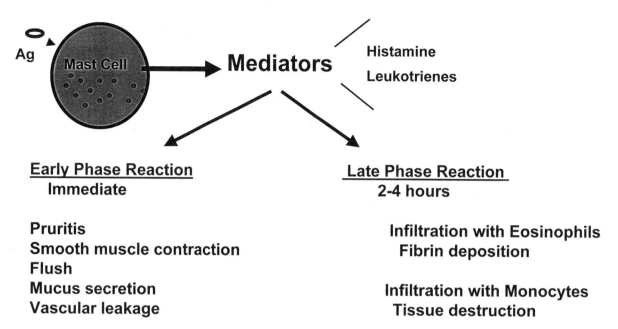

**FIG. 2.17.** Consequences of mediator release.

fetal circulation. If the fetus has an incompatible blood type, the antibodies stimulate destruction of the red blood cells.

Drug-induced reactions also may be the result of type II hypersensitivity reactions. Other types of type II reactions include Goodpasture's syndrome, pemphigus, myasthenia gravis, and Lambert-Eaton syndrome

## Type III: Immune Complex–mediated Hypersensitivity

Excess antibody–antigen complexes may be deposited in tissues when they are not removed effectively by the phago-cyte system. Complement is activated with attraction of neutrophils to the site of inflammation, causing local tissue damage. The sites of immune complex deposition are determined by location of the antigen in tissues (Fig. 2.19).

Immune complexes can trigger a great variety of inflammatory reactions. Interaction with complement generates production of C3a and C5a. These complexes act directly on basophils and platelets to produce vasoactive amines such as histamine and 5-hydroxytryptamine. Platelet aggregation occurs and stimulates complement activation. These aggregated platelets may form microthrombi on the basement membrane and are not effectively removed by neutrophils.

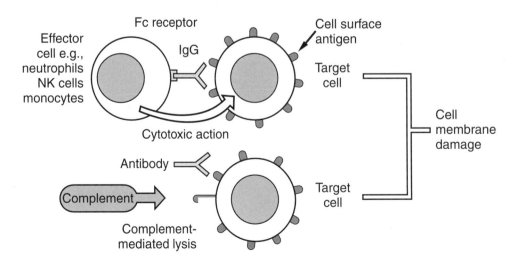

**FIG. 2.18.** Type II hypersensitivity reaction. (From Mudge-Grout C. *Immunologic disorders.* St. Louis: Mosby Year Book, 1993:26, with permission.)

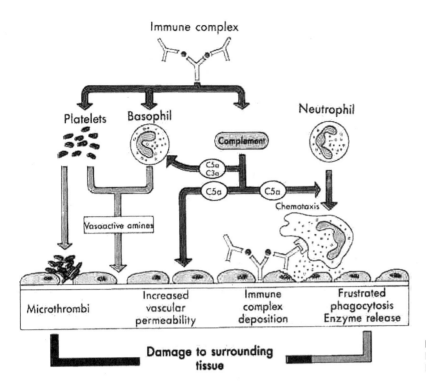

**FIG. 2.19.** Type III hypersensitivity reaction. (From Mudge-Grout C. *Immunologic disorders.* St. Louis: Mosby Year Book, 1993:26, with permission.)

Enzyme release by the neutrophils results in further cell wall damage.

## Type IV: Cell-mediated Hypersensitivity

Delayed hypersensitivity reactions take more than 12 hours to appear. Antigen-sensitized T cells may release cytokines after a second contact with antigen. The cytokines released induce an inflammatory reaction. There are three variants of this type reactions: contact hypersensitivity, tuberculin hypersensitivity, and granulomatous hypersensitivity (Fig. 2.20).

Contact hypersensitivity is characterized by an eczematous reaction at the point of contact with the allergen, often produced by agents such as nickel, chromate, latex, or poison ivy. Langerhans' cells in the skin participate in generation and recruitment of CD4[+] lymphocytes.

Tuberculin hypersensitivity (originally described by Koch) is an example of cell-mediated hypersensitivity. T cells are activated to secrete cytokines that mediate this reaction at the site of injection, usually within 48 hours.

Granulomatous hypersensitivity causes the most severe pathologic effects of this form of inflammation. Its results form the persistence of microorganisms or other particles in the macrophage that the cell is unable to destroy. Exam-

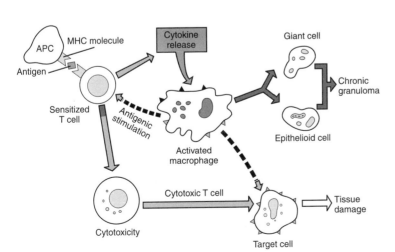

**FIG. 2.20.** Type IV hypersensitivity reaction. (From Mudge-Grout C. *Immunologic disorders.* St. Louis: Mosby Year Book, 1993:27, with permission.)

ples of granulomatous hypersensitivity reactions include the Kveim test for sarcoidosis and the Mitsuda reaction to *Mycoplasma leprae* antigens. Important diseases characterized by granulomatous hypersensitivity reactions are leprosy, tuberculosis, sarcoidosis, and Crohn's disease (Table 2.4).

## IMMUNOPATHOLOGY

Under normal circumstances, the immune system functions well to protect the organism; however, there are occasions when the immune system fails, and this failure may lead to immune deficiencies.

Autoimmunity may develop when the immune system no longer recognizes one or several self-components and reacts against them. The distinction between self and nonself breaks down, and autoimmune disease occurs. Examples include rheumatoid arthritis and pernicious anemia.

Immunodeficiency results when some elements of the immune system become ineffective. Immunodeficiency may be either congenital (X-linked agammaglobulinemia, IgA

deficiency, or severe combined immunodeficiency) or acquired (AIDS).

In the case of hypersensitivity, the immune system mounts a response out of proportion to the damage caused by the pathogen and the immune reactions cause more damage than the pathogen. The symptoms related to both rhinitis and asthma are characteristic of inflammatory hypersensitivity.

## BIBLIOGRAPHY

Abbas AK, Lichtman AH, Pober JS. *Cellular and molecular immunology.* Philadelphia: WB Saunders, 2000.

Claman HA. The biology of the immune response. *JAMA* 1992;8: 2790–2796.

King HC. *An otolaryngologist's guide to allergy.* New York: Thieme Medical, 1990.

Krause HF. *Otolaryngic allergy and immunology.* Philadelphia: WB Saunders, 1989.

Naclerio RM, Durham SR, Mygind N. *Rhinitis mechanisms and management.* New York: Marcel Dekker, 1999.

Roitt I, Brostoff J, Male D. *Immunology,* 5th ed. London: Mosby, 1998.

Stites DP, Terr AI. *Basic and clinical immunology,* 7th ed. Norwalk, CT: Appleton & Lange, 1991.

# 3

# INHALANT ALLERGY

## JOHN H. KROUSE
## BRUCE R. GORDON
## MICHAEL J. PARKER

In the practice of allergy, the selection of the appropriate antigens for testing and treatment is a critical component of the clinical approach to the patient. Because allergy represents a hypersensitive response to an environmental substance to which the person is exposed, effective treatment involves an understanding of the range of those substances capable of provoking sensitivity. Because patients may encounter environmental antigens through various sources, allergens usually are classified by their routes of exposure: inhalants, ingestants (foods), contactants, and injectants. This chapter focuses on the wide range of substances involved in inhalant allergy. In addition, it discusses the cross-reactivity between various inhalant allergens, and between inhalant allergens and foods.

## CROSS-REACTIVITY OF ANTIGENS

Cross-reactive allergens are different antigenic substances that act as though they are the same substance in triggering allergic responses. Cross-reactivity exists when the specific antibody synthesized in response to one antigen is able also to react with one or more other antigens. The portion of the antigen that is recognized by the antibody and is able to evoke the allergic response is known as the *epitope*. Epitopes can be shared among antigens from genetically related species, as well as among distantly related species.

Knowledge of cross-reactivity is useful to the allergist in several ways. Once allergy testing has been completed, knowledge of cross-reactivity assists in the prediction of what other substances may produce allergic responses.

J. H. Krouse: Department of Otolaryngology, Wayne State University, Detroit, Michigan.

B. R. Gordon: Department of Otology and Laryngology, Harvard University, Cambridge; Associate Surgeon, Massachusetts Eye and Ear Infirmary, Boston; Chief of Otolaryngology, Cape Cod Hospital, Hyannis, Massachusetts.

M. J. Parker: Department of Ear, Nose, and Throat, Community General Hospital, Syracuse, New York.

Cross-reactivity information also assists by allowing testing for fewer antigens, thus simplifying and shortening the testing procedure. In addition, knowledge of cross-reactivity between pollens and foods allows education of the allergic person in avoidance of concomitant foods during periods of high pollen prevalence in the environment. Finally, testing and treatment only for non–cross-reacting allergens avoids duplicated tests and treatments and helps keep therapeutic antigen exposure to the necessary minimum, therefore helping to prevent administration of excess antigen loads.

## Measuring Cross-reactivity

Before the development of assays for immunoglobulin E (IgE), all cross-reactivity studies were done by clinical correlation. Cross-reactivity was noted very early in the 20th century, when allergists recognized that treatment with one specific antigen was able to desensitize patients to other antigens as well. This observation was especially noted among grasses because patients who were positive for one grass usually were positive to all grasses tested. Also, treatment with one grass often was found to be just as effective as treatment with several grasses, and was less likely to cause serious reactions.

Cross-reactivity studies now are most commonly done using a technique known as radioallergosorbent test (RAST) inhibition. In this in vitro competition assay, a second antigen, varying in concentration, is placed into a series of assay tubes or wells that contain identical amounts of a reference antigen. As increasing amounts of the second antigen are added, the degree to which the binding of the reference antigen to a specific IgE antibody is inhibited is measured. The more cross-reactivity exists between the two substances, the more the reference antigen is displaced.

## Food-inhalant Cross-reactivity

Cross-reactivity between inhalant allergens and inhaled or ingested foods has been observed for many years. This cross-reactivity is often called *concomitant food sensitivity*. At times this relationship is obvious, such as between wheat flour and inhaled wheat pollen. Some food–inhalant relationships, however, are not so intuitively obvious. Four food–inhalant cross-reactions have been well studied and documented. One such interaction is the oral allergy syndrome observed between birch pollen and various fruits and nuts. Birch is known to cross-react with hazelnuts, potatoes, rose family fruits (especially apples), and with carrots and celery (1). Up to 90% of patients with in vitro-proven birch allergy also are positive to apples (2). In these cross-reactions, birch pollen contains all of the fruit epitopes, whereas the fruits do not contain all birch epitopes (3). A similar cross-reaction has been noted between timothy grass pollen and apple, carrot, and celery. Common mugwort pollen is known partially to cross-react with celery, coriander, and chamomile tea (4,5). Finally, there is a significant cross-reaction between allergenic epitopes on ragweeds and those on cantaloupe, watermelon, and banana (6). Many other food–inhalant cross-reactions have been suspected from clinical observations, but have not yet been confirmed by laboratory studies.

## CATEGORIES OF INHALANT ALLERGENS

Inhalant allergens usually are divided into two varieties on the basis of their persistence in the environment: perennial and seasonal. Perennial allergens are those substances that are present throughout the year, with little variation as a function of season. Seasonal allergens, on the other hand, have distinct periods in which they are present in greater quantities in the environment, usually related to the pollination or sporulation patterns of various organisms. Seasonal allergens are responsible for the commonly recognized "hay fever" of seasonal allergic rhinitis. In certain situations, a single allergen can act as both a perennial and a seasonal allergen. For example, in a temperate climate, house dust is typically a winter seasonal allergen, yet, in closed, climate-controlled buildings, house dust normally becomes a perennial allergen. And, in the north, grass pollination is clearly seasonal, whereas closer to the equator, it becomes perennial. Inhalant allergens also can be grouped into basic categories based on structure. These categories are plant pollens, fungi and fungal spores, animal danders, insect antigens, and environmental dusts. Each of these broad categories is examined in this chapter.

### Pollens

Pollen represents the viable male germinal cells of higher plants, released in the process of sexual reproduction. Grasses, trees, and weeds all produce pollens, and these pollens can be released into the environment, usually on a seasonal basis.

### Allergenicity of Pollens

Two factors are critical in determining whether a particular species produces a pollen that is of allergenic significance. First, the pollen antigens must be sensitizing. Fortunately, plant pollens vary widely in their sensitizing potential, and relatively few species cause major reactions. The second determining factor is the physical structure of the plant flower and of the pollen it produces. The relationship between the physical characteristics of a pollen and its ability to create allergic reactions was first described by Thommen, and these principles are known as *Thommen's postulates* (7) (Table 3.1). Thommen noted that for a pollen to cause significant inhalant allergy, it must be able to be dispersed widely and in large quantity. This dispersal depends heavily on the size, structure, and buoyancy of pollen grains, as well as on the ability of wind to dislodge pollen from its flower.

Two types of plants, anemophilous plants and entomophilous plants, differ in their mode of fertilization and, as a result, vary in their ability to produce widespread allergy. Anemophilous, wind-pollinated plants such as oak trees, ragweed, and grasses have specialized male flowers that produce huge amounts of buoyant pollen, and easily release this material into the wind from exposed anthers. Entomophilous, insect-pollinated plants such as locust trees, palm trees, roses, and other plants with easily visible flowers produce heavy, sticky pollen that is contained within flowers and is poorly dispersed into the air. As a result, anemophilous plants usually meet Thommen's postulates and can be significant allergenic plants, whereas most entomophilous plants cannot. Exceptions primarily occur when entomophilous plants are planted very close to human habitations, or are handled by humans.

Pollen grains of distinct species differ widely in size, shape, and weight, and these variables also affect their dispersal. Allergenically important plants typically produce pollens of approximately 20 to 40 μm in diameter, although some trees produce pollen grains as large as 160 μm. Pollen is most often released by plants in the mornings, and is dispersed widely by the wind on being released. Pollen-allergic patients therefore often are more symptomatic in the morning than later in the day. With increased winds, pollen is held in the air for a longer time, and is more widely dispersed, than on calm days. During rain, pollen is washed

**TABLE 3.1. THOMMEN'S POSTULATES**

1. The plant must be seed bearing, with pollen wind-borne for wide distribution.
2. The pollen must be produced in large quantities.
3. The pollen must be buoyant to be distributed over a wide area.
4. The plant must be widely and abundantly distributed, preferably close to human habitation.
5. The pollen must be allergenic.

to the ground, but often becomes airborne again after the rain ceases and the ground dries. Because light, buoyant pollens are very easily dispersed, it is not uncommon to find significant amounts of pollen transported long distances from the source.

### Distribution of Pollens

Allergenic pollens, especially from grasses, are widely present throughout the world and can be found in any region in which plants can grow. In the temperate regions of the world, three seasons are noted in which plants typically pollinate. These seasons vary in length as a function of the growing season in any given locale, but three broad categories are described for pollination. In the spring, trees pollinate. Then, in the summer months, especially in early summer, grasses pollinate. Finally, in late summer and into autumn, weeds pollinate. Pollen production ceases in winter owing to reduced light and cold temperatures, but small amounts of pollen may remain in dead catkins, to be dispersed by severe winter winds.

In general, allergenic plants are distributed throughout rather distinct climactic regions. The United States is divided into eleven pollen regions, or zones, on the basis of the climate and assemblage of indigenous flora found in each area (Table 3.2; Fig. 3.1). The best reference source for distribution of pollens in the United States and southern Canada is the text by Lewis, Vinay, and Zenger (8). Although flora maps and pollen surveys are useful, there can be local variations in climate and flora that might significantly affect local pollen sources. Local agricultural extension services or universities often can be an excellent source of pollen data for a specific city or county. Occasionally, there are published reports of the frequency of allergic reactions to large numbers of inhalant allergens in a defined geographic region. These reports also are very useful. A recent example,

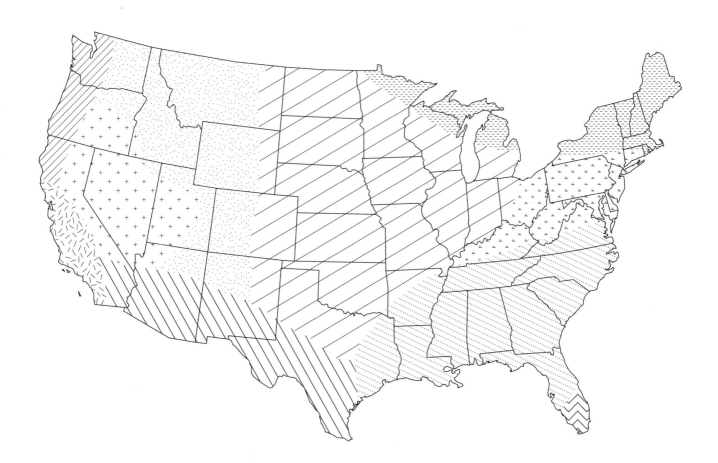

# The United States
(not to scale)

**FIG. 3.1.** Pollen zones in the continental United States.

## TABLE 3.2. U.S. POLLEN ZONES

Northern Forest
Eastern Agricultural
Southeast Coast
Subtropical Florida/Caribbean
Central Plains
Rocky Mountains
Great Basin
Arid Southwest
Northwest Coast
California Coast
Tropical Hawaii

## TABLE 3.3. TREE FAMILIES

Gymnosperms
  Cupressaceae
    Cypress, false cypress, juniper, arborvitae
  Pinaceae
    Firs, larch, spruce, hemlock
  Taxaceae
    Yews
  Taxodiaceae
    Redwood, bald cypress
  Ginkoceae
    Ginkgos
Angiosperms
  Aceraceae
    Box elder, red maple, sugar maple
  Anacardiaceae
    Cashew, mango, pistachio, sumac, poison ivy
  Arecaceae
    Palms, palmetto, date palm
  Betulaceae
    Birches, alders, hornbeams, hazelnut
  Casuarinaceae
    Australian pine
  Fagaceae
    Oaks, beeches
  Juglandaceae
    Walnuts, hickories
  Moraceae
    Mulberry
  Oleaceae
    Olive, ash, jasmine, privet, lilac
  Platanaceae
    Sycamore, plane trees
  Salicaceae
    Aspens, cottonwoods, poplars, willows
  Ulmaceae
    Elm, hackberry
  Vitaceae
    Ivy, grapes, Virginia creepers

for California, where there are high numbers of sensitizing plant species, has tried to simplify the number of inhalant allergens that should be tested (9). Testing 58 aeroallergens was found to be sufficient to detect approximately 90% of sensitivities (2 dust mites, cat, cockroach, 2 grasses, 9 molds, 16 weeds, and 27 trees). In addition, pollen sampling and measurement can be conducted by individual practices by using either impact or volumetric methods. Devices such as the Rotorod sampler (Sampling Technologies, Minnetonka, MN) or the Burkard sampler (Burkard Manufacturing, Rickmansworth, Hertfordshire, United Kingdom) can be used, along with microscopic identification, for accurate information regarding current local prevalence of various pollens and molds.

### Trees

In general, trees pollinate in the United States from the late winter months through the early spring. There is variability in the pollination of trees, however, in that in certain areas of the South and Southwest, trees may pollinate in the fall, and may overlap grass or weed seasons. Even in the Northeast, the end of the tree season often overlaps the beginning of the grass season. The highest pollen counts often are encountered in spring as numerous species of trees produce copious amounts of airborne pollen (10). Unlike weeds and grasses, most trees have very short and distinct seasons of pollination. Because of its appearance and abundance, tree pollen often is readily observed by patients, and they often are able to correlate the onset of tree pollen season with the exacerbation of their allergies.

In certain regions, the number of tree species can be as many as 300 (11). It is very important, therefore, to be clearly aware of the specific allergenic trees that are indigenous to a discrete geographic region. Unfortunately, with the abundant variation of tree families, there is little cross-reactivity between most families, subfamilies, and genera. However, there usually is substantial cross-reactivity within each genus. Two large classes of trees are discussed here, the gymnosperms, or coniferous trees, and the angiosperms, or flowering trees (Table 3.3).

### Tree Families

*Gymnospermae.* The gymnosperms consist of coniferous, primarily evergreen, trees such as cedars and pines. These are the most numerous and widespread trees in North America. They are found close to human habitation, are heavy pollinators, and are exclusively wind pollinated. It might be thought, therefore, that gymnosperms would be significant stimulators of allergy. Of this large class, however, only members of the cypress family, Cupressaceae, are always clinically important.

The family Cupressaceae includes species of cypress, false cypress, juniper, cedar, and arborvitae. They produce copious amounts of light, buoyant, allergenically potent pollen late in fall, winter, or early spring. A particularly important member of this family is mountain cedar (*Juniper ashei*), a small tree that grows abundantly in Texas and areas of the southwestern United States. Mountain cedar pollen is highly allergenic and produces a very severe seasonal rhinitis in middle to late winter. There is very little cross-reactivity noted among most gymnosperms, with the exception of the cypress family, where useful cross-reactivity does allow a single representative species to be tested.

Pollens of most other gymnosperms have been considered to be unimportant allergens. However, little actually is known about the allergenicity and clinical importance of even common gymnosperms, such as yews and gingkos. Bald cypress, a common southern tree, is known to produce a sensitizing pollen, but has not been identified as an allergic problem.

Family Pinaceae contains the other potentially significant gymnosperms. Pines are the largest family of gymnosperms, including species of fir, larch, spruce, hemlock, Douglas fir, and pines. Together, pines produce huge quantities of pollen. However, pine pollen is large and falls to the ground rapidly. Despite this, it still can be transported for long distances. Pollen from many pines is low in allergenicity, so it may not be an important allergen. Patients, however, often believe that they have pine allergy because they observe the heavy coat of yellow-green pollen on their cars and driveways during pollen season, and correlate it with the very visible pollen on pines. It usually is the other accompanying tree pollens, such as oak, that are clinically significant. Patients also frequently react to Pinaceae species brought into the house for use as Christmas trees. These reactions are believed to be caused both by pine resins and by grass, weed, and mold allergens present on the needles and bark (12). In certain regions, however, where pine pollen is present in extremely large quantities, enough pollen may be available to create significant exposure and symptoms. Pine pollen can be a particular problem in areas, like the Northeast coastal region, where pitch pine (*Pinus rigida*) pollination occurs at the end of the tree season, and earlier-blooming species, like ash, cedar, elm, birch, maple, and oak, have primed patients to high levels of reactivity. Pine pollen allergy should not be assumed always to be insignificant.

**Angiospermae.** Angiosperms, in terms of number of species, are the largest tree class. Angiosperms are primarily deciduous flowering trees, and are widely distributed in North America. Like gymnosperms, angiosperms vary significantly in both their degree of antigenicity and in the geographic distribution of allergenically important species. Of all the pollen-producing plants, trees show the greatest diversity and the least cross-reactivity.

*Oaks.* The single most important type of allergenic tree pollen in the United States is that from the family Fagaceae, the oaks. Over 50 important species exist, with the white oak (*Quercus alba*) and the northern red oak (*Quercus rubra*) being very common in the eastern half of the country. The large number of western oak species have more restricted distributions, but are equally important pollen sources in their regions. Oak pollen is produced in large amounts, and

for prolonged periods, from the late winter to early summer, most typically in April and May. Oak pollen is both profuse and moderately allergenic, and is of major clinical importance to most atopic patients. Beech trees are closely related to oaks, and are allergenic, but in most areas are of secondary importance to oak. Substantial cross-reactivity in this family allows treatment with a single species.

*Birches.* A second group of angiosperms that is of great importance is the family Betulaceae, the birches. Birch pollen has been well studied and is among the most potent of tree pollens. Other significant members of this family include alders, hornbeams, and hazelnuts. There is strong cross-reactivity between all members of the birch family. Members of this family are widespread throughout the northern United States, Canada, and in mountain ranges, but also are found in most nonarid parts of North America. Birch pollen normally is shed in great quantities in early spring. Birch allergy is the cause of the best-documented example of inhalant–food cross-reactivity, the oral allergy syndrome.

*Maples.* The third major angiosperm family is Aceraceae, or the maples. Maples are very common on both the east and west coasts, but also are widely planted ornamentals in all parts of the United States and Canada. The most widespread, and also most allergenic, maple is the box elder (*Acer negundo*), a hardy shade tree. Maples are easily recognized by their distinctive, lobed leaves (as on the Canadian flag), except for box elder, which has pinnately compound leaves that resemble the leaves of ash or hickory trees. In lieu of adequate data, box elder usually is chosen as the representative maple for testing.

*Olive—Ash.* The fourth important family, Oleaceae, consists of olive trees and related species. Olive pollen is buoyant and highly allergenic, and these trees are now widely cultivated in the Southwest, especially in urban areas, where mid-spring olive-induced symptoms are commonly seen. In other parts of the country, other members of the family may be important. For example, in the Southeast and in California, jasmine pollen may cause symptoms in the late winter and early spring. Rarely, even *Forsythia* and lilacs are troublesome for individual patients. In many areas, ash and privet are important causes of allergy. Different ash species may pollinate from mid-winter through late spring, but usually, ash is one of the earliest important pollinators. The last Oleaceae species to bloom are normally the widely planted hedge privets (*Ligustrum*), which flower in late spring and summer. Olive and privet pollens significantly cross-react, but ash pollen is less cross-reactive, and may require separate treatment.

Several other angiosperm families often are clinically important, but are less universally distributed than the previous four families. One such family is the Moraceae, or the mulberry family. Mulberry pollen is small, easily distributed by the wind, and produced in abundant quantity. It is found in large amounts in the East and Southwest, and locally, throughout the United States, where it has been planted as an ornamental. Because of this frequent planting, mulberry appears to be growing in importance (13). The family Salicaceae, which includes the cottonwoods, poplars, aspens, and willows, also is of importance. These common trees produce their pollen in middle to late spring and are abundant pollinators throughout their range. There is good cross-reactivity among Salicaceae species, and because the percentage of patients testing positive to this family is greatest for poplar, poplar often is used as the representative species for this family. Members of the walnut family, Juglandaceae, are very important in the South and West, particularly in agricultural areas. In the Southeast, pecan allergy is similar in importance to ragweed allergy. Hickory and pecan trees produce the most potent pollen, but all members of the family are significant, heavy pollinators. Cross-reactivity is extensive in the Juglandacea family. Ulmaceae, the elms and hackberries *(Celtis)*, also are important pollinators in late winter and early spring. In the South, and particularly in California, some elm species bloom in fall, where they often are more of a problem than are spring-blooming species. Cross-reactivity between elms and hackberries is incomplete, so *Celtis* species may require separate testing where they are common.

Still other tree families are not general sources of allergic symptoms, but may be important in certain locales. Sycamore and plane trees are sources of abundant, but only moderately allergenic pollen in middle to late spring. Because these trees tolerate urban conditions well and are frequently planted, they may contribute to tree symptoms in larger cities. During much of the year, *Acacia* species are potent allergenic pollinators in the Southwest and South Central states, but with such broad pollination seasons, they may not always be identified as significant causes of allergy. The introduced species of *Eucalyptus* can sensitize, and have been observed occasionally to be clinically important. *Eucalyptus* pollen is commonly captured in Florida and in Southern California. Finally, in Florida and California, individual patients may become highly sensitive to the pollen of several species of ornamental Australian pines *(Casuarina)* or several species of palm trees, including the commercial date palm *(Phoenix dactylifera)*.

Cross-reactivity is strong between the species in most of the angiosperm genera, and also is significant between genera, within each angiosperm family. This means that in a local region, it usually is not necessary to treat every species of oak, birch, or maple; rather, the most common local species of each family for which there is an available allergen extract may be used.

## Grasses

Grasses are ubiquitous plants in nearly all ecologic zones, with over a thousand species in North America. Grass pollen

### TABLE 3.4. GRASS FAMILIES

**Pooideae**
  Grasses
    Bluegrass, June grass, brome, canary, orchard, fescue, foxtail, quack, redtop, rye, timothy, vernal grass
  Cereal grains
    Barley, oats, rye, wheat, triticale, spelt
  Cross-reactivity is strong
**Panicoideae**
  Grasses
    Bahia, barnyard, bluestem, crabgrass, elephant, gamma, Johnson, St. Augustine
  Cereal grains
    Corn, millet, sugarcane, sorghum
  Cross-reactivity is strong
**Chloridoideae**
  Grasses
    Bermuda, buffalo, cord, zoysia
  Cross-reactivity is strong
**Bambusoideae**
  Grasses
    Bamboo
  Cereal grains
    Rice, wild rice
**Arundinoideae**
  Grasses
    Common reed, giant reed

has been extensively studied for many years, and there is a great deal of information available regarding its antigenicity. In most parts of North America, grass is second only to ragweed in symptom production, and in much of the western United States, Puerto Rico, and in subtropical areas, grass is the primary aeroallergen. In the Northeast and other temperate climates, grass pollination occurs in a relatively distinct season beginning in late May or early June. Peak grass season is normally in August, but grasses are still very active during fall, along with ragweed. In warmer climates, however, grass pollination begins earlier, is prolonged into late fall, and can become perennial in areas such as Southern California and South Florida. Grass pollens are the most potent allergens known, and are highly allergenic even at very low levels in the environment. One study has shown that grass pollen is able to stimulate allergic rhinitis even at concentrations as low as 20 pollen grains per m$^3$ (14). Three grass subfamilies contain the most important antigenic grasses in North America: Pooideae, Panicoideae, and Chloreidoideae (Table 3.4). Most of the grasses in each of these subfamilies are highly cross-reactive, although some unique antigens have been observed.

### Pooideae

Most of the wind-borne grass pollen in the United States is produced by members of this common subfamily. Rye, blue, brome, fescue, June, orchard, saltgrass, and timothy grasses are the most common allergenic grasses of this family. The grains, barley, oats, rye, and wheat, also are in this family, but, except for rye, are self-pollinators and so are not major sources of pollen. It is clinically important to recognize that the pollens of this family are the most potent allergens known. Given this potency, and the strong cross-reactivity of these grasses, testing and treatment should be done with only a single representative species from this subfamily, so that patients are not inadvertently given antigen overloads. Timothy grass often is chosen as the representative pooid. Because of substantial inhalant–food cross-reactivity, this subfamily is very important both as a source of inhalant and of food allergies.

## Panicoideae

Panicoid grasses also are widely distributed in North America, especially in more southern areas. The most common of these grasses include Bahia, barnyard, crabgrass, gamma, Johnson, and St. Augustine. The foods sugarcane, sorghum (cultivated Johnson grass), corn, and millet are in this group. Sugarcane normally is cut before flowering, but corn and millet produce significant, potent pollen in agricultural areas, and sorghum is both cultivated as well as an important weed grass. Bahia grass has some unique antigens, and because of the strong cross-reactivity among panicoid species, it can be used as the representative grass for testing this group. Johnson grass may not be fully cross-reactive with Bahia, and it may be necessary to test it separately when it is locally important.

## Chloridoideae

The third important grass subfamily in the United States is the chloridoids. The primary representative of this group is Bermuda grass, which is commonly found in the southern half of North America. Other subfamily members are grama and zoysia. Again, because of strong cross-reactivity, Bermuda grass is useful for testing and treatment as the antigen representative of the chloridoid family.

## Bambusoideae and Arundinoideae

Two additional subfamilies of grasses are common throughout the world, yet are not considered to be allergenically important in the United States. Members of subfamily Bambusoideae, which includes bamboos, rice, and wild rice, are found in some parts of the United States, but are self-pollinators. Because their pollen is not widely dispersed, they are of little clinical significance. Members of the Arundinoideae subfamily, including the common reeds and giant reeds, are known to be allergenic, but are fall pollinators that produce only moderate amounts of pollen. Their importance in most regions is thought to be minor, with the concurrent pollens of ragweed and other fall weeds being more clinically significant.

## Grass-like Plants

Several small families of grass-like plants may sometimes produce allergic symptoms. Sedges, rushes, and cattails have caused symptoms in widely separated areas of the United States and are potentially sensitizing anywhere near marshes and wetlands. If these plants are common in a particular region, testing may be warranted.

## Weeds

Weed seasons also tend to occur at a distinct times of the year, although blooming may be somewhat prolonged and irregular, especially in southern areas (10). Weeds bloom intermittently or continuously from mid-spring through mid-fall in many areas of the country. As a result, weed seasons overlap with grass seasons, and present a significant problem for many patients throughout the United States. Ragweed, the most clinically important allergenic weed in most locations, is the predominant cause of allergy symptoms where it is common. Three major, and several minor, allergenic weed families are present in the United States. (Table 3.5).

## Asteraceae

This large family has three tribes that contain significant allergenic species. Ragweed *(Ambrosia)*, the most clinically significant weed in the United States and southern Canada, is a member of tribe Heliantheae. Ragweed pollen has a very distinct season, from late summer through mid-fall, and is the predominant cause of allergy symptoms during this season east of the Rocky Mountains. Although the duration of sunlight appears to be the key factor, in areas of the

**TABLE 3.5. WEED FAMILIES**

**Amaranthaceae**
  Amaranths, waterhemps, pigweeds, careless weed, cockscomb
**Asteraceae**
  *Heliantheae*
    Ragweed (*Ambrosia*), Marsh elder (*Iva*), Cocklebur (*Xanthium*)
  *Astereae*
    Goldenrod (*Solidago*), Baccharis
  *Anthemideae*
    Sagebrush, wormwoods, mugworts (*Artemesia*), chamomile
**Brassicaceae**
  Mustard, rape
**Cannabaceae**
  Hemp, marijuana, hops
**Chenopodiaceae**
  Burning bush (*Kochia*), Russian thistle (tumbleweed), lamb's quarters
**Plantaginaceae**
  English plantain (*Plantago*)
**Polygonaceae**
  Dock, sorrel (*Rumex*)
**Urticaceae**
  pellitory (*Parietaria*), nettles (*Urtica*)

United States that are subject to colder temperatures, the first frost usually occurs at approximately the time of the end of ragweed pollination. In more southern regions, ragweed may continue to pollinate through the winter months. Although 17 species of ragweed have been identified, short, giant, and western ragweed are the most widespread species, and all completely cross-react with each other, and with southern ragweed. Short ragweed usually is chosen for testing and treatment.

Other members of the helianth tribe are also clinically important. The *Iva* genus, which includes marsh elders, and the *Xanthium* genus, which includes cocklebur, both elicit significant allergic responses. Although these plants are not commonly found in the Great Lakes region and the Appalachian Mountains, they are important on the East Coast, in the Great Plains, and the West as far north as Canada. Given the strong cross-reactivity among members of the helianth tribe, testing and treatment may be conducted with short ragweed as a representative of the entire family, unless other species are very common in the local area.

The other two important Asteraceae are genera *Baccharis* and *Artemesia* (sages). *Baccharis* often grows as large, woody shrubs with tiny, thistle-like flowers, and is most common in the Southwest, as far north as Colorado and Nebraska. Other *Baccharis* species range along the Gulf, East, and West coasts as far north as Cape Cod and the Columbia River. *Artemesia* species, including great basin sagebrush, wormwoods, and mugworts, grow in all parts of the United States and Canada except the lower Mississippi Valley and South Florida. Because *Bacharis* and *Artemesia* are in different tribes, they may not fully cross-react, either with each other or with helianths. Therefore, they should be tested individually, when locally common.

Although goldenrod *(Solidago)* also is a member of the Asteraceae, in the same tribe as *Baccharis,* it is primarily entomophilous, so is not a significant allergen in most people. Nevertheless, it may be incriminated by patients because goldenrod blooms at the same time that ragweed pollinates. Even so, some physicians do routinely test for goldenrod.

### Amaranthaceae

A second major group of allergenic weeds is represented by the amaranth family. These weeds are widely distributed in the United States and Southern Canada, and consist of approximately 65 species, including waterhemps, pigweeds, careless weed, amaranths, *Tidestromia,* and cultivated flowering cockscomb *(Celiosa).* Cultivated edible amaranth (quinoa) is used as a cereal substitute. Amaranth pollination usually is severe in the Midwest and West, and less so in the East. Among common amaranths there is strong cross-reactivity, and a single species may be used as representative of the group (14).

### Chenopodaceae

The chenopod family is closely related to the amaranths, and consists of 22 genera, most of which are adapted to living in saline soils. Chenopods grow in almost all regions of North America south of the Arctic. Representative species include cultivated sugar beets, spinach, New Zealand spinach, burning bush *(Kochia),* Russian thistle (tumbleweed), goosefoot, lamb's quarters, and Mexican tea. There is little cross-reactivity among chenopods, with the exception of the *Atriplex* genus (saltbush, shadscale, spearscale, wingscale). For that reason, common chenopods should be tested and treated individually, except for a single representative of the *Atriplex* genus.

### Minor Weed Families

Minor weed families are not as universally significant as the major families, but may be of local or individual importance.

***Plantaginaceae.*** There are many plantain species growing throughout the United States and Southern Canada, with greater concentrations in the middle part of the continent. English plantain *(Plantago lanceolata)* is common and tends to pollinate earlier in the summer than other weeds, producing copious amounts of potent pollen. It usually produces symptoms in patients who are skin-test positive for this antigen. It should be tested and treated individually.

***Polygonaceae.*** The major members of this family include cultivated buckwheat and rhubarb, and sorrels. Sorrels grow in all parts of North America and are particularly common in the West. Sheep sorrel and dock sorrel can produce large amounts of highly allergenic pollen in mid-summer, and may be clinically important. Sorrels should be tested if locally common.

***Urticaceae.*** Although nettle allergy is widespread in Europe, it is of only potential clinical importance in the United States. High levels of nettle pollen have been detected in Michigan and Florida, and the plants are relatively widely distributed in the United States, so that reactions to nettle pollen might be observable. The important European allergenic plant, wall pellitory *(Parietaria),* is cultivated in the United States and could become a problem if it naturalizes. The genera *Urtica* (stinging nettles) and *Parietaria* (pellitories) do not significantly cross-react, and require separate testing when both are present in a region.

***Cannabaceae.*** Members of this family include hemp, marijuana, and hops. Heavy pollinators, these plants can be clinically important in some regions, especially in the Midwest, Northern Plains, and Northwest, where hemp grows wild, and in other areas where they are cultivated.

***Brassicaceae.*** Wild and cultivated mustard and rape plants produce potent pollen, but are primarily entomophilous. However, they may be important for some individuals on the West coast and in Southern Canada, where these plants are common.

***Fabaceae.*** Legumes, except for the *Acacia* tree (discussed previously), are entomophilous and usually not sensitizing by inhalation. However, farmers and ranchers who handle hay made from legumes like clover, alfalfa, and vetch often become strongly sensitized to these plants.

***Pteridophytes.*** Ferns and fern-like plants grow in all non-arid parts of North America and produce large amounts of spores. The common bracken fern, horsetails, and club mosses all have been suggested to be significant sources of allergy, but only the club moss, *Lycopodium,* has been known to be a problem, owing to use of its spores in cosmetics. Asiatic and, recently, European species of fern are known to be definitely allergenic, and appear to be major allergens in tropical countries (15).

## Fungi

Fungi are primarily saprophytic eukaryotic organisms that are universally present throughout the world. They thrive in moist, dark environments, and live by digesting organic debris or by parasitizing plants or animals. Molds are able to grow throughout the temperature range that humans find comfortable, and are not killed by freezing. Available moisture usually is the key factor restricting mold growth, especially inside buildings. However, fungi are not quickly killed by dry conditions, and normally thrive above 60% relative humidity. Growth is especially profuse in contact with free water, so that leaks and condensation are major factors encouraging indoor mold growth. In many fungi, ejection of spores requires free water, so that rain, dew, and fog commonly trigger massive spore releases (16). In other species, spores break loose only under dry and windy conditions. Although approximately 100,000 species of fungi exist, only a few hundred are responsible for human diseases (17) (Table 3.6), and only approximately 70 of these are

## TABLE 3.6. COMMON ALLERGENIC FUNGI

*Alternaria*
*Aspergillus*
*Cladosporium (Hormodendrum)*
*Candida*
*Helminthosporium*
*Epicoccum*
*Fusarium*
*Penicillium*
*Phoma*
*Mucor*
*Rhizopus*
*Bipolaris*
*Curvularia*

known allergens (18). Fungi may be both seasonal and perennial allergens, and commonly stimulate not only immediate hypersensitivity reactions of Gell and Coombs type I, but type IV delayed hypersensitivity reactions.

Fungi grow in two different forms, as yeasts and as molds. Molds are characterized by growth through the production of multicellular, filamentous colonies composed of branching, tubular cells referred to as *hyphae*. These hyphae can be divided by cross-walls, otherwise known as *septae*. The manner of growth is specific to various species of molds, and their colonies have characteristic features, including color, branching patterns, fruiting body types, spore shapes, and presence or absence of septa. Yeasts, on the other hand, are single cells, either ellipsoid or spherical. Yeasts reproduce by budding and can form chains of yeast cells known as *pseudohyphae*. Some species of fungi are dimorphic in that they can reproduce either by mycelial colony formation and sporulation, or by growing as a yeast and budding.

### Complexity of Fungal Studies

Fungal taxonomy is complex and species identification is confused. One entire group of "fungi" has been reclassified as protists (19), and some fungi that had been thought to be different species have been shown to be different stages of a single species. Many fungi also cannot be easily classified because they have never been observed to form distinctive fruiting bodies or spores. Different isolates of a single fungal species often are given different scientific names, and may not be appreciated as being identical. Misidentification of fungal species by antigen supply companies also has been observed (20). Finally, many fungi are difficult to culture, requiring specific environmental growth factors that cannot yet be duplicated in a laboratory environment. For all of these reasons, it is difficult to be certain exactly what fungus is actually being tested for, and comparative studies on fungal allergy are difficult to carry out unless all participants are using materials obtained from the same source. Thus, research on fungal allergy has lagged appreciably behind research on other, more easily characterized, inhalant allergens. In the future, advances in DNA genotyping are anticipated to clarify fungal taxonomy.

All fungi have a rigid external cell wall composed of the polysaccharide, chitin, as well as other long-chain polysaccharides, glycoproteins, proteins, and lipids. Most fungal allergens are polysaccharides and glycoproteins (18), and their carbohydrate components make them chemically distinctive compared with most other common allergens. This distinctive structure has made it more difficult to test for fungal allergy because the fungal antigens usually do not produce as strong reactions as do pollens, in either in vitro or in vivo testing. In addition to their vegetative growth as molds or yeasts, many fungi can reproduce by sexual or nonsexual sporulation. Spores readily become airborne and also are antigenic. Whether spores or vegetative mycelia and yeasts are the most appropriate antigens to use for testing often is debated, but patients normally are exposed to both types of antigens in the air. A further complicating factor is that many fungi produce volatile or soluble toxins, and these may produce nonallergic symptoms.

Mold spores are common airborne antigens. They are very buoyant, usually measure from 2 to 20 μm in diameter, and, because of their small size, are easily inhaled into the tracheobronchial tree, with the smallest spores being capable of reaching the alveoli (21). They rise high in the atmosphere during the warming of the day, falling back to the ground with the cool of the evening. During the summer, counts of mold spores can outnumber pollen grains by approximately 1,000 to 1. In temperate climates, mold spores also normally are high in middle to late fall, after ragweed season is over, and increase again as soon as the ground warms in spring, often coincident with early tree pollination (22). Spore counts normally decrease in temperate climates when the ground is covered with snow, although low levels of spores continue to be produced on trees, homes, and other sun-warmed surfaces. Also, during winter, spores can be blown in by storms that have passed through more southerly regions.

### Allergenic Fungi

The importance of fungi in the causation of respiratory allergy has been controversial, primarily because of the taxonomic and technical problems encountered with fungal antigen testing (see earlier). However, most clinicians have found fungal allergy to be important. Approximately 20 common fungi with worldwide distribution are believed to be primarily responsible for most fungal allergic reactions, although many additional fungi are capable of contributing to allergic diseases. The fungi that most commonly cause positive skin test reactions are from the genera *Alternaria, Cladosporium, Helminthosporium, Fusarium, Penicillium, Phoma, Aspergillus, Rhizopus,* and *Mucor* (22). A national summary of fungal aeroallergen survey data was published in 1964 and is a useful guide to approximate regional fungal prevalences (23). A 1984 summary of many aeroallergen surveys found the most prevalent fungi to be from the genera *Cladosporium, Alternaria, Aspergillus, Penicillium, Helminthosporium, Aureobasidium, Phoma, Nigrospora, Rhizopus, Mucor, Epicoccum, Stemphylium, Curvularia, Fusarium, Scopulariopsis, Cephalosporium, Chaetomium, Trichoderma, Streptomycetes, Candida, Cryptococcus,* and *Rhodotorula,* as well as the rusts and smuts (24). Corey et al. studied molds in Chicago (25), and found that positive in vitro mold tests were nearly as prevalent as those to ragweed, dust mites, or cat. The most prevalent mold sensitivity was to *Alternaria,* which was positive in 40% of patients. *Helminthosporium* and *Candida* were less prevalent, but still frequent. Even the least prevalent of the 14 tested molds were positive in 10% of cases.

*Alternaria.* This is the most completely studied of the allergenic mold genera, and contains at least 14 important species. *Alternaria* has been considered to be the third most important allergen in parts of the United States, after ragweed and grasses (20). Spores of *Alternaria alternaria* (previously *Alternaria tenuis*) are highly allergenic, and are one of the most potent fungal provokers of asthma (12). *Alternaria* spore counts peak in middle to late summer, but minor peaks can occur at any time, even during winter. *Alternaria* spores are one of the most prevalent fungi identified, worldwide, both on aeroallergen surveys and by allergy testing. For example, in Italy, *Alternaria* tests were positive in 2% to 30% (average 10%) of patients from various regions (26). Twelve percent of patients reacted only to *Alternaria,* and 80% of all *Alternaria*-positive patients had symptomatic rhinitis and 53% had asthma. *Alternaria* allergy had a 20% prevalence in asthmatic American children (27). Furthermore, highly symptomatic patients were more likely to be *Alternaria* positive, and, the degree of bronchial hyperreactivity was correlated with the severity of *Alternaria* sensitization. *Alternaria* also has been identified as the most common airborne fungal contaminant in modern, closed office buildings (28).

*Aspergillus.* This is one of the most prevalent fungal genera found both in indoor and outdoor environments. *Aspergillus niger* is the most common representative of the genus, and also grows as a skin saprophyte in the external auditory canal. *Aspergillus* species are highly allergenic and in rare cases severe sensitization occurs, causing diseases such as pulmonary aspergillosis. There are many identified *Aspergillus* species, and the predominant species frequently varies in different geographic regions. The major *Aspergillus fumigatus* antigen, Asp f I, is a potent cell toxin (19), and other species, such as *Aspergillus flavus,* which is widely used in industry (12), also produce aflatoxins. *Aspergillus oryzae* is used to ferment sake and soy sauce.

*Aureobasidium.* One of the most common fungi found in the United States by culture plate surveys, *Aureobasidium* (formerly *Pullularia*) causes less severe bronchial reactions than *Alternaria* but does produce positive skin reactions in some patients.

*Cladosporium.* The genus *Cladosporium* (formerly *Hormodendrum*) produces very large amounts of airborne spores, which are the most prevalent fungal spores found in aeroallergen surveys in most of the temperate zones of the world (20). *Cladosporium* spores move with weather fronts and are capable of crossing the Atlantic ocean (12). Like *Alternaria,* but less antigenic, *Cladosporium herbarum* and *Cladosporium cladosporoides* also peak in late summer, and are common both indoors and out.

*Curvularia.* This genus has recently been recognized to be an important allergen because of its role as a cause of allergic fungal sinusitis. It often is found on aeroallergen surveys, but is less prevalent than *Cladosporium.*

**Epiccocum.** Growing on common plants, such as cedar trees, *Epicoccum nigrum* produces highly allergenic spores that peak in early autumn, after the peak of ragweed season.

**Fusarium.** Although capable of causing significant skin re-actions, and frequently producing high spore counts, the importance of the common agricultural pest genus, *Fusarium,* in human allergy is not well documented.

**Helminthosporium.** The fungal genus *Helminthosporium* is a recently recognized, common allergen that causes significant human allergy. It is highly allergenic, being as potent in bronchoprovocation tests as *Alternaria,* although it is not as widely distributed. In the Midwest, skin sensitization to *Helminthosporium solani* is almost as frequent as to *Alternaria* (16).

**Penicillium.** *Penicillium* is one of the most common indoor fungi, and commonly is cultured in basements. Although laboratory strains of *Penicillium* are the source of the antibiotic penicillin, there is no known cross-reactivity between allergy to the fungi and allergy to the antibiotic. Like *Aspergillus,* the numerous *Penicillium* species vary in prevalence by geographic locale, and even from home to home. *Penicillium* strains are used to ferment blue, Camembert, and Roquefort cheeses.

**Mucor, Rhizopus, and Stemphylium.** These fungal genera are potentially significant allergenic fungi that are found in moist environments. *Mucor* is best known for causing fatal invasive fungal infections, but is also a moderately common aeroallergen. In some allergy test series, sensitivity to *Mucor* is only slightly less common than to *Alternaria* (16). *Rhizopus* species frequently are positive on skin testing, and *Stemphylium,* where present, causes very strong skin test reactions (12).

**Smuts and Rusts.** These parasitic basidiomycetous fungi grow on living plants, especially on grains and grasses. They produce very high numbers of spores during the late summer and autumn months, and can be a significant cause of allergy. Mowing releases smuts, causing them to be airborne, and triggering acute allergic symptoms in the people who are mowing their lawns or harvesting grains. Smuts are very prevalent in grain-producing agricultural areas, and, at their peak, can exceed the spore counts of all other fungi. Several smut and rust species, such as *Puccinia graminis* and *Ustilago maydis,* may be present in any local area, and decisions about which to test for and treat normally are based on a comparison of the frequency and severity of skin test reactions.

**Yeasts.** There are many unrelated species of airborne yeasts, which may be difficult to differentiate on impact or volumetric detectors, but can often be identified from environmental culture plates. Some, like *Rhodotorula, Saccharomycetes,* and *Sporobolomyces,* are suspected of being significant allergens, whereas others, like *Candida albicans,* may be both allergens and pathogens; the allergic status of *Monilia sitophila* remains undetermined.

**Basidiomycetes (Mushrooms).** Very important in terms of late summer and fall aeroallergen levels, but little recognized, mushroom spores, such as from *Agaricus, Coprinus, Fomes,* and *Ganoderma,* are known to be significant allergens and have been implicated as causes of fall asthma attacks. In one study, 10% of allergic patients were sensitized to at least one of three common mushrooms, and confirming nasal challenges were positive (29). However, few allergen extracts are available for mushrooms because of technical difficulties in their culture.

### Testing for Common Fungi

There is very little significant cross-reactivity among fungal species, even within a genus. For that reason, one or more representatives from each prevalent, sensitizing genus of fungi must be individually tested and treated. Whenever possible, local information from aeroallergen and plate culture surveys should be used to improve the selection of test species for a given practice locale. The suggested primary testing board for fungi, therefore, should be chosen from the genera known commonly to be positive: *Alternaria, Aspergillus, Cladosporium, Epicoccum, Fusarium, Helminthosporium, Mucor, Penicillium, Phoma,* and *Rhizopus. C. albicans* normally is tested and treated separately because of its special role as a commensal, and sometimes pathogenic fungus (see Chapter 13).

### Testing for Less Prevalent Fungi

In cases of allergic fungal sinusitis, when the seasonal timing of symptoms suggests unknown fungal sensitivities, or when a patient has not responded to immunotherapy and fungi are suspected to play a role in symptoms, additional fungi should be tested. More extensive testing often is necessary to determine the precise profile of fungal allergies among very sensitive patients. Second-tier test antigens often include representatives of *Aureobasidium, Cephalosporium, Chaetomium, Cryptococcus, Curvularia, Nigrospora, Puccinia, Rhodotorula, Saccharomycetes, Scopulariopsis, Sporobolomyces, Stemphylium, Streptomycetes, Trichoderma, Ustilago,* and the mushrooms, if available. The most useful method to develop a secondary fungal test panel for an individual practice is to purchase small quantities of many fungal extracts and use these for additional testing of mold-sensitive patients. Skin tests identify the local prevalence and range of severity of skin reactions to each extract, and any extract that either causes strong reactions or is frequently positive should be considered for the secondary panel. In more severe cases, as an aid to identifying unsuspected, possibly significant fungal allergens, home or office environmental mold culture plates always should be considered.

## Bacteria

Allergy to bacteria has been demonstrated and treatment of bacterial allergy was formerly in common use, but now is rare in clinical practice. One of the reasons bacterial allergy treatment has fallen out of favor is because bacterial antigens are potent and can cause severe local or systemic reactions. However, Dolowitz has shown that untoward reactions in the treatment of bacterial allergies result from treatment overdoses (30,31). He found, using quantitative studies with skin endpoint titration (SET), and evaluating both immediate and delayed skin reactions, that there was an optimal dose level at which bacterial therapy can be used safely and successfully. Few, if any, reactions occur as long as therapy is confined to this safe dose range. A second major reason bacterial allergy has fallen out of favor is that few good efficacy studies were published, leading to questions about the value of bacterial therapy. Finally, bacteria are not identified by standard aeroallergen collection methods, as are fungal spores and pollen, so that the extent of human exposure is not appreciated. Despite this, bacteria commonly are identified on environmental culture plates from home and office environments and widely contaminate water faucets, humidifiers, and air conditioners. Certain species, particularly the mycelia-forming, heat-tolerant actinomycetes, also are known to induce hypersensitivity pneumonitis.

Dolowitz observed that most otolaryngic allergy patients had bacterial sensitivities. He reviewed a random sample of 200 allergy charts in 1976 and found positive bacterial skin tests in 95%. This compared with 93% positive to fungi, 75% to pollens, and 65% to house dust and animal danders. Bacterial allergy also has been identified in cases of nasal polyps, and has been proposed to be an etiologic factor (32, 33). Dolowitz attempted to determine the effectiveness of bacterial allergy treatment by using patient satisfaction as the measured variable (30). To determine whether there was any improvement with added bacterial antigens, patients treated in 1969 and 1970 without these antigens in their treatment serum were studied and compared with patients treated in the same way, but with bacterial antigens added. A total of 118 (19.9%) dropped out of allergy treatment in the belief that the degree of improvement was not sufficient to warrant continuing injections. In contrast, only 142 (12.5%) of patients treated in 1971 to 1973, with the addition of bacterial antigens, dropped out of treatment. The decrease of 37.2% after the addition of bacterial antigens was a statistically highly significant improvement.

Except for vaccines, there are no commercial bacterial antigen sources currently being produced in the United States. Bacterial antigens still can be obtained abroad by individual patients, or can be prepared by individual physicians for use in their own practices.

## House Dust

House dust is a potent antigen, and is not simply composed of soil tracked into the home. House dust is a mixture of many organic and inorganic substances found in home environments (34). It is composed of the antigenic portions of insects such as cockroach, dust mites, and food storage mites, as well as mineral, wood, and food dusts, cat and dog hair, hemp, cotton, wool, and synthetic fibers, fungi, pollens, chemicals, and many other substances. In older homes, mouse and rat antigens can be significant, and horse antigens can be present because of antique furniture or plaster. Horse antigens also can be brought into the home from ranching or riding activities, as can antigens from other farm animals. Feathers in clothing and home furnishings do not need to be tested separately because this type of feather allergy has been shown to be due to the presence of house dust mites that feed on the feathers (35). Finally, other insects, such as flies, beetles, or moths, occasionally can cause sensitization (36,37).

Although house dust is a composite substance, it tends to behave in testing and treatment as if it were a single antigen. The home age and local home climate directly correlate with house dust antigenicity, with dust from older homes being more potent than more recent dust, and dust from humid climates normally being more allergenic than dust from arid regions. Like house dust, other allergenic dusts can be formed from organic substances that collect in farms, industrial buildings, libraries, and other structures, and each dust has a unique mix of components. Because total avoidance of house dust and other dusts often is impractical, people allergic to any dust usually require immunotherapy with either the composite dust antigen or with its major components. Because the major components of house dust now are recognized, there is a trend to treat these separately, rather than use house dust antigen. However, if the important constituent allergens of any other dust either are not known or are not available as single antigens, then that dust should be considered for use as an antigen.

## Dust Mites

The major allergenic substance in house dust was unknown until the 1960s, when house dust mites were first linked to allergic reactions, and especially to asthma. Dust mites are microscopic arthropods that feed on human and animal dander. They live primarily in mattresses, pillows, thick carpets, and upholstered furniture, and require temperatures between 25°C and 30°C for maximum propagation. Mites thrive in high humidity and rarely are found in large numbers in arid climates or at high elevations, except in human habitats that maintain appropriate climatic conditions. In some areas, such as northern Scandinavia, northern Canada, and mountainous areas, mite growth is reduced enough that animal danders become the primary allergens in house dust. Two species of house dust mites commonly are found in the United States, *Dermatophagoides farinae* and *Dermatophagoides pteronyssinus*. Of the two major mite species, *D. pteronyssinus* is more dependent on high humidity and is less common in drier homes. All dust mite populations wax and wane with seasonal variations in humidity, with a summer peak and winter nadir in temperate climates (38). Normally, both *D. farinae* and *D. pteronyssinus* are present in homes, and although significantly cross-reactive, are antigenically distinct enough to require individual testing and treatment. Two additional dust mites, *Dermatophagoides microceras* and *Euroglyphus maynei,* also are found in North America, and may be significant in specific homes, but their prevalence is not accurately known. The major antigenic element of dust mites is their fecal particles, which are similar in size to pollens, measuring approximately 10 to 40 $\mu$m in diameter. Other antigens are produced by decomposing mite bodies (39). As these allergenic particles dry, they become airborne and are easily inhaled. Besides their critical role in triggering asthma (16), mite allergen particles also are important in causation of eczema (40).

## Storage Mites

Other mites also live in homes, feeding on food debris and other organic remains. Storage mites from the genera *Blomia, Tyrophagus, Glycophagus, Lepidoglyphus,* and *Acarus* may comprise a significant fraction of the mite flora in some homes, particularly in the South or in coastal locales, and can be a factor in the indoor allergy load.

## Cockroaches

Over the past several decades, cockroach has become increasingly recognized as an important source of inhalant allergen. Cockroach allergy has been linked to asthma, especially among inner-city children. In crowded urban areas where cockroach populations are the highest, allergy to cockroach is very common. Older homes and inner-city homes are especially likely to have significant cockroach infestation. The major antigenic component of the cockroach is crumbled debris from the desiccated bodies. Of the eight common types of indoor cockroaches, the American *(Periplaneta americana)* and German *(Blattella germanica)* types are most common in the United States. There is substantial cross-reactivity between American and Oriental *(Blatta orientalis)* species, and also with German cockroaches (39,41), but American cockroaches have some unique antigens not found in the other species.

## Animal Danders

The proteins of animals' skin, urine, hair or feathers, and saliva form dry airborne particles that are collectively known as *dander.* Domestic animal allergy is common, with over 57% of asthmatic children reactive to at least one pet species (42). Allergy from occupational exposure to animals also is frequent, especially from farm and laboratory species.

### Cats

Of all allergenic animals, cat is the most thoroughly studied. Approximately 28% of U.S. homes have at least one cat (39). Cat dander is recognized as an extremely potent antigen, and is widely distributed in the environment because of its small, buoyant particles. The major antigenic protein of cat dander is Fel d I, but cat-allergic people also can be allergic to other minor cat proteins. Cat dander particles are primarily believed to arise from sebaceous gland secretions, and are very small, ranging in size from 10 to less than 1 $\mu$m, small enough to penetrate into the peripheral lung and alveoli. This property probably accounts for the immediate and substantial impact that the mere presence of a cat has on most asthmatic patients. The particles also are sticky and can persist for many months, even after removal of the cat. Cat dander is easily transported on clothing from location to location, introducing cat antigen into homes, schools, or offices in which no cat is present. In fact, random sampling has shown that up to 70% of homes contain cat allergen. Therefore, most patients, including those who do not own a cat, should be tested for cat allergy.

### Dogs

Dog dander in general is thought to be less allergenic than that of cat (42). It can be a significant allergen, however, and should be tested if allergy to dog is suspected. Dog antigens are more varied than those in cats. Multiple major antigens are present, and these vary in relative concentration from breed to breed, so that some breeds may appear to be more or less allergenic for specific individuals. However, there is no generally hypoallergenic dog breed. Some cross-reactivity has been shown between dog and cat allergens, but not enough to obviate the need for testing both species.

### Other Danders

Allergy to other animal species also is possible, and should be considered when people are exposed to other mammals or birds on a regular basis. For example, allergies to horses and cattle are frequent among people living on farms or ranches. Allergy to sheep wool also has been observed in weavers, as well as among the general population. Finally, laboratory animals, wild rodents or birds, small pet mammals, and pet birds all can be significant sources of allergic symptoms. Rodent antigens are a special problem because, like cat dander, the particle sizes are less than 10 μm, which allows deep inhalation, and the antigens also are chemically very stable. Therefore, potentially significant rodent allergen levels could build up in older dwellings.

## CONCLUSION

This chapter has described major elements of inhalant allergy as applied to allergy testing and treatment. Major allergens have been discussed in enough depth to assist in selection of relevant allergens for testing. Inhalant allergens are not all of equal sensitivity in provoking an allergic response. Also, not every potential inhalant allergen is found in any individual's specific environment. It is important, therefore, to be judicious in the use of testing for inhalant allergy, guiding practice on the basis of such factors as geographic distribution, relative antigenicity, and cross-reactivity. Testing too many antigens at one time, especially ones that cross-react, may subject a patient to a dangerous antigen overload. In addition, testing hundreds of antigens on any patient is unnecessary and wasteful. Through an understanding of these basic principles, the otolaryngic allergist can successfully apply this knowledge to clinical practice.

## ACKNOWLEDGMENTS

The authors thank June L. Bianchi, Sally C. Schumann, and Jeanie M. Vander Pyl, Cape Cod Hospital Medical Library, for their expertise in medical literature research.

## REFERENCES

1. Dreborg S, Foucard T. Allergy to apple, carrot, and potato in children with birch pollen allergy. *Allergy* 1983;38:167–172.
2. Halmepuro L, Vuontela K, Kalimo K, et al. Cross-reactivity of IgE antibodies with allergens in birch pollen, fruits, and vegetables. *Int Arch Allergy Appl Immunol* 1984;74:235–240.
3. Kazemi-Shirazi L, Pauli G, Purohit A, et al. Quantitative IgE inhibition experiments with purified recombinant allergens indicate pollen-derived allergens as the sensitizing agents responsible for many forms of plant food allergy. *J Allergy Clin Immunol* 2000;105:116–125.
4. Reider N, Sepp N, Fritsch P, et al. Anaphylaxis to camomile: clinical features and allergen cross-reactivity. *Clin Exp Allergy* 2000;30:1436–1443.
5. Luttkopf D, Ballmer-Weber BK, Wuthrich B, et al. Celery allergens in patients with positive double-blind placebo-controlled food challenge. *J Allergy Clin Immunol* 2000;106:390–399.
6. Anderson LB Jr, Dreyfuss EM, Logan J, et al. Melon and banana sensitivity coincident with ragweed pollinosis. *J Allergy* 1970;45:310–319.
7. Coca AF, Thommen AA, Walzer M. *Asthma and hay fever in theory and practice.* Springfield, IL: Charles C Thomas, 1931.
8. Lewis WH, Vinay P, Zenger VE. *Airborne and allergenic pollen of North America.* Baltimore: Johns Hopkins University Press, 1983.
9. Galant S, Berger W, Gillman S, et al. Prevalence of sensitization to aeroallergens in California patients with respiratory allergy. *Ann Allergy Asthma Immunol* 1998;81:203–210.
10. Lewis WH, Dixit AB, Ward WA. Distribution and incidence of North American pollen aeroallergens. *Am J Otolaryngol* 1991;12:205–226.
11. Jelks ML. Aeroallergens of Florida. *Immunol Allergy Clin North Am* 1989;9:381–397.
12. Bassett IJ, Crompton CW, Parmelee JA. *An atlas of airborne pollen grains and common fungus spores of Canada.* Hull, Quebec: Printing and Supply Services Canada, 1978.
13. Dzul AI. Selecting allergenic extracts for inhalant allergy testing and immunotherapy. *Otolaryngol Clin North Am* 1998;31:11–25.
14. Wodehouse RP. Pollens of the amaranth-chenopod group. *Ann Allergy* 1957;15:527–536.
15. Rodriguez A, DeBarrio M, DeFrutos C, et al. Occupational allergy to fern. *Allergy* 2001;56:89.
16. Platts-Mills TAE, Solomon WR. Aerobiology and inhalant allergens. In: Middleton E, ed. *Allergy principles and practice,* 4th ed. St. Louis: Mosby, 1993:57–80.
17. Mitchell TG. Overview of basic medical mycology. *Otolaryngol Clin North Am* 2000;33:237–249.
18. Burge HA. Airborne allergenic fungi. *Immunol Allergy Clin North Am* 1989;9:307–319.
19. Horner WE, Lehrer SB, Salvaggio JE. Fungi. *Immunol Allergy Clin North Am* 1994;14:551–566.
20. Hoffman DR. Mould allergens. In: Al-Doory Y, Domson JF, eds. *Mould allergy.* Philadelphia: Lea & Febiger, 1984:104–116.
21. Cole GT, Samson RA. The conidia. In: Al-Doory Y, Domson JF, eds. *Mould allergy.* Philadelphia: Lea & Febiger, 1984:66–103.
22. Howard WA. Incidence and clinical characteristics of mould allergy. In: Al-Doory Y, Domson JF, eds. *Mould allergy.* Philadelphia: Lea & Febiger, 1984:147–156.
23. Morrow MB, Meyer GH, Prince HE. A summary of air-borne mold surveys. *Ann Allergy* 1964;22:575–587.
24. Al-Doory Y. Airborne fungi. In: Al-Doory Y, Domson JF, eds. *Mould allergy.* Philadelphia: Lea & Febiger, 1984:27–40.
25. Corey JP, Kaiseruddin S, Gungor A. Prevalence of mold-specific immunoglobulins in a Midwestern allergy practice. *Otolaryngol Head Neck Surg* 1997;117:516–520.
26. Corsico R, Cinti B, Feliziana V, et al. Prevalence of sensitization to *Alternaria* in allergic patients in Italy. *Ann Allergy Asthma Immunol* 1998;80:71–76.
27. Perzanowski MS, Sporik R, Squillace SP, et al. Association of sensitization to *Alternaria* allergens with asthma among school-age children. *J Allergy Clin Immunol* 1998;101:626–632.
28. Menzies D, Comtois P, Pasztor J, et al. Aeroallergens and work-related respiratory symptoms among office workers. *J Allergy Clin Immunol* 1998;101:38–44.
29. Helbling A, Gayer F, Pichler WJ, et al. Mushroom (Basidiomycete) allergy: diagnosis established by skin test and nasal challenge. *J Allergy Clin Immunol* 1998;102:853–858.
30. Dolowitz DA. Inhalant and ingestant bacterial allergy. *Trans Am Soc Ophthalmol Otolaryngol Allergy* 1977;17:36–41.
31. Dolowitz DA, David A. Bacterial allergy. In: King HC, ed. *Otolaryngologic allergy.* New York: Elsevier, 1981:163–177.
32. Calenoff E, McMahan JT, Herzon GD, et al. Bacterial allergy in nasal polyposis. *Arch Otolaryngol Head Neck Surg* 1993;119:830–836.
33. Calenoff E, Guilford FT, Green J, et al. Bacteria-specific IgE in patients with nasal polyposis. *Arch Otolaryngol* 1983;109:372–375.

34. Pollart SM, Ward GW Jr, Platts-Mills TAE. House dust sensitivity and environmental control. *Immunol Allergy Clin North Am* 1987;7:447–462.

35. Kilpio K, Makinen-Kiljunen S, Haatela T, et al. Allergy to feathers. *Allergy* 1998;53:159–164.

36. Mathews KP. Inhalant insect-derived allergens. *Immunol Allergy Clin North Am* 1989;9:321–338.

37. Cuesta-Herranz J, de las Heras M, Sastre J, et al. Asthma caused by Dermestidae (black carpet beetle): a new allergen in house dust. *J Allergy Clin Immunol* 1997;99:147–149.

38. Arlian LC. Biology and ecology of house dust mites, *Dermatophagoides* spp. and *Euroglyphus* spp. *Immunol Allergy Clin North Am* 1989;9:339–356.

39. Thien FCK, Leung RCC, Czarny D, et al. Indoor allergens and IgE-mediated respiratory illness. *Immunol Allergy Clin North Am* 1994;14:567–590.

40. Darsow U, Vieluf D, Ring J. Evaluating the relevance of aeroallergen sensitization in atopic eczema with the atopy patch test: a randomized, double-blind multicenter study. *J Am Acad Dermatol* 1999;40:187–193.

41. Tsai JJ, Kao MH, Wu CH. Hypersensitivity of bronchial asthmatics to cockroach in Taiwan: comparative study between American and German cockroaches. *Int Arch Allergy Immunol* 1998;117:180–186.

42. Kyysak D. Animal aeroallergens. *Immunol Allergy Clin North Am* 1989;9:357–364.

# FOOD ALLERGY AND HYPERSENSITIVITY

RICHARD J. TREVINO
BRUCE R. GORDON
MARIA C. VELING

*Allergy* refers to those diseases in which immune responses to environmental antigens cause tissue inflammation and organ dysfunction. Food allergy is further defined as the immune-mediated production of symptoms brought on by the ingestion of a food antigen. This chapter presents the history of food allergy and describes the immunology involved, including the concept that food antigens potentially activate the entire immune system, and that all immune effectors contribute to the production of symptoms. The clinical concept of two distinct patterns of food allergy, including diagnostic and treatment methods for both types, is stressed.

## HISTORY OF FOOD ALLERGY

Evidence of food sensitivities can be found dating back to the Old Testament, which describes the Hebrews' efforts to prevent disease. Cutaneous reactions caused by food also were recorded in China in approximately 3000 B.C. Later, Hippocrates (1) observed that milk could cause gastric distress and urticaria. Reports of adverse reactions to foods such as milk, eggs, almonds, and oatmeal finally began to appear in modern medical literature early in the 20th century, but were not reported with any frequency until after Von Pirquet (2) introduced the concept of allergy in 1906. After this, scratch, single intradermal, and, finally, prick skin tests were used to detect food allergies. Because these simple skin tests easily detect food allergies caused by immediate allergic reactions, but require special attention to technique to detect delayed-type food allergies, the prevalence

of food sensitivities often has been underestimated. Smith (3) described buckwheat allergy associated with gastrointestinal symptoms in 1909, and Schloss (4) in 1912 reported on a child with asthma induced by egg white, almond, and oatmeal. In this case, Schloss demonstrated a positive scratch test in the patient, but was unable to detect serum antibodies. Coke (5), in 1932, recognized that people could be sensitized by ingestion of wheat or wheat products during infancy, or by inhaling flour later in life.

At approximately the same time, Herbert Rinkel, a classically trained American internist-allergist, first described a second clinical pattern of food sensitivity that was distinctly different from the classic immediate anaphylactic reaction (6). Rinkel realized the limitations of simple skin testing, and by 1934 had developed the basic procedure for the deliberate individual food test, which is now usually known as the *oral food challenge*. He described symptoms that occurred hours to days after food ingestion, and that could be relieved, or masked, by eating more of the offending food. Previous researchers such as Schloss (4), Rowe (7), and Coca (8) had alluded to this type of delayed food sensitivity, but Rinkel described the masking and unmasking of symptoms as developmental phases of a single process, which he called *cyclic food allergy*. The fortunate combination of Rinkel's studies of skin testing for food allergy, his interest in dietary management of food allergy, his astute clinical observations of his patients with allergy, and his own personal suffering from food allergies, eventually led to this new concept of cyclic food allergy (see later). Between 1936, when his first paper was published, and 1964, Rinkel and colleagues (6,9–14) further described cyclic food allergy in a series of papers and a book. In addition, without knowing specific biochemical mechanisms, he accurately described the clinical behavior of cyclic food sensitization, including the masking phenomenon and the development of tolerance. He also developed a standard method of oral food challenge, compared and correlated skin and oral challenge testing for food allergies, and developed the rotary, diver-

**R. J. Trevino:** Ear, Nose, and Throat Allergy, San Jose, California.

**B. R. Gordon:** Department of Otology and Laryngology, Harvard University, Cambridge; Associate Surgeon, Massachusetts Eye and Ear Infirmary, Boston; Chief of Otolaryngology, Cape Cod Hospital, Hyannis, Massachusetts.

**M. C. Veling:** Department of Surgery, Division of Otolaryngology, University of Louisville School of Medicine, Louisville, Kentucky.

| Food Antigen<br>Dilution | Skin Wheal<br>Size (mm) | Symptoms<br>Provoked | Wheal<br>Interpretation |
|:---:|:---:|:---:|:---:|
| # 1 | 11 | strong | positive |
| # 2 | 9 | slight | positive |
| # 3 | 7 | feels well | endpoint |
| # 4 | 7 | feels well | negative |
| # 5 | 7 | slight | underdose |
| # 6 | 9 | strong | underdose |

**FIG. 4.1.** Carleton Lee's observations of cyclic food allergy skin tests.

sified diet as a treatment modality for this type of food sensitivity.

In 1958, Dr. Carleton Lee was studying the serial endpoint skin testing responses to single food antigens in an attempt to find ways to desensitize patients with food allergy. He knew, from Rinkel's work, that large intradermal doses of food antigen often could provoke symptoms in sensitive patients, and that these symptoms could be replicated by oral challenge feedings. He also knew that attempts at food allergy desensitization by high-dose escalation, as was done for inhalant allergy, frequently led to serious anaphylactic reactions. Then, Lee adapted Rinkel's technique for treatment of pathogenic fungal allergy, by using doses weaker than the skin testing endpoint, and made the observation that when symptoms were produced by food extract injection (provocation), subsequent injection of a weaker dilution could extinguish those symptoms (neutralization). In the next 2 years of studies, he learned that administering even weaker dilutions, below the neutralizing dose, also could provoke symptoms (underdosing) (Fig. 4.1). He then began to apply this knowledge to treatment, and found that neutralizing dose injections frequently helped patients with food allergy feel better (15).

Rinkel et al. (14), and subsequently Rinkel's colleagues and students, elaborated on Lee's procedure to develop several other variations of intradermal food testing, some of which are still in use. Rinkel was primarily interested in the diagnostic use of skin testing for food allergy because he believed strongly that diet manipulation was the answer to food allergy treatment. However, since his death in 1963, provocation and neutralization techniques also have become widely used for treatment of food allergies, especially when combined with dietary management (16). The details of this period in Rinkel's career have been summarized in Dr. Theron Randolph's eulogy (17).

## REVIEW OF BASIC IMMUNOLOGY OF ALLERGY

### Immune System

The immune system differentiates between self and nonself. It is made up of a variety of cells that are present in the circulation and the body tissues. Numerous types of chemical substances are produced by these cells that are capable of interacting with and affecting foreign molecules or organisms, other cells of the immune system, and, at times, other cells of the body. A foreign substance (an *antigen*) can produce two types of responses: *nonspecific*—no targeted response occurs (e.g., a reaction to a generic gram-negative bacterium), or *specific*—recognition of nonself antigens occurs, with generation of specific antibodies and sensitized cells in response to the specific antigen. The nonspecific, or innate immune response, is genetically specified for an entire species, and reacts to broad categories of antigens (18). The specific immune response develops differently in every individual, reacts to very small differences in antigen structure, and consists of two phases. First, antigen activates specific lymphocytes that recognize it, and second, in the effector phase, these lymphocytes coordinate an immune response that eliminates the foreign antigen. The immune response is traditionally categorized by response time and reaction type as *humoral* (B-lymphocyte–mediated, immediate—minutes to hours) or *cell mediated* (T-lymphocyte–mediated, delayed—hours to days).

## Lymphocytes

Immune responses are mediated by a variety of cells and by the effector molecules they secrete. Most important are the *lymphocytes,* the leukocytes that are capable of recognition and thus can generate the exquisite specificity of the immune system. Lymphocytes make up 20% of total circulating leukocytes. All lymphocytes are derived from bone marrow stem cells, but T lymphocytes (T cells) then develop in the thymus, whereas B lymphocytes (B cells) develop in the bone marrow. Natural killer cells, also known as *large granular lymphocytes,* are a third type of lymphocyte. B cells are defined by the presence of specific surface antibody produced by the cell itself. Antibodies anchored to the cell surface act as antigen receptors by binding specific antigen. Each lymphocyte is capable of generating only a single antibody specificity. Having recognized its specific antigen, a B cell multiplies and differentiates into a clone of identical *plasma cells,* which secrete large amounts of specific antibody known as *immunoglobulin.*

T cells are effectors of both cell-mediated immunity and cytotoxicity, and also regulate the immune system through cytokine production and cell-to-cell contact. One group, helper cells, interacts with B cells and stimulates them to divide, differentiate, and make specific antibody. Other T cells have an antigen-specific suppressor role, and inhibit B-cell functions. A third group, cytotoxic T cells, is responsible for the destruction of infected or malignant cells. In every case, T cells recognize antigen, but only in association with self-markers on cell surfaces. The specific T-cell antigen receptor is related, both in function and structure, to the surface antibody that B cells use as their antigen receptors.

## Immunoglobulins

*Immunoglobulins* are the primary effectors of the humoral immune response, and all types share a common basic structure composed of two pairs of proteins known as *light chains* and *heavy chains,* linked by disulfide bonds. The heavy chain determines the ability of an antibody to bind to cells and participate in specific types of immune responses, and confers immunoglobulin class (G, M, A, D, and E). Each B cell ultimately becomes committed to producing only a sin-

gle class of heavy chain, and thus just a single type of antibody. Light chains determine the specific antigen-binding site of each antibody molecule, and an almost infinite number of specificities can be generated by genetic recombination during lymphocyte development. Immunoglobulin D (IgD) functions only as a cell surface marker, but IgG, IgM, IgA, and IgE all are involved in the mechanisms of food allergy.

Immunoglobulin G comprises 70% to 75% of the total serum immunoglobulin pool, and is the major immunoglobulin of the antiinfection anamnestic secondary immune response. IgG also is produced after allergen exposure, and is believed normally to be protective, by complexing with and helping to clear foreign substances from the circulation. However, IgG appears to have a significant pathologic role in certain cases of food allergy (see later). IgG also forms protective blocking antibodies during immunotherapy for treatment of inhalant and insect venom allergic disease.

Immunoglobulin M comprises approximately 10% of serum immunoglobulin, activates the classic complement pathway, and is the predominant antibody in the primary antiinfective immune response. IgM and IgG both contribute to the formation of immune complexes that assist in clearing circulating antigens, and IgM also assists IgA in defending external surfaces.

Immunoglobulin A makes up most of the remaining immunoglobulin pool. It is the predominant secreted antibody, and is found in saliva, colostrum, and the seromucous secretions of the sinobronchial, gastrointestinal, and genitourinary tracts. IgA is the major immune barrier to antigen penetration into the body, and, when deficient, leads to increased gastrointestinal food antigen absorption.

Immunoglobulin E is the primary antibody responsible for triggering acute allergic hypersensitivity reactions, although it is present only in minute amounts in serum. IgE is primarily found bound to the surface membranes of basophils and mast cells. When specific antigen binds to and cross-links adjacent surface IgE receptors, degranulation and release of multiple allergic mediators occurs. IgE is unable to fix complement.

## Antigen-processing Cells

Phagocytes function actively to engulf and destroy, or phagocytose, organisms, macromolecules, and tumor cells. *Macrophages,* the best-known phagocyte type, function as antigen-presenting cells, where they have a pivotal role in digesting antigens into smaller fragments, or epitopes, and presenting these antigen fragments to lymphocytes. When a foreign substance enters the body, it is picked up by a macrophage and ingested, then processed and displayed on the cell surface. When the macrophage interacts with an appropriate lymphocyte capable of recognizing one of the bound epitopes, that lymphocyte is activated. If a B cell is activated, it goes on to form a clone of identical plasma cells, each of which produces and secretes antibody specific to the antigen producing the sensitization. If a T cell is activated, it may become a helper, suppressor, or cytotoxic cell, depending on the circumstances. Specialized cells with antigen-presenting capacity can be found in all tissues.

## Mediator Cells

Mediator cells mediate allergic inflammation by releasing molecules, such as histamine and chemotactic factors, that attract other leukocytes and affect local tissues, especially blood vessels, glands, and smooth muscles. *Basophils* and *mast cells* both have granules containing a variety of preformed mediators that produce inflammation in surrounding tissues. Mediator cells also can synthesize and secrete other mediators, such as leukotrienes, that control the development and duration of immune reactions. These regulatory mediators also are released when the cells are triggered by an allergic reaction. Mast cells and basophils strongly bind IgE of various antigen specificities, sensitizing the cells to trigger when exposed to appropriate antigens. *Platelets* also can release inflammatory mediators when activated by means of antigen–antibody complexes.

## Complement

Another component of the immune system is the complement system, with its classic and alternative pathways. When bound to antibodies, complement has a major role in the amplification and regulation of immune inflammation, and also enhances uptake and removal of immune complexes by phagocytosis. Complement activation occurs during some, and possibly many, allergic food reactions.

## TYPES OF ADVERSE REACTIONS TO FOODS

Adverse reactions to food ingestion can be divided into immunologic (food hypersensitivity) and nonimmunologic (food intolerance) types. The first requirement of any immunologic reaction is the penetration of antigenic molecules into the body, with resultant stimulation of immunologically competent cells to elicit an immune response. Antigenic food molecules are known to be capable of crossing the mature mammalian gut and then triggering the formation of specific antibodies of all types (19–21).

## Immunologic Reactions to Foods (Food Hypersensitivity)

Allergy is a malfunction of the immune system that may involve any immune effector cells and that frequently involves more than one mechanism. These hypersensitivity reactions are the result of normally beneficial immune responses acting inappropriately, and sometimes cause inflammatory reactions and tissue damage. Hypersensitivity is not manifested on first contact with the antigen, but usually appears on subsequent contact. Gell and Coombs (22) classified the different types of immune reactions into four classes.

### Type I Reactions (Immediate Hypersensitivity)

On exposure to an antigen, IgE bound to mast cells becomes cross-linked, leading to degranulation and mediator release. The onset of symptoms usually occurs within seconds to minutes after antigen exposure, but the entire reaction may take many hours to subside. The initial physiologic response to histamine and other preformed mediators includes vasodilatation, increased vascular permeability, stimulation of the mucous glands, and smooth muscle contraction. The late-phase response, stimulated by release of newly synthesized mediators such as leukotrienes, includes attraction of an inflammatory cell infiltrate and chronic tissue edema. Clinically, type I reactions can result in urticaria, rhinitis, angioedema, diarrhea, and asthma, and can progress to anaphylaxis. Once sensitized, most patients retain this type of allergy for many years, often for a lifetime. Although type I reactions to foods are uncommon, they usually are easily detected because each exposure to the offending food produces an immediate symptom response. These reactions are often severe and can be life threatening, involving one or more shock organs with predictable and consistent severity. Type I reactions to food antigens are thought to have approximately a 5% prevalence in the general population, and are the second most commonly observed clinical expression of food hypersensitivity. Susceptibility to food-induced type I reactions can be easily and safely identified by specific in vitro blood IgE measurement.

### Type II Reactions

Cytotoxic reactions occur when antibody binds to either self-antigen or foreign antigen on cells and leads to phagocytosis, killer cell activity, or complement-mediated lysis. Clinical examples include hemolytic anemia, Goodpasture's syndrome, transfusion reactions, and rare cases of food reactions, such as thrombocytopenia from allergy to cow's milk. Detection of type II reactions currently is performed only in research laboratories.

### Type III Reactions

Also known as *immune complex disease,* these reactions involve the formation of antigen–antibody complexes with subsequent tissue damage. Antibody molecules (primarily IgG) bind to circulating antigens, producing macromolecular complexes that can precipitate in capillary beds, binding and activating complement to produce tissue inflammation.

If the target organ is the intestinal tract, cramps or diarrhea may result. If the target organ is the cerebral arteries, migraine may be triggered. Similarly, if the target organ is the nose, congestion or rhinorrhea may develop. Maximum immune complex formation may not occur for hours or days after challenge, and complete clearance of immune complexes from the circulation may take as long as several days, so it is evident how type III reactions may be both delayed in onset and prolonged in terms of symptom production. Clinical examples include serum sickness, acute poststreptococcal glomerulonephritis, and some drug reactions. Type III allergy is believed to be the most common form of immune reaction causing food hypersensitivity. Although circulating immune complexes have been detected in many food allergy studies, the identification of food-specific complexes is technically difficult and limited to research laboratories. Detection of immune complexes rarely is necessary in clinical practice, but when it is, single serologic tests are of limited reliability, so usually more than one complementary test is required. The only available clinical tests for immune complexes are an indirect method, by measurement of low C3 complement levels or by the presence of complement split fragments, and direct cell binding assays, using the Raji lymphocyte cell line to detect binding of complexes to C3b and Fc receptors.

### Type IV Reactions

Delayed-type hypersensitivity is T-cell mediated, with a response occurring 24 to 48 hours after contact. Type IV reactions represent the most delayed−onset group of immune reactions, and are therefore suspected of participating in the development of chronic allergic conditions. T-cell receptors react with specific antigens in the same manner as those of B cells. As with the IgE-producing B cell in type I allergy, previous sensitization also is required to establish the necessary primed condition on the T-cell surface. Once sensitization has been established and the cell activated by a new contact with the antigen, T cells release a variety of cytokines that mobilize other inflammatory cells, which in turn produce a direct effect on the target organ. This is the basis for the tuberculin skin test, poison ivy reactions, and some drug and food reactions. Some cases of delayed, type IV cell-mediated allergic reactions due to cow's milk have been demonstrated in the research laboratory by showing milk-specific lymphocyte blastogenesis.

### Mixed-type Reactions

Symptoms that suggest mixtures of Gel and Coombs reaction types often are observed in clinical situations, and laboratory studies have shown circulating complexes with mixed immunoglobulin types, particularly IgE and IgG (23), and complement activation during allergic reactions to foods. It is likely that multiple reactions are usual and that, for convenience, the predominant symptoms observed are used to classify a particular immunologic reaction to food in a specific individual patient.

## Nonimmunologic Reactions to Foods (Food Intolerance)

These adverse reactions to foods can be confused with true immunologic reactions, but if correctly diagnosed, usually can be readily treated. Important types of these reactions are briefly described. *Anaphylactoid* reactions are anaphylaxis-like reactions due to the nonimmune release of chemical mediators such as histamine, either contained in foods like spoiled fish or released from cellular stores by foods like tomatoes and strawberries. *Idiosyncratic* reactions are due to abnormal responses that occur in genetically predisposed patients. An example would be an asthmatic patient reacting to salicylates in food by development of an acute asthma attack. *Digestive enzyme deficiencies* commonly cause gastrointestinal symptoms, such as those associated with lactase deficiency. *Toxic reactions* result from food components or additives, such as lectins, monosodium glutamate, food dyes, bisulfites, and toxins released by microbes in food (24). Finally, *pharmacologic reactions* occur when chemicals in foods produce drug-like effects. Examples include phentolamine in chocolate, tyramine in red wine, methylxanthines in tea, and vasoactive amines in bananas and avocados. Many food additives, including various food dyes and preservatives, also are suspected of having neurotransmitter activity.

## SENSITIZATION TO FOODS

Although some food antigens are absorbed from the mouth and respiratory tract, the amount of food allergen reaching the immune system depends primarily on the permeability of the gut mucosa. In newborns and infants (25), significant intestinal macromolecular permeability is common, accounting for the increased incidence of food allergy in youth. As the gut matures, there is progressive diminution of antigen uptake. At any age, conditions promoting dysfunction of the gastrointestinal tract that allow increased absorption of antigenic foods can give rise to increased food allergy. One example is the intestinal inflammation due to existing food allergy (26) creating the conditions for additional allergies to arise. Other factors influencing food allergies include concomitant food and inhalant allergy with cross-reactivity between a food and an inhalant allergen. This explains why some usually well tolerated foods cause allergic symptoms during a specific pollen season. Clinically, allergic food hypersensitivity can be divided into fixed and cyclic types.

## Fixed Food Allergy

This term applies to IgE-mediated responses manifesting as an immediate reaction within seconds to hours after contact with the allergen. Some patients also describe late-occurring symptoms of pruritus up to 24 hours after the exposure. Sensitivity to the food usually persists for years and may last indefinitely. The reaction is prompt, obvious, and frequently severe. Once sensitization has occurred, it occurs every time the patient is exposed to the allergen. Symptom production does *not* depend on the quantity of food eaten, and may occur from very small exposures. Once IgE was discovered in 1966, it became obvious that fixed food reactions are actually IgE-mediated type I reactions, and in many respects resemble IgE-mediated inhalant allergies. Fixed food allergy may present in various ways, including atopic dermatitis or eczema, asthma, allergic rhinitis, urticaria, angioedema, oral allergy syndrome, gastrointestinal distress, or severe anaphylactic reactions. These symptoms can present simultaneously with different degrees of severity.

*Atopic dermatitis* or *eczema* usually presents in the first few years of life. In one study, 37% of children with moderate to severe atopic dermatitis were found to have type I food allergy (27). The most common IgE-mediated food allergies in infants with atopic dermatitis are cow's milk, fish, and eggs (28,29). It is believed that mechanisms unrelated to IgE-mediated histamine release also can trigger mast cell degranulation after the ingestion of alcohol, spicy foods, or additives, and this can exacerbate atopic dermatitis.

*Immunoglobulin E–mediated asthma* can be exacerbated by the inhalation of airborne food antigens, as in baker's asthma. Asthmatic reactions caused by airborne foods have been reported in cases where susceptible individuals are exposed to dusts, vapors, or steam emitted from cooking food. This has been observed on a large scale in the food processing industry (30). In addition to asthma, symptoms may include rhinoconjunctivitis, urticaria, laryngeal edema, and, rarely, shock. Foods often implicated in occupational asthma include eggs, grain flour, coffee bean, cocoa, peanut, soy, cottonseed, sunflower, garlic, tea, fish, poultry, and shellfish. Food-related asthma also can be triggered by ingestion of the offending food (31).

*Urticaria* is a wheal-and-flare cutaneous reaction, usually to ingested foods or drugs. Each individual wheal normally lasts less than 24 hours, but new ones continue to form as long as antigen exposure continues. Contact urticaria also can occur with cutaneous contact with food (32). Contact reactions usually are seen with prolonged handling of raw food, and also occur around the mouth in children. Angioedema produces areas of cutaneous or mucosal, nonpruritic swelling, sometimes painful, developing suddenly and usually lasting no more than 3 days. Urticaria is present in association with angioedema in more than 45% of the cases, and these mixed presentations are believed to be among the most common manifestations of food-induced allergic reactions. When urticaria and angioedema are so extensive and severe that systemic symptoms are present, such as headache, cough, hoarseness, wheezing, vomiting, abdominal pain, diarrhea, dizziness, and syncope, the term *anaphylaxis* is appropriate. Foods often implicated in urticaria and angioedema include shellfish, fish, milk, nuts, beans, potatoes, celery, parsley, spices, peanuts, and soy (33).

The *oral allergy syndrome* is another common form of IgE-mediated food allergy (34,35). In oral allergy syndrome, the correlation between the offending food and the immediacy of the local reaction is readily made by the patients, who therefore may never seek medical attention. Local IgE-mediated mast cell activation results in immediate swelling of the lips, tingling of the tongue and throat, and blistering of the oral mucosa. Symptoms usually are short-lived and most commonly are associated with the ingestion of various fresh fruits and vegetables that cross-react with their specific allergic rhinitis-inducing pollen (36). Cross-reactivity between inhalant and contactant allergens and foods is common because the oral allergy syndrome is estimated to affect up to 40% of patients with pollen allergy, especially to birch, ragweed, and mugwort pollens (37). Major cross-reactions include:

Birch with apple, carrot, celery, hazelnut, kiwi, peach, pear, and potato

Dust mites with shrimp and snail

Grass with kiwi, melon, tomato, watermelon, wheat, and other grains

Latex with avocado, banana, chestnut, kiwi, and rose family fruits such as cherry and peach

Mugwort with carrot and celery

Ragweed with banana, cucumbers, lettuce, melons, and watermelon

The *gastrointestinal anaphylactic syndrome* is an IgE-mediated gastrointestinal reaction that often accompanies allergic manifestations in other target organs, but it may be seen without other signs of immediate allergy. Symptoms typically develop within minutes of consuming the responsible food, and consist of some combination of abdominal cramps, nausea, vomiting, and watery diarrhea. In some cases, intestinal fluid loss can cause hypotension.

### Anaphylaxis

Food allergies are the single most common cause of anaphylaxis seen in hospital emergency departments (38). In addition to the cutaneous, respiratory, and gastrointestinal symptoms noted previously, patients may have cardiovascular symptoms caused by direct cardiac effects of massive mast cell mediator release. Anaphylaxis may lead to death in minutes from irreversible respiratory or cardiac failure. In the early stages of anaphylaxis, urticaria, angioedema, and respiratory symptoms of coughing and bronchospasm are common, and laryngeal edema may subsequently develop. The gastrointestinal tract may react with nausea, vomiting, and diarrhea. If the cardiovascular system becomes involved, with hypotension, dysrhythmia, and vascular collapse, the patient often has an intense feeling of impending doom. Diaphoresis, palm and groin pruritus, severe headache, and faintness also may occur. Milder reactions may cause only profuse epiphora, rhinorrhea, drooling, cutaneous tingling, and anxiety. Anaphylaxis usually presents soon after exposure to the offending food, but onset may be delayed by medications or illness that slow down peristalsis. Factors associated with severe or fatal allergic food reactions include concomitant asthma, history of previous severe reactions, and failure to initiate therapy expeditiously. Prevention for IgE-mediated fixed food sensitivity is dietary elimination of the offending food.

## Cyclic Food Allergy

All types of food allergy, other than fixed, are designated *cyclic allergy.* Cyclic food allergy reactions may occur shortly after food ingestion, or many hours later. This non–IgE-mediated delayed sensitivity probably accounts for 60% to 80% of food sensitivity seen in clinical practice. Cyclic allergy is believed to be primarily the result of IgG-mediated, type III immune complex disease, although all three other Gel and Coombs types of reactions may contribute. Even type I reactions may contribute because low levels of specific IgE sometimes are detected by in vitro tests in patients with classic cyclic symptoms to a particular food. Cyclic food allergy differs strongly from fixed food allergy because it is *both* dose and frequency related. In many cases, only large or repeated ingestions of a food are observed to be required for symptom production with cyclic food allergy, probably because only large amounts of ingested food antigens are capable of forming enough immune complexes to cause detectable symptom production. Increased frequency of ingestion is observed to lead to increased sensitivity, probably because the more often the food is eaten, the higher the concentration of specific IgG forms, and therefore the greater the immune complex formation and the greater the potential there is for symptom production. Conversely, omission of the food from the diet decreases sensitization, probably because as antibody levels drop, immune complexes become fewer.

### Stages of Cyclic Food Sensitivity

The concept of cyclic food sensitivity was conceived by Rinkel (6), based on clinical observations of the results of dietary manipulation (12). Trevino delineated the probable immunologic basis, namely, the concept of immune complex disease (39). A brief review of the stages of cyclic food sensitiv-

ity follows (12). Figure 4.2, modified from Rinkel's, depicts the idealized stages that a patient with a cyclic food allergy passes through, and the symptoms produced, as he or she varies the frequency of eating that allergenic food. Not every patient will show all stages clearly, but the general progression of stages is constant for all cyclic-type food reactions.

***Stage 1: Masked Sensitization.*** When they first come to the office, most patients are eating allergic foods regularly and feeling chronically ill without suspecting that they are allergic. Rarely, they are eating a food intermittently (see stage 3, later) and experiencing intermittent acute symptoms that they can identify with a particular food. The sensitized food is eaten frequently, leading to immune complex disease with continuous, chronic symptoms. During this stage, there is a phenomenon called *masking,* in which small and frequent exposures to the offending food result in brief symptom relief. Masking may be explained in at least two ways (see later). Dependence on this masking action for continued well-being often results in food craving or addiction.

***Stage 2: Omission.*** If the antigen or the food is omitted for a period of 4 to 5 days, the food antigen is cleared from the body, both from the gut and from the circulation. However, a high level of specific anti-food IgG is still circulating. This can lead to clinical symptoms of withdrawal, which can be severe and last up to 4 days, as antigen decreases and immune complexes equilibrate and change their properties. If no antigenic food is consumed, antibody levels remain high during this phase, but without symptoms once withdrawal has ended.

***Stage 3: Hyperacute Sensitization.*** At this stage there is a large amount of circulating antibody. If the antigenic food is then consumed, it leads to a large amount of immune complex formation with provocation of symptoms. This is the basis of the oral challenge test in which a person experiences exaggerated symptoms after a 4- to 5-day fast from the suspected food allergen, followed by its oral ingestion. This stage lasts 4 to 12 days. Waiting too long to do the challenge, after eliminating the suspect food, makes reactions milder and harder to identify. On the other hand, doing the challenge without elimination of the suspect food for at least 4 days runs the risk also of missing a reaction due to the masking phenomenon. These are two common errors in food challenge testing that are made by persons who do not understand cyclic food allergy concepts. When critically reading journal articles, the clinician always should note the methodology used for any food challenges because the method used markedly influences the percentage of positive results observed.

***Stage 4: Active Sensitization.*** Symptoms are produced if the antigenic food is consumed during this stage, but usually

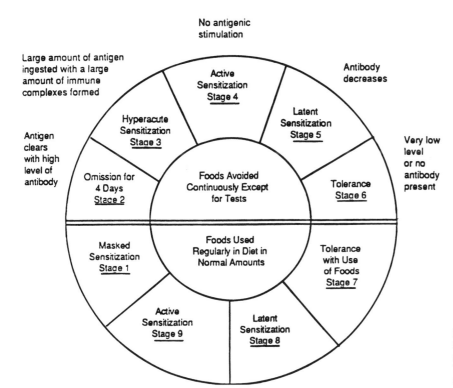

**FIG. 4.2.** Cyclic food allergy. Increased immune complex disease occurs with increased antigen exposure. (From Rinkel HJ, Randolph TG, Zeller M. *Food allergy.* Springfield, IL: Charles C Thomas, 1951, with permission.)

are less severe. For this reason, for greatest sensitivity, oral food challenges should be performed only during the 5- to 12-day period after food omission.

***Stage 5: Latent Sensitization.*** With no antigen stimulation, the antibody levels decrease and continued antigen elimination leads to tolerance. An antigenic food ingestion at this stage may cause either mild symptoms or no symptoms, unless several exposures occur.

***Stages 6 and 7: Tolerance to Foods.*** This stage usually is attained after 4 to 5 months of continuous antigen avoidance. At this point, there are very low levels of antibody production and food ingestion no longer produces symptoms. Foods must then be added back to the diet as rotated foods (see later) to avoid increased antibody formation with recurrence of symptoms. If tolerance cannot be attained, lifelong avoidance is required.

***Stages 8 and 9: Sensitization.*** If the person again ingests the food frequently (stage 8), the increased antigen exposure results in anamnestic stimulation of memory lymphocytes, renewed antibody production, increased immune complex formation, and increased symptoms (stage 9). Ultimately, unless the patient realizes the food allergy is again causing symptoms and resumes a rotation diet, masking reoccurs, and the cycle is complete. Resensitization often occurs because of human nature. Patients who are doing well on a

rotation diet often feel that "a bit more won't hurt," and slowly increase their use of certain rotated foods. When they do, they slip back into sensitization. If the symptoms are noticed, often patients again adhere strictly to their diet and again become tolerant. But because the symptoms of resensitization are mild, patients may not notice, and so they may complete the circle and again enter the stage of masked sensitization, where a food is eaten often enough that symptoms never have a chance to clear. The resensitization process may take only a week or two to complete, yet regaining tolerance may again take many months. In some persons, the process repeats over and over, giving rise to the term *cyclic food allergy.*

### Masked Sensitization and Food Addiction

One facet of cyclic food allergy needs to be examined in more detail: the phenomenon of masking. Masked food allergy is the counterintuitive clinical finding of a *decrease* in symptoms after eating a food to which a patient is allergic. Masking arises when an allergic food is consumed often enough that the symptoms created by one ingestion never completely subside before the food is eaten again. Usually, the second ingestion results in a temporary improvement in symptoms, followed hours later by worsening. The masking phenomenon can be explained in two complementary ways. In a serum sickness model (type III reaction), altering the size of the circulating food–antibody complexes by adding antigen (eating more food) changes the ability of the complexes to deposit in target organ capillary beds, and thus affects symptom production. In the prostaglandin release model (see later), small doses of food ingestion cause release of protective prostaglandins that attenuate the response to a subsequent, larger ingestion. Because this waning and waxing of symptoms is not obviously related to the food ingestion, identification of cyclic food allergies is difficult for patients and their physicians unless the stages of cyclic food allergy that Dr. Rinkel identified are understood. Even attempts to correlate symptoms with ingestion (as recorded in a diet diary), or attempts to provoke symptoms by oral challenge, often fail unless the concepts of cyclic food allergy are taken into account. The transient improvement in chronic allergy symptoms that occurs with masking often leads patients to eat an allergic food very often. This attempt to feel better by eating an allergic food is known as *food addiction,* and the foods being craved the most are usually the ones causing a patient's symptoms. Therefore, key factors in the dietary history that suggest probable cyclic food allergy are food cravings, symptom improvement shortly after eating, symptom worsening hours after eating (for example, awakening from sleep with symptoms), and symptom improvement after prolonged fasting.

## Summary of Fixed and Cyclic Food Allergy Concepts

Immunologic food hypersensitivity reactions can be clinically categorized as fixed or cyclic. Patients with fixed food allergy have an immediate, easily identifiable adverse response whenever the offending food is consumed. Tolerance usually is not achieved, even after years of avoidance. In contrast, cyclic food allergy produces symptoms that are directly related to the quantity and frequency of ingestion of the antigenic food. Patients usually experience chronic symptoms and may initially experience the masked stage of cyclic sensitivity, where the offending food temporarily improves the adverse reaction from a previous ingestion of that food. It therefore may be a difficult diagnosis to make, and a careful history, including the use of a food diary, can become an invaluable diagnostic tool.

## USE OF THE HISTORY AND PHYSICAL EXAMINATION IN FOOD ALLERGY

Diagnosis of food allergy depends primarily on a patient's history. Food allergies of either fixed or cyclic type should be suspected in patients with childhood symptoms of formula intolerance, colic, or gastroesophageal reflux; severe diaper rashes or perirectal inflammation; asthma; recurrent croup or bronchitis; hyperactivity; chronic or frequent otitis media or sinusitis; red, patchy cheeks, red ears, and other signs of eczema; or gastrointestinal symptoms without a specific pathologic diagnosis (e.g., irritable bowel syndrome). Chronic constitutional symptoms, such as fatigue, poor-quality sleep, nonspecific pruritus, frequent respiratory illnesses, frequent gastrointestinal complaints, and the "many syndrome" (many complaints, many physicians, many failed treatments) also should raise suspicion of food allergy. Parents occasionally observe that these symptoms improve or resolve with changes in diet or fasting, and recurrence is noted when the previous diet is resumed. Children often appear to "outgrow" these problems as they consume less food per kilogram of body mass, but frequently they experience the same, or other, allergic symptoms later in life because of allergies to the same foods. The food-allergic patient often has many symptoms and many organ systems involved, so a thorough review of systems also should be an integral part of the initial history. Obtaining a careful history helps to select patients who require food allergy testing, and may identify whether fixed or cyclic food allergy is more likely. Use of preprinted forms or computerized data collection can be helpful in obtaining both pertinent history and a diary of current food consumption.

## Signs and Symptoms of Food Allergy

Signs and symptoms of food allergy depend somewhat on whether the allergy is fixed or cyclic, but there is overlap. IgE-mediated, fixed allergy usually produces obvious signs and symptoms whenever the food is consumed, even if it has been avoided for a prolonged time. Symptoms are secondary to both the rapid release of histamine and other preformed mediators, and also to the slow development of the late-phase reaction. Patients often can identify what food is causing their problem, except in two situations. One is when they have eaten a mixture of foods before the reaction. In this situation, the fixed allergy is evident, but the specific food allergy is unknown. The other exception is for chronic allergy conditions, such as eczema and asthma, where the late-phase reaction plays a prominent role. In these situations, it is not always evident that a fixed allergy is responsible because the increase in symptoms after a meal may be too small, compared with the ongoing chronic symptoms, to be easily noticed. In both of these exceptions, there should be high suspicion for fixed food allergy, and specific testing for IgE food allergy should be done.

In non–IgE-mediated, cyclic food allergy, the signs and symptoms usually are more complex and difficult to recognize than in fixed food allergy. Symptoms are secondary to the slow accumulation of immune complexes in the capillary beds of target organs, with damage to the vessels and leakage of fluid and inflammatory substances into the tissues of that organ. The presence of symptoms depends on both the frequency of eating and the amount of antigen consumed because these factors determine the quantity, quality, and persistence of immune complexes. Because any organ system can be involved, and because symptom production regularly occurs long after meals, patients normally do not connect their chronic symptoms with food ingestion. The sole exception is when patients realize that they have a food "addiction," and feel better when regularly eating a particular food.

There are many common symptoms and signs that may be caused by cyclic food allergies. Rowe recognized this, early in the 20th century, but at that time there was wide disbelief that food allergy could have such varied expression. Presence of any of these symptoms, signs, or conditions in the review of systems should include cyclic food allergy in the differential diagnosis, but it is important to remember that food allergy is not the only possible explanation. Potentially serious alternate diagnoses always must be evaluated, such as in the exclusion of a brain tumor as an explanation for headaches, or hepatitis C as a cause of fatigue.

*Neurologic* symptoms include headaches, especially weather-dependent headaches and migraine, cluster, and histamine types (40), learning disabilities, behavioral problems or hyperactivity (especially in children), forgetfulness, short attention span, cognitive problems ("brain fog"), insomnia, depression, and chronic fatigue (41–43). Rarely, even seizures can be food triggered.

*Ophthalmologic* symptoms often are greater than signs, and may be unilateral or affect only one lid. Mild symptoms are pruritus, stinging, and irritation, often with scleral injection, or mild conjunctival or eyelid edema that feels like a foreign body is present. Periorbital or lid edema or eczema, with itching, scaling, and erythema, is common. Severe symptoms are tearing, burning, thick mucoid discharge, and photophobia, frequently accompanied by rough tarsal mucosa, with visible inflammatory papules that feel like sand. Episodic blurred vision may be due to either epiphora or edema, but the cornea should *not* be inflamed, eroded, or misshapen, or the globe hard. Ophthalmologic consultation is important when any corneal abnormality is noted, or if symptoms fail to improve with treatment.

*Otologic* symptoms include external conditions such as chronic otitis externa, with narrowed ear canals, red auricles, scaling or cracking, especially in the concha, behind, and beneath the ear, and eczematous otitis externa. The ear is the most common site of an "Id" reaction (see later discussion of skin symptoms). Middle ear conditions include clicking, popping, pressure sensation, lancinating pains, or other eustachian complaints, recurrent otitis media, chronic serous otitis media with effusion (44,45), persistent otorrhea after myringotomy tubes, and failed ear surgery in a nonsmoker. Inner ear conditions are dizziness or disequilibrium, Meniere's syndrome (46–48), cochlear hydrops, tinnitus, and dull ear pain.

*Nasal* obstruction is common, sometimes with voice change, snoring, or sleep disturbance, and often is due to edema of the turbinates. Common symptoms are clear rhinorrhea, thick postnasal discharge, crusting, pruritus, sneezing, sniffing, snorting, or clucking, decreased olfaction (and

taste), allergic salute, "sinus" headaches, facial fullness, pain, and pressure. Associated diagnoses are nasal polyps, allergic fungal sinusitis, chronic or recurrent sinus infections (49), and recurrent adenoiditis.

*Oral* symptoms are oral, perioral, and palatal pruritus, dry mouth and halitosis (subjective) from mouth breathing, nocturnal bruxism (to open eustachian tube), and dysphagia or respiratory difficulty due to adenotonsillar hypertrophy. Signs are geographic tongue, aphthous ulcers, and angioedema of the lips and oral mucosa (34).

*Pharyngeal and laryngeal* allergy-related conditions include chronic sore throat, recurrent pharyngitis, tonsillitis, or lingual tonsillitis, chronic throat clearing, perception of a lump in throat (globus pharyngicus), and itching. Signs are enlarged lateral pharyngeal bands and posterior pharyngeal lymphoid islands (due to postnasal drip), laryngeal edema with intermittent hoarseness, and angioedema of the laryngopharynx (50).

In the *neck,* fluctuating adenopathy or edema of major or minor salivary glands may be due to allergy.

*Pulmonary* symptoms usually are nonspecific and include chronic cough, especially multiple or strong enough to cause nausea, shortness of breath, chest tightness, chest pain with breathing, and wheezing (51). Sometimes exercise-induced symptoms, or hard to clear, thick, tenacious, colorless sputum are clues. Allergy often is involved in recurrent bronchitis or croup, and may be a factor in recurrent pneumonia or chronic obstructive disease. Symptoms are on a continuum from allergic bronchitis to exercise-induced asthma to asthma. Pulmonary consultation is important when symptoms are severe.

*Cardiovascular* effects from food and chemical exposures can include vasculitis and arrhythmias (52).

*Gastrointestinal* food-induced symptoms are very common, but nonspecific, such as intermittent abdominal pain, vomiting, or diarrhea, constipation or alternating constipation and diarrhea, gastroesophageal reflux, abdominal distention, gas, belching, and fatigue after meals. Symptoms may or may not be obviously related to food ingestion, but pruritus ani or perirectal inflammation ("burned butt") and acute cramps and diarrhea may be more easily identified with specific ingestions.

*Genitourinary* signs and symptoms commonly include enuresis, due to allergic bladder irritation, and pruritic vaginitis or balanitis. Rarely, food- or inhalant-induced allergic nephrotic syndrome is seen. This is a common site of the "Id" reaction, especially in female patients (see discussion of skin, later).

*Musculoskeletal* effects such as arthralgias, myalgias, stiffness, and erythema or edema over joints can have an allergic cause, but this seldom is suspected (53).

*Skin* has three major allergy symptom complexes: atopic dermatitis or eczema, urticaria and angioedema, and the dermatophytid (termed the *Id* ) reaction. Atopic dermatitis/eczema is not a rash that itches, but an itch that rashes, because persistent pruritus causes chronic scratching. The rash may come and go, usually in the same locations, or may be constant, typically on the extensor or flexor surfaces of the limbs, and face. Skin is dry, rough, red, and thick, with scaling and edema, and fissuring, weeping, and crusting occur when secondary staphylococcal infection occurs (54). Contact dermatitis and eczema have overlapping symptoms and appearance. Urticaria and angioedema differ primarily in the depth of skin inflammation, with urticarial wheals developing more superficially, and causing more itch than pain. Both produce more edema than other allergic skin problems. Some angioedema is nonallergic, caused by defects in kinin pathways, such as deficient function of C1 esterase inhibitor. The Id reaction appears superficially similar to eczema, but usually has small, itchy, punctate lesions, rather than large areas of itchy skin. Id reactions usually are the result of allergy to cutaneous fungi, but may worsen from cross-reacting food ingestion. The clear dermal vesicles are most evident on hands, feet, external ears, and genitalia, and usually are smaller than 1 mm. Raised, rough, "goose-flesh" bumps on lateral arms, thighs, or trunk also may occur. As in eczema, if the Id reaction is not treated effectively, scaling, erythema, cracking, and superficial infection subsequently develop. With all skin rashes thought to be allergic, dermatologic consultation is helpful for nonclassic skin findings or treatment resistance.

## Food Consumption History and Diet Diary

To evaluate further the potential for cyclic food allergy, the patient is asked to keep a food diary for a 2-week period. It is important that all items consumed be recorded, including medications, vitamins, herbal remedies, all nonwater beverages, chewing gum, junk foods, and candies. Emphasis is placed on recording actual diet habits and on being truthful. The patient should record the time of ingestion, as well as the time of any symptoms observed. It is essential that entries be made throughout the day, instead of waiting until the end of the day. Symptoms should be recorded whenever they occur. It also is important to record any improvement of symptoms or cravings. The allergy care provider then analyzes this information for frequently eaten foods and whether any pattern can be seen in symptom production. Most people tend to be habit eaters, regularly eating only approximately ten foods. Favorite foods are eaten over and over, often at several meals a day, just by changing the form or method of preparation a little so that the foods seem different. The hidden foods (corn, milk, soy, wheat, and yeast) that are used in packaged or processed foods are an almost universal problem. The problem of repetitious eating is made more complex by the presence of allergic cross-reactions between closely related foods. For example, people with wheat allergy often also react to closely related grains such as rye and barley, so that there is even less variety in

most diets. The suspect cyclic allergy foods are those eaten at least twice weekly, and especially those eaten daily or several times a day. Craved foods, or foods eaten during the night, also are highly suspect. Once the diary is reviewed, then the definitive diagnosis is made by appropriate in vitro or in vivo tests.

## DIAGNOSTIC TECHNIQUES FOR FIXED FOOD ALLERGY

### In Vitro Tests

#### Specific Immunoglobulin E Testing

In vitro specific IgE testing is preferred whenever there is a history of prior serious reaction to a food, or when the patient has a "brittle" history of high sensitivity or significant asthma. Over 30 years of specific IgE testing have resulted in a very sensitive, specific, and reliable technology (55,56). High sensitivity results (class 3 and higher) from IgE in vitro tests indicate that significant symptoms will likely be produced if that food is ingested, and therefore those foods should be permanently avoided. On the other hand, low sensitivity results (class 2 and lower) from IgE in vitro tests require clinical correlation before making dietary recommendations. In young children, who typically have low levels of serum IgE, low-class IgE scores may indicate very significant sensitization and a need for avoidance. In adults, low-class specific IgE food results commonly are seen without a history of immediate food reactions, and in conjunction with classic cyclic food allergy symptoms. Therefore, these low-class results may reflect mixed-type food allergy reactions and often can be treated like cyclic food allergy, rather than by permanent exclusion (see later section on Oral Challenge Test).

#### Basophil Histamine Release

Histamine is detectable both in the blood, after eating an allergic food, and after mixing food antigens ex vivo with basophils obtained from an allergic person. Several methods for an ex vivo assay have been developed, using radioimmunoassay, fluorometry, or high-pressure liquid chromatography (57–59). Current methods using glass microfiber adsorption of histamine require only small quantities of blood per test, comparable with specific IgE determinations (60). Histamine release results correlate well with results from skin tests, provocation tests, and specific IgE tests (61,62) for IgE-mediated allergy, but also may detect some non–IgE-mediated food reactions (61). The principal advantage of measuring histamine release is that it allows detection of both allergic and anaphylactoid reactions and can be applied to any antigen or substance, including those that are not currently available for specific IgE assays. The chief disadvantage of this test is the small number of clinical laboratories where it is available, and the consequent need for shipping whole-blood samples.

## Skin Tests

In patients who have no history of serious reactions, skin tests (prick or patch) may be cautiously performed. *Deaths have occurred from attempting to skin test patients with severe, anaphylactic, fixed food allergies.* Prick tests were first described by Lewis and Grant in 1926 (63) and were popularized in the 1970s by Pepys (64). Prick tests are specific and easily performed, and infrequently cause systemic allergic reactions (65,66). However, prick test variations greatly influence testing results owing to the difficulty of precisely reproducing the depth of penetration, amount of force used, and the amount of skin lifting. The vertical prick puncture is more reproducible because a guard prevents penetration beyond a predetermined depth (67). Most prick puncture test devices now use single, 1-mm tips (68–70). Prick puncture devices reduce testing variability, yet there are detectable differences in reproducibility between them (68,71,72). In comparisons between prick, intradermal, and specific IgE in vitro tests, correlations of 85% to 90% between prick and in vivo tests (66) and 81% to 89% between prick puncture tests and intradermal skin endpoint titration tests have been reported (73).

### Modified Prick Tests

The prick puncture test has been further modified by adding multiple, longer tips to introduce greater quantities of antigen and thereby increase sensitivity. Lengthening the tips beyond 1 mm often allows antigen to enter the dermis, as occurs during intradermal testing (65). An example is the Multi-Test I device, with an array of eight clusters, each using nine 1.9-mm tips, to test eight antigens simultaneously (74). Several similar devices are available. The increase in antigen dose makes modified prick test devices more similar to intradermal tests than to single-prick tests (74–76), but it also makes them less comfortable for patients and decreases their reproducibility (71). In one study, Multi-Test I, 1:1,000 w/v single intradermal tests, fivefold skin endpoint titration, and IgE in vitro tests were found to be comparable test techniques (75). In another study, Multi-Test I was compared with fivefold skin endpoint titration, and was found to be approximately 5 to 25 times less sensitive than 1:1,000 w/v intradermal tests (74).

With any prick test method, very careful adherence to technique is needed (77). Because of the possibility for false-positive reactions when tests are placed closely together, prick tests should be separated by approximately 2 cm (68, 78). Because the variability in reaction size is less for larger wheals (79), weaker prick responses are the most likely to be in error. With all prick techniques, the greater the experi-

ence of the testing personnel, the lower the test variability (80,81).

### Patch Tests

In patch testing, allergens are applied to the intact skin, under an occlusive dressing, and allowed to react for times ranging from minutes to days. Antigens as large as 30,000 daltons can penetrate intact skin (82). There are many variations of patch testing, depending on skin preparation technique, antigen dose, method of antigen solubilization, and the type of occlusion. Patch tests usually detect delayed allergic reactions due to either the late phase of type I reactions (83) or to type IV reactions (84), although, when applied for only 30 minutes, patch tests also can detect early-phase type I reactions (85,86). When dimethyl sulfoxide is used to dissolve food antigens, patch tests may be capable of detecting all four Gel and Coombs reaction types (87). Patch tests have the advantages of being nonpainful (88) and rarely causing systemic reactions (89). The chief disadvantage of patch testing is that it is less reproducible than other skin tests, with both false-negative and false-positive reactions. However, when carefully performed, sensitivity is approximately 61% to 77% and specificity is approximately 71% to 81% (84,90), which is comparable with other skin tests. One of the reasons for poor patch test performance is the difficulty in differentiating irritative reactions from true allergic responses (89,91). When used for diagnosis of food allergies, patch tests may be either more or less sensitive than prick tests, depending on the specific antigen and method used (84,92,93).

## DIAGNOSTIC TECHNIQUES FOR CYCLIC FOOD ALLERGY

## Oral Challenge Test

Once the dietary analysis is complete and the potential offending foods have been identified, the next step is to prepare the patient for elimination and challenge tests. The oral challenge test involves elimination of a specific food for 4 to 5 days, followed by ingestion of that food in large amounts. If the patient has a cyclic type of sensitivity to this food, he or she will respond in an exaggerated symptomatic manner. This can be explained by the fact that after 4 days of antigen elimination, the amount of free antibodies in the circulation is high (94), and the reintroduction of the antigen leads to a large amount of immune complex formation that produces a strong onset of symptoms. The principal difficulty with this type of testing is that only one food can be tested at a time, so that testing can be prolonged if multiple foods need to be evaluated.

The oral food challenge is the standard for complete detection of food allergies. Oral challenges can detect all Gel and Coombs reaction types but, in usual practice, because of the safety risk, are *not* used to confirm fixed, anaphylactic food allergies. However, oral challenges, even when done as open procedures, are slow to perform and require considerable willpower from patients. The double-blind, placebo-controlled elimination and challenge test (95) is the most difficult oral challenge to do because it uses dehydrated food capsules or liquified food given by feeding tube, or mixes the food with a nonallergenic substance to mask flavor, texture, and aroma. Problems with the blinded test are that dehydrated food may not react like fresh foods, and the food may not be given in sufficient quantity to trigger symptoms. Also, interpretation of symptoms from both kinds of oral challenge may be subjective, and all oral feedings require a major clinician time commitment. Because it is easier to perform and more closely mimics normal food exposure, the open, unblinded oral challenge is normally used in clinical practice. For patients without a history of serious food reaction, oral food challenges may be done at home, but whenever there is any concern, the office setting is preferred.

## Elimination

To perform the oral challenge test properly, care must be taken to eliminate the food to be tested from the body as completely as possible. Any amount of that particular food that is not eliminated from the diet results in attenuation of the response in proportion to the amount of the food consumed. Following are patient instructions in preparation for the oral challenge test:

> Before elimination, the test food should be eaten at least every day for 2 weeks. Then, eliminate the test food completely for 4 days. On the day of the test (fifth day), it is easiest to do the challenge on an empty stomach, after arising. Alternatively, eat an early breakfast of known safe foods, while still omitting the food to be tested, and plan the test for approximately 5 hours later, while avoiding any further food or liquids (except for water) before the test. Also avoid all nonessential medicines, and avoid smoking for 3 hours.

## Challenge

Baseline symptoms and pulse are recorded before oral challenge. The patient is fed an average portion of the pure food within a 5-minute period; it is very important to feed only one pure food, prepared simply. Specific suggestions as to what to test and how to prepare the foods are essential if accurate tests are desired. For example, to test wheat, a large serving of cream of wheat is cooked only with water and sea salt, then eaten plain, without milk or sweetener. If no symptoms are noted within 1 hour, a second feeding can be given. Symptoms are recorded over the first hour and the patient is observed for a minimum of 2 hours. Subjective and objective symptoms are recorded, as well as pulse changes. Symptom development within the first hour, or

within an hour of the second feeding, indicates that the test food probably is allergenic. Symptoms developing several hours after the test indicate a delayed positive reaction. Taking Alka-Seltzer Gold, unflavored milk of magnesia, or 2 to 3 g of vitamin C may relieve provoked symptoms. In cases where symptoms are weak, entirely subjective, or not clearly related to the challenge, the test can be repeated the following day. Identical symptoms should occur after each challenge with the same food. If the challenge correctly identifies an allergenic food, avoidance of that food should eliminate the triggered symptoms.

## Rechallenge

For cyclic allergies, to determine when a food can be put back into the diet as a rotated food, rechallenge must produce no symptoms. Symptoms of cyclic allergy typically decrease quickly with continued avoidance, so rechallenge commonly is done after an initial avoidance period of 2 or more months. If the first rechallenge is positive, that food should be avoided for another several months before attempting another challenge. Periodic rechallenges are continued until either there is no reaction, or until 2 years of avoidance. Any food that still produces symptoms after 2 years should be considered to be a fixed food allergen requiring lifelong avoidance.

## Skin Tests

Cyclic food allergies also may be accurately diagnosed by injecting food antigen into the skin, using the intradermal progressive dilution food test (IPDFT) technique. This test is a type of titration test using the sequential injection of several different dilutions of each food allergen, and is similar in principle to skin endpoint titration, as used for inhalant testing. It was initially conceived by Rinkel et al. (12) and further developed by Lee et al. (96). Rinkel and colleagues observed that intradermal injection of large amounts of food allergens caused whealing and, in some cases, also produced symptoms that mimicked those seen in oral food challenges. There are numerous published double-blind studies confirming the diagnostic efficacy of this test (97). The most definitive work is the double-blind, crossover, placebo-controlled, multicenter study by William King and colleagues (98,99). The basis for skin testing for non–IgE-mediated allergies is that substances other than IgE, including immune complexes and complement, cause mast cell degranulation. Studies by Breneman et al. (100) and Kuwabara et al. (101) demonstrated that immune complexes, together with complement, cause mast cell degranulation when food antigens are applied to the dermis. The resulting wheal-and-flare reaction of the skin is both predictable and reproducible, making this method of diagnosis an efficacious option.

## Comparison of IPDFT Effectiveness with Other Food Allergy Tests

The King study directly compared the oral food challenge, IPDFT (using both provocation and whealing responses), modified prick (Multi-Test), and in vitro (both IgE and IgG) tests in the same patients. The major study result was that only the IPDFT correlated highly with the oral food challenge. Compared with the oral food challenge, the IPDFT, by skin whealing response, was 78% reliable, and by provocation response 61% reliable. When symptom provocation was observed, it was highly specific, but the skin whealing response was found to be the more sensitive means of detecting an allergenic food. Results were significant at the 0.01 confidence level (skin whealing) and 0.05 confidence level (provocation). Weaknesses of the IPDFT primarily consisted of some false-positive whealing and some false-negative provocation, approximately 20% of the responses in each group. Weaknesses of the other food allergy tests included the following: modified prick tests and in vitro IgE tests were insensitive, detecting only a small percentage of positive oral challenges, and in vitro IgG tests had extensive overlap between the results for allergic and nonallergic foods.

## Food Skin Testing Safety Guidelines

In deciding when to skin test for food allergy, the clinician should keep in mind these safety guidelines:

1. Never test a food to which the patient has a known IgE-mediated fixed allergy. If needed, IgE in vitro tests can confirm the allergy.
2. Test only for foods that are in the diet on a regular basis. If the food is not consumed at least twice per week, it is unlikely to cause allergic symptoms, and testing is unnecessary. Moreover, if a food has been omitted from the diet, it could be a possible anaphylactic food.
3. Patients should be carefully questioned for a history of any past serious allergic reaction. Test sensitive patients, such as those with brittle asthma, with caution. Consider initial IgE in vitro testing.
4. All foods to be tested must have been eaten within 24 hours of testing to minimize risk of provocation.
5. Consider IgE in vitro testing before intradermal tests for all known potent allergens like peanuts or cottonseed.

## Performing the IPDFT Cyclic Food Allergy Skin Test

The method used for the IPDFT takes each food antigen concentrate (1:20 w/v) and dilutes it fivefold by taking 1 mL of antigen and diluting it in 4 mL of phenolated saline, calling this the #1 dilution (1:100 w/v). Serial fivefold dilutions are then made by taking 1 mL of the previous dilution and adding it to 4 mL of phenolated saline to come up with

**TABLE 4.1. IPDFT SKIN ENDPOINT TITRATION DILUTIONS**

| Dilution | Antigen (w/v) Concentration | Glycerin (%) Concentration |
|---|---|---|
| Concentrate | 1:20[a] | 50[a] |
| #1 | 1:100 | 10 |
| #2 | 1:500 | 2 |
| #3 | 1:2,500 | 0.4 |
| #4 | 1:12,500 | 0.08 |
| #5 | 1:62,500 | 0.016 |
| #6 | 1:312,500 | 0.003 |

IPDFT, intradermal progressive dilution food test
[a] Concentrates are not normally used for intradermal testing.

the next weaker dilution. These are labeled consecutively as #2 to #6 dilutions. Similar dilutions are made from 50% glycerin to serve as negative controls (Table 4.1). On rare occasion, dilutions weaker than #6 may be required. Alternatively, some physicians use 1:10 w/v food antigen concentrates, and perform a tenfold initial dilution to prepare the #1, 1:100 w/v antigen solutions. In this case, the glycerin concentration in each antigen dilution is one-half as great as when 1:20 w/v concentrates are used, and the glycerin controls must be diluted in the same way.

After first checking skin reactivity with a positive histamine control and a negative control of phenolated saline, testing is started by applying 0.05-mL wheals of both a food antigen and a corresponding dilution of glycerin. This is done because all extracts, except lyophilized ones, are made with 50% glycerin, a preservative used to maintain potency for shelf life. High concentrations of glycerin cause irritative wheals to form, so antigen-containing tests must be placed simultaneously with comparable glycerin controls to determine if the wheal growth observed is caused by glycerin rather than antigen. Glycerin wheals at #1 dilution frequently show growth, #2 wheals sometimes do, and, rarely, so do #3 or #4 glycerin wheals.

Antigen testing for nonbrittle patients is started with injection of 0.05 mL of the #1 dilution, this volume usually producing a 7-mm wheal (Fig. 4.3). Wheals are observed for up to 10 minutes and commonly spread to 8 or 9 mm. If there is no size difference between the control and antigen wheals, and if no symptoms are produced, the test is negative. In these patients, it is necessary to use diagnostic oral food challenges to be certain allergy is not missed. If the antigen wheal grows larger than the negative glycerin control by 2 mm or more, with or without symptoms, it is a positive response and the next weaker dilution (#2) is applied immediately, regardless of time lapsed. A matching #2 glycerin also is applied. If symptoms occur but there is no wheal growth, the test also is positive, and the #2 dilution also should be applied. This titration is continued to

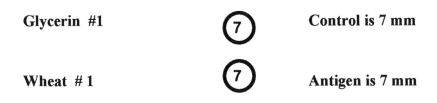

## 7 mm wheals made

Glycerin  #1                    (7)                    Control is 7 mm

Wheat  # 1                      (7)                    Antigen is 7 mm

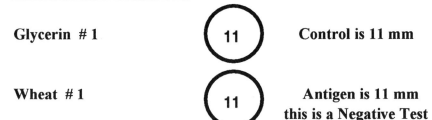

## Wheals read in 10 minutes

Glycerin  # 1                   (11)                   Control is 11 mm

Wheat  # 1                      (11)                   **Antigen is 11 mm
                                                        this is a Negative Test**

**FIG. 4.3.** Example of a single intradermal progressive dilution food test on a nonbrittle cyclic food-allergic patient.

weaker antigen and glycerin dilutions until no growth occurs during the 10-minute observation time, and, if symptoms had been produced, until they are relieved. After the initial positive wheal, the dilution at which no symptoms or growth occur (negative response) is considered the endpoint of the titration.

Most endpoints in nonbrittle patients range from dilutions #1 to #4. Rarely, in single IPDFT testing, symptom-relieving endpoints are not clear, and intermediate amounts of antigen between the standard fivefold dilutions may be identified. For example, when titrating to more dilute concentrations, a point may be reached where the wheal is negative but symptoms are not completely cleared. Sometimes, repeating the injection of that dilution once or twice relieves the symptoms, and if so, that endpoint is called a *multiple,* and the neutralizing dose to use in therapy is 0.10 or 0.15 mL instead of the usual 0.05 mL.

Judgment is required in testing patients who may be more sensitive. Depending on the clinical assessment, IPDFT may be started with dilution #3 (Figs. 4.4, 4.5). Rarely, in very brittle patients, testing may start with dilution #5 or #7, but these dilutions also can provoke an underdose reaction. In these cases, if symptoms are provoked by the initial test wheal, it may be due either to an overdose *or* an underdose. In either situation, the initial wheal size is not useful in deciding the next step. To be conservative, the next wheal applied should be *more* dilute. But, if symptoms are not rapidly improved by the more dilute antigen, and especially if the more dilute wheal is

larger than the initial wheal, the direction of titration should be reversed, and a stronger dilution should be applied in an effort to neutralize the symptoms.

During the testing procedure, symptoms can be transiently produced and the patient needs to be observed carefully. If no symptoms occur, but positive whealing occurs, that food may still cause symptoms when ingested in sufficient quantity. If no wheal growth or symptoms occur with the #1 dilution, than that food is considered nonallergenic for that patient. When patients have a good history for food allergy but antigen and control wheals are of similar sizes, symptoms are not clearly defined, and no clear positives are found, it will be necessary to use diagnostic oral food challenges instead of skin tests.

There are three differences between intradermal IPDFT food testing and intradermal skin endpoint titration inhalant testing. Food testing injects five times more antigen solution volume (0.05 vs. 0.01 mL) and therefore produces larger wheals (7 vs. 4 mm). Food testing also uses much stronger initial antigen solutions, normally beginning testing at #1 (1:100 w/v) instead of #4 (1:12,500 w/v) or #6 (1:312,500 w/v). Finally, the definition of the endpoint is different. In food testing, the endpoint is the first nonreactive wheal, whereas in inhalant testing, the endpoint is the first reactive wheal that initiates progressive whealing. Although both types of testing are based on the titration concept of quantification of sensitivity, and the quantity of allergen injected into the endpoint wheal is identical, these specific technique differences must be kept in mind while

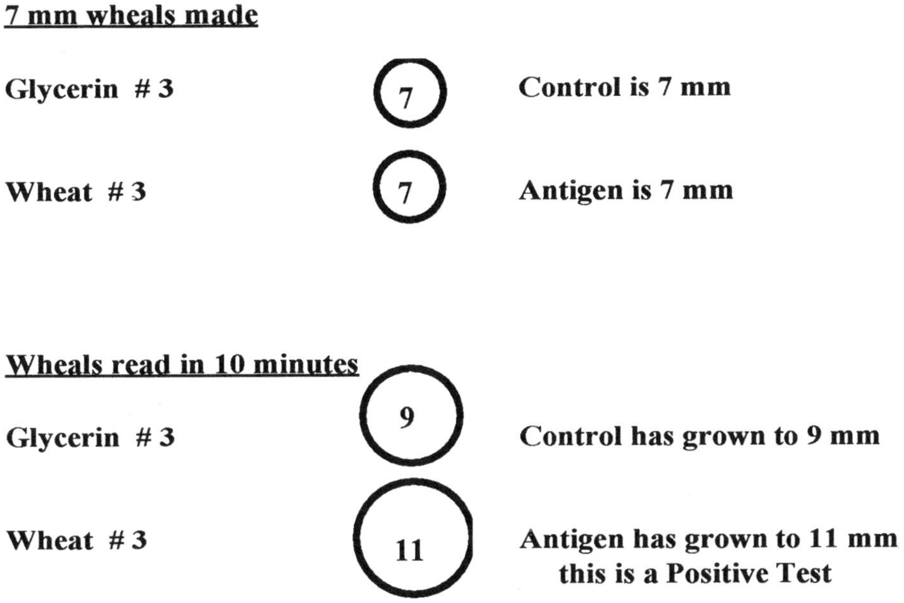

**7 mm wheals made**

Glycerin # 3          (7)          **Control is 7 mm**

Wheat # 3          (7)          **Antigen is 7 mm**

**Wheals read in 10 minutes**

Glycerin # 3          (9)          **Control has grown to 9 mm**

Wheat # 3          (11)          **Antigen has grown to 11 mm
this is a Positive Test**

**FIG. 4.4.** Example of a single positive intradermal progressive dilution food test on an asthmatic cyclic food-allergic patient.

performing and interpreting allergy skin tests. The IPDFT technique must *never* be used to test for inhalant allergy or for fixed, anaphylactic food allergy because it is *not safe* to test for these IgE-mediated allergies with initial strong antigen concentrations.

The IPDFT endpoint also is the therapeutic neutralizing dose. Successful neutralization stops the allergic reaction, makes the positive wheal disappear, reverses any symptoms produced, and determines a treatment dose for cyclic food immunotherapy. As described below, the neutralizing dose is the dose of the antigen that triggers the prostaglandin protective mechanism, and also places the specific lympho-

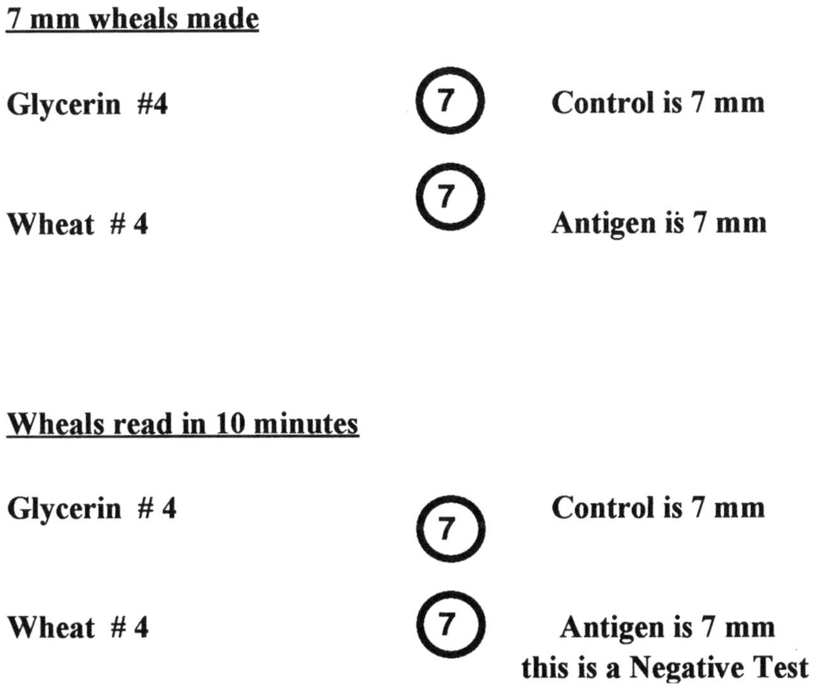

**7 mm wheals made**

Glycerin #4          (7)          **Control is 7 mm**

Wheat # 4          (7)          **Antigen is 7 mm**

**Wheals read in 10 minutes**

Glycerin # 4          (7)          **Control is 7 mm**

Wheat # 4          (7)          **Antigen is 7 mm
this is a Negative Test**

**FIG. 4.5.** Example of a single negative intradermal progressive dilution food test. Continue testing weaker dilutions to find the endpoint. Dilution #4 is the endpoint for wheat in this example.

cytes into low dose tolerance to stop the production of IgG. The IPDFT is able to verify which foods a patient is sensitive to, and also identifies therapeutic doses that can be applied for treatment purposes.

### Skin Testing Multiple Foods Simultaneously

It is possible for experienced testers to use the IPDFT technique to test more than one food simultaneously. This multitest technique was developed in the late 1980s by Walter Ward and William King (102). Normally, novices to multiple food tests should test only three foods at once, and prior experience with single IPDFT testing is very helpful. Experienced testers may perform as many as ten simultaneous food tests, but normally from three to six are tested, depending on clinical assessment of the patient's degree of sensitivity and the experience level of the tester. Whenever many allergen skin tests are done, the total allergen load may be large enough to produce systemic symptoms; consequently, experience is needed to enable the tester to know when to stop testing. Provocation of symptoms is seen less commonly when multiple foods are tested than when single food tests are done, so endpoints are determined from the relative wheal sizes alone.

For novice testers, testing begins with application of #3 food dilutions and the corresponding #3 glycerin control. Experienced testers may begin with #1 dilutions. Sensitive patients should begin testing with #5 dilutions, or single IPDFT tests should be considered. Standard food wheals of 7-mm diameter, produced by injection of 0.05 mL of antigen solution, are used. As in the single-food IPDFT, 10 minutes is allowed for wheal development, after which antigen wheals are measured and compared with the control glycerin wheal.

As an example, consider a multitest begun with #3 dilutions. To be positive, an antigen wheal must exceed the glycerin wheal size by 2 mm or more. Because the #3 glycerin rarely shows wheal growth, most wheals that show growth are true positives. Any antigen wheals that are less than 2 mm larger than the control are negative, but this does *not* indicate that these are not allergenic foods because these negative tests must be completed. A food cannot be said to be nonallergenic unless it is negative at the strongest (#1) dilution. We know from inhalant testing that, after a negative test, it is safe to jump up two dilutions, or 25-fold. Consequently, the negative #3 tests are followed by antigen dilution #1 tests and a corresponding #1 glycerin control. Negative #1 wheals are now completed tests, and indicate no allergy. Positive #1 wheals now require the application of #2 antigen and glycerin wheals, to identify possible endpoints. In some cases, the #3 dilution proves to be the true endpoint, and may be reapplied.

After completing the initial negative tests, the initial positive food tests now are completed. Any #3 antigen wheals that are 2 mm or larger than the control are positive, that is,

indicating an allergenic food. To determine the endpoints of these positive tests, the next most dilute antigen solutions (#4) are placed, allowed to develop for 10 minutes, and again compared with the appropriate glycerin control. Any #4 antigen wheals that are less than 2 mm larger than the #4 control are negative, indicating a completed test and the endpoint. Successively weaker dilutions must continue to be applied for each positive food until a negative endpoint wheal finally is obtained.

In the unlikely event that symptoms are provoked during a multitest, the first priority always should be to try to determine neutralizing doses for all positive tests. Only if good neutralization is obtained, and the patient is clinically stable, should initially negative tests be completed by injecting stronger antigen dilutions. If symptoms persist despite neutralization efforts, it always is wisest to postpone additional testing to another day.

### In Vitro Food Tests

Many in vitro food allergy tests have been available over the years (103,104), starting with the original cytotoxic test (105). Although this test has theoretic validity, its clinical use has been restricted because of poor reproducibility. Among the several more recent in vitro tests for cyclic food allergy that are available are IgG and IgG4 in vitro assays (106), the antigen leukocyte antibody test (107), and the enzyme-linked immunosorbent assay—activated cell test (108). Basophil histamine release tests also appear to detect some cyclic food allergies (see earlier, in section on Fixed Food Allergy). These tests are more reproducible, but the last three depend on live blood cells remaining normally functional after being shipped to a diagnostic laboratory. Also, there is substantial overlap of specific IgG levels between normal and food-allergic patients. And, when these in vitro tests are used, high immunoglobulin levels or reactive leucocytes do not necessarily guarantee clinical disease is present. Positive results obtained with these tests therefore should be corroborated by successful dietary manipulation or oral food challenge.

### THEORY OF ACTION OF NEUTRALIZATION TREATMENT

At least three mechanisms may explain the neutralization phenomenon, two immunologic and one nonimmunologic. One possibility is immune system negative feedback regulation by idiotypes and antiidiotype antibodies. Jerne (109) proposed a hypothesis to explain the complex interactions that regulate antibody formation (Fig. 4.6). According to this theory, an antigen elicits the production of an antibody (Ab1) that creates a unique sequence of amino acids, the idiotype, in its antigen-binding region, distinguishing it from other antibodies. The unique sequence displayed by

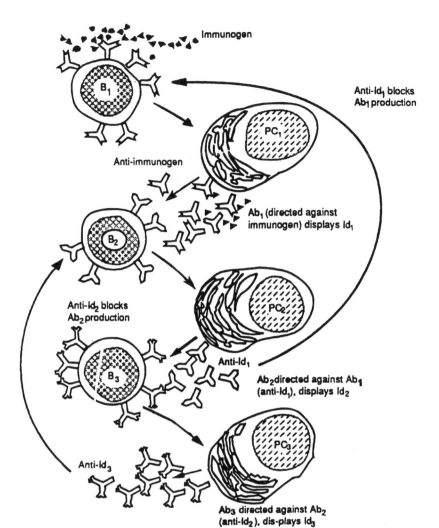

**Immunogen**

Anti-Id₁ blocks
Ab₁ production

$B_1$

$PC_1$

Anti-immunogen

Ab₁ (directed against
immunogen) displays Id₁

$B_2$

$PC_2$

Anti-Id₂ blocks
Ab₂ production

Anti-Id₁

Ab₂ directed against Ab₁
(anti-Id₁), displays Id₂

$B_3$

$PC_3$

Anti-Id₃

Ab₃ directed against Ab₂
(anti-Id₂), dis-plays Id₃

**FIG. 4.6.** Schematic representation of idio-type–antiidiotype regulation of antibody formation. (From Jerne NK. Towards a network theory of the immune system. *Ann Immunol* 1974;125C:373–389, with permission.)

idiotype 1 (Id1) also may function as an immunogen in the same host, because this new array of amino acids is not recognized as self and stimulates the production of another antibody (Ab2) that has antiidiotype specificity for Ab1. At the same time, it displays another unique idiotype, idiotype 2 (Id2). Ab2 suppresses the production of Ab1. In a similar manner, Ab2 stimulates the production of Ab3, and its own unique idiotype 3 (Id3), displaying anti-antiidiotype antibody against Ab2. Each idiotype that is expressed stimulates the production of a corresponding antiidiotype antibody to suppress the production of the antibody against which it was produced. This network of idiotypes, antiidiotypes, and anti-antiidiotypes either turns on or turns off antibody formation and the activities of the various subsets of immunoregulatory T cells. With low doses of antigen exposure, this regulatory system is shifted toward shutting off Ab1 to the original immunogen, and the patient moves into the low-dose tolerance phase.

A second possible mechanism involves the direct effect of antigen on T cells. Presentation of an antigen by antigen-presenting cells results in the activation of helper T cells, which cooperate with B cells to initiate antibody formation. At the same time, the suppressor T-cell population is activated to exert its regulatory effect. With low-dose antigen administration, the T-cell regulatory mechanism favors the suppression of antibody production.

The nonimmunologic mechanism involves prostaglandin production. Robert et al. (110) reported on the cytoprotective effects of prostaglandin. These investigators orally administered caustic substances to rats, inducing gastric necrosis. Prior administration of small, nontoxic doses of the caustic material prevented subsequent gastric injury when injurious doses of the caustics were given. Pretreatment with indomethacin completely ablated this cytoprotective effect, leading to the discovery that this is a prostaglandin-mediated effect. The cytoprotective effect also has been observed with antigen-induced asthma in humans, when patients were pretreated with neutralizing doses of antigen determined by IPDFT (111). Other studies documented antigen-specific desensitization of basophils for histamine release by low-dose antigen preincubation (112,113). This mechanism of neutralization also is supported by a double-blind study of low-dose house dust mite treatment (114).

In summary, low-dose antigen therapy appears to affect the immune system by downregulating both B-cell antibody production and T-cell function. Prostaglandin E, another nonimmunologic mechanism, also probably is involved by increasing intracellular cyclic adenosine monophosphate levels, decreasing cell metabolism, and increasing short-term resistance to injury.

## DIETARY TREATMENT OF FOOD ALLERGY

As Rinkel taught, the most effective method of treating any type of food sensitivity is elimination of the offending food from the diet. Success depends on several factors that include patient compliance and the ability properly to identify and avoid all food offenders. Elimination diets may lead to malnutrition, and patients unable to consume basic foods, such as milk or eggs, may need monitoring for nutritional inadequacies. Once immediate IgE-mediated food sensitivity has been demonstrated, the only proven mode of therapy is strict elimination of the offending allergen. Patient education is an integral part of managing this type of allergy, and if the reaction is severe, the patient also should be instructed on how to respond to a life-threatening reaction, including having a readily available dose of autoinjectable epinephrine. Research continues on high-dose desensitization, either oral or by injection, for fixed food allergies. This treatment can be contemplated in academic centers as part of a regulated clinical investigation. For cyclic food allergies, treatment can begin after the offending foods have been identified using the techniques described. Rotation diet manipulation to control the major offenders can be very effective in relieving the patient's symptoms. However, the more foods that must be avoided, the more complicated the dietary manipulation will be, and the more easily the patient can become discouraged.

### Elimination, Reintroduction, and Rotation of Foods

Treatment of cyclic food allergy consists of elimination of the food for 5 to 6 months, or longer, until the tolerance stage, at which time the food may be reintroduced into the diet on a rotating basis so that it is not consumed more than once or twice per week. Limited and infrequent exposure to these foods is aimed at preventing an increased production of specific IgG so that symptomatic levels of immune complexes are not sustained.

One of the earliest consequences of Rinkel's developing concept of cyclic food allergy was his perfection of the modern rotary diet in the mid-1930s. He first tried this form of diet treatment in an attempt to avoid cumulative food

reactions in food-allergic patients. At that time, it was known that recovery after an acute food allergic reaction might take several days. It also was known that exclusion diets, such as those of Dr. Albert Rowe, were effective in some food-allergic patients. Rinkel had several patients with multiple food allergies and almost constant symptoms, who had improved briefly on exclusion diets, and then had relapsed. He realized that the relapses were due to development of new food allergies in the patients to the foods they were allowed to eat on their elimination diets. He then tried a periodic exclusion diet by making sensitive foods appear in the diet less often in proportion to the severity of the reactions they produced. These patients improved, and stayed improved, on the new periodic diet. Encouraged by these results, Rinkel continued to modify the diet until he understood, by trial and clinical correlation, the essential features of successful periodic diets, which we now know as *diversified rotary diets* or *rotation diets*. His food allergy discoveries during the 1930s and 1940s, combined with those of his colleagues Michael Zeller and Theron Randolph, were ultimately published in book form as *Food Allergy* (12). Fifty years later, this is still a very useful reference text.

If prominent symptoms are produced on elimination and challenge, that food is then omitted from the diet for a prolonged period. How long to omit a food depends on loss of symptoms on rechallenge. In general, rechallenge is first attempted after 2 or 3 months. A reaction of decreased severity indicates a decrease in sensitized cells and antibody levels. If, after further time, rechallenge produces no symptoms, there has been further decline in sensitized cells and antibody levels below the threshold levels for mediator release to produce symptoms (tolerance). If, after 2 years of omission, challenge still produces symptoms, then that food is considered to be a fixed allergen and should be permanently avoided.

Once tolerance is reached, the food may be reintroduced into the diet as part of a rotation diet. Most foods can be rotated every 4 days, that is, eaten at one meal once every 4 days without causing resensitization. However, some sensitive people may require a longer rotation period. Almost all foods that are eaten more often than every 3 days *will* cause resensitization. It also has been observed that the same quantity of food, if eaten in several meals on the same day instead of at one meal only, is more likely to cause resensitization. Occasionally, one challenge is negative, but on reintroduction of the food and attempted rotation, symptoms occur. In this situation, continued omission usually allows tolerance to develop.

### Uses of the Rotary Diet in Cyclic Food Allergy

The rotary diet has three primary uses in managing cyclic food allergy. First, understanding cyclic food allergy enables accurate diagnosis by dietary manipulation. Oral challenge testing while the patient is masked, or after long periods of abstinence, usually does not identify cyclic food allergens. Knowledge of the stage of hyperacute sensitization permits appropriately timed food challenge tests to be done during the period of maximum sensitivity after food omission. The use of diagnostic oral challenge tests is very important because it convincingly shows the patient what his or her problem is, and helps the patient associate certain allergy symptoms with food reactions. Further, the oral challenge confirms the importance of any food that is thought to be allergenic based on skin tests, in vitro tests, or food diary analysis. Also, with a rotary diet, diagnosis is ongoing because the fact that foods are being rotated means that some previously unsuspected foods may become unmasked by short periods of omission, cause acute symptoms, and be recognized as problems. Thus, the rotary diet is continually diagnostic.

Second, understanding cyclic food allergy allows construction of an individualized therapeutic rotary diet for each patient. Initially, the diet is a combination of exclusion for both fixed and cyclic sensitizing foods, and rotation of all tolerated foods. As tolerance develops to cyclic sensitizing foods, these are included in the rotation plan until, finally, only fixed allergenic foods are omitted. The diet is never immutable because some foods may become resensitized from too-frequent use, and other problem foods may be identified after beginning the diet. These foods need omission until tolerance is reached, after which they can be added to the rotation diet. The therapeutic effect of the diet improves in proportion to the number of significant sensitizing foods that are identified and treated, so in properly instructed, intelligent, and compliant patients, results continue to improve with time. Eventually, knowledge of cyclic foods and the rotary diet gives a patient control over his or her symptoms and therapy.

Understanding cyclic food allergy also has a third benefit apart from diagnosis and therapy, that of prevention. Foods to which the patient is not already sensitized, if placed into a rotation diet, probably will not be eaten frequently enough to cause sensitization. This concept is particularly important to teach to patients because one of the most common mistakes made in dietary therapy of food allergies is simply to substitute one food for another. The classic example is the cow's-milk–allergic infant who is switched to soy formula, improves, and then a few weeks later is again covered with eczema and has serous otitis, only now from the new soy allergy. It therefore is important to rotate all foods, not just the ones to which tolerance has been achieved.

## Essential Features of the Maintenance Rotary Diet

1. Patients must permanently avoid all fixed food allergens.

2. The list of suspected cyclic allergy foods is drawn from IPDFT-positive foods, foods the patient craves, the diet diary (any foods eaten more often than every 3 days, especially foods eaten every day), and the top ten most commonly allergic foods in your area. Each region or ethnic group has a unique list of suspect foods.

3. Patients must avoid all challenge-positive foods for at least 2 or 3 months before rechallenge. If a food still causes symptoms, continue avoidance, and rechallenge every few months until either there is no reaction or 2 years pass. Before placing any food into the rotation, it must not produce any symptoms on rechallenge.

4. How often each reintroduced food can be safely eaten varies. A 4-day rotation works for many people, but more sensitive people may have to use a 5-day, or longer, rotation plan. Rarely, foods that sensitize easily may not be tolerated more often than once every few weeks. Foods eaten more often than every 3 days usually cause resensitization.

5. Patients must avoid all forms of sensitizing foods until testing proves certain forms to be tolerated. For some foods, components or derivatives of that food may not cause symptoms because the relevant antigen is not present. For example, a vegetable oil may be tolerated, whereas the vegetable will not. Similarly, the method of food preparation may determine sensitivity. For example, cooking a food may denature the relevant antigens and prevent sensitivity. Finally, the stage of maturation of the food may be important. For example, ripening of a fruit may convert a tolerated food to a sensitizing one. Occasionally, tolerance may depend on extremely fine distinctions. For example, in the processing of oils, the type of extraction, clarification, and storage technology used determine whether any protein, carbohydrate, or chemical antigens remain in the final product. This means that even the brand of food purchased may be of importance in determining if a food is tolerated.

6. Patients must avoid all amounts of sensitizing foods (no matter how small) until testing proves lack of sensitivity to small quantities. Some patients' immune systems are so exquisitely sensitive that cross-contamination by different foods cooked in the same container, or even from vapors given off from cooking, may be sufficient to produce symptoms.

7. All other (nonsuspect) foods should be rotated on a 4-day schedule. This is very important to prevent new food allergies from developing in sensitive persons, especially those with many other food allergies. Prophylactic rotation also is useful in managing the early feeding of infants who have allergic parents, in the very worthwhile effort to prevent these potentially allergic children from acquiring major food allergies. The common pediatric feeding practice of feeding one new food at a time for a few weeks "to see if it is tolerated well" is a poor way to feed an allergic child, and probably unnecessarily sensitizes many infants.

8. Patients should eat a normal serving of a food only once on a permitted day. Rinkel observed more frequent problems with resensitization when multiple feedings were allowed. He also observed that related foods from the same food family should not be eaten on the same day, and preferably should be separated by at least 2 days to avoid development of cross-sensitivity.

9. Stress the importance of not eating too many foods on any one day, so that something is left to eat on the next 3 days. The best way to do this is for the patient to avoid eating mixtures. As an example, it is better to drink pure grape juice, apple juice, orange juice, and pineapple juice on different days, than to drink a multijuice fruit punch, which eliminates all of its components from being consumed over the next 3 days. Reading labels is crucial to avoiding mixtures because so many products contain multiple ingredients. Emphasize that a dinner composed of a meat, a vegetable, and a fruit can be just as delicious and nourishing as a meal with 20 ingredients. Discuss breakfast and lunch as examples of problem meals where people tend to eat repetitiously and use mixtures, and how to solve this. For example, at breakfast, alternate between single-grain wheat, corn, and rice cereals, or eggs, or meat leftovers from dinner. The liquid put on cereals also should be alternated: pure fruit juices, milk, soy milk, and rice milk can be used, and hot cereals can be eaten with only added sweetener. Even sweeteners can be varied: pure maple syrup, cane sugar, beet sugar, corn syrup, honey, and the several kinds of artificial sweeteners. People need both an explanation of the dietary concepts and concrete examples of how to change their old habits in an acceptable way.

10. Patients should use the purest foods and water obtainable. Contamination with unknown additives may cause symptoms. People with chemical sensitivities must be particularly careful. Processed foods and "junk" foods should be avoided. Organically grown food is desirable, if it is affordable and available. Food storage also is important because food can absorb residues from waxes, plastic, treated paper, and lined metal containers—glass is safest. Fresh-frozen foods and local farm or fishery products are least likely to contain extra additives. Pure water should be either glass-bottled from a reliable company, or resin and charcoal filtered at home. Contacts with additives in cosmetics, toothpaste, vitamins, and drugs also must be minimized, and strong efforts put into smoking cessation.

11. Patients should keep a continuing diary of foods eaten and symptoms present. This is vital if additional food allergies are to be diagnosed and resensitizations detected. If symptoms increase, check for possible masking of previously tolerant foods. When a rotary diet has been faithfully followed for a long time, continuing the diary may not be necessary. However, whenever symptoms arise, starting the diary again helps sort out what is giving trouble.

12. Patients should keep written instructions for the diet, including information on food families, hidden sources of sensitive foods, and how to construct an allowed food chart for home use. There is simply too much information that must be imparted to patients to depend on verbal instructions alone. They need a list of foods to avoid, and if that is a large list, they also need a list of allowed foods. Psychologically, it is better to stress what *can* be eaten, rather than focusing on what cannot. A list of food families is essential to help with possible cross-reaction avoidance, as well as to reinforce that there are many permitted foods. Lists of hidden sources of food contacts are very helpful for sensitive patients and for those having difficulty reaching tolerance. Allergic patients have to become good label readers, and they need their allergist's expert help in interpreting food ingredients, components, derivatives, and additives. Finally, patients need some guidance in how to construct a simple chart for the kitchen to guide daily food choices. As the diet becomes strict or involves many omitted foods, deciding what to eat what can become a major emotional barrier to compliance. This is where one of the paperback allergy rotation diet books can be a help. Provide references or a food allergy lending library for patients' use.

13. Check diet for adequate nutrition. Supplements and nutritionist consultation may be required. Many nutritionists are not well versed in either food allergy or in rotation diets, so that you may have to educate them before they work with your patients. Calcium supplements are critical for patients on milk restriction. Vitamins A and D, extra calcium, and more protein may be needed for growing patients. Vitamin C supplements are needed if many fruits are restricted, and B complex supplements if grains or vegetables are restricted. In young children, combined egg and milk restriction may cause protein malnutrition. Essential fatty acids, iron, iodine, and other nutrients also may be depleted. There also may be local environmental factors (e.g., smog) that may indicate the need for higher doses of antioxidants. Some vitamin and mineral preparations contain significant amounts of hidden foods, especially corn and yeast.

14. Do not allow deviations from the prescribed diet unless the patient discusses them with you first. Until patients have become well educated in dietary management, they are not capable of analyzing their problems and formulating a corrective plan. If they are allowed to do so, successful therapy is unlikely, and you will have an unnecessary failure to contend with.

15. Review progress at regular intervals. Especially early in dietary management, regular feedback to analyze failures and to identify and pinpoint problems is important for getting the diet successfully established. Without

regular review, patients often suffer in silence, eventually become discouraged, and drop out of treatment. Nursing personnel can handle some of this follow-up, individually or in groups, but it is important for the physician to remain involved.

16. Stress the fact that success is up to the patient: it is his or her responsibility. Food allergy treatment results depend heavily on patient understanding and cooperation. Ensure that patients are given the necessary instructions and support, but be perfectly clear that if they want to get better, it is up to them. If they cooperate and learn the rotary diet, they gain control over their symptoms and are no longer helpless victims. They may then choose to cheat, but they also can recover.

17. Also stress that no one is perfect, that patients should be satisfied with their honest efforts and whatever symptom improvement they can achieve. Therapy must be realistic and consonant with a patient's abilities and lifestyle. In some cases, easy forms of the rotary diet may be needed, or dietary management may not even be feasible. Medications such as once-daily antihistamines, leukotriene inhibitors, and oral cromolyn may be used as adjuncts. Neutralization should be considered for foods that are hard to avoid. The physician must be flexible and work to devise the most helpful approach for the individual patient.

## Food Allergy Diagnosis by a Rotary Diet

In addition to beginning a maintenance rotary diet (see earlier), there are three other ways to start the diagnostic aspects of a rotary diet: by single-food eliminations, by use of a restricted, oligoallergenic diet, or by fasting. There are advantages and disadvantages to each.

*Single-food eliminations* are simple to do, but work best when there are only a few suspect foods (Tables 4.2, 4.3). One food at a time is totally eliminated for 4 days, then challenged. The major disadvantage of this approach is that eliminating all the common hidden sources of ubiquitous foods like milk, corn, wheat, or soy is very demanding be-

cause it requires knowledge of what ingredients are in foods, and also means that food labels must be read and understood. Also, it is necessary completely to avoid commercial processed foods and restaurant foods. Second, there is a risk that if multiple food reactions are causing the symptoms, challenge for only one food may not produce symptoms different from the background symptoms, so that the food will be falsely thought negative. However, for major allergenic foods like milk, wheat, corn, or eggs, single-food elimination often works very well. This is the strategy most often used in small children being evaluated for allergic serous otitis. After identifying the few problem foods, a treatment elimination and rotation diet is begun.

*Oligoallergenic diets* focus on permitted foods, rather than on eliminating foods, and so do not demand so much attention to detail (Table 4.4). The allowed foods are selected from those foods that are not common allergens in the patient's area, and may be customized by eliminating any foods that occur frequently in a given patient's normal diet. A well known example is the lamb and rice diet, which

### TABLE 4.2. COMMON ALLERGENIC FOODS FOR U.S. ADULTS

| | | |
|---|---|---|
| Alcoholic beverages | Coffee | Pineapple |
| Apple | Corn | Pork/ham |
| Banana | Egg | Potato |
| Beans | Fish | Rice |
| Beef | Lettuce | Soybean |
| Berries | Milk products | Sugar (cane) |
| Buckwheat | Mustard | Sugar (corn) |
| Chicken | Nuts | Tea |
| Chocolate | Oat | Tomato |
| Citrus fruit | Onion | Vinegar |
| Cola drinks | Peanut | Wheat |
| Coconut | Peas | Yeasts |

### TABLE 4.3. COMMON ALLERGENIC FOODS FOR U.S. CHILDREN

| | | |
|---|---|---|
| Apple | Egg | Rice |
| Banana | Milk | Soy |
| Barley | Oat | Sugar (cane) |
| Beef | Orange | Sugar (corn) |
| Carrot | Peach | Tomato |
| Chicken | Pear | Wheat |
| Chocolate | Pork/ham | Yeasts |
| Corn | | |

### TABLE 4.4. EXAMPLE OF AN OLIGOALLERGENIC DIET (ALLOWED FOODS)

Proteins: Duck, lamb, ostrich, venison

Grains: Bamboo, quinoa, rice

Fruits: Apricot, blueberry, cranberry, guava, kiwi

Nuts: Macadamia, pine

Vegetables: Artichoke, avocado, beet, okra, sweet potato, turnip, yam, yucca

Greens: Swiss chard, spinach, New Zealand spinach

Oils: Avocado oil, olive oil, safflower oil

Spices: Sea salt

Sweets: Honey, maple sugar, artificial sweeteners (if tolerated)

Desserts: Tapioca, frozen juice from above fruits

Beverages: Pure water, fresh juice from above fruits

works well in the United States, but would not be helpful in the Middle East. Uncommon foods that often can be used in the United States are lamb, duck, rice, yams, apricots, artichokes, avocados, beets, Swiss chard, okra, olives or olive oil, safflower oil, honey, and tapioca. One of the best ways to choose foods that will probably be safe (nonallergenic) is by asking patients to list foods that they will eat, but only rarely do eat (less often than weekly). A second advantage of an oligoallergenic diet is that it does eliminate most common allergens, so patients usually do get significant withdrawal symptoms, and then feel much better within 4 or 5 days. They can then begin a diagnostic one-food-per-meal rotation diet (see later). These dramatic changes, which also are seen during fasting, are very helpful in convincing patients to continue with the evaluation. Patients should be warned in advance that they might go through withdrawal, and that if they do, it is a good sign that they *can* be helped.

The most rigorous method, and the only one suitable for those with severe symptoms, such as continuous urticaria or severe asthma, is *supervised fasting*. This can be done safely with most healthy patients on an outpatient basis. Use of commercial elemental diets usually is not tolerated as well as fasting because of poor taste and high expense. Patients must be very cooperative (or very tired of being ill) to fast. A complete physical and laboratory examination is recommended before fasting. Patients with significant other medical problems should have internal medicine consultation before fasting. Only pure water is allowed until symptoms subside (usually approximately 5 days), and mild laxatives, in the form of milk of magnesia, vitamin C, magnesium citrate, or sodium bicarbonate are used to clear food residues from the gut. In some chronic allergic conditions, such as eczema, chronic inflammation that requires

healing does not heal in 5 days, but the acute symptoms, like erythema and itching, should show improvement with elimination of the responsible antigens. As soon as major symptom improvement occurs, move directly to the one-food-per-meal diagnostic rotation diet so that the problem foods can be identified. If symptoms do not subside after 4 or 5 days of fasting, either the diagnosis of food allergy is wrong and there is another cause for the symptoms, or there are uncontrolled problems with the environment or with inhalant, fungal, or chemical allergies.

## The One-Food-per-Meal Rotation Diet

This strict diet is used for diagnosis of patients with serious symptoms, or when a simple maintenance rotation diet has failed to produce sufficient improvement (Table 4.5). Before starting, lists of suspect, safe, and uncertain foods are prepared with the patient. All foods that are skin test positive, suspect from the diet diary, eaten daily, or low-level IgE in vitro test positive (but do *not* cause anaphylactic symptoms when eaten) are put on the suspect list. All foods that are acceptable, but are eaten less than weekly, are put on the safe list. Uncertain foods are those eaten less often than daily, but more often than weekly.

After either an oligoallergenic diet or fasting, once symptoms improve, each food that is suspected of possible cyclic food allergy is challenged, one at a time, by being eaten as the only food at one meal in a day. The other meals that day are made up of foods that are believed to be safe. In the case of the oligoallergenic diet, the safe list is composed of all foods on the allowed list for that particular diet, in addition to foods eaten less often than weekly. A very strict 4-day rotation diet, made up from the safe list of foods, is

## TABLE 4.5. EXAMPLE OF A SINGLE-FOOD-PER-MEAL, 4-DAY ROTARY DIVERSIFIED DIET

| Day | Morning | Noon | Afternoon | Evening |
|-----|---------|------|-----------|---------|
| 1 | Apple | Walnut | Asparagus | Salmon |
| 2 | Pumpkin/pepitas | Avocado | Sweet potato | Pork/ham |
| 3 | Apricot | Cashew | Broccoli | Scallops |
| 4 | Chicken egg | Artichoke | Banana | Rabbit |
| 5 | Blueberry | Almond | Carrot | Red snapper |
| 6 | Cantaloupe | Tuna fish | Zucchini squash | Shrimp |
| 7 | Pineapple | Macadamia | Yam | Turkey |
| 8 | Sunflower seed | Tangerine | White potato | Deer (venison) |
| 9 | Papaya | Navy bean | Brussels sprout | Halibut |
| 10 | Kiwi fruit | Olive | Beet | Lamb |

Stone Age–type diet, single food, four feedings per day, with only one member of a food family every 4 days, and no grains, refined or processed foods, or milk products.
Many alternatives are available. Over 40 edible fish families provide excellent choices for obtaining protein variety. Also, alligator, buffalo, duck, elk, frog's leg, llama, moose, ostrich, rabbit, and rattlesnake may be available. Seasonal fruits such as breadfruit, mango, passion fruit, star fruit, and cherimoya (custard apple), as well as persimmon, pomegranate, quince, and gooseberry can be used. Alternate starches are amaranth (quinoa), yucca root, and taro. Less common vegetables are collard greens, dandelion greens, purselane, spinach, Swiss chard, turnips, and New Zealand spinach.

then begun. Usually, four feedings a day are given, each consisting of a serving of a single pure food that is large enough to prevent hunger. Each food is prepared simply, without sauces, fats, or spices, using ceramic, glass, or stainless steel cookware. Any positive food challenge is followed immediately with a mild laxative, and only known safe foods are given until symptoms clear and testing new foods can resume. Symptoms from a positive oral challenge usually occur from minutes to a few hours after eating, and are replicable. If a challenge is positive, that food is eliminated from the diet. If the challenge is negative, however, that food is added to the list of safe foods and may be included in the rotation diet. The most suspect foods are tested one per day in succession, until all suspect foods have been tested. If many foods must be tested, it is important to remember that omission for too long can produce a false-negative challenge. To counter this, after 10 days on the diet, any additional foods to be tested should be reintroduced and eaten daily for several days, and then omitted again for 4 days before testing. After all suspect foods have been tested, uncertain foods may be tested, or they may be included in a rotation diet without testing. Once all foods have been tested, revised lists of safe and allergic foods are prepared, and the diet is broadened into a general maintenance rotary diet, avoiding the allergic foods until tolerance is attained.

The many variations of rotary diets used today all share essential features that were worked out from clinical experimentation by Rinkel and other pioneering allergists. Only now, with modern immunologic techniques, are we beginning actually to understand the molecular mechanisms involved. Lack of this mechanistic knowledge, combined with failure to understand the complex clinical behavior of cyclic food allergies, has resulted in many allergists refusing to acknowledge that any diet other than one of strict exclusion could possibly have any benefits. The same reasons have led these same allergists even to deny the existence of food allergies, excepting only obvious, immediate IgE-mediated reactions (115).

## COMBINING DIETS AND NEUTRALIZATION

Once the diagnosis of food allergy is made, the best treatment always is elimination of the food from the diet. For immediate anaphylactic, fixed food allergy, the food must be eliminated indefinitely. For delayed cyclic IgG food allergy, the food should be eliminated for several months, with attempted reintroduction of the food after that time as part of a rotary, diversified diet. Only in those patients who have cyclic food allergies to ubiquitous foods, such as corn, soy, and wheat, and cannot eliminate those foods from the diet, is treatment with neutralization immunotherapy instituted. Other common foods may be difficult to rotate in the diet or to eliminate for a period of months, particu-

larly for a person who travels frequently and depends on restaurants. In these cases, neutralization may be used in conjunction with the best possible diet.

## Mixing Food Neutralization Treatment Vials

Food antigen multiple-dose vials are mixed much like vials for inhalant treatment. If there are four or fewer foods requiring treatment, a 20-dose injection treatment vial may be made from the endpoint dilutions by placing 1 mL (20 × 0.05 mL) of each food endpoint dilution into the vial. The vial is completed by adding enough glycerin and phenolated saline to achieve 5.00 mL total volume, containing a final concentration of approximately 10% glycerin as preservative. Vials mixed primarily from concentrates or #1 dilutions do not need any added glycerin. When 20-dose vials are mixed with more than 4 antigens, 0.20 mL of the next stronger dilution (stronger than the endpoint) of each food is added (Table 4.6).

## Neutralization Dosing Schedules

The method that is preferred by Trevino is that of giving a neutralizing dose (0.05 mL of the endpoint dilution) by injection, every day for 2 weeks, then twice a week for 2 months, then once a week for 6 to 7 months. King prefers injections twice weekly for 1 month, then weekly for 1 month, and then every other week (116). Gordon prefers twice weekly injections for as long as required. These three regimens all clinically appear to attenuate reactions to the treated foods. Note that treatment doses are not escalated, as in inhalant treatment, but are kept always at the same neutralizing dose. Patients who initially benefit from food neutralization, but then relapse, should be retested to detect possible endpoint shifts. Patients who tolerate food injections well in the office, meet safety criteria (117), and can be successfully instructed in self-injection, are allowed to go on home injections. At the end of 6 to 12 months, specific IgG is expected to be at a low level, and symptoms should be well controlled, if low-dose tolerance has been achieved. Also, as patients learn better dietary habits, clean up their environment, and escalate to effective inhalant therapy, they are less bothered by food-induced symptoms. For these two reasons, most patients eventually are able to stop food injections.

## Sublingual Neutralization

At the same time food injection therapy is begun, patients may be given a dropper vial containing the same food antigens, mixed in 50% glycerin, at neutralizing dose strength (Table 4.7). The high glycerin concentration masks the peppery phenol taste and makes the drops palatable. Before

## TABLE 4.6. EXAMPLE OF A MULTIANTIGEN, 20-DOSE, FOOD NEUTRALIZATION TREATMENT VIAL

| Food | Neutralizing Dose (mL) | 20-Dose Volume (mL) | Next Stronger Dilution (mL) |
|------|------------------------|---------------------|------------------------------|
| Apple | 0.05 #1 | 1.00 #1 | 0.20 Concentrate |
| Beef | 0.05 #2 | 1.00 #2 | 0.20 #1 |
| Chicken | 0.05 #4 | 1.00 #4 | 0.20 #3 |
| Corn | 0.05 #7 | 1.00 #7 | 0.20 #6 |
| Egg | 0.05 #5 | 1.00 #5 | 0.20 #4 |
| Milk | 0.10 #3[a] | 2.00 #3 | 0.40 #2 |
| Soy | 0.05 #6 | 1.00 #6 | 0.20 #5 |
| Sugarcane | 0.15 #2[a] | 3.00 #2 | 0.60 #1 |
| Tomato | 0.05 #1 | 1.00 #1 | 0.20 Concentrate |
| Wheat | 0.05 #6 | 1.00 #6 | 0.20 #5 |
| Baker's yeast | 0.05 #4 | 1.00 #4 | 0.20 #3 |
| **Antigen volume** | | **14.00** | **2.80** |
| 50% Glycerin | | | 1.00 |
| Phenol saline | | | 1.20 |
| **20-Dose vial** | | | **5.00** |

[a] These endpoints were "multiples" (see text).

## TABLE 4.7. EXAMPLE OF A MULTIANTIGEN, 100-DOSE, SUBLINGUAL TREATMENT BOTTLE

| Food | Neutralizing Dose (mL) | 100-Dose Volume (mL) | Two Dilutions Stronger (mL) |
|------|------------------------|----------------------|------------------------------|
| Apple | 0.05 #1 | 5.00 #1 | 1.00 Concentrate |
| Beef | 0.05 #2 | 5.00 #2 | 0.20 Concentrate |
| Chicken | 0.05 #4 | 5.00 #4 | 0.20 #2 |
| Corn | 0.05 #7 | 5.00 #7 | 0.20 #5 |
| Egg | 0.05 #5 | 5.00 #5 | 0.20 #3 |
| Milk | 0.10 #3[a] | 10.00 #3 | 0.40 #1 |
| Soy | 0.05 #6 | 5.00 #6 | 0.20 #4 |
| Sugarcane | 0.15 #2[a] | 15.00 #2 | 0.60 Concentrate |
| Tomato | 0.05 #1 | 5.00 #1 | 1.00 Concentrate |
| Wheat | 0.05 #6 | 5.00 #6 | 0.20 #4 |
| Baker's yeast | 0.05 #4 | 5.00 #4 | 0.20 #2 |
| **Antigen volume** | | **70.00** | **4.40** |
| 50% Glycerin[b] | | | 1.60 |
| Phenol saline | | | 0 |
| **100 dose bottle**[c] | | | **6.00** |

[a] These endpoints were "multiples" (see text).
[b] Add up to 4.00 mL per 6.00 mL total volume.
[c] Determine number of drops to equal 0.06 mL, the neutralizing dose.

meals, patients can take the neutralizing dose in drop form, sublingually, to produce prostaglandins that prevent symptoms until the injection therapy becomes fully effective. The specific dropper bottle used determines the number of drops given because drop volume varies, and must be determined for each new lot of bottles. Clinicians use many different combinations and treatment schedules of neutralization injection and sublingual therapy, but no comparative efficacy studies have been performed. Normally in young children, and as an option in adults, the entire neutralization treatment program may be given sublingually. Neutralization appears to be more effective when combined with a rotation diet, so the best dietary management possible should be the goal, even when using neutralization therapy.

## CONCLUSION

True food allergies are those reactions that occur because of the activity of the immune system when exposed to sensitizing foods. Clinically, true food allergies occur in two very different types: immediate, fixed reactions, and delayed, cyclic reactions. Fixed food allergies develop rapidly after food exposure, and therefore usually are easy to diagnose. Conversely, cyclic food allergies often develop slowly and vary with both the quantity and frequency with which allergenic foods are eaten. They therefore may be difficult to diagnose. Despite this difficulty, it is important to learn about cyclic food allergies because they represent most of the clinically observed food allergies, and are a very important cause of treatable chronic allergy symptoms. Understanding the clinical behavior of cyclic food allergies allows the physician and patient to cooperate for both diagnosis and successful intervention. Learning the necessary skills to evaluate and treat food-allergic patients takes time and requires thoughtful study, but the benefits to allergic patients are great with the successful treatment of previously intractable chronic allergies.

## ACKNOWLEDGMENTS

The authors thank June L. Bianchi, Sally C. Schumann, and Jeanie M. Vander Pyl, Cape Cod Hospital Medical Library, for their expertise in medical literature research.

## REFERENCES

1. Chobot R. *Pediatric allergy.* New York: McGraw-Hill, 1951.
2. Von Pirquet C. Allergie. *Munch Med Wochenschr* 1906;53:1457.
3. Smith HC. Buckwheat poisoning. *Arch Intern Med* 1909;3:350.
4. Schloss OM. Case of allergy to common foods. *Am J Dis Child* 1912;3:241.
5. Coke F. Sensitization to wheat. *Practitioner* 1932;129:408.
6. Rinkel HJ. Food allergy. *J Kans Med Soc* 1936;37:177–184.
7. Rowe AH. *Clinical allergy due to foods, inhalants, contactants, fungi, bacteria, and other causes: manifestations, diagnosis, and treatment.* Philadelphia: Lea & Febiger, 1937.
8. Coca AF. *Familial nonreaginic food-allergy.* Springfield, IL: Charles C Thomas, 1943.
9. Rinkel HJ. Food allergy II: the technique and clinical application of individual food tests. *Ann Allergy* 1944;2:504–514.
10. Rinkel HJ. The role of food allergy in internal medicine. *Ann Allergy* 1944;2:115–124.
11. Rinkel HJ. Food allergy IV: the function and clinical application of the rotating diversified diet. *J Pediatr* 1948;82:266–274.
12. Rinkel HJ, Randolph TG, Zeller M. *Food allergy.* Springfield, IL: Charles C Thomas, 1951.
13. Rinkel HJ. The management of clinical allergy, part IV: food and mold allergy. *Arch Otolaryngol* 1963;77:302–326.
14. Rinkel HJ, Lee CH, Brown DW Jr, et al. The diagnosis of food allergy. *Arch Otolaryngol* 1964;79:71–79.
15. Lee CH. A new test for detection of food allergies, pollen and mold incompatibilities. *Buchanan Co Med Bull* 1961;25:9.
16. Miller JB. *Food allergy: provocative testing and injection therapy.* Springfield, IL: Charles C Thomas, 1972.
17. Randolph TG. Biographical sketch of Herbert J. Rinkel, MD, emphasizing his medical contributions. In: Johnson F, ed. *Allergy: including IgE in diagnosis and treatment.* Chicago: Yearbook Medical, 1979:1–9.
18. Medzhitov R, Janeway C Jr. Innate immunity. *N Engl J Med* 2000;343:338–344.
19. Majamaa H, Isolauri E. Evaluation of the gut mucosal barrier: evidence for increased antigen transfer in children with atopic eczema. *J Allergy Clin Immunol* 1996;97:985–990.
20. Knutson TW, Bengtsson U, Dannaeus A, et al. Effects of luminal antigen on intestinal albumin and hyaluronan permeability and ion transport in atopic patients. *J Allergy Clin Immunol* 1996;97:1225–1232.
21. Benard A, Desreumeaux P, Huglo D, et al. Increased intestinal permeability in bronchial asthma. *J Allergy Clin Immunol* 1996;97:1173–1178.
22. Gell PG, Coombs RR, Lachman PJ. *Classification of allergic reactions responsible for clinical hypersensitivity and disease: clinical aspects of immunology.* Oxford: Blackwell, 1975.
23. Brostoff J. Mechanisms: an introduction. In: Brostoff J, Challacombe SJ, eds. *Food allergy and intolerance.* London: Bailliere Tindall, 1987:433–455.
24. Strong FM, Atkin L, Coon JM, et al. *Toxicants occurring naturally in foods.* Washington, DC: National Academy of Sciences, 1973.
25. Soothill JF, Stokes CR, Turner MW, et al. Predisposing factors and the development of reaginic allergy in infancy. *Clin Allergy* 1976;6:305–319.
26. Majamaa H, Laine S, Mietinen A. Eosinophilic protein X and eosinophil cationic protein as indicators of intestinal inflammation in infants with atopic eczema and food allergy. *Clin Exp Allergy* 1999;29:1502–1506.
27. Eigenmann PA, Sicherer SH, Borkowski TA, et al. Prevalence of IgE-mediated food allergy among children with atopic dermatitis. *Pediatrics* 1998;101:E8.
28. Blaylock WK. Atopic dermatitis: diagnosis and pathobiology. *J Allergy Clin Immunol* 1976;57:62–79.
29. Burks AW, Mallory SB, Williams LW, et al. Atopic dermatitis: clinical relevance of food hypersensitivity reactions. *J Pediatr* 1988;113:447–451.
30. Chan-Yeung M, Malo JL. Occupational asthma. *N Engl J Med* 1995;333:107–112.
31. Onorato J, Merland N, Terral C, et al. Placebo-controlled double-blind food challenge in asthma. *J Allergy Clin Immunol* 1986;78:1139–1146.

32. Winton GB, Lewis CW. Contact urticaria. *Int J Dermatol* 1982; 21:573–578.

33. Fisher AA. Contact urticaria from handling meats and fowl. *Cutis* 1982;30:726–729.

34. Enberg RN. Food-induced oropharyngeal symptoms: the oral allergy syndrome. *Immunol Allergy Clin North Am* 1991;11: 767–772.

35. Ortolani C, Ispano M, Pastorello EA, et al. The oral allergy syndrome. *Ann Allergy* 1988;61:47–52.

36. Amlot PL, Kemeny DM, Zachary C, et al. Oral allergy syndrome (OAS): symptoms of IgE-mediated hypersensitivity to foods. *Clin Allergy* 1987;17:33–42.

37. Bircher AJ, Van Melle G, Haller E, et al. IgE to food allergens are highly prevalent in patients allergic to pollens, with and without symptoms of food allergy. *Clin Exp Allergy* 1994;24: 367–374.

38. Yocum MW, Khan DA. Assessment of patients who have experienced anaphylaxis: a 3-year survey. *Mayo Clin Proc* 1994;69: 16–23.

39. Trevino RJ. Immunologic mechanisms in the production of food sensitivities. *Laryngoscope* 1981;91:1913–1936.

40. Monro J. Food induced migraine. In: Brostoff J, Challacombe SJ, eds. *Food allergy and intolerance.* London: Bailliere Tindall, 1987:633–665.

41. Uhlig T, Merkenschlager A, Brandmaier R, et al. Topographic mapping of brain electrical activity in children with food-induced attention deficit hyperkinetic disorder. *Eur J Pediatr* 1997;156:557–561.

42. Pearson DJ, Rix KJB. Psychological effects of food allergy. In: Brostoff J, Challacombe SJ, eds. *Food allergy and intolerance.* London: Bailliere Tindall, 1987:688–708.

43. Bell IR. Effects of food on the central nervous system. In: Brostoff J, Challacombe SJ, eds. *Food allergy and intolerance.* London: Bailliere Tindall, 1987:709–721.

44. Viscomi GJ. The relationship between allergy and otitis media. In: King HC, ed. *Otolaryngic allergy.* New York: Elsevier North-Holland, 1981:409–424.

45. Draper WL. Secretory otitis media in children: a study of 540 children. *Laryngoscope* 1967;77:636–653.

46. Derebery MJ, Valenzuela S. Meniere's syndrome and allergy. *Otolaryngol Clin North Am* 1992;25:213–224.

47. Derebery MJ, Rao VS, Siglock TJ, et al. Meniere's disease: an immune-complex mediated illness? *Laryngoscope* 1991;101: 225–229.

48. Derebery MJ. Allergic and immunologic aspects of Meniere's disease. *Otolaryngol Head Neck Surg* 1996;114:360–365.

49. Knops JL, McCaffrey TV, Kern EB. Inflammatory diseases of the sinuses: physiology, clinical applications. *Otolaryngol Clin North Am* 1993;26:517–534.

50. Dixon HS. Allergy and laryngeal disease. *Otolaryngol Clin North Am* 1992;25:239–250.

51. Wraith DG. Asthma. In: Brostoff J, Challacombe SJ, eds. *Food allergy and intolerance.* London: Bailliere Tindall, 1987: 486–497.

52. Rae WJ, Brown OD. Cardiovascular disease in response to chemicals and foods. In: Brostoff J, Challacombe SJ, eds. *Food allergy and intolerance.* London: Bailliere Tindall, 1987: 737–753.

53. Panush RS, Stroud RM, Webster EM. Food-induced (allergic) arthritis: inflammatory arthritis exacerbated by milk. *Arthritis Rheum* 1986;29:220–226.

54. Strobel S. Mechanisms of tolerance and sensitization in the intestine and other organs of the body. *Allergy* 1995;50[Suppl 20]:18–25.

55. Nalebuff DJ. In vitro testing methodologies: evolution and current status. *Otolaryngol Clin North Am* 1992;25:27–42.

56. Emanuel IA. In vitro testing for allergy diagnosis: comparison of methods in common use. *Otolaryngol Clin North Am* 1998; 31:27–34.

57. Harvima RJ, Harvima IT, Tuomisto L, et al. Comparison of histamine assay methods in measuring in vitro-induced histamine release in patients with allergic rhinitis. *Allergy* 1989;44: 235–239.

58. van Toorenenbergen AW, Vermeulen AM. Histamine release from human peripheral blood leukocytes analyzed by histamine radioimmunoassay. *Agents Actions* 1990;30:278–280.

59. Clinton PM, Murdoch RD, Kemeny DM. Development of a microassay for histamine release. *Clin Allergy* 1987;17:181–189.

60. Nolte H, Schiotz O, Skov PS. A new glass microfibre-based histamine analysis for allergy testing in children: results compared with conventional leukocyte histamine release assay, skin prick test, bronchial provocation test, and RAST. *Allergy* 1987; 42:366–373.

61. Du Buske LM. Introduction: basophil histamine release and the diagnosis of food allergy. *Allergy Proc* 1993;14:243–249.

62. Kordash TR, Freshwater LL, Amend MJ. Standardization of allergenic extracts by basophil histamine release. *Ann Allergy Asthma Immunol* 1995;75:101–106.

63. Lewis T, Grant RT. Vascular reactions of the skin to injury. *Heart* 1926;13:219–225.

64. Pepys J. Skin tests for immediate, type I, allergic reactions. *Proc R Soc Med* 1972;65:271–272.

65. Bosquet J, Michel FB. In vivo methods for study of allergy: skin tests, techniques, and interpretation. In: Middleton E, Reed CE, Ellis EF, et al., eds. *Allergy principles and practice,* 4th ed. St. Louis: Mosby, 1993:573–594.

66. Mangi RJ. Allergy skin tests: an overview. *Otolaryngol Clin North Am* 1985;18:719–723.

67. Brown HM, Su S, Thantrey N. Prick testing for allergens standardized by using a precision needle. *Clin Allergy* 1981;11: 95–98.

68. Demoly P, Bosquet J, Manderscheid JC, et al. precision of skin prick and puncture tests with nine methods. *J Allergy Clin Immunol* 1991;88:758–762.

69. Malling HJ, Andersen CE, Boas MB, et al. The allergy pricker. *Allergy* 1982;37:563–567.

70. Osterballe O, Weeke B. A new lancet for skin prick testing. *Allergy* 1979;34:209–212.

71. Adinoff AD, Rosloniec DM, McCall LL, et al. A comparison of six epicutaneous devices in the performance of immediate hypersensitivity skin testing. *J Allergy Clin Immunol* 1989;84: 168–174.

72. Nielsen NH, Dirksen A, Mosbech H, et al. Skin prick testing with standardized extracts from 3 different manufacturers. *Allergol Immunopathol* 1992;20:246–248.

73. Norman PS. In vivo methods of study of allergy. In: Middleton E Jr, ed. *Allergy principles and practice.* St. Louis: Mosby, 1983: 295–302.

74. Kniker WT. Multi-test skin testing in allergy: a review of published findings. *Ann Allergy* 1993;71:485–491.

75. Kniker WT, Hales SW, Lee LK. Diagnostic methods to demonstrate IgE antibodies: skin testing techniques. *Bull NY Acad Med* 1981;57:524–548.

76. Menardo JL, Bousquet J, Michel FB. Comparison of three prick test methods with the intradermal test and with the RAST in the diagnosis of mite allergy. *Ann Allergy* 1982;48:235–239.

77. Nelson HS. Variables in allergy skin testing. *Allergy Proc* 1994; 15:265–268.

78. Nelson HS, Knoetzer J, Bucher B. Effect of distance between sites and region of the body on results of skin prick tests. *J Allergy Clin Immunol* 1996;97:596–601.

79. Berkowitz RB, Tinkelman DG, Lutz C, et al. Evaluation of the

multi-test device for immediate hypersensitivity skin testing. *J Allergy Clin Immunol* 1992;90:979–985.

80. Dirksen A, Misbech H, Soborg M, et al. Comparison of a new lancet and a hypodermic needle for skin prick testing. *Allergy* 1983;38:359–362.

81. Nelson HS, Rosloniec DM, McCall LI, et al. comparative performance of five commercial prick skin test devices. *J Allergy Clin Immunol* 1993;92:750–756.

82. Remy W, Siebenwirth J, Rakoski J. Skin test of inhalant allergens by topical iontophoretic delivery in comparison to common skin prick tests. *Dermatology* 1995;190:87.

83. Bruijnzeel PLB, Kuijper PHM, Kapp A, et al. the involvement of eosinophils in the patch test reaction to aeroallergens in atopic dermatitis: its relevance for the pathogenesis of atopic dermatitis. *Clin Exp Allergy* 1993;23:97–109.

84. Isolauri E, Turjanmaa K. Combined skin prick and patch testing enhances identification of food allergy in infants with atopic dermatitis. *J Allergy Clin Immunol* 1996;97:9–15.

85. Lahti A, Maibach HI. Immediate contact reactions. In: Middleton E, Reed CE, Ellis EF, et al., eds. *Allergy principles and practice,* 4th ed. St. Louis: Mosby, 1993:1641–1647.

86. Oranje AP, Van Gysel D, Mulder PGH, et al. Food-induced contact urticaria syndrome in atopic dermatitis: reproducibility of repeated and duplicate testing with a skin provocation test, the skin application food test (SAFT). *Contact Dermatitis* 1994; 31:314–318.

87. King HC, King WP. Alternatives in the diagnosis and treatment of food allergies. *Otolaryngol Clin North Am* 1998;31:141–156.

88. Oranje AP. Skin provocation test (SAFT) based on contact urticaria: a marker of dermal food allergy. *Curr Probl Dermatol* 1991;20:228–231.

89. Maibach HI, Dannaker CJ, Lahti A. Allergic contact dermatitis. In: Middleton E, Reed CE, Ellis EF, et al., eds. *Allergy principles and practice,* 4th ed. St. Louis: Mosby, 1993:1605–1640.

90. Nethercott J. The positive predictive accuracy of patch tests. *Immunol Allergy Clin North Am* 1989;9:549–553.

91. Gawkrodger DJ, McDonagh JG, Wright AL. Quantification of allergic and irritant patch test reactions using laser-Doppler flowmetry and erythema index. *Contact Dermatitis* 1991;24: 172–177.

92. Gaddoni G, Baldassari L, Zucchini A. A new patch test preparation of dust mites for atopic dermatitis. *Contact Dermatitis* 1994; 31:132–133.

93. Langeland T, Braathen LB, Borch M. Studies of atopic patch tests. *Acta Derm Venerol Suppl (Stockh)* 1989;144:105–109.

94. Trevino RJ. Food allergies and hypersensitivities. In: Donald PJ, Gluckman JL, Rice DH, eds. *The sinuses.* New York: Raven Press, 1995:126.

95. Bock SA, Sampson HA, Atkins FJ, et al. Double-blind, placebo-controlled food challenge (DBPCFC) as an office procedure: a manual. *J Allergy Clin Immunol* 1988;82:986–997.

96. Lee CH, Shepherd EM, Scala LS. Foods. In: Lee CH, Shepherd EM, Scala LS, eds. *Allergy neutralization: the Lee method.* St. Joseph, MO: Tri Sigma Press, 1987:67–88.

97. King HC. Double-blind controlled studies of food allergy published in the literature: an otolaryngologist's guide to allergy. In: *An otolaryngologist's guide to allergy.* New York: Thieme Medical, 1990:239.

98. King WP, Rubin WA, Fadal RG, et al. Provocation-neutraliza-tion: a two-part study. Part I: the intracutaneous provocative food test: a multi-center comparison study. *Otolaryngol Head Neck Surg* 1988;99:263–271.

99. King WP, Fadal RG, Ward WA, et al. Provocation-neutralization: a two-part study. Part II: subcutaneous neutralization therapy: a multi-center study. *Otolaryngol Head Neck Surg* 1988; 99:272–277.

100. Breneman JC, Sweeney M, Robert A. Patch tests demonstrating immune (antibody and cell-mediated) reactions to foods. *Ann Allergy* 1989;62:461–469.

101. Kuwabara N, et al. Evaluation of patch test with dimethylsulfoxide in association with lymphocyte proliferation in food sensitive atopic dermatitis. *Pediatr Asthma Allergy Immunol* 1993;7: 173–178.

102. King WP, Motes JM. The intracutaneous progressive dilution multi-food test. *Otolaryngol Head Neck Surg* 1991;104: 235–238.

103. King WP, Rubin WA, Fadal RG, et al. Efficacy of alternative tests for delayed-cyclic food hypersensitivity. *Otolaryngol Head Neck Surg* 1989;101:385–391.

104. King HC. *Food allergy diagnosis: an otolaryngologist's guide to allergy.* New York: Thieme Medical, 1990:104–119.

105. Black AB. A new diagnostic method in allergic disease. *Pediatrics* 1956;7:716–724.

106. el Rafei A, Peters SM, Harris N, et al. Diagnostic value of IgG4 measurements in patients with food allergy. *Ann Allergy* 1989; 62:94–99.

107. Fell PJ, Soulsby S, Brostoff J. Cellular responses to food in irritable bowel syndrome: an investigation of the ALCAT test. *J Nutr Med* 1991;2:143–149.

108. Donovan PM. The ELISA/ACT test—parts I and II: its role in identifying time-delayed reactive environmental toxicants. In: Collin J, ed. *Townsend letter for doctors and patients.* Port Townsend, WA: 1991:8–11.

109. Jerne NK. Towards a network theory of the immune system. *Ann Immunol* 1974;125C:373–389.

110. Robert A, Nezamis JE, Lancaster C, et al. Cytoprotection by prostaglandins in rats: prevention of gastric necrosis produced by alcohol, HCL, NaOH, hypertonic NaCl and thermal injury. *Gastroenterology* 1979;77:433–443.

111. Boris M, Schiff M, Weindorf S. Injection of low dose antigen attenuates the response to subsequent bronchoprovocative challenge. *Otolaryngol Head Neck Surg* 1988;98:539–545.

112. Sobotka AK, Dembo M, Goldstein B, et al. Antigen specific desensitization of human basophils. *Ann Immunol* 1979;122: 511–517.

113. Mendoza GR, Minagawa K. Subthreshold and suboptimal desensitization of human basophils. *Int Arch Allergy Immunol* 1982;65:101–107.

114. Scadding GK, Brostoff J. Low dose sublingual therapy in patients with allergic rhinitis due to house dust mite. *Clin Allergy* 1986;16:483–491.

115. King WP, King HC. The evolution of otolaryngic allergy practices. *Ear Nose Throat J* 1990;69:11–26.

116. King WP. Food hypersensitivity in otolaryngology: manifestations, diagnosis, and treatment. *Otolaryngol Clin North Am* 1992;25:163–179.

117. Hurst DS, Gordon BR, Fornadley JA, et al. Safety of home based and office allergy immunotherapy: a multicenter prospective study. *Otolaryngol Head Neck Surg* 1999;121:553–561.

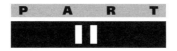

# DIAGNOSIS OF ALLERGIC DISEASE

# PATIENT HISTORY

## EDWYN L. BOYD

The history is the most useful and economic diagnostic tool available to physicians engaged in the diagnosis and management of allergic patients. Contrary to popular lay belief, the diagnosis of allergic disease is not made on the basis of skin testing or blood testing results. The diagnosis is made on the basis of the patient's chief complaint (CC), history of present illness (HPI), past, family, and social history (PFSH), review of systems (ROS), and physical examination (PE). The purpose of the history is to establish that the patient is indeed manifesting symptoms related to allergic disease, and to try to incriminate what specific allergens are contributing to the patient's symptom complex. The initial history should never be considered complete or totally accurate, and should be reviewed frequently because the patient often remembers pertinent information after the initial visit is over. The interview may stimulate the patient to ask other family members for answers to questions for which no answer was known at the time. Allergy testing should be reserved for those patients in whom medical therapy and environmental control have failed. Under these circumstances, testing is performed to determine, based on the history, what specific allergens may be contributing to the patient's symptoms and, more important, to determine at what dosage treatment with allergenic extract injection immunotherapy may safely begin.

It is very unfortunate in today's high-technology medical arena that the art of obtaining a thorough and detailed medical history has for the most part been lost. It is much easier and time efficient to ask patients to fill out a questionnaire and draw some laboratory tests than it is to sit down and spend time with patients face to face to obtain their history in their own words. Allergy questionnaires serve a very useful purpose but cannot take the place of time spent with the patient. Before the development of the sophisticated tests that now are at our disposal, our medical forefathers had nothing to rely on other than their ability to question, examine, and observe. Their decisions and medical recommendations were made on the basis of acquired clinical acumen and observations of fact. As science grew, their observations were either validated or disproved.

## THE CHIEF COMPLAINT

The CC should be a concise description of the patient's symptoms, problem, or condition that motivated them to make an appointment to see the physician. When the CC is being documented, this author asks the patient to report the problem in his or her own words without using the word "sinus." Patients should not use technical or diagnostic terms when reporting their complaint, but rather should report specific symptoms that generated the appointment. Reported symptoms may be subjective, objective, or both. Examples of subjective symptoms would be headache, ringing in the ears, or itching. Examples of objective symptoms include hives, watery eyes, or swelling. Objective and subjective symptoms would be itching and hives.

## HISTORY OF PRESENT ILLNESS

The HPI is then developed from the CC. The HPI should detail a chronologic description of the patient's present illness from the very first sign or symptom to the present. This description should involve the present illness only, and not any other peripheral medical history that is more appropriately included in another element of the history, such as the ROS.

Documentation of the history is not just limited to what the problem is and when it started but must also include location, quality, severity, duration, timing, context, factors that modify the problem, and associated signs and symptoms. Location of the problem is self-explanatory; that is, where is the pain or problem? Quality, as it applies to the HPI, refers, for example, to the color of the expectorant or nasal discharge, if present. Duration of the problem initially seems obvious, but the examiner must go back in the patient's history to when the problem first began. In the case of allergic disease, the patient might reply "for as long as I

E. L. Boyd: Hoover Ear, Nose, and Throat Associates, Hoover, Alabama.

can remember." The severity of the problem is recorded in terms of mild, moderate, or severe to document how it affects the patient's occupational, familial, and social interactions. Timing of the problem is exceptionally important for incriminating the specific allergens that may be contributing to the patient's symptoms. The context in which the problem occurred also might incriminate suspect allergens. For example, if the patient is typically worse after mowing the lawn, mold spores or grass pollen are suspect. If they are worse within 30 minutes of retiring for the night, then dust or dust mites are suspect. Modifying factors that make the problem better or worse also help to narrow the field of differential diagnoses. If antihistamines or decongestants improve the symptoms, then allergy as a likely diagnosis should be considered. If the patient is better indoors in air conditioning, then the patient may be pollen sensitive.

Next, any associated symptoms or problems that coexist with the CC should be identified. Knowledge of all of these domains of the HPI are paramount to the critical analysis of the CC as it relates to allergic disease.

Finally, this author finds it extremely useful to ask the patient to report and rank according to severity the three symptoms that bother him or her most. Recording this answer allows the physician to inquire of the patient the continued presence or severity of these specific symptoms when returning after the initiation of treatment—whether environmental control, pharmacotherapy, immunotherapy, or any combination of these treatment modalities.

## REVIEW OF SYSTEMS

The ROS is an inventory of systems obtained through a series of questions to identify any other symptoms that the patient may be having or may have had in the past that may contribute to the his or her current illness. The patient is asked to answer "yes" or "no" to the questions. Analysis of the CC can then be developed more specifically, correlating it with the "yes" answers from the ROS. The ROS helps define the problem and clarify the possibility of other diagnoses. Otolaryngologists practicing allergy must remember that allergic disease affects the entire body and not just the head and neck; a detailed ROS must be obtained.

It is essential to inquire about constitutional symptoms related to the body as a whole when developing the ROS. It is important to know if the patient has chronic weakness, persistent unexplainable fatigue, or insomnia. Of all symptoms reported by allergic patients, fatigue is probably recorded most frequently. Chronic insomnia is an important symptom because it may be a result of food allergy, and insomnia of course perpetuates fatigue. An assessment of the patient's general nutritional status also must be made because a poor diet can be the cause of a variety of different symptoms. It also is useful to know if the patient eats out frequently at restaurants or fast-food establishments. People

who do so both have a limited perspective on what foods actually are included in their diet, and may have difficulty in following an elimination/rotation diet.

The respiratory system should be assessed and questions should be specifically addressed concerning general symptoms, sneezing, cough, and nasal complaints. General questions about the respiratory system should determine the presence or absence of pain, fever, sore throat, frequent colds, epistaxis, weight loss, or night sweats. Epistaxis is not specific to allergic disease, but probably occurs with an increased frequency in allergic patients. Night sweats in the absence of any other pathologic process are common manifestations of allergic disease (1). The presence of fever does not always mean infection; acute allergic exacerbations have been associated with temperature elevation. If sneezing is present, it is extremely important to know if it is seasonal, perennial, at a specific time of day, with a specific contact, with a specific location, or during or after meals. Sneezing and other associated nasal symptoms that are present on awakening and that last until breakfast are a reminder of the total allergic load of the previous day and will be the last symptoms to be controlled (1). Patients who complain of sneezing with exposure to smoke suffer from its effects as an irritant. Smoke, as a rule, is not an allergen. Nasal airway obstruction is a very common symptom of allergic disease and the examiner should know if it is alternating, constant, or seasonal, or experienced at day, night, or after meals. Chronic unilateral obstruction should alert the examiner to the possibility of an intranasal mechanical defect. Dust-sensitive patients typically are worse both at night and during the winter and better during the day. Seasonal nasal symptoms are frequent in the allergic person. Increased nasal congestion during the spring, summer, or fall is primarily due to pollens and secondarily to molds. Clear, watery rhinorrhea is typical of allergic disease, whereas thick, ropy, discolored nasal drainage more likely represents infection with a possible concomitant allergic factor. Report of cough by allergic patients is second in frequency only to the complaint of fatigue. If there is an associated cough, the examiner should question whether it is seasonal or perennial, worse at a particular time of day, productive or nonproductive, associated with an expectorant, and, if so, what color. Seasonal cough represents pollen sensitivity and winter cough suggests dust allergy. Productive coughs typically are of allergic origin and the color and consistency of the expectoration is of clinical importance. "Thin, frothy mucous represents recent irritation; a stringy, semi-brown or tenacious expectoration is typical of a reaction 6 to 12 hours in duration; whereas, a purulent expectoration means that it is at least 48 hours old" (1).

Pruritus could almost be considered a pathognomonic sign of allergic disease. Pruritus of the eyes typically is associated with pollens, especially tree, and less commonly with dust. Pruritus of the ears may be caused by allergy, but other pathologic conditions such as otitis externa also cause this common symptom. The pathogenic fungi *Trichophyton,* Oidiomycetes, and *Epidermophyton* almost always cause ear itching. Inquire if the patient has frequent or chronic itching between the shoulder blades. The patient during the HPI often does not volunteer this symptom, but its presence is an important positive finding, suggesting a referred symptom from allergic irritation of the tracheobronchial tree (1). Palatal itching is a very common symptom of food allergy; the patient who complains of persistent itching of the roof of the mouth after successful treatment of other symptoms probably has concomitant food sensitization.

Every symptom in the respiratory system that has been mentioned thus far can be attributed either to chronic food sensitization or inhalant allergy (1). In fact, no organ system in the body is exempt from the effects of food sensitization in the genetically predisposed patient.

The next anatomic area considered for the occurrence of symptoms in the ROS is integumentary. The skin provides the major protective barrier between the immune system and the environment. Foods, inhalants, and contactants all have the potential to cause allergic dermatologic reactions. The patient should be questioned about chronic or recurrent urticaria, pruritus, angioedema, or eczematous eruptions. Contactants cause skin manifestations that usually are limited anatomically to the exposed areas. Atopic eczema may occur at any age, whereas dust must be considered a prime suspect in infantile eczema (1). Collagen vascular diseases such as systemic lupus erythematosus must be evaluated in any adult with an idiopathic dermatologic condition.

The ROS for the gastrointestinal system should include questions relating to both general symptoms and bowel reactions. Symptoms may occur anywhere from the beginning to the end of the alimentary canal. In the oral cavity, manifestations include recurrent aphthous stomatitis as well as edema of the tongue and epiglottis. Esophageal spasm and a constellation of gastric symptoms, including nausea, vomiting, belching, bloating, or retasting of foods several hours after a meal, are frequent complaints. Abdominal pain is a very common symptom and can affect any quadrant. Hypermotility is probably the most commonly reported gastrointestinal symptom (1). The examiner should inquire if the patient's appetite is good, poor, or selective, and whether there are any suspect foods or foods that are avoided for specific reasons. Children with very selective appetites typically are avoiding foods that make them feel bad. Bowel reactions also must be questioned. A patient's recent change in bowel habits should not be assumed to be due to allergy. These patients must be evaluated for bowel diseases of nonallergic origin before pursuing a possible allergic etiology. It must be known if the patient has ever been diagnosed with Crohn's disease, irritable bowel syndrome, colitis, or spastic colon. Other important pertinent symptoms include the presence of stinging after defecation, perianal itching, or constipation.

The cardiac system also may be affected by allergic disease. These symptoms typically are related to sensory disturbances such as tachycardia, palpitations, irregularity of heart rate, and pseudoangina (1).

The ROS for the genitourinary system should include questions relating to both urgency and frequency of urination. These symptoms, particularly in women, can be the most annoying of the allergic manifestations (1). Edema of the prostate may occur as a result of food sensitization, and enuresis also may have an allergic factor (1). Food sensitization may account for albuminuria up to $4+$ as well as hematuria, both occult and obvious (1).

The most common allergic symptom related to the neurologic system is headache. The examiner should ask how long the headaches have been present, the age at onset, the duration, and if there are any known triggers. Duration is extremely important because headaches caused by food sensitization may last up to 72 hours, and occur with a frequency of two to three per week (1). Other neurologic symptoms include the presence or absence of vertigo, tinnitus, deafness, or epilepsy (2). Insomnia also may be present and is a very common symptom related to food allergy (1).

In the musculoskeletal system, foods and inhalants may cause painful, swollen joints with limitation of motion. Foods also may cause bursitis and myalgias (1).

The final element of the ROS to be developed is the psychiatric, or behavioral. It is essential to know if the patient has a history of psychiatric illness because allergic disease with the brain as the shock organ may imitate a variety of psychiatric conditions (2). Parents or guardians should be questioned about behavioral disorders in their children. Allergic disease affects behavior; the first reference to allergy altering behavior and sleep patterns in children was in 1916 (3). In 1947, Randolph proposed that any food could cause behavioral problems in children (4). Unfortunately, his work was largely ignored until his hypothesis withstood a double-blind, placebo-controlled, crossover trial some 37 years after publication (5). In 1975, 27 years after Randolph's hypothesis but before its validation in 1985, Feingold described that some children with behavioral disorders improved when food colorings were removed from their diet (6). Controlled studies to test his hypothesis were not supportive of his claim, possibly because those children who did not improve were allergic to the foods as opposed to the dyes contained in the foods (7).

## PAST, FAMILY, AND SOCIAL HISTORY

The past medical history for allergy should go back to the third trimester of the patient's *in utero* history if this information is readily available. If the patient is a child, the mother usually is present and able to provide the answers to these questions. The examiner should inquire if the child was exceptionally active *in utero,* with a lot of movement, kicking, or hiccoughs. During infancy, was the patient breast-fed or bottle-fed? Was there colic, whether breast-fed or bottle-fed? If bottle-fed, what was the formula? Was it milk based? Was the patient a happy child or always fussy? Did the patient have frequent colds or ear infections during childhood? Was there a history of dermatitis, hives, or eczema during infancy or childhood? Did the child have unusual problems with diaper rash? Was the child a good or poor sleeper? Were there behavioral problems during childhood? Answers to all of these questions, if available, are invaluable to the evaluation of the allergic patient.

The patient's personal past medical history must also include any past surgeries, resolved or continuing medical illnesses, the presence of known allergic reactions to medications, and medications the patient is currently taking. The past surgical history is extremely important for patients who have had multiple sinus, nasal, or turbinate surgeries, as well as abdominal procedures. Surgery does not correct allergic problems but sometimes is necessary to treat the long-term consequences of unrecognized and untreated allergic disease. In these particular patients, food and inhalant allergy, as well as immune deficiencies, must be considered as the underlying cause of their resistant surgical disease. Patients who describe chronic gastrointestinal problems, have been diagnosed with Crohn's disease, ulcerative colitis, spastic colon, or colitis, have had abdominal surgery, and who continue to have problems in spite of conventional treatment should be of particular interest to the physician. These patients must be evaluated for food sensitization as the underlying cause for their chronic symptoms. The aforementioned chronic intestinal conditions are inflammatory. Allergy also is an inflammatory disease. It is reasonable to assume that if a food to which the patient is sensitive is ingested regularly, then that food, as it passes over the mucosa of the gastrointestinal system, has the potential to cause degranulation of mucosal mast cells. The physiologic response of the gastrointestinal system to mast cell mediators is smooth muscle contraction, resulting in chronic pain, and hypersecretion of mucus, causing diarrhea. The late-phase allergic reaction attracts eosinophils that erode the mucosa, cause ulceration, and result in bleeding. Unfortunately, until the food culprit is identified, the patient will continue to have problems until he or she or the physician suspects a dietary cause.

Chronic, persistent dermatologic conditions also should alert the physician to the possibility of food and inhalant sensitivity. We should keep in mind that allergic disease affects all organ systems of the body, and some allergic patients may not demonstrate the classical upper respiratory symptoms of sneezing, itching, nasal congestion, and drainage. These patients have a different shock organ or target organ serving as the Achilles heel of their allergic disease.

An accurate review of the medications taken daily is essential in history taking. There are many commonly prescribed medications that either have side effects mimicking allergy or that actually reduce the allergic patient's threshold of tolerance, aggravating his or her symptoms. In today's medical world, many patients see multiple specialists who treat specific organ systems. It is not uncommon to trace the onset or aggravation of symptoms to the institution of a new medication prescribed by a specialist unfamiliar with the patient's underlying allergic predisposition.

Antihypertensive and antiarrhythmic medications in the form of angiotensin-converting enzyme (ACE) inhibitors and β-adrenergic blockers are the most notorious of these drugs. The side effect profiles of ACE inhibitors and β-blockers listed in the *Physician's Desk Reference* describe myriad side effects consistent with food and inhalant sensitivity.

There is published evidence indicating that $\beta_2$ receptor hyporesponsiveness may contribute to the pathogenesis of atopic disease (7–15). Stimulation of β receptors inhibits the degranulation of mast cells (16), whereas cholinergic and α-adrenergic stimulation enhances degranulation (17–19). β-Blockade results in unopposed α-adrenergic activity (20) and lowers the threshold for mediator release from basophils and mast cells (19). Consequently, the release of histamine and other chemical mediators requires a weaker stimulus than would be necessary under normal conditions (17,21–23). β-Blockade also amplifies end-organ responsiveness to the mediators of allergic reactions (19,24–26), increases the blood eosinophil count by approximately 30% (27), increases the size of the skin whealing response (19), increases total immunoglobulin E (IgE) production (28–30), and can reverse the inhibitory effect on specific IgE that usually is seen with immunotherapy (30). Topical β-blockers used for the treatment of glaucoma have the same effects as oral β-blockers because as much as 80% of an eyedrop's volume is systemically absorbed as it passes over the mucosa of the nasolacrimal system (31–43). Patients often forget about eyedrops when asked what medications they take on a regular basis, so they must be asked specifically if they have glaucoma and, if so, what medication they take.

Angiotensin-converting enzyme inhibitors have specific side effects that mimic symptoms associated with food and inhalant allergic disease, such as cough and migratory angioedema. The physiologic mechanism for ACE inhibitor side effects is unknown.

Review of the patient's family history is another essential element in history taking. If one parent is allergic, 35% of the offspring will have some form of allergy, and if both parents are allergic, the incidence is 65% (1). Although most allergic patients have a positive family history for allergic disease, it may be described as "sinus" or some other anatomic or diagnostic term. The physician must ask if there is a positive family history for hay fever, asthma, chronic skin conditions, headache, or chronic bowel problems, and in whom. The examiner also should know if any other family members have had allergy testing performed and, if possible, the results of those tests. This is important because children inherit sensitivity to 80% of the same allergens to which the parent is allergic, and knowledge of this information may be of great benefit to the examiner (1).

Personal living accommodations, occupational environment, and personal habits play a significant role in the allergic patient's symptoms and must be developed in detail. The physician must know if the patient lives in a house, apartment, or manufactured home, as well as the age of the residence and how long the patient has lived there. Is there a basement? If so, has it been converted to a living area? Is there a moisture problem in the basement? Is there a particular room in the house in which the patient is worse? Are there or have there been pets in the residence and, if so, what kind? If recently moved, did the previous occupants have pets and, if so, what kind? Did the patient's symptoms begin with the move? If so, did the patient move from another geographic region of the country? Has the residence had previous fire damage? Did the patient's symptoms begin after recent home remodeling? Is the dwelling urban, suburban, or rural? Is the patient employed? Does he or she work indoors, outdoors, around chemicals, dust, animals, grains, stables, or barns? Has there been a recent occupational change or remodeling in the work environment? If the patient is a smoker, the allergic symptoms will not likely subside significantly if he or she continues to use tobacco. The amount and frequency of alcohol consumption is essential information to the physician. Many patients state that they become symptomatic when they consume alcohol with meals; alcohol accelerates the absorption of food. It may not be the alcohol that is the culprit, but one or more of the foods that are consumed with the alcohol.

## ANALYSIS OF THE CHIEF COMPLAINT

After all of the previously described elements have been obtained, and the onset and course of the CC have been detailed, the examiner should then attempt to incriminate specific factors as a cause of the patient's symptoms. Symptoms resulting from pollen exposure should be worse outdoors between 7 and 11 A.M., as well as on windy days, and should improve indoors in air conditioning. These patients may be worse on a clear day after a storm. Tree pollens affect susceptible allergic patients in the spring, grass pollens in the summer, and weed pollens in the fall. Some areas of the country, such as southern California, have grass pollen present throughout most of the year.

If dust is the responsible allergen, the patient will is worse indoors and better outdoors. They experience an aggravation of symptoms with house cleaning or other situations with an increased exposure to dust. Symptoms increase during the winter months with increased time spent indoors. Of utmost importance in the dust-sensitive patient is the typical complaint of symptoms within 30 minutes of going to bed, usually resulting from dust mite sensitivity. Dust

mites are harbored in bedding; it is the airborne fecal material rather than the mite itself that is the culprit.

The patient who has mold spores as the etiologic agent may have symptoms year round. They often are worse in the warmth and humidity of the summer months, around freshly cut grass, in low-lying damp areas, and outdoors in the evening between 5:30 and 8:30 P.M. Mold-sensitive patients also may notice an aggravation of symptoms during the Christmas holidays if they celebrate the season with a live tree or garland in the house. They often are worse around wood-burning fireplaces, in stables or barns with stored hay, or if their home contains many potted plants.

Food-sensitive patients may have a symptom flare within an hour after lunch or dinner and possibly around 4:30 P.M. each afternoon.

## SUMMARY

The atopic patient's history is never complete because allergy is not a static disease, but rather a dynamic one with the capacity for constant change. Allergic patients are exposed to different allergens in different concentrations through different routes of exposure on a daily basis. Knowing how to take an accurate and complete history is the key to establishing the diagnosis and narrowing down what specific suspect allergens may be contributing to the patient's symptoms.

## REFERENCES

1. Rinkel HJ. The management of clinical allergy. *Archives of Otolaryngology* 1976;76:491.
2. Speer F, ed. *Allergy of the nervous system.* Springfield, IL: Charles C Thomas, 1977.
3. Hoobler BR. Some early symptoms suggesting protein sensitization in infancy. *Am J Dis Child* 1916;12:129.
4. Randolph TG. Allergy as a causative factor of fatigue, irritability, and behavior problems of children. *J Pediatrics* 1947;31:560.
5. Egger J, Carter CM, Graham PJ, et al. Controlled trial of oligoantigenic diet treatment in the hyperkinetic syndrome. *Lancet* 1985;1:540.
6. Feingold BP. Hyperkinesis and learning disabilities linked to artificial food flavours and colors. *Am J Nurs* 1975;75:797.
7. Szentivanyi A. The beta adrenergic theory of the atopic abnormality in bronchial asthma. *J Allergy* 1968;42:203.
8. Calnan CD. An atopic theorem. *Trans St Johns Hosp Dermatol Soc* 1969;55:105.
9. Hemels HG. The effect of propranolol on the acetylcholine-induced sweat gland response in atopic and non-atopic subjects. *Br J Dermatol* 1970;83:312.
10. Warndorff JA. The response of the sweat gland to acetylcholine in atopic subjects. *Br J Dermatology* 1970;83:306.
11. McNeill RS. Effect of beta-blocking agent, propranolol, on asthmatics. *Lancet* 1964;2:1101.
12. McNeill RS, Ingram CG. Effect of propranolol in ventilatory function. *Am J Cardiol* 1966;18:473.
13. Zaid G, Beal GN. Bronchial response to beta adrenergic blockade. *N Engl J Med* 1966;275:580.

14. Kaplan AP, ed. *Allergy.* New York: Churchill Livingstone, 1985.
15. Kaliner M, Shelhamer JH, David PB, et al. Autonomic nervous system abnormalities and allergy. *Ann Intern Med* 1982;96:349.
16. Orange RP, Kaliner MA, LaRasa PJ, et al. Immunological release of histamine and slow reacting substance of anaphylaxis from human lung: II. influence of cellular levels of cyclic AMP. *Fed Proc* 1971;30:1725.
17. Kaliner M, Orange RP, Austen KF. Immunological release of histamine and slow reacting substance of anaphylaxis from human lung: IV. enhancement by cholinergic and alpha adrenergic stimulation. *J Exp Med* 1972;136:556.
18. Kaliner M. Human lung tissue and anaphylaxis: the role of cyclic GMP as a modulator of the immunologically involved secretory process. *J Allergy Clin Immunol* 1972;60:204.
19. Sherett RH, Harwell W, Lieberman P, et al. Effect of beta-adrenergic stimulation and blockade on immediate hypersensitivity skin test reactions. *J Allergy Clin Immunol* 1973;52:328.
20. Awai LW, Mekori YA. Insect sting anaphylaxis and beta-adrenergic blockade: a relative contraindication. *Ann Allergy* 1984;53:48.
21. Assem ESK. Adrenergic mechanisms and immediate type allergy. *Clin Allergy* 1974;4:185.
22. Mjorndal TO, Chesnown SE, Frey MJ, et al. Effect of beta-adrenergic stimulation on experimental canine anaphylaxis in vivo. *J Allergy Clin Immunol* 1983;71:62.
23. Assem ESK, Schild HO. Antagonism by beta-adrenoreceptor blocking agents of the antianaphylactic effect of isoprenaline. *Br J Pharmacol* 1971;42:620.
24. Matsumura Y, Tan EM, Vaughan JH. Hypersensitivity to histamine and systemic anaphylaxis in mice with pharmacologic beta-adrenergic blockade: protection by nucleotides. *J Allergy Clin Immunol* 1976;58:387.
25. Nisam MR, Zhinden Z, Chesrown S, et al. Distribution and pharmacologic release of histamine in canine lung in vivo. *J Appl Physiol* 1978;44:455.
26. Matsumura Y, Tan EM, Vaughan JH. Histamine hypersensitivity in mice induced by *Bordetella pertussis* or pharmacological beta-adrenergic blockade. *J Allergy Clin Immunol* 1976;58:395.
27. Koch-Weser J. Beta-adrenergic blockade and circulating eosinophils. *Arch Intern Med* 1968;121:255.
28. Homer JT, Cain WA. Enhancement of IgE antibody formation in the rabbit by adrenergic antagonists. *Int Arch Allergy Appl Immunol* 1979;59:212.
29. Pauwels R, Bazin H, Platteau B, et al. Influence of adrenergic drugs on IgE production. *Int Arch Allergy Appl Immunol* 1980;61:347.
30. Houmark A, Asbrink E. Effects of a beta receptor blocking agent (propranolol) on synthesis of IgE in vitro by peripheral blood lymphocytes from atopic patients. *Allergy* 1981;36:391.
31. Dunn TL, Gerber MJ, Shen AS, et al. The effect of topical ophthalmic instillation of timolol and betaxolol on lung function in asthmatic subjects. *Am Rev Respir Dis* 1986;133:264.
32. Charan NB, Lakshminarayan S. Pulmonary effects of topical timolol. *Arch Intern Med* 1980;140:183.
33. Noyes JH, Chervinsky P. Case report: exacerbation of asthma by timolol. *Ann Allergy* 1980;45:301.
34. Prince DC, Carliner NH. Respiratory arrest following first dose of timolol ophthalmic solution. *Chest* 1983;84:640.
35. Jones FL Jr, Ekberg NL. Exacerbation of obstructive airway disease by timolol. *JAMA* 1980;244:2730.
36. Jones FL Jr, Ekberg NL. Exacerbation of asthma by timolol. *N Engl J Med* 1979;301:270.
37. Schoene RB, Martin RT, Charan NB, et al. Timolol-induced bronchospasm in asthmatic bronchitis. *JAMA* 1981;245:11460.
38. Laursen SO, Bjerrum P. Timolol eyedrop-induced severe bronchospasm. *Acta Med Scand* 1982;211:505.
39. McMahon CD, Shaffer RN, Hoskins HD Jr, et al. Adverse effects experienced by patients taking timolol. *Am J Ophthalmol* 1979;88:736.
40. Lockey SD Sr. Bronchospasm precipitated by ophthalmic instillations of timolol. *Ann Allergy* 1981;46:267.
41. Williams T, Ginther WH. Hazards of ophthalmic timolol. *N Engl J Med* 1984;311:1441.
42. Guzman CA. Exacerbation of bronchorrhea induced by topical timolol. *Am Rev Respir Dis* 1980;121:899.
43. Shell JW. Pharmacokinetics of topically applied ophthalmic drugs. *Surv Ophthalmol* 1982;26:207.

# PHYSICAL EXAMINATION OF THE ALLERGIC PATIENT

## JEFFREY J. MILLER
## JOHN DAVID OSGUTHORPE

Coupled with a detailed history, the physical examination completes the initial evaluation of the patient suspected of having allergies. Although many of the signs and symptoms of allergy are systemic, and a thorough evaluation from head to toe of a patient is necessary, most of the abnormalities are related to structures in the head and neck region and the emphasis of the examination should be so directed (1). A methodical and complete physical examination elucidates findings that can confirm a diagnosis of atopy, disclosing body-wide manifestations as directed by facts derived from a thorough history.

## GENERAL

The physical examination should begin as the patient or the clinician walks into the examination room, and introductions occur. It may be as straightforward as observing a handkerchief in the patient's hand, a facial eczema, an apparent inattentiveness that may turn out to be an auditory deficit, or an altered gait that may serve to alert the clinician to the possibility of inner ear disease (2,3). Observation may reveal a chronically fatigued adult, worn from persistent symptoms of perennial allergies, or a child with recurrent behavioral problems secondary to environmental allergies (1). Sitting in the office, the patient may exhibit signs of a chronic, nagging cough, mouth breathing or wheezing, or an intermittent but persistent throat clearing or even hoarseness, all potentially related to the continuous posterior nasal drainage and inflammation of the upper aerodigestive track secondary to allergies. The younger patient may exhibit classic "adenoid facies" consisting of flattened malar eminences, a widened nasal bridge, and a retracted upper lip (1,4,5)

**J. J. Miller and J. D. Osguthorpe:** Department of Otolaryngology and Communicative Sciences, Medical University of South Carolina, Charleston, South Carolina.

(Fig. 6.1). Such findings are due to chronic nasal obstruction from enlarged adenoids or hypertrophic turbinates. Further examination of this patient also may reveal a shortened mandible with an irregular dental pattern and protrusion of the front teeth (1,6). A young patient also may demonstrate the "allergic salute," an action in response not only to nasal obstruction, but pruritus of the nasal mucosa and soft palate. Typically the patient uses the palm of his or her hand to lift the nasal tip superiorly, temporarily opening and improving the nasal airway as well as ameliorating the itch. Repetitive saluting may result in the formation of a transverse nasal crease just superior to the nasal tip, referred to as the *supratip crease* (7). Some patients with an itchy nasal mucosa do not use their hands to relieve symptoms, but rely instead on facial grimacing to alleviate nasal irritation, an action often elicited in children by restraining their hands to prohibit saluting (1) (Fig. 6.2).

## SKIN

Examination of the skin may disclose one or more of several changes characteristically found in the allergic patient. Indeed, something so simple as a pallor not accounted for by the ethnic background manifested by the parents who usually accompany young patients (as do siblings) is suggestive of allergies, particularly with chronic nasal airway compromise or bronchospasm (8). The vasomotor instability typical of chronic allergy may manifest as variations in cutaneous turgor, with areas of erythemic blotching or blushing of the skin as well as blanching. The patient also may exhibit easy bruising or even petechiae secondary to capillary fragility. Urticaria, an intensely pruritic whealing with surrounding erythema, may be noted over any aspect of the body, although is more common on the trunk area (9). Angioedema caused by edema of the deeper dermal layers and subcutaneous tissue may be noted in any location. Dry, scaly lesions of atopic dermatitis are the classic skin manifestations of allergy. Pruritus is the hallmark characteristic of these lesions

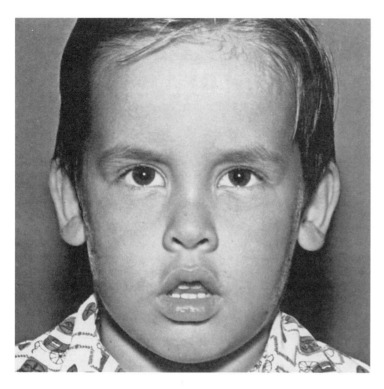

**FIG. 6.1.** Classic "adenoid facies" of allergic patient with chronic nasal obstruction. Note also Dennie's lines bilaterally. (Reprinted with permission from Marks MB. *Stigmata of respiratory tract allergies.* Kalamazoo, MI: Upjohn Company, 1977:17.)

and may even lead to self-inflicted injury caused by scratching to relieve the itching (8). On the scalp, atopic dermatitis may manifest as dandruff. A classic eczematous eruption in the antecubital and popliteal fossae is typical of eczema secondary to food allergies, and can spread to the head and neck as disease worsens (4). The erythemic, and sometimes macular progressing to vesicular, eruptions of contact dermatitis occur in distributions that point to the source, such as circumorally or on the eyelids if due to cosmetics; on the fingers, wrists, or neck if due to the metal in jewelry; or around the waist or bra area if due to latex or similar materials (Fig. 6.3). When checking the skin, the examiner should note any areas of fungal infection, most commonly in the finger or toenails, or scalp (as dandruff).

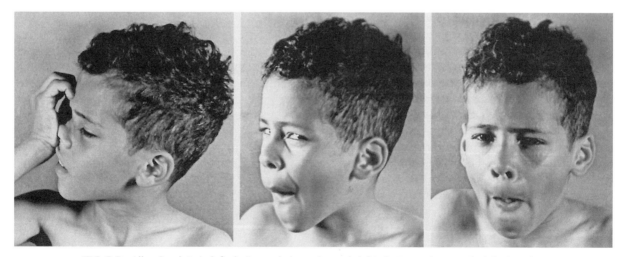

**FIG. 6.2.** Allergic salute in *left* photograph; in *center* and *right* photographs, note facial grimacing when hands are restrained to alleviate nasal irritation and obstruction. (Reprinted with permission from Marks MB. *Stigmata of respiratory tract allergies.* Kalamazoo, MI: Upjohn Company, 1977: 9.)

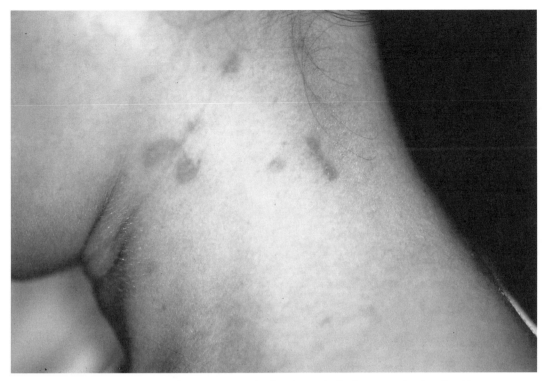

**FIG. 6.3.** Contact dermatitis patches on neck of patient who had contacted poison ivy. (Courtesy of B. J. Ferguson, MD, University of Pittsburgh, Pittsburgh, PA.)

## CHEST

In the chest, the most common clinical manifestation of atopy is asthma. Inspection of adults with long-standing disease may reveal a barrel chest with enlarged anteroposterior size, rounding of the shoulders, and stooping, whereas children with severe asthma may be pigeon breasted (4). Percussion of the chest in an older asthmatic patient may produce hyperresonance (8). Subjectively, patients may complain of cough, shortness of breath, or even substernal pressure. "Cough variant" asthma is a mild form of the disease in children, whose history is that of a chronic, dry cough, especially with exertion (when mild wheezing can sometimes be heard) or when around allergens to which they are sensitive (e.g., cat, pollens). Reflux sometimes is misinterpreted as cough variant asthma, and must be considered in a child with a chronic, dry cough and occasional mild wheezing.

Auscultation of the chest in an asthmatic patient may reveal the classic expiratory wheezes in all lung fields, although in mild bronchospasm, wheezing may be heard only on the anterior chest a few inches below the clavicles and just lateral to the sternum. If substantial wheezing is heard, the clinician should inspect the fingers for cyanosis and the lower neck for distended veins. Patients with allergy or asthma do not routinely exhibit the signs or symptoms of infection such as fever or purulent, productive cough, so if such is present medical attention should be directed toward control of infection before proceeding with the elective allergy evaluation.

## CARDIAC

No typical findings on cardiac examination are pathognomonic for allergies; however, murmurs, gallops, or thrills heard on auscultation may suggest pulmonary congestion caused by allergies in these patients (8). In those with acute manifestations of allergy, especially if food related or associated with a mild bronchospastic component, tachycardia is present.

## EYES

Periorbital examination may reveal classic "allergic shiners" in the atopic patient (Fig. 6.4). These markings are dark discolorations of the lower eyelids caused by the deposition of hemosiderin in the epidermis secondary to chronic venous stasis. Normally, venous drainage in these tissues proceeds through the palpebral and angular veins to the plexus of the sphenopalatine veins just beneath the nasal mucosa.

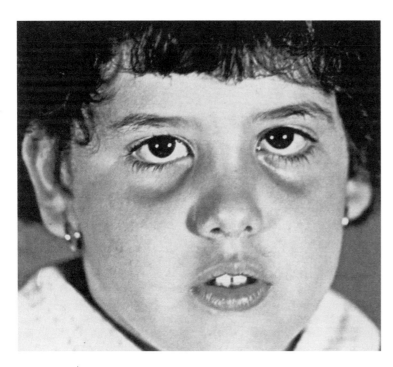

**FIG. 6.4.** "Allergic shiners" in young patient. Note also the classic adenoid facies with widened nasal bridge and retracted upper lip. (Reprinted with permission from Marks MB. *Stigmata of respiratory tract allergies.* Kalamazoo, MI: Upjohn Company, 1977:12.)

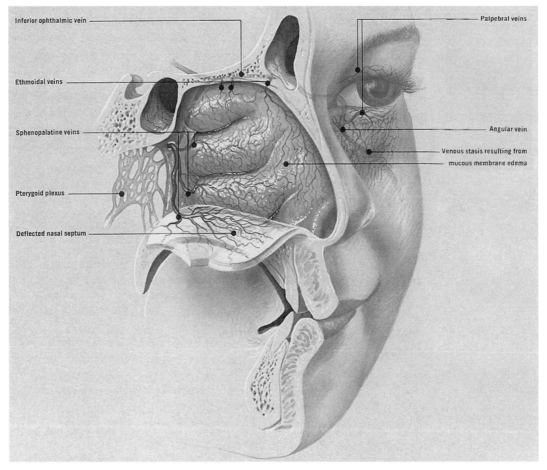

**FIG. 6.5.** Venous drainage pattern of the lower periorbital area. Chronic nasal congestion obstructs drainage of the sphenopalatine veins, resulting in engorgement of the angular and palpebral veins. (Reprinted with permission from Marks MB. *Stigmata of respiratory tract allergies.* Kalamazoo, MI: Upjohn Company, 1977:14.)

Chronic nasal congestion in the allergic patient leads to obstruction of the sphenopalatine plexus and resultant venous stasis in the tissues of the lower eyelids (1,10) (Fig. 6.5). Further inspection also may reveal Dennie's lines, which are semihorizontal, concentric creases in the lower eyelid skin. These creases are produced by persistent spasm of the unstriated muscle of Müller in the eyelid as a result of poor oxygenation, again resulting from venostasis in this region as described previously. Lower lid swelling from lymphedema draining from the nasal mucosa also may contribute to this finding. Over time, these creases can become fixed and permanent (1). Inspection of the eyelashes may reveal long, silky eyelashes of uneven length, classic for the allergic patient, but whose etiology is unknown (1) (Fig. 6.6). The discoloration and edema of the eyelids also may be accompanied by scaling as well as secondary infections caused by opportunistic bacteria. Inspection of the globe and conjunctiva may reveal watery, itchy eyes with scleral injection and mild to moderate conjunctival edema. Allergic eye diseases usually are secondary to inhaled allergens and consist of atopic keratoconjunctivitis, vernal keratoconjunctivitis, acute allergic conjunctivitis, and contact dermatoconjunctivitis (11).

Acute allergic conjunctivitis is a type I hypersensitivity reaction involving the eyes. Itching is prominent bilaterally, and examination reveals an injected and edematous conjunctiva (Fig. 6.7). The signs and symptoms of allergic conjunctivitis almost always are noted in conjunction with allergic rhinitis, and a thorough history elucidates the causal relationship of a potential aeroallergen (11).

Contact dermatoconjunctivitis is a form of contact dermatitis seen more often in women secondary to the applica-

tion of facial makeup. Classic findings reveal eyelids that are thickened and red with chronic inflammation and vesiculation (12). Examination of the conjunctiva reveals erythema and tearing (from pruritus and burning), as well as vasodilation of the scleral circulation and possibly even chemosis.

Atopic keratoconjunctivitis may manifest as lid dermatitis, blepharitis, conjunctivitis, keratoconjunctivitis, and keratoconus (a conical protrusion in the center of the cornea) (13). Cataracts develop in approximately 10% of patients as they age, and most patients tend toward dry eyes from the gradual destruction of mucous glands in the conjunctiva and lids (which become thickened and lichenified) by low-grade yet chronic staphylococcal infection (13). There also is predisposition to other ocular infections such as herpes simplex and vaccinia viruses.

The cause of vernal keratoconjunctivitis is obscure, but results in chronic bilateral catarrhal inflammation of the conjunctiva. It usually is seen in children and younger adults 5 to 35 years of age and is most pronounced during the spring and summer. Symptoms include intense itching, burning, and even photophobia. Vernal keratoconjunctivitis can be further divided into two groups. The first is palpebral, which is the more common and consists of inflammation of the tarsal conjunctiva of the upper eyelid. Examination of the inner surface of the upper eyelid reveals a thickened, gelatinous vegetation produced by marked papillary hypertrophy. This hypertrophy causes the classic cobblestoning of the upper lid conjunctiva (Fig. 6.8). The limbal form has similar gelatinous cobblestoning, but most is located at the corneal and scleral junction. The patient also may have Trantas' dots, which are small white dots com-

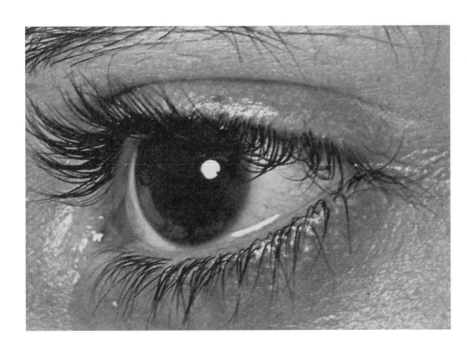

**FIG. 6.6.** Long, silky eyelashes in young allergic patient. (Reprinted with permission from Marks MB. *Stigmata of respiratory tract allergies.* Kalamazoo, MI: Upjohn Company, 1977:23.)

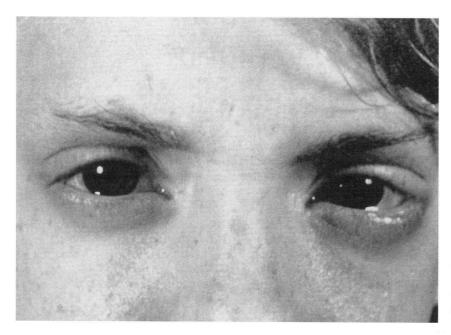

**FIG. 6.7.** Patient with acute allergic conjunctivitis secondary to airborne allergen exposure. Note the edematous upper and lower lids bilaterally with watery conjunctiva. (Courtesy of Richard Mabry, MD, University of Texas–Southwestern Medical Center, Dallas, TX.)

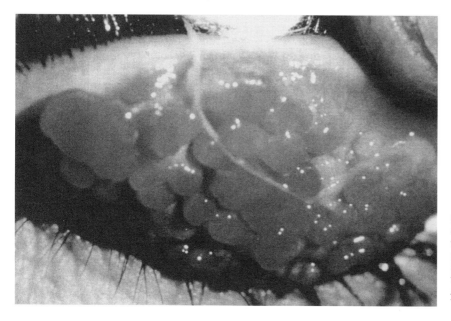

**FIG. 6.8.** Papillary hypertrophy resulting in cobblestoning of upper lid conjunctiva in patient with vernal keratoconjunctivitis. (Reprinted with permission from Abelson M. Diagnosis and treatment of allergic diseases of the eye. In: Lieberman P, Anderson JA, eds. *Allergic diseases: diagnosis and treatment.* Totowa, NJ: Humana Press, 1996:165.)

posed of an aggregation of eosinophils, located at the sclerocorneal junction. A thick, stringy exudate of eosinophils also may be present (11,14).

## EARS

Examination of the ears involves close inspection of the external pinna as well as the external auditory canal and the tympanic membrane. Close examination of the pinna may reveal contact dermatitis from perfume, shampoo, or the metal in an earring, or the postauricular fissures typical in patients with mold sensitivities (a dermatophytid or id reaction). The id reaction is a secondary allergic skin eruption that occurs in specifically sensitized people and is a result of the hematologic spread of fungi or their allergenic products from a primary focus of fungal infection. Typical sites of the id reaction are the auricle, external auditory canal, or the hands or feet (Fig. 6.9). Classic sites of the primary infection may be the nails, skin, or vagina. The most common fungi responsible for dermatophytid reactions are *Trichophyton,* Oidiomycetes *(Candida),* and *Epidermophyton*

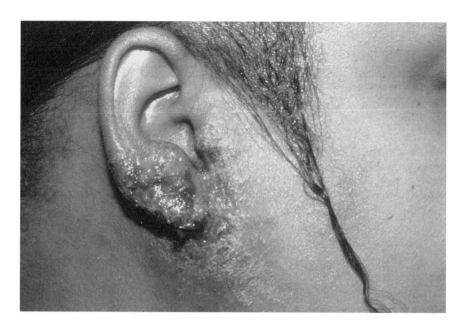

**FIG. 6.9.** Patient with external otitis from id reaction to fungi. (Courtesy of B. J. Ferguson, MD, University of Pittsburgh, Pittsburgh, PA.)

(collectively referred to as TOE) (1,3). Food allergies can produce an intense vasodilation of the ears, resulting in a bright red pinna that can be mistaken for an acute auricular chondritis (3). Examination of the external auditory canal may reveal chronic otitis externa with erythematous, scaling, and pruritic skin, yet no evidence of infection (1). Besides a mold-mediated reaction, a dermatitis on the auricle or external auditory canal may be caused by a reaction to ear drops, usually containing neomycin, and often presents as an acute otitis externa that has worsened with topical therapy (i.e., otic drops) (4). Auricular contact dermatitis (Gell and Coombs type IV delayed hypersensitivity and cell-mediated reaction) also may be due to the plastic on hearing aids or other offending agents (3). Metals on earrings often result in contact sensitivity, particularly the nickel or chromium that frequently is used in the posts. This sensitivity results in edema, erythema, and scaling localized to the earlobes. Avoidance of earrings is the definitive treatment, although most patients respond well to posts made of gold, titanium, or surgical steel (3).

Continuing the examination of the ear, the tympanic membrane may reveal a thickened membrane secondary to repeated middle ear infections as well as possible tympanosclerosis, calcified scar tissue deposited in the middle ear cleft, or myringosclerosis, the same deposits in the layers of the tympanic membrane. Allergies play a role in eustachian tube dysfunction owing to the increased nasal mucus production and inflammatory mediators associated with inhalant sensitivities causing adenoid hypertrophy, or food allergens causing the same plus a poorly understood but well documented middle ear "shock organ" response (15,16). Examination may reveal a membrane that is retracted, possibly with a retraction pocket in the posterior superior quadrant, or even

atelectasis of the membrane. Pneumatoscopy often reveals a serous effusion that, if unilateral, warrants close inspection of the nasopharynx to exclude a nasopharyngeal carcinoma, although in patients with allergy is most likely due to eustachian tube dysfunction from allergies or the sequelae of upper respiratory infections. As in patients who complain of a decrement in auditory acuity or problems with balance, those with significant abnormalities discovered on otoscopy should have an audiogram.

In those complaining of dizziness, unsteadiness, vertigo, or episodic hearing decrements, assessment of the function of the vestibular system should include inspection for spontaneous nystagmus in all three directions of gaze, an appraisal of gait, a Romberg test, and a fistula test with pneumatic otoscopy.

## NOSE

The paranasal region is the most common area in the head and neck affected by allergy and usually is the center of complaints of most allergic patients. As described earlier, the patient with chronic allergies may exhibit classic facial grimacing to relieve nasal itching, or a supratip crease secondary to repetitive allergic saluting (which can become permanent if practiced for more than a year or two) (1) (Fig. 6.10). In addition, the patient may demonstrate chronic sneezing with obvious nasal congestion, and moist, irritated, and erythemic skin about the nostrils and philtrum from persistent rubbing, or from the direct irritation of chronic drainage (1). Anterior rhinoscopy performed with a nasal speculum and adequate illumination with a headlight reveals classic edematous (frequently called *boggy*), pale, and

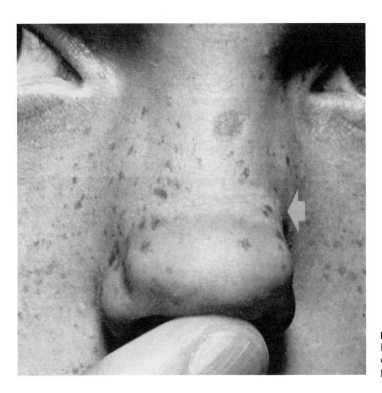

**FIG. 6.10.** Supratip crease caused by repetitive allergic saluting. (Reprinted with permission from Marks MB. *Stigmata of respiratory tract allergies.* Kalamazoo, MI: Upjohn Company, 1977:11.)

bluish mucosa overlying enlarged inferior and middle turbinates, plus an elevated level of nasal secretions, particularly during pollen seasons, that characteristically are clear and watery unless there is a concomitant infection (6). This picture is different from the erythemic, dry, and atrophic, even to the point of friability, nasal mucosa in those with rhinitis medicamentosa, whether from the commonly abused over-the-counter topical decongestants or from cocaine (4). Note that those with inhalant allergies have an increased incidence of nasal and sinus infections because of the poor aeration and mobilization of excess secretions, which creates an inviting environment for opportunistic organisms (1). The purplish-blue color of the mucosa is secondary to venous engorgement of the mucosal blood vessels throughout the nasal cavity, and usually is most noticeable on the anterior portions of the inferior turbinates (1). The mucosa of the turbinates and septum may show surface irregularity with polypoid changes referred to as *cobblestoning,* or the mucosa may be dry and red, particularly in dust-sensitive patients or those with chronic exposure to airborne irritants such as tobacco or work-related substances (woodworking, milling, weaving, welding, baking, and printing are some examples) (1). Dilated blood vessels may result in recurrent epistaxis with evidence of dry, crusted blood or eschars in the anterior nasal cavity. Before applying a topical vasoconstrictor such as oxymetazoline or phenylephrine, which is necessary for a more posterior nasal examination or the passage of an endoscope, the clinician should note whether the patient is

having a normal cycling of nasal mucosal turgor, in which one nasal passage is more open than the other. Fixed anatomic obstructions such as from a septal deviation, a concha bullosa, or polyps also should be noted (4,8). Usually, the nasal mucosal cycle alternates from side to side approximately every 30 to 120 minutes. With the application of a topical vasoconstrictor, the mucosa of the allergic nose typically shrinks dramatically within 5 to 10 minutes. This can be contrasted to the response of irritated or infected mucosa, which may respond slowly or not at all to application of a topical vasoconstrictor (8).

Examination of the posterior nasal cavity with a rigid or flexible endoscope may reveal cobblestoning of the mucosa with enlargement of the posterior tips of the inferior turbinates, termed *mulberry tips.* Flesh-colored or whitish, edematous, and grapelike polyps may be seen in the middle meatus and can spill out into the nasal cavity and even protrude out the anterior nose or proliferate in a posterior direction, causing partial or even complete obstruction of the choana (Figs. 6.11 and 6.12). Although common in the allergic patient, nasal polyposis is not pathognomonic for allergic disease (4). Typically, allergic nasal polyposis is bilateral owing to the generalized nasal process of allergies, and unilateral polyposis raises concerns for other disease processes such as a foreign body reaction, particularly in children, inverting papilloma, or allergic fungal sinusitis. In the latter, the "allergic mucin" (inspissated mucus, fungi, and degenerated eosinophils in Charcot-Leyden crystals) pathogno-

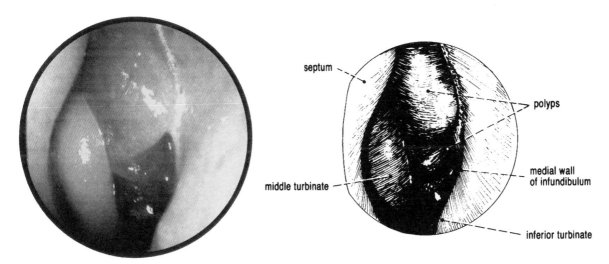

**FIG. 6.11.** Endoscopic view of left nasal cavity with polyps occluding left middle meatus in a patient with allergies. (Reprinted with permission from Baker W, Buckingham RA, Holinger PH, et al. *Atlas of ear, nose, and throat diseases including bronchoesophagology,* 2nd ed. Stuttgart, New York: Thieme Medical, 1984:115.)

monic of allergic fungal sinusitis sometimes can be seen emanating from affected sinuses. Obtaining a sample of this material on an endoscopically guided nasal swab allows the diagnosis on histologic examination, and identification of the offending fungus through culture (most commonly *Aspergillus, Bipolaris,* or *Alternaria*). Nasal polyps also are a component of Samter's triad, which consists of aspirin sensitivity, asthma, and nasal polyposis. Visualization of the nasopharynx also may be partially or completely obstructed by an enlarged adenoidal pad, especially in children. Enlarged adenoids also may impinge on the tori tubarius and are a common cause eustachian tube dysfunction.

## ORAL CAVITY/OROPHARYNX

Proceeding on to the examination of the oral cavity/oropharynx, inspection may reveal several findings secondary to chronic mouth breathing caused by the persistent nasal obstruction of allergies. Externally, the oral airflow of chronic mouth breathing in a patient with nasal obstruction may result in dry, scaling, chapped lips. Chronic obligate mouth breathing also may result in a retracted upper lip and a high-arched hard palate (Fig. 6.13), as well as pH changes that can cause foul breath and hypertrophic gingiva, periodontal disease, or dental caries (1,6). The patient may

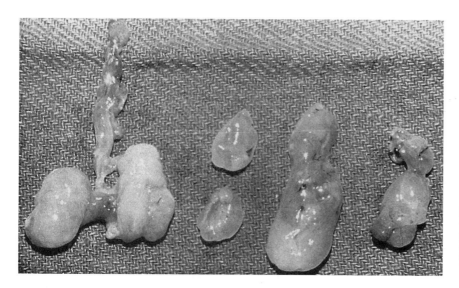

**FIG. 6.12.** Multiple nasal polyps removed from patient with diffuse bilateral nasal polyposis secondary to allergic disease. (Reprinted with permission from Slavin RG. Nasal polyps and sinusitis. *JAMA* 1997;8:1850.)

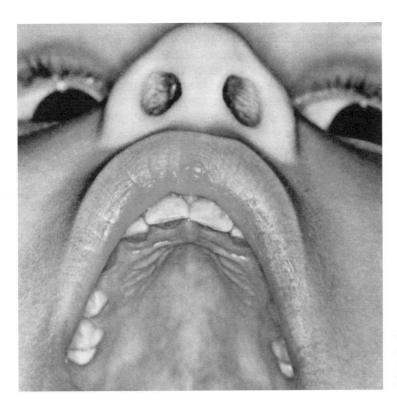

**FIG. 6.13.** High-arched palate in patient with chronic mouth breathing secondary to nasal obstruction. (Reprinted with permission from Marks MB. *Stigmata of respiratory tract allergies.* Kalamazoo, MI: Upjohn Company, 1977:17.)

exhibit flattened molars secondary to nocturnal bruxism to relieve intermittent eustachian tube obstruction, particularly in children (17). The tongue may be fissured as a direct result of allergic reaction, which is rare, or the patient may have a geographic tongue, which occurs more commonly in the allergic population (1,3).

More posteriorly, enlarged and fissured or cryptic tonsils with prominent lateral pharyngeal bands may be observed (8). The etiology is that chronic irritation from continuous posterior nasal drainage frequently causes recurrent infectious episodes, and hence hypertrophy of regional lymphoid tissue (i.e., the tonsils, the adenoids, the base of tongue lymphatic follicles, and the submucosal follicles located in the pharyngeal walls). The chronic posterior nasal drainage

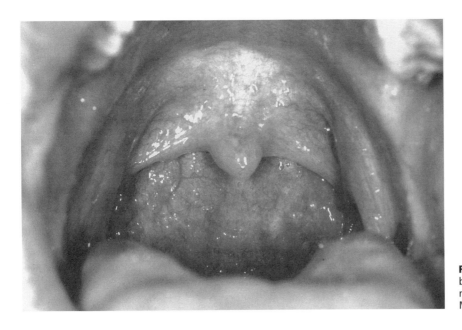

**FIG. 6.14.** Posterior pharyngeal wall cobblestoning secondary to chronic posterior nasal drainage. (Courtesy of B. J. Ferguson, MD, University of Pittsburgh, Pittsburgh, PA.)

also can incite hypertrophy of the many small patches of submucosal lymphoid tissue, most prominent in the posterior pharyngeal wall, referred to as *cobblestoning* (Fig. 6.14), or in a confluence of adjacent follicles such as can occur on the posterior lateral pharyngeal walls, the "gutter" for most nasal secretions, termed *lateral pharyngeal bands* (8).

## LARYNX

The most notable involvement of the larynx with allergies is with an acute anaphylactic reaction causing angioneurotic edema of the upper airway. This edema can involve the tongue, oropharynx, hypopharynx, epiglottis, arytenoids, ventricular bands, vocal folds, and subglottic airway, and can be so pronounced as to cause complete airway obstruction (9)

More commonly, involvement of the larynx by allergies results in a low-grade global edema of the laryngeal structures (1). The patient may complain of frequent throat clearing with chronic posterior nasal drainage, chronic

cough, or even a globus sensation. On physical examination with videostroboscopy, patients have minimal physical abnormalities such as thick, viscid mucus bridging the vocal folds with abduction, mild edema of the vocal folds, slightly reddened arytenoids, and a "twitchy" larynx (17,18) (Fig. 6.15). Allergies also may be manifested in the larynx as vocal fold nodules, polyps, chronic Reinke's edema, chronic non specific laryngitis, and contact granulomas (18).

## NECK

Inspection of the skin overlying the neck may reveal manifestations of allergies as previously described (eczema, contact dermatitis, excessive erythema or pallor). Palpation of the neck may reveal regional lymphadenopathy, particularly along the jugulodigastric chains, consistent with chronic infections of the skin, pharynx, or nose/sinuses caused by the underlying allergies. Palpation also may reveal hypertrophy of the neck muscles and strap muscles, which can be caused by the increased swallowing necessary to clear the throat of nasal secretions.

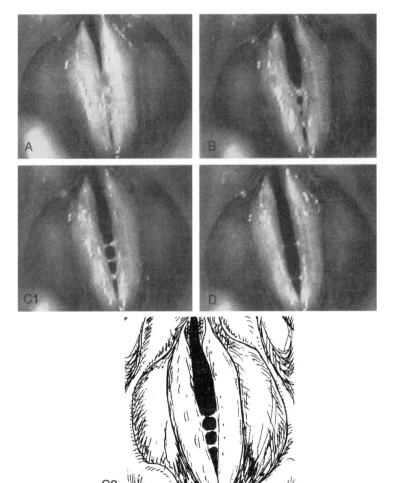

**FIG. 6.15.** A, B, C1, D: Videostrobographic prints of vibratory cycle in allergic patient with chronic hoarseness and cough showing global edema of true vocal cords with mucus bridging. **C2:** Diagrammatic representation of mucus bridging seen in **C1.** (Reprinted with permission from Corey JP, Gunger A, Karnell M. Allergy for the laryngologist. *Otolaryngol Clin North Am* 1998;31:194.)

## REFERENCES

1. King HC, Mabry RL, Mabry CS. *Allergy in ENT practice: a basic guide.* New York: Thieme Medical, 1998.
2. Derebery MJ, Valenzuela S. Meniere's syndrome and allergy. *Otolaryngol Clin North Am* 1992;25:213–224.
3. Derebery MJ, Berliner KI. Allergy for the otologist: external canal to inner ear. *Otolaryngol Clin North Am* 1998;31:157–173.
4. Lieberman PL, Crawford LV. *Management of the allergic patient: a text for the primary care physician.* New York: Appleton-Century-Crofts, 1982.
5. Sly RM. *Pediatric allergy.* Flushing, NY: Medical Examination Publishing, 1977.
6. Ricketti AJ. Allergic rhinitis. In: Patterson R, Grammer LC, Greenberger PA, eds. *Allergic diseases: diagnosis and management,* 5th ed. Philadelphia: Lippincott–Raven, 1997:183–207.
7. Marks MB. Physical signs of allergy on the respiratory tract in children. *Ann Allergy* 1969;25:310.
8. Rinkel HJ. The management of clinical allergy. *Arch Otolaryngol* 1962;76:491–508.
9. Weiss NS, Rubin JM. *Practical points in allergy,* 2nd ed. Garden City, NY: Medical Examination Publishing, 1980.
10. King HC. *An otolaryngologist's guide to allergy.* New York: Thieme Medical, 1990.
11. Lieberman PL, Blaus MS. Allergic diseases of the eye and ear. In: Patterson R, Grammer LC, Greenberger PA, eds. *Allergic diseases: diagnosis and management,* 5th ed. Philadelphia: Lippincott–Raven, 1997:223–251.
12. Fisher AA. Cutaneous reactions to cosmetics. In: Fisher AA, ed. *Contact dermatitis,* 3rd ed. Philadelphia: Lea & Febiger, 1986:77.
13. Foster CS, Calonge M. Atopic keratoconjunctivitis. *Ophthalmology* 1990;97:92.
14. Abelson MB, George MA, Garofalo C. Differential diagnosis of ocular allergic disorders. *Ann Allergy* 1993;70:95.
15. Hurst DS. Association of otitis media with effusion with allergy as demonstrated by intradermal skin testing and eosinophil cationic protein levels in both middle ear effusions and mucosal biopsies. *Laryngoscope* 1996;106:1128–1137.
16. Bernstein JM. The role of IgE-mediated hypersensitivity in the development of otitis media with effusion: a review. *Otolaryngol Head Neck Surg* 1993;109:611.
17. Krause HF. Diagnostic patterns of otolaryngic allergy: symptoms. In: Krause HF, ed. *Otolaryngic allergy and immunology.* Philadelphia: WB Saunders, 1989:51–65.
18. Corey JP, Gunger A, Karnell M. Allergy for the laryngologist. *Otolaryngol Clin North Am* 1998;31:189–205.

# ANAPHYLAXIS: PREVENTION AND TREATMENT

## BRUCE R. GORDON

When thinking about possible anaphylaxis, some physicians adopt the attitude of the fabled ostrich with its head in the sand. However, fate favors the prepared, and every professional who treats allergies must be trained to act quickly if the need should arise. This chapter summarizes information about the prevention and management of allergy emergencies that is essential to the safe practice of office- and home-based allergy treatment. The information contained in this chapter is as complete and accurate as possible. However, emergency treatment is an area of both controversy and constant change. In addition, the clinical approach must be tailored to the unique situation of each patient. Consequently, the clinician should not use this chapter as a dogmatic, inflexible treatment guide. The reader should use multiple reference sources to broaden his or her knowledge, including recent articles and editions of texts on allergy, pharmacology, and advanced cardiac life support.

Anaphylaxis cases appear to be increasing (1), and currently account for approximately 500 deaths annually in the United States, with an estimated incidence among hospital inpatients of 0.03%, and a fatality rate of 3% (2,3). The incidence in the general population is unknown, but has been estimated to be as high as 1 case per 3,500 persons per year (1). A retrospective analysis of patients with anaphylaxis treated at the Mayo Clinic found that the most frequent causes were food (33%), unknown (20%), insect sting (14%), drugs (13%), and exercise (7%) (4). In Europe, drug allergy was the most common cause, followed by insect stings and food (5). Fortunately, emergencies rarely occur during care of otolaryngic allergy patients (6). Major systemic reactions were reported after approximately 0.005% of immunotherapy injections, and all were successfully treated (7). This very low reaction rate is due largely to the inherent safety of the techniques taught by the American Academy of Otolaryngic Allergy (AAOA) (7): skin endpoint

titration (8), in vitro testing (9,10), and the intracutaneous progressive dilution food test (11). It is far more likely that knowledge of emergency procedures will be used to treat acute asthma attacks, drug reactions, or insect stings, than anaphylactic reactions to allergy testing or treatment.

## PREVENTION OF REACTIONS

### Diagnosis and Treatment

Because administering an excessive antigen dose remains one of the most common reasons for triggering anaphylaxis (12), prevention begins with proper use of diagnostic and treatment techniques (13). Excess antigen can be given by high doses of immunotherapy during peak pollen (12) or mold (14) seasons, or whenever there is high natural allergen exposure or increased allergy symptoms (15). Overdoses also can be given by inexperienced physicians (16), by error, by skin testing too many reactive antigens at one time, or by beginning immunotherapy at too high a dose. The great advantage of titration testing by skin or by in vitro methods is that it directly and accurately measures the patient's degree of sensitivity to each allergen (17). The desensitizing treatment mix can then be made up and treatment initiated with high confidence that it will not cause a reaction (18). However, great care must be used in preparation and maintenance of the allergen testing and treatment sets to ensure both potency and accuracy. Testing and treatment sets must contain identical allergens at identical concentrations. Also, whenever the manufacturer or strength of an antigen is changed, it is wise to retest the patient to that allergen and mix a new treatment set (19). Use of glycerin preservative, refrigeration, and dated treatment vials helps to preserve antigen potency, and reduces potency variations between treatment vials. During the buildup phase of immunotherapy, excess antigen can be given (7,14) by too rapid an escalation, by giving injections too frequently (14,20), or by a rush technique (19). When immunotherapy is administered at home or in the office of a physician who is not specially trained in allergy, additional safety measures

---

**B. R. Gordon:** Department of Otology and Laryngology, Harvard University, Cambridge; Associate Surgeon, Massachusetts Eye and Ear Infirmary, Boston; Chief of Otolaryngology, Cape Cod Hospital, Hyannis, Massachusetts.

should be considered (7). Finally, errors in patient identification, dose calculations, diluting, mixing, or injecting can have serious consequences (7,21,22), and thus all allergy personnel must be intelligent, well trained, and continually alert.

## Potent Antigens

Second, certain antigens are known to have potential for causing severe reactions (22) and should be skin tested with caution, or in vitro testing should be used. Examples are cottonseed, flaxseed, castor bean, peanut, and any allergen the patient suspects of causing serious reactions (23–27). Insect venoms and locally abundant pollens in season (e.g., grass) also can cause problems, and should be screened at a high dilution before proceeding with further testing (28). When in doubt, it always is safest to begin with more dilute testing solutions than usual. This is especially true during early clinical experience, or when practicing in a new geographic locale.

## Sensitive Patients

Third, testing and treatment must be more conservative when dealing with a highly sensitive, brittle, or allergen-loaded patient (12,29). For example, young children (30), patients with a history of prior anaphylaxis (12), and patients who are taking a β-adrenergic blocker (29) are at increased risk, as are asthmatic patients with active or uncontrolled disease (7,15,31). In these patients, multiple short diagnostic skin testing sessions and a slow treatment buildup may be required to prevent worsening of symptoms or anaphylaxis. Consideration also must be given to having asthmatic or other brittle patients wait in the office longer than the traditional 20 to 30 minutes after allergen injections (32) because significant late-onset reactions may occur over as long as 60 minutes (33). Thus, taking a good history helps prevent potential problems in patients with allergy. And, when history or testing has identified a severely reacting allergen, obtaining a Medic Alert identification from the Medic Alert Foundation (Turlock, CA 95382) is advisable.

## In Vivo Safety Test (Vial Test)

Fourth, a safety check always can be run on any treatment mix by doing a vial test (34). This initial skin test from the treatment vial (before starting dose escalation) must *always* be done when therapy is based on in vitro testing. A vial test also may be used to check treatment mix potency or to help determine the source of arm reactions, or done whenever a new vial is made up. Because the first injection from a treatment vial is more likely than subsequent injections to trigger anaphylaxis (7), as an added safety factor, some physicians prefer to give either a vial test or the first dose from any new vial in the office.

## Home Immunotherapy

Fifth, safety recommendations from the large office- and home-based immunotherapy study of Hurst et al. can be summarized (7):

Adhere to recommended AAOA procedures for diagnosis and treatment, obtain written consent, and carefully train both staff and patients to diagnose and treat reactions.

Use caution when treating asthmatic patients, patients who have had previous anaphylaxis, and patients who are taking β-blockers.

Use a vial test, or reduce the first dose, from every new treatment vial.

Consider using antihistamine premedication before treatment injections, have epinephrine available wherever injections are given, and, promptly use epinephrine for systemic reactions. Thorough training in use of epinephrine injectors is critical for proper home or school use (35–38).

Use distinctively marked vials for different family members, and verify the vial and patient identity at every encounter.

Insist that at least one adult, capable of rendering emergency aid, is present during treatment and during 20 minutes of observation after any antigen injection.

## Clinical Follow-up

Finally, good follow-up and careful attention to a patient's clinical course result in the safest possible advancement of treatment doses. Patients must be encouraged to report any unusual symptoms because reactions are most likely to occur when patients are having either unresolved symptoms or are experiencing exacerbation of symptoms after injections. Timely reassessment with modification of dosage, vial tests, remixing of treatment vials, partial or complete retesting, or attention to other allergens such as foods or chemicals may be needed. Also critically important, but seldom stressed, is the continuing search for significant environmental exposures that can be controlled. Allergy care is dynamic, and cannot be safely practiced by a "hands-off" technique.

## DIAGNOSIS OF REACTIONS
## Nonallergic Events

Occasionally, patients with concomitant illnesses have symptoms that can be confused with anaphylaxis (3,39,40). Examples are acute anxiety attack, cutaneous flushing syndromes (pheochromocytoma or carcinoid), diabetic hypoglycemia, cardiac arrhythmia, angina or myocardial infarction, cerebral transient ischemic attack, seizure, hereditary or acquired angioedema, nonallergic airway obstruction, and acute pulmonary embolism. Recommendations for diagnosis of some of these office medical emergencies have been made (41,42). Whenever significant symptoms occur in the period after antigen exposure, even if they are not clearly those expected from an allergic reaction, the wisest course always is to arrange for a prompt medical evaluation. In confusing or fatal cases, serum tryptase, total immunoglobulin E (IgE), and specific IgE values usually can be detected in serum between 45 minutes and 6 hours after the initial symptoms, confirming that anaphylaxis did occur (1,39,43).

## Vasovagal Events

Most allergy-related reactions fall into three categories: vasovagal events, delayed allergic reactions, and immediate allergic reactions. Vasovagal events are the most common and least dangerous reactions, but must be quickly diagnosed to differentiate them from potentially fatal anaphylaxis. Vasovagal reactions arise from fear or anxiety, and may range in severity from unease to fainting. Most of the so-called allergic reactions to local anesthetics in the dental office, as well as most of the reactions in the allergy office, fall into this category. Characteristic features of vasovagal events are pale skin, cold sweating, slow pulse, and normal recumbent blood pressure (BP). Anaphylaxis features are usually the opposite: red or flushed, warm, dry skin, rapid pulse, and low recumbent BP. In addition, patients with anaphylaxis often have itching or respiratory distress early in the reaction, but these are not seen during vasovagal events. Anxious or panicked patients can appear to have respiratory distress, but this is due to hyperventilation rather than to a measurable drop in peak flow. Close examination of the skin is particularly important because over 90% of patients with anaphylaxis have distinctive skin signs or symptoms of urticaria, angioedema, or pruritus (43), and do not show diaphoresis. Cyanosis or pallor may develop later in anaphylaxis, but by then, the diagnosis usually is obvious (1). Some patients with vasovagal faints may lose consciousness, and, rarely, they may seize or become bradyarrhythmic, but always rapidly recover when placed head down. Patients who are taking β-blockers, or patients with a large local or general allergic reaction *and* panic or anxiety, may initially be difficult to identify as definitely not having anaphylaxis. Tables 7.1 and 7.2 compare signs and symptoms of anaphylaxis with those of vasovagal and panic attacks.

## Anaphylactoid Reactions

Severe reactions can be triggered, without allergen exposure, by contact with allergic mediators or with substances capable of chemically releasing allergic mediators. Anaphylactoid reactions are observed most commonly as scombroid poisoning after ingestion of spoiled fish (44), or after exposure to narcotics, vancomycin, anesthetics, muscle depolarizing drugs (45), hyperosmolar solutions, or radiologic contrast

**TABLE 7.1. COMPARISON OF SIGNS AND SYMPTOMS: VASOVAGAL EVENTS AND ANAPHYLAXIS**

| Sign or Symptom | Vasovagal Event | Anaphylaxis |
|---|---|---|
| Pulse | Slow | Fast[a] |
| Blood pressure (recumbent) | Normal | Usually low |
| Feeling of doom | Absent | May be present |
| Itching, urticaria, or edema | Absent | Usually present |
| Skin color/ temperature | Pale/cool | Red/warm[b] |
| Sweating | Present | Absent |
| Respiratory distress | Absent | May be present |
| Cough or wheeze | Absent | May be present |

[a] May be slow with β-blockade (67).
[b] Cyanosis or pallor may develop subsequently (1).

agents (39). Contrast agents are estimated to cause approximately 1 anaphylactoid reaction for every 5,000 exposures (39), whereas anaphylaxis or anaphylactoid reactions during general anesthesia occur in from 1 in 6,000 to 20,000 cases (46). Anaphylactoid reactions present exactly like allergen-induced anaphylaxis, and their treatment is identical (43, 47,48). After a particular reaction is treated, it subsequently may be possible to determine the exact cause and whether the trigger was an allergen (49).

## Delayed Allergic Reactions

Delayed, immune complex– or T-cell–mediated reactions, usually with mold or food antigens, are relatively common.

**TABLE 7.2. COMPARISON OF SIGNS AND SYMPTOMS: PANIC ATTACK AND ANAPHYLAXIS**

| Sign or Symptom | Panic Attack | Anaphylaxis |
|---|---|---|
| Pulse | Fast | Fast[a] |
| Blood pressure (recumbent) | Normal or high | Usually low |
| Feeling of doom | May be present | May be present |
| Itching, urticaria, or edema | Absent | Usually present |
| Flat skin rash | May be present | May be present |
| Skin color | Normal or red | Red[b] |
| Sweating | Present | Absent |
| Reduced peak flow | Absent | May be present |
| Cough or wheeze | Absent | May be present |
| Hyperventilation | May be present | Absent |

[a] May be slow with β-blockade (67).
[b] Cyanosis or pallor may develop subsequently (1).

The immediate skin reactions, which had faded away, reappear in 6 or more hours, usually peaking at 1 to 2 days (50). Patients should be asked to report delayed skin reactions because these antigens may cause problems with dose advancement. Delayed arm reactions due to treatment injections sometimes may be reduced by prior use of antihistamines, but often require dose adjustment to minimize discomfort. Delayed systemic reactions, usually in the form of worsening of allergic symptoms, also occasionally occur with or without delayed local arm reactions. These usually require symptomatic treatment, as well as a dosage decrease, but seldom are severe enough to require emergency treatment unless asthma is provoked.

## Immediate Allergic Reactions

There are four types, or grades, of immediate reactions: local, large (severe) local, general (systemic), and anaphylaxis. These immediate reactions differ in their degree of severity, and only anaphylaxis is uniformly life threatening. Immediate reactions may occur within seconds, minutes, or up to several hours after antigen exposure, owing to the combination of immunologic mechanisms of Gell and Coombs types I, II, and III and the development of late-phase inflammation, all of which may be taking place simultaneously (51). A history of prior large local or general reactions is not statistically linked with increased risk of anaphylaxis (22,52), but their occurrence does indicate need for caution and patient reevaluation.

### Local Reactions

Local reactions are frequent, normal events during allergy treatment, where a local patch of itching, erythema, or swelling smaller than a half-dollar (3 cm) develops after injection. Local reactions merely indicate the administration of an antigen dose capable of eliciting a skin reaction. These often may be avoided by good subcutaneous injection technique and by use of preinjection oral antihistamine.

### Large Local Reactions

Large local reactions may vary from silver dollar–sized (4 cm) lumps to swelling that prevents raising the arm. If a large local reaction occurs during testing, it usually indicates a very sensitive patient, and testing should be stopped at that point, to be continued another day. Such large reactions after treatment injections usually indicate either overdose of at least one antigen in the mix, or concomitant exposure to a strong environmental or food allergen. Recurring large local reactions are not necessary to successful treatment of inhalant allergy (53), and should be eliminated by reducing the dose. If a lower dose and cautious readvancement is not successful, and the patient has not reached an effective immunotherapy dose, retesting is required to identify the responsible allergen(s). In this case, the use of a quantitative testing technique, such as skin endpoint titration or an in vitro method, helps to minimize future problems with dose advancement (17).

### General Reactions

General, systemic reactions include exacerbation of preexisting allergic symptoms, bronchospasm, urticaria, and angioedema. These reactions occur when the patient already has a high antigen load and testing or treatment adds enough antigen to exceed the symptom-producing threshold. Although general reactions usually do not progress to anaphylaxis, symptomatic treatment and careful observation are advisable. Even if anaphylaxis does not occur, a general reaction may initiate a troublesome, and potentially dangerous, asthma flare. Late-phase general reactions also may occur for up to 6 hours after allergen injection, although serious reactions, such as asthma or laryngeal edema, have not been observed after 1 hour (33). These late-onset general reactions sometimes may be difficult to treat because of the persistent nature of late-phase inflammation (54). For this reason, patients always should be advised of the possibility of delayed reactions, and the physician should specify where they should go if problems do arise out of the office.

Like large local reactions, the occurrence of a general reaction is an indication to reevaluate the allergy treatment plan and, in particular, to try to identify and control any known, but untreated allergens or any new sources of allergen exposure. While seeking other allergens, the treatment dose should be reduced significantly below the dose that caused the reaction. Often, once exposure to allergic foods or other environmental allergens is curtailed, the immunotherapy plan may be continued without further change (21).

### Anaphylaxis

True anaphylaxis may begin like a general reaction, but instead of being self-limited, continues to evolve rapidly to respiratory or circulatory collapse. Organs rich in mast cells are most affected (55), so typical early symptoms include marked exacerbation of allergic symptoms, especially nasal, throat, and ocular itching, facial flushing, and throat tightness. These usually are accompanied by tachycardia, which normally is a reliable sign that anaphylaxis, and not a vasovagal event, is occurring (56). Tachycardia may not occur in patients who are on β-blockers, complicating the diagnosis as well as subsequent treatment (57,58). Other common early symptoms are bronchospasm and cough, urticaria or pruritus, angioedema, or a feeling of impending doom. Less often, abdominal symptoms such as diarrhea, cramps, vomiting, and urinary urgency may develop. Respiratory difficulty (often with laryngeal edema), hypotension, and arrhythmias may precede collapse. Ultimately, most cases progress to hypotension and cardiovascular compromise

(57), with death occurring in minutes if appropriate measures are not undertaken rapidly.

### Biphasic Anaphylaxis

Anaphylaxis may be instantaneous, and usually starts within 15 minutes after antigen exposure (31). In general, the longer the delay from exposure to onset of anaphylaxis, the less severe the reaction. In two studies, no anaphylaxis began beyond 45 to 60 minutes after parenteral antigen exposure (31,33). But, because of slow absorption of antigens from oral exposure, anaphylaxis symptoms due to drugs or foods may not occur until several hours after ingestion (59).

After apparently successful initial treatment of anaphylaxis, up to 20% of patients subsequently may relapse, hours later, into protracted, stubborn, late-phase reactions, including angioedema, laryngeal edema, pulmonary edema, gastrointestinal or pulmonary tract hemorrhage, shock, and severe, persistent bronchospasm (2,59,60). These biphasic, or multiphasic, anaphylaxis cases are more likely to occur when the antigen exposure has been by the oral route, and often require greater total doses of epinephrine in the initial treatment phase, but otherwise are indistinguishable from anaphylaxis in patients who do not relapse (61). Because of the possibility of a biphasic reaction, after initial treatment of anaphylaxis, the clinician always should consider hospitalizing patients for up to 12 to 24 hours of further observation (57,62).

### Recurrent or Multiple Anaphylaxis Episodes

Recurrent anaphylaxis is most likely to occur with idiopathic anaphylaxis, which is estimated to occur in as many as 47,000 people in the United States (63). Patients with this disorder, where a specific allergic trigger cannot be identified, often must be placed on a prophylactic treatment program to prevent dangerous and expensive repeated acute anaphylactic attacks (64). Patients with presumed idiopathic anaphylaxis should have a careful evaluation for allergies, including foods and environmental exposures such as latex and formaldehyde, and should be evaluated for possible systemic mastocytosis and progesterone-induced anaphylaxis (59). Less frequently, recurrent anaphylaxis occurs after exercise alone, or after postprandial exercise (65). These patients may have identifiable triggers, especially foods, that, if avoided, prevent the anaphylaxis episodes. However, prophylactic medical treatment of exercise-triggered anaphylaxis has not always been helpful, and these patients must be trained in emergency treatment measures. The final circumstances in which multiple anaphylaxis episodes may occur are during allergy immunotherapy. In this situation, patients may undergo rush therapy, with injections being given in very close succession, or are treated with the maximal dose method and pushed to very high allergen doses in an attempt to adhere to a rigid immunotherapy advancement schedule. In such situations, the treat-

ment staff always must be on highest alert for possible anaphylaxis.

## BEING PREPARED TO TREAT ANAPHYLAXIS

Every office, even those next door to a hospital, must be ready to handle the most critical first minutes of emergency care. Preparedness begins with ensuring that all office personnel are currently trained in basic cardiopulmonary resuscitation (CPR). This is vitally important because failure to institute CPR when there is no effective cardiac output is one of the most critical errors made during anaphylaxis treatment (57). Physician and nursing supervisors also may wish to become certified in advanced cardiac life support (ACLS), particularly if it will take 8 minutes or longer for an emergency medical service (EMS) ambulance to arrive (41). The individual practice locale determines how extensive other preparations must be. This discussion assumes the typical urban or suburban office with nearby definitive hospital care. Rural practitioners may need to function at a more advanced level. The treatment goal always is to stabilize the patient for immediate transport to a hospital. The physician practicing allergy care sees serious reactions so rarely that his or her experience cannot compare with that of hospital-based emergency care specialists. Therefore, the physician's responsibility is to diagnose the problem rapidly, promptly initiate treatment, and stabilize the patient to allow EMS transport to the hospital as quickly, and in as good a condition, as possible.

The second aspect of being prepared is to understand what anaphylaxis symptoms are most likely to become life threatening, and what complicating circumstances may influence the choice of treatment options. Anaphylaxis victims with a fatal course die 75% of the time from hypoxia caused by upper airway edema or intractable asthma (66). This means that equipment and training must emphasize establishing and maintaining the airway, and that early, aggressive asthma therapy is essential. The remaining 25% of victims die from circulatory failure primarily related to plasma volume loss with hypotension, or from myocardial pump failure. This means that rapid volume replacement and effective cardiac protection also are of critical importance. Complicating factors primarily relate to drug interactions that affect how anaphylaxis is treated, and special circumstances that may arise during anaphylaxis treatment and require intensive, but narrowly targeted treatment.

## DRUG INTERACTIONS COMPLICATING ANAPHYLAXIS

### β-Blockers

Drug interactions may complicate treatment of anaphylaxis, especially from β-adrenergic blockers (67), tricyclic antidepressants, and monoamine oxidase (MAO) inhibitors (8). β-Blockers are the drug class most likely to be encountered. β-Blockade has two major types of adverse effects during anaphylaxis treatment. First, β-blockade is proallergic because it both blocks smooth muscle relaxation and amplifies the production of anaphylactic mediators (67), thus increasing the severity of any allergic reaction (68). This proallergic effect may render standard anaphylaxis therapy ineffective (69). Second, β-blockade may cause hypertensive crisis because of the unopposed α-adrenergic effects of epinephrine given to treat the anaphylaxis (59,68). Presence of β-blockade has been estimated to increase the risk of radiocontrast anaphylactoid reactions by approximately 2.7-fold (70), and probably enhances allergically mediated reactions to a similar degree. β-Blockers are available in three subclasses: nonselective, $\beta_1$ selective, and combination α-blocker and β-blocker. $\beta_1$-Selective drugs have relatively less bronchoconstricting effects (mediated by $\beta_2$ receptors) than effects on the heart (mediated by $\beta_1$ receptors), and theoretically should be less likely to cause harm when used in allergic patients. However, the effects of β-blockers on mediator production are nonselective, and thus even $\beta_1$-selective drugs are proallergic (67). There also is a drug, labetalol, that combines α-blockade and β-blockade. Because of intrinsic $\alpha_1$-blocking action, labetalol should be less prone to cause hypertension during anaphylaxis treatment, but could still cause bronchoconstriction and mediator production problems.

## Tricyclic Antidepressants and Monoamine Oxidase Inhibitors

These two classes of antidepressants also may cause adverse effects during anaphylaxis treatment. Tricyclic antidepressants block reuptake of catecholamines, causing both hypertension and sensitizing patients to arrhythmias, and also have α-adrenergic blocking effects, which can further complicate pressor use (71). Reduced initial epinephrine or dopamine doses, with close monitoring, should be considered, and intravenous (IV) magnesium is specifically recommended if ventricular arrhythmias occur (71). MAO inhibitors, on the other hand, prevent degradation of catecholamines, thus allowing their buildup to levels that can cause symptoms ranging from severe headache to hypertensive crisis (72). Dopamine, and probably also epinephrine, should be given in 10% or less of usual doses (71,72). Both classes of drugs are now used much less frequently since development of the newest class of antidepressants, the selective serotonin reuptake inhibitors (SSRIs). The SSRIs all have some potential for causing cardiovascular side effects and drug allergy, but have not been observed to complicate anaphylaxis treatment.

## Other Drugs with Potential Side Effects During Anaphylaxis

It is not known if the antihypertensive angiotensin-converting enzyme inhibitors, which can trigger angioedema in some patients (73), complicate treatment of anaphylaxis. It is possible that angiotensin-converting enzyme inhibitors have some adverse effects because they enhance kinin-mediated reactions (4,74), and kinins are known to be active during anaphylaxis. α-Adrenergic blocking drugs are another potential problem. Phenothiazine antipsychotic drugs have antihistamine activity and can be used as antiallergic drugs (75); however, both phenothiazines and tricyclic antidepressants, as well as some popular antihypertensive agents, have α-adrenergic blocking activity, and have been proposed to have adverse effects during anaphylaxis treatment (76). If this suggestion is correct, during anaphylaxis, α-blockade can cause refractory hypotension that is not improved by epinephrine and might be better treated by use of a pure α-adrenergic agonist, such as phenylephrine (77). Finally, it also is not known if the selective MAO inhibitor, selegiline, used for Parkinson's disease, complicates treatment of anaphylaxis. Until more data are available, patients using any of these drugs should be treated with caution.

## SPECIAL CIRCUMSTANCES DURING TREATMENT

### Risk of Hypertensive Crisis

β-Blockers, tricyclic antidepressants, and MAO inhibitors all increase the likelihood of arrhythmias and serious hypertension when epinephrine or other pressor drugs are used (8). If the hypertension becomes severe, intracranial bleeding may occur (78), or vagal reflexes may cause asystole. Caution and close monitoring therefore must be used when treating anaphylaxis in patients taking these drugs. Epinephrine and other pressors should be used initially at reduced doses until the degree of response is known, and the clinician should be prepared to use phentolamine to control hypertension, atropine to increase heart rate, and lidocaine and magnesium to control ventricular arrhythmias. In adult patients taking MAO inhibitors, based on the recommended 90% reduction in dopamine doses during cardiac resuscitation (71), an initial epinephrine dose probably should be only 0.05 mL (0.05 mg), or less. Even in patients who are not taking any conflicting drug, hypertensive crisis may occur from epinephrine overdose, especially if vital signs are not monitored regularly or if excessively aggressive IV doses are given.

### Overcoming β-Blockade

For patients on β-blockers who are not responding to initial epinephrine treatment, inhalation or IV infusion of a pure β-agonist, isoproterenol, has been suggested to be superior to continued use of epinephrine (40,59). Low-dose IV dopamine also can be used in this situation. Isoproterenol is contraindicated in coronary disease. The recommended initial dosage is 0.1 μg/kg/minute, titrated by clinical response. A 10-μg/mL solution is prepared by adding a 5.0-mL ampoule of 1:5,000 weight/volume (w/v) isoproterenol to 100 mL normal saline (NS) (40). Other drugs for treatment of anaphylaxis, especially ipratropium, heparin, and glucagon, always should be considered for use in these difficult cases. According to the American Heart Association, glucagon should be used (71).

## β-Agonist Treatment of Poorly Responsive Bronchospasm

Nonselective β-blockers worsen bronchospasm, but albuterol, metaproterenol, terbutaline, isoproterenol, or other β-agonist inhalations usually can overcome the effect (79), although multiple inhalations with close monitoring may be needed. Similar problems with poor treatment response also occur when a patient has been using β-agonists regularly, and has some tachyphylaxis. These patients also may respond to multiple inhalations (56,80). Higher-than-usual doses and frequent or continuous administration of inhaled albuterol may be effective in relieving bronchospasm when usual doses or frequency are not (81). Albuterol updraft doses of up to 10 mg were found, in a small study, to be much more effective than standard doses for bronchospasm treatment, and did not increase arrhythmias (82). Inhaled epinephrine (1.5 to 3 mg, 10 to 20 puffs at 150 μg/puff) also may be effective in relieving bronchospasm when intramuscular (IM) epinephrine has not been effective (66,83).

## Reversible Myocardial Pump Failure

Some cases have been reported of reversible myocardial dysfunction during anaphylaxis (84), due to both direct heart muscle effects of mediators released during local cardiac mast cell degranulation as well as effects of systemic histamine on sympathetic effector nerves that innervate the heart and vessels (85). This situation is improved by giving both $H_1$ and $H_2$ antihistamines (55,59,66). Because $H_1$ and $H_2$ receptors mediate opposing effects on cardiac conduction and coronary artery tone, with $H_1$ receptor stimulation causing conduction delay and coronary constriction, treatment with $H_2$ antihistamines alone is likely to be detrimental during anaphylaxis, and this has been observed in one clinical case (86). However, several studies have shown superior results with use of combined $H_1$ and $H_2$ blockade (66). Recent animal studies also support the use of experimental $H_3$ antihistamines, and indicate that otherwise favorable effects of $H_1$ antihistamines in anaphylaxis can be overwhelmed by high antigen exposures, whereas the helpful effects of $H_3$ antihistamines are not (85). If anaphylaxis progresses to myocardial pump failure, trial of an intraaortic balloon pump is indicated, as is use of glucagon, amrinone, and all other possible therapies, because eventual recovery of myocardial function is possible (57,87). Inflatable military antishock trousers may raise BP (88).

## Disseminated Intravascular Coagulation

This clotting disorder may complicate the treatment of anaphylaxis. Optimal therapy of disseminated intravascular coagulation (DIC) is still uncertain, but effective treatment of the anaphylaxis probably is the most useful therapy. Heparinization may be useful (89), and it also has beneficial antiallergic effects (see later). If serious bleeding develops, or if an invasive procedure is required while a patient has DIC, fresh plasma and platelet transfusions have been shown to be effective (89).

## ADJUNCTIVE DRUGS FOR ASTHMA TREATMENT
### Anticholinergics, Glucagon, Magnesium, and Vitamin C

Asthma is a major component of many anaphylaxis reactions, and these compounds have been shown to be of benefit in acute asthma therapy. Ipratropium (90) or other anticholinergic drugs, such as glycopyrrolate, always should be tried in refractory bronchospasm because bronchodilation by anticholinergics is not blocked by β-blockers (91), and inhaled anticholinergics are low in toxicity. More severely obstructed patients benefit the most, and most studies show that combined treatment with β-agonists and anticholinergic drugs is synergistic (91). In fact, a recent meta-analysis of combined treatment in acute asthma showed statistically significant improvements in peak expiratory flow and forced expiratory volume, and a reduced risk of hospitalization (92). Once venous access is established, IV glucagon, magnesium, and vitamin C can be used further to improve asthma. Animal studies and human case reports (69,93) show that the hormone glucagon is helpful in anaphylaxis treatment of β-blockaded patients. Glucagon is a positive inotrope (66), works better during β-blockade, and appears to reverse the adverse cardiac effects of anaphylaxis. Glucagon has also been recommended for use in protracted anaphylaxis (94,95) and for β-blocker overdose (71). Magnesium is necessary both for normal energy metabolism and for neuromuscular function, and probably acts to improve striated respiratory muscle efficiency as well as relaxing bronchial smooth muscle. Magnesium has been shown to improve respiratory function above that due to β-agonists alone (96). Vitamin C probably acts to limit bronchoalveolar inflammation and damage caused by reactive oxygen metabolites, which are released during the allergic reaction (97).

## Naloxone, Atrial Natriuretic Factor, and Eicosanoid Antagonists

These agents may be helpful in treating acute asthma and are unlikely to be harmful, but studies are limited. Naloxone, the opiate antagonist, was beneficial in one reported case of anaphylaxis with bronchospasm and shock (98). Because naloxone is nontoxic, it is reasonable to try in refractory cases at the same doses as for narcotic overdose, 2 mg every 2 minutes, up to 10 mg maximum (71). Children can receive up to 0.1 mg/kg, and naloxone can be given intratracheally. In a small series, atrial natriuretic factor (ANF) was as effective as β-agonist treatment, and no side effects were observed (99). The effective dose of ANF is 0.1 μg/kg/minute, given by continuous infusion. Antileukotriene drugs are known to be beneficial in chronic asthma (100) by blocking the late-phase reaction. Animal studies support a beneficial effect when leukotriene antagonists are used before anaphylaxis (85) or before β-blockade (101). Because leukotriene antagonists are known to have significant activity soon after ingestion, some emergency physicians now include them as part of standard therapy for acute asthma. Other eicosanoid hormones, including prostaglandins and thromboxanes, also are known to be active during anaphylaxis. However, although thromboxane $A_2$ antagonists are known to be effective for chronic asthma control (101), it is not known if any of these agents are effective for acute care.

## Aminophylline

Although IV aminophylline has long been used to treat bronchospasm (66), some reports now question the efficacy of theophyllines in emergency treatment (102,103). There are no controlled trials of the use of theophylline in anaphylaxis, and it confers no proven additional effectiveness when added to optimal β-agonist and corticosteroid therapy (104). Because theophyllines have significant toxicity and no proven effectiveness, they should not be used in acute anaphylaxis.

## RECOMMENDED EMERGENCY SUPPLIES

What emergency supplies are stocked is determined by many factors, especially the distance from hospital care. Examples of suggested items are given in many anaphylaxis treatment reviews (41,43,70,105). These lists should be used as a general guide, and modified to suit the circumstances of each office.

1. *Cot, examination table, or examination chair with drop back.* Anyone showing possible reaction signs should be laid down promptly and vital signs checked. Quick action can prevent vasovagal fainting and a possible fall. Tight clothing should be loosened, and oxygen may be administered while the situation is assessed.

2. *Monitoring equipment.* Have a sphygmomanometer and stethoscope at a minimum, plus an electrocardiograph (ECG)/defibrillator or an automated external defibrillator (AED) if a significant distance from help. An oximeter also is extremely helpful. Early monitoring of pulse and BP distinguishes vasovagal from true immediate allergic reactions. Continuous monitoring is critical during life-threatening or protracted reactions, and while giving IV epinephrine or other pressors.

3. *Tourniquets.* When possible, place one between injection site and the heart to slow absorption of antigen. Loosen every 5 minutes (106). Also used for starting IV lines.

4. *Epinephrine 1:1,000 (1 mg/mL). This is the single most valuable drug* (56). It should be immediately at hand in office test and treatment areas, as well as in the homes of sensitive patients with allergy (4,107). At the first suspicion of real trouble, give epinephrine. The decision to give epinephrine is like the decision to do a tracheotomy: if you think of it, you should do it! A prolonged resuscitation effort with a poor or fatal outcome from anaphylaxis treatment is seen when epinephrine is not used early in the reaction (1,2,25,57,108). The Canadian Laboratory Centre for Disease Control states, "failure to use epinephrine promptly is more dangerous than using it improperly" (62), and, according to the United Kingdom Resuscitation Council, "epinephrine is greatly under-used . . . and when given intramuscularly is very safe" (1). However, as critical as epinephrine is, it should be used carefully because a large overdose or aggressive IV use can cause a potentially serious hypertensive crisis (1,48,66,70).

The previous sections detail the possible drug interactions when using epinephrine.

If a tourniquet cannot be applied, the initial dose of epinephrine may be infiltrated around the allergen injection site to delay absorption (107).

a. *Adult use:* The use of prefilled, 0.3-mL, dual-dose syringes (Ana-Kit; Hollister-Stier, Spokane, WA) or self-injecting 0.3- or 0.15-mL syringes (EpiPen, EpiPen Jr., EpiE-Z Pen, EpiE-Z Pen Jr.; Dey Laboratories, Napa, CA) is recommended because they can be used quickly. The usual adult dose is 0.3 to 1.0 mL (0.3 to 1.0 mg) IM. The English consensus recommendation is to use 0.5 mL IM (1). IM use is now *always* preferred over subcutaneous because of more rapid action (1,62,109). Higher doses of epinephrine have been given to healthy adults, but are not routinely recommended (71,110).

b. *Pediatric use:* The usual IM child dose is 0.01 mL/kg (up to 0.3 to 0.5 mL maximum) (109). Typical doses of 1:1,000 w/v epinephrine are as follows: 2 to 6 months, 0.07 mL; 1 year, 0.1 mL; 1.5 to 4 years, 0.15 mL; 5 years, 0.2 mL (62), 6 to 11 years, 0.25 mL; and older than 11 years, 0.5 mL (1). For infants, to measure small doses accurately, 1:1,000 w/v epinephrine should be diluted 1:10 (111). Because of variable absorption (83), more epinephrine may be required, and should be given with vital sign monitoring. Tachycardia is common from epinephrine, but cardiac dysrhythmias are rare in otherwise healthy children (62). Epinephrine 1:1,000 w/v can be given intratracheally, 0.1 mL/kg (71).

c. *Reduced doses:* Seniors, especially those with cerebrovascular disease, cardiovascular disease, or hypertension, and persons taking β-blockers, may not tolerate usual adult doses. Therefore, consider starting at 0.2 mL (41). Precautions for epinephrine use with antidepressants and other drugs were previously discussed.

d. *Inhaled doses:* Epinephrine can be administered by metered-dose inhaler or updraft, provided respirations are sufficiently deep and the patient is able to cooperate. Ten to 15 puffs in a child, or more than 20 puffs in an adult produce blood epinephrine levels similar to those with recommended IM doses (4).

e. *Repeated doses:* The liver in adults ordinarily rapidly inactivates epinephrine, so that one dose is clinically effective only for approximately 3 to 5 minutes. Therefore, repeat epinephrine, as needed, with careful monitoring, every 3 to 5 minutes until clinical stability is attained (1,71). In children, epinephrine's half-life is much longer, approximately 40 minutes (109).

f. *Circulatory collapse:* To be effective during severe shock, *epinephrine (diluted to 1:10,000 or 1:100,000) must be given centrally* by IV (94) or endotracheal routes (71), or, if no airway or IV access is established, given IM into the tongue or through transtracheal puncture. IV epinephrine should be used only for immediately life-threatening shock. The initial IV dose (children or adults) is 5 µg/kg (94), up to a maximum adult dose of 1 mg in 10 mL (71). Give half the calculated dose by *slow* IV push, then *slowly* give the remainder in small amounts, while monitoring rhythm and BP. Monitoring by ECG is strongly suggested whenever IV epinephrine is used (1). British authorities prefer using even more dilute 1:100,000 solutions, starting at 1 to 2 mL/minute (66). Endotracheal or IM routes may require 2 to 2.5 times greater doses.

5. *Oxygen and ventilation support.* Oxygen is *the second key drug* because hypoxemia is what often triggers cardiovascular collapse during anaphylaxis. Oxygen is available in small tanks for office use. Start low flow (1 to 2 L/minute) at once by face mask with a bag reservoir, for both psychological and physiologic effects. Maintain low-flow oxygen during initial treatment of anaphylaxis to improve oxygenation without causing hypercarbia (112). But if shock develops, the patient is intubated, or CPR is started, give high-flow oxygen (10 to 15 L/minute) (1). If oximetry is available, maintain greater than 90% oxygen saturation. If artificial ventilation becomes necessary, a face mask with a one-way valve is safer than using mouth-to-mouth technique.

A bag–valve device, used with either a plastic anesthesia mask or endotracheal tube, also is useful for assisted ventilation. Various sizes of masks and oral airways should be stocked. Also, a laryngoscope (with fresh batteries), endotracheal tubes, and cricothyrotomy instruments such as Nu-Trake and Pedia-Trake (Armstrong Medical Industries, Lincolnshire, IL), or tracheotomy instruments, should be available in case airway edema or cardiorespiratory collapse develops.

6. *Intravenous supplies.* In every significant reaction, early IV access is necessary for administering both drugs and fluids. If the patient is vasoconstricted, good options are the external jugular vein or greater saphenous vein, or, if the clinician is experienced, subclavian or internal jugular veins, or scalp vein or intraosseous IV in children. The largest possible IV catheter should be inserted in case shock develops and large fluid volumes must be given quickly. Stock IV catheters, syringes and needles, 1% lidocaine, alcohol wipes, connecting tubing, IV fluids, tape, second tourniquet, and IV pole. Major plasma loss does not occur in all patients, but when it does, it can be rapid and massive, and crystalloid IV solutions may not be effective in restoring intravascular volume. In severe shock, colloids must be given (57,66). Therefore, both types of IV solutions are recommended [NS or 5% dextrose ($D_5W$), and 5% albumin, 5% plasma protein solution, or a dextran plasma volume expander solution]. If hypotension develops, give a fluid bolus *before* starting pressors. As a rough guide, give approximately 20 mL/kg of IV fluid as initial therapy for hypotension in adults or children (1,94). During fluid resuscitation, do not neglect to continue periodic epinephrine injections or an epinephrine infusion because epinephrine is synergistic with fluid therapy (66).

7. *Suction and catheters.* Without strong suction, thick secretions may make ventilation or intubation impossible. Check that your suction catheters fit into your endotracheal and cricothyrotomy tubes, and that your suction reaches wherever it is needed and is strong enough ($> -120$ mm Hg) (71).

8. *Albuterol inhaler,* or equivalent β-agonist. Use two or more inhalations, every 2 to 4 hours, for bronchospasm treatment (106). In some patients, multiple inhalations may be required, particularly if the patient is β-blockaded or has been using β-agonists regularly (see earlier).

9. *Ipratropium inhaler.* Use 15 to 30 inhalations, every 4 hours, for maximum bronchospasm treatment. This is the dose found to be effective in experimental asthma studies (81,90). The only alternate is glycopyrrolate, an injectable anticholinergic. Use 2 mg in adults or, in children, 0.05 mg/kg by nebulizer every 4 hours (81).

10. *Dopamine.* This is the most useful pressor because it is primarily a β-adrenergic agonist at doses below 10 µg/kg/minute. Start at 1 µg/kg/minute IV and titrate up to a maximum of 20 µg/kg/minute to support BP. Reduce initial dose to 0.1 µg/kg/minute in patients on MAO inhibi-

tors (71). Before starting dopamine, give a fluid challenge, and continue to administer fluids during dopamine infusion to support intravascular volume. Dopamine must be diluted for use: add one 400-mg ampoule to 250 mL of $D_5W$ or NS to make 1,600 µg/mL (71). For an average adult, begin at approximately 0.05 mL/minute. An alternative drug for patients on β-blockers requiring high pressor doses is isoproterenol (see earlier).

11. *Phentolamine.* This is a pure α-adrenergic blocker that is used in 5- to 10-mg IV increments (child: 1 mg) every 5 to 15 minutes, or as often as needed to control BP in catecholamine-excess hypertensive crisis (113). If phentolamine is unavailable, the vasodilator sodium nitroprusside is an effective alternative, and labetalol also can be used (113), but creates or increases a β-blockade. Be sure to stop pressors (e.g., dopamine) before using phentolamine. Excessive use of phentolamine can overcorrect hypertension and induce shock.

Phentolamine also is used for local infiltration to prevent ischemic necrosis in the event of extravasation of dopamine or other pressor drugs. For this use, dilute 5 to 10 mg with 10 to 15 mL NS and infiltrate around the area (71).

12. *Nitroglycerin.* Sublingual 0.4-mg tablets are used for coronary vasodilation if angina develops. Give one tablet every 5 minutes, up to three doses, or until relief occurs (71). Repeat every half hour, as needed. Store tightly sealed.

13. *Lidocaine.* This is the drug of choice for ventricular ectopy. Give an IV bolus of 1.0 to 1.5 mg/kg IV, then repeat every 3 to 5 minutes until ectopy is controlled, or to 3 mg/kg maximum; then start IV drip at 2 to 4 mg/minute (71). The intratracheal dose is 2.5 times the IV dose.

14. *Atropine.* This is the primary drug for treatment of bradyarrhythmias and heart block, and also may have some bronchodilator activity (67). Give in 0.5- to 1-mg increments IV, intratracheal, or IM intralingual, repeating every 5 minutes until effective, or to 2 to 3 mg maximum (71).

15. *Antihistamines.* Because the human myocardium is very sensitive to histamine (58), block further histamine effects by giving an $H_1$ antihistamine by mouth or IV push, such as diphenhydramine 100 mg (child: 12.5 to 100 mg) (62) or chlorpheniramine 10 mg. Then give an $H_2$ antihistamine like ranitidine 50 mg or cimetidine 300 mg. Give diluted $H_2$ drugs IV, slowly over 5 minutes to minimize risk of hypotension, arrhythmia, or asystole (59). There is evidence that both $H_1$ and $H_2$ agents are helpful (114), particularly in β-blockaded patients (115) or in refractory cases of anaphylaxis (66). When IV nonsedating $H_1$ agents become available, they will be preferred because of their minimal side effects and added antiinflammatory activities. When $H_3$ agents are available, they also may be of value. Always give an $H_1$ antihistamine *before* any $H_2$ antihistamine to prevent adverse cardiac effects (see earlier).

16. *Corticosteroids.* In seriously ill patients, IV steroids are used. In less ill patients, oral steroids are safer and preferred. By either route, steroids take up to 4 to 6 hours to become fully effective (66), but probably shorten the course of anaphylaxis and usually prevent late-onset reactions. For oral use, 40 to 50 mg prednisone is sufficient (66). For IV therapy, give dexamethasone sodium phosphate 20 mg, or hydrocortisone sodium succinate 500 mg (1,116). If the patient is sulfite allergic, substitute IV methylprednisolone sodium succinate 40 mg, unless patient has known succinate ester allergy (55) or allergy to benzyl alcohol. Corticosteroid doses may be reduced for children, but this is more related to severity of the reaction being treated than to age or size. Use a minimum methylprednisolone dosage of 0.5 mg/kg/24 hours in children. Corticosteroids probably should be given to every patient with a general or anaphylactic reaction (56), and *always* should be given if severe asthma is present (117). Corticosteroids also should *always* be given to patients who are already taking systemic corticosteroids because it must be assumed that such patients have hypothalamic–pituitary–adrenal axis suppression (108). Oral corticosteroids may be as effective as IV forms (117) if swallowing and absorption are normal. Administration of a corticosteroid, however, is no guarantee that a delayed or recrudescent reaction will not occur (118).

Corticosteroids also are used at very high doses as adjunctive treatment for shock: dexamethasone up to 1 mg/kg, or methylprednisolone up to 30 mg/kg. Oral or parenteral steroids occasionally can cause anaphylaxis, and parenteral steroids, if not given slowly, can cause coronary spasm, ischemia, or sudden death (66). Doses of methylprednisolone over 500 mg should be given over 30 minutes to prevent arrhythmias; smaller doses may be given by slow IV push.

17. *Heparin.* After epinephrine, next consider giving heparin. Heparin adsorbs and inactivates histamine and other mediators of inflammation (119,120), and releases diamine oxidase (histaminase) into the circulation, lowering histamine levels (121). Heparin also improves the coagulopathy that occurs during anaphylaxis (122), treats DIC, stabilizes coronary thrombosis, and has beneficial antiinflammatory effects (123). Heparin ameliorates or prevents experimental anaphylaxis in animal models (124). Heparin also has been successfully used in small clinical trials of several serious allergic conditions, including obstructive croup and acute asthma (125,126). Its use in anaphylaxis treatment, according to experienced clinicians, is very helpful, especially in β-blockaded or refractory patients. The usual adult dose is 10,000 U IV, the same dose used for initiating anticoagulation therapy. In children, use 50 to 75 U/kg (127). If there is a favorable response, a constant heparin IV infusion can be initiated at 1,000 U/hour (child: 25 U/kg/hour), with monitoring of partial thromboplastin times to prevent overanticoagulation (71,127). Heparin is contraindicated if the patient has severe thrombocytopenia, uncontrolled active bleeding, or recent neurosurgery. Caution is needed in patients who are taking aspirin or other anticoagulants, or who have had recent surgery or CPR. Carefully read and understand the package insert before

using heparin. Low–molecular-weight fractionated heparins have not yet been tested for clinical efficacy in anaphylaxis.

18. *Glucagon.* Used for treatment of acute hypoglycemia or to relax gastrointestinal smooth muscle, glucagon should be added to initial therapy in cases of β-blockade or refractory anaphylaxis. Suggested doses are from 1 to 5 mg IV push (71), followed by continuous infusion at 50 μg/hour (128), or repeat boluses every 5 minutes (40). Use 0.5 mg for children (129). Because glucagon stimulates release of endogenous catecholamines and insulin, it could trigger hypertension or hypoglycemia, and thus is contraindicated in known or suspected insulinoma or pheochromocytoma. Side effects normally are minor, although vomiting can occur.

19. *Magnesium.* Intravenous magnesium has been shown to be effective in treatment of acute bronchospasm (130,131). Like ipratropium, it may be of special benefit in β-blockaded patients, and should be considered in any case not responding well to other bronchodilators. Because magnesium has been used extensively for treatment of eclampsia and arrhythmias, its safety and tolerated doses are well known (71,72). The initial IV dose is 1 g magnesium sulfate (2 mL of 50% solution), diluted with 50 mL NS. Up to 4 g may be given over 20 minutes, and up to 1 g/hour thereafter, with frequent monitoring of deep tendon reflexes to detect overdose. Calcium is the antidote for magnesium intoxication. In renal insufficiency, magnesium doses must be reduced and blood levels checked.

20. *Vitamin C (ascorbic acid).* After standard therapy has been given, consider administration of 2 g IV vitamin C. Vitamin C has a significant effect in reducing acute allergic bronchospasm (132), and because it is very nontoxic (133, 134) it is worth adding as adjunctive therapy.

21. *Flash cards and maintenance.* Type on index cards brief, clear descriptions of how to mix each drug, contraindications, how much to give, and how often. Keep the cards with your emergency kit, and store the kit in an easily accessible place. Schedule regular kit checks for missing or outdated items. Plan periodic readiness drills.

## ALLERGY EMERGENCY EVALUATION AND TREATMENT SAMPLE PROTOCOLS

I. Initial Evaluation of Possible Allergic Reaction
   A. Cease administration of allergenic extracts.
   B. Record symptoms.
   C. Record vital signs: pulse, BP, respirations, skin color, temperature, and moisture.
   D. Quickly assess type of reaction.
   E. Consult other clinicians in office.
   F. If allergic, proceed with treatment.
   G. If not allergic, refer.

II. Office Treatment of Allergic Reactions
   A. Vasovagal reaction or panic attack
      1. Lower head, loosen clothing.
      2. Confirm diagnosis.
      3. Low-flow oxygen by mask.
      4. Provide postreaction teaching and reassurance.
   B. Local reaction
      1. Check injection technique.
      2. Consider antihistamine before each injection.
      3. Reduce dose if bothersome reactions continue.
      4. Provide postreaction teaching and reassurance.
   C. Large local reaction
      1. Confirm there is *no* general reaction.
      2. Consider oral $H_1$ antihistamine.
      3. Reduce next dose, then consider slow readvancement.
      4. For repeat large local reactions, retest allergen sensitivities.
      5. Provide postreaction teaching and reassurance.
   D. General reaction
      1. Lower head, loosen clothing.
      2. Confirm diagnosis.
      3. Notify supervisor physician.
      4. Give oral $H_1$ antihistamine.
      5. If respiratory symptoms, check peak flow, start low-flow oxygen.
      6. If bronchospasm, albuterol inhaler, two puffs, repeat if not effective.
      7. If continued bronchospasm, ipratropium inhaler, 15 to 30 puffs.
      8. *If severe symptoms, give epinephrine* (note precautions):
         a. 1:1,000, 0.3 to 0.5 mL IM (adult)
         b. or, epinephrine 1:1,000, 0.2 mL IM (elderly or on β-blocker)
         c. or, epinephrine 1:1,000, 0.05 mL IM (on MAO inhibitor)
         d. or, epinephrine 1:1,000, 0.01 mg/kg, up to 0.3 mL IM (child).
      9. Consider oral or IM corticosteroid to abort late-phase reaction.
      10. Before any future treatment: plan nurse/physician conference.
      11. Provide postreaction teaching and reassurance.
      12. *If symptoms progress, change diagnosis to anaphylaxis.*
   E. Anaphylaxis
      1. Lower head, loosen clothing.
      2. Confirm diagnosis.
      3. Apply tourniquet proximal to allergen injection site.
      4. Assess reaction severity and review patient's medical and medication history.
      5. *Always give epinephrine* (note precautions):
         a. 1:1,000, 0.3 to 1.0 mL IM (adult)

b. or, epinephrine 1:1,000, 0.2 mL IM (elderly or on β-blocker)

c. or, epinephrine 1:1,000, 0.05 mL IM (on MAO inhibitor)

d. or, epinephrine 1:1,000, 0.01 mg/kg, up to 0.3 mL IM (child).

6. Call for help and notify supervisor physician.

7. Consider local injection of epinephrine 1:1,000 around antigen entry site.

8. *If severe hypotension (shock), give epinephrine 1:10,000 centrally:*
   a. 1 mg in 10 mL (71), slow IV, transtracheal, or intralingual IM
   b. for children, use 0.1 mg/kg in 5 mL (56).

9. Call ambulance, request crash cart, defibrillator, suction machine, and oximeter.

10. Check peak flow; if reduced, albuterol inhaler, two puffs, repeat if not effective.

11. If continued bronchospasm, ipratropium inhaler, 15 to 30 puffs.

12. Start 100% oxygen by mask. If oximeter available, keep the oxygen saturation above 90%.

13. Assign duties, record personnel, symptoms, vital signs, and treatment given.

14. *If severe,* establish IV as soon as possible *and* consider heparin 10,000 U IV.

15. *If β-blocked,* consider heparin 10,000 U IV *and* give glucagon 1 to 2 mg IV.

16. If angina, nitroglycerin 0.4 mg sublingually, every 3 minutes to relief or to three doses maximum, repeat every 30 minutes. If no relief, consider aspirin and heparin per ACLS protocol.

17. *If no respirations, begin CPR,* bag–mask, intubate or cricothyrotomy, suction.

18. *If no pulse, begin CPR,* attach ECG monitor, defibrillator, or AED.

19. *Consider epinephrine second dose;* continue to repeat at least every 3 to 5 minutes in adults until satisfactory clinical improvement occurs (71). In children, monitoring is required to determine if subsequent doses are required. Give third and subsequent doses to all patients depending on clinical need.

20. Check, loosen tourniquet every 5 minutes.

21. Give IV $H_1$ antihistamine: diphenhydramine 50 to 100 mg, or chlorpheniramine 10 mg.

22. Give IV $H_2$ antihistamine: ranitidine 50 mg, or cimetidine 300 mg, in 20 mL NS, slowly over 5 minutes.

23. Give corticosteroid. If able to take oral drugs, prednisone 40 to 50 mg. If very ill, IV dexamethasone 20 mg, or methylprednisolone 40 mg, or hydrocortisone sodium succinate 500 mg. If shock, increase dexamethasone up to 1 mg/kg, or methylprednisolone up to 30 mg/kg.

24. If continued bronchospasm, magnesium sulfate IV, 1 to 4 g over 20 minutes with reflex monitoring.

25. Reconsider heparin 10,000 U IV, then infusion at 1,000 U/hour (note precautions).

26. Reconsider glucagon 1 to 2 mg IV, then infusion at 50 μg/hour. Use 0.5 mg for children.

27. If hypotension, administer IV fluid, up to 1,000 mL every 20 minutes (106).

28. Start second IV.

29. If hypotension persists, mix 1 ampoule (400 mg) of dopamine in 250 mL $D_5W$, making 1,600 μg/mL. Start dopamine IV drip at 1 μg/kg/minute, increase as needed, up to 20 μg/kg/minute per ACLS protocol.

30. If hypotension persists, administer IV *colloid* solution wide open.

31. If hypertension occurs, turn off dopamine, then, if persistent, give phentolamine 5 to 10 mg IV, repeat every 5 minutes until BP normal.

32. If hypertensive asystole, use ACLS protocol, including atropine 1 mg IV every 5 minutes to 3 mg total.

33. If ventricular ectopy, use ACLS protocol, including lidocaine bolus 1.0 to 1.5 mg/kg IV, then 0.5 mg/kg every 5 to 10 minutes until ectopy controlled, or to 3 mg/kg maximum, then start IV drip at 2 to 4 mg/minute.

34. If ventricular fibrillation, or pulseless ventricular tachycardia, immediately defibrillate per ACLS protocol.

35. If respiratory obstruction requires artificial ventilation, but lungs cannot deflate, add external end-inspiratory thoracic compressions (requires two people).

36. When stable, consider vitamin C, 2 g IV.

37. Transport by EMS ambulance to hospital as soon as possible, communicate with emergency department physician, consider cardiology consult.

38. Post-code debriefing of personnel, completion of records, replenish supplies.

39. Before any future treatment: plan nurse/physician conference.

## CONCLUSION

Acute anaphylaxis is a rare, potentially fatal, multisystem allergic reaction that every allergy office must be prepared to treat. Key points are reaction prevention, diagnosing the serious reaction, proper staff training, and keeping on hand, readily accessible and in functioning condition, adequate supplies to provide emergency treatment appropriate to the office locale. The diagnosis and treatment of each common type of allergic reaction is discussed. Equipment and medicines suggested for office use are reviewed, and a sample allergy reaction management protocol is outlined.

Office treatment of anaphylaxis is directed at stabilizing the patient for early transport to a hospital. *Early administration of epinephrine is the most crucial step.* The airway is maintained, oxygen given, circulation supported, and further mediator effects blocked. *Cardiopulmonary resuscitation is used whenever respiration or circulation is insufficient.* Cardiac monitoring and defibrillation capability are helpful in the event of a severe reaction. Similarly, the ability to intubate or create a cricothyrotomy may be lifesaving. Stabilized patients should be transported as soon as possible, by the most medically capable method available, preferably by ambulance with medical personnel in attendance. Because of the risk of subsequent delayed-onset, late-phase, or biphasic reactions, and the possibility of multiorgan injury, patients with anaphylaxis should be considered for admission to the hospital, and some authorities would make admission mandatory for all patients with anaphylaxis who receive epinephrine (66). Hospitalized patients should be monitored and observed for a minimum of 6 to 8 hours (66,41), and appropriate specialist consultations arranged.

## ACKNOWLEDGMENTS

The author thanks June L. Bianchi, Beverly J. Flynn, Nancy E. Frazier, Sally C. Schumann, and Jeanie M. Vander Pyl, Cape Cod Hospital Medical Library, for their expertise in medical literature research.

## REFERENCES

1. Chamberlain D, Fisher J, Ward M, and the Project Team of the Resuscitation Council (UK). Consensus guidelines: emergency medical treatment of anaphylactic reactions. *Resuscitation* 1999; 41:93–99.
2. Brady WJ Jr, Luber S, Joyce TP. Multiphasic anaphylaxis: report of a case with prehospital and emergency department considerations. *J Emerg Med* 1997;15:477–481.
3. Heffner D. Anaphylaxis. *Lippincott's primary care practice* 1997; 1:220–223.
4. Sampson HA. Fatal food-induced anaphylaxis. *Allergy* 1998; 53[Suppl 46]:125–130.
5. Sorensen HT, Nielsen B, Ostergaard-Nielsen J. Anaphylactic shock occurring outside hospitals. *Allergy* 1989;44:288–290.
6. Hunsaker DH. Approaches to otolaryngic allergy emergencies. *Otolaryngol Clin North Am* 1998;31:207–219.
7. Hurst DS, Gordon BR, Fornadley JA, et al. Safety of home based and office allergy immunotherapy: a multicenter prospective study *Otolaryngol Head Neck Surg* 1999;121:553–561.
8. Mabry RL, ed. *Skin endpoint titration manual.* Silver Spring, MD: American Academy of Otolaryngic Allergy, 1990.
9. Anon JB. Introduction to in vivo allergy testing. *Otolaryngol Head Neck Surg* 1993;109:593–600.
10. Fadal RG. Experience with RAST-based immunotherapy. *Otolaryngol Clin North Am* 1992;25:43–60.
11. King WP. *The intracutaneous provocative food test and neutralization treatment.* Silver Spring, MD: American Academy of Otolaryngic Allergy, 1989.
12. VanArsdel PP Jr, Sherman WB. The risk of inducing constitutional reactions in allergic patients. *J Allergy* 1957;28:251–261.
13. Norman PS, Van Metre TE Jr. The safety of allergenic immunotherapy. *J Allergy Clin Immunol* 1990;85:522–525.
14. Tinkelman DG, Cole WQ, Tunno J. Immunotherapy: a one-year prospective study to evaluate risk factors of systemic reactions. *J Allergy Clin Immunol* 1995;95:8–14.
15. Gibofsky A. Legal issues in allergy and clinical immunology. *J Allergy Clin Immunol* 1996;98:S334–S338.
16. Norman PS. Editorial: safety of allergen immunotherapy. *J Allergy Clin Immunol* 1989;84:438–439.
17. Gordon BR. Allergy skin tests and immunotherapy: comparison of methods in common use. *Ear Nose Throat J* 1990;69:47–62.
18. AMA Council on Scientific Affairs, Panel on Allergy. In vivo diagnostic testing and immunotherapy for allergy. *JAMA* 1987; 258:1363–1367.
19. Bosquet J, Michel FB. Safety considerations in assessing the role of immunotherapy in allergic disorders. *Drug Safety* 1994;10: 5–17.
20. Vervloet D, Khairallah E, Arnaud A, et al. A prospective national study of the safety of immunotherapy. *Clin Allergy* 1980;10: 59–64.
21. King HC. *An otolaryngologist's guide to allergy.* New York: Thieme Medical, 1990:175–177.
22. Lockey RF, Benedict LM, Turkeltaub PC, et al. Fatalities from immunotherapy and skin testing. *J Allergy Clin Immunol* 1987; 79:660–667.
23. U.S. Food and Drug Administration. *Reports of deaths with allergenic extracts.* FDA Drug Bulletin. Washington, DC: U.S. Government Printing Office, November 1988.
24. Hansel FK. *Allergy and immunology in otolaryngology.* Rochester, MN: American Academy of Ophthalmology and Otolaryngology, 1975.
25. Sampson HA. Peanut anaphylaxis. *J Allergy Clin Immunol* 1990; 86:1–3.
26. Sampson HA, Mendelson L, Rosen JP. Fatal and near-fatal anaphylactic reactions to food in children and adolescents. *N Engl J Med* 1992;327:380–384.
27. Settipane GA. Anaphylactic deaths in asthmatic patients. *Allergy Proc* 1989;10:271–274.
28. Ward WA Jr. Diagnostic skin testing: skin endpoint titration. In: Krause HF, ed. *Otolaryngic allergy and immunology.* Philadelphia: WB Saunders, 1989:133–140.
29. Greineder DK. Risk management in allergen immunotherapy. *J Allergy Clin Immunol* 1996;98:S330–S334.
30. Hejjaoui A, Dhivert H, Michel FB, et al. Immunotherapy with a standardized *Dermatophagoides pteronyssinus* extract: IV. systemic reactions according to the immunotherapy schedule. *J Allergy Clin Immunol* 1990;85:473–479.
31. Bousquet J, Hejjaoui A, Dhivert H, et al. Immunotherapy with a standardized *Dermatophagoides pteronyssinus* extract: III. systemic reactions during the rush protocol in patients suffering from asthma. *J Allergy Clin Immunol* 1989;83:797–802.
32. American Academy of Allergy and Immunology. The waiting period after allergen skin testing and immunotherapy. *J Allergy Clin Immunol* 1990;85:526–527.
33. Greenberg MA, Kaufman CR, Gonzalez GE, et al. Late systemic-allergic reactions to inhalant allergen immunotherapy. *J Allergy Clin Immunol* 1988;82:287–290.
34. King HC. *An otolaryngologist's guide to allergy.* New York: Thieme Medical, 1990:103.
35. Grouhi M, Alshehri M, Hummel D, et al. Anaphylaxis and epinephrine auto-injector training: who will teach the teachers? *J Allergy Clin Immunol* 1999;103:190–193.
36. Huang SW. A survey of EpiPen use in patients with a history of anaphylaxis. *J Allergy Clin Immunol* 1998;102:525–526.

37. Vickers DW, Maynard L, Ewan PW. Management of children with potential anaphylactic reactions in the community: a training package and proposal for good practice. *Clin Exp Allergy* 1997;27:898–903.

38. Sicherer SH, Forman JA, Noone SA. Use assessment of self-administered epinephrine among food-allergic children and adolescents. *Pediatrics* 2000;105:359–362.

39. James JM. Anaphylaxis: multiple etiologies—focused therapy. *J Ark Med Soc* 1996;93:281–287.

40. Wyatt R. Anaphylaxis. *Postgrad Med* 1996;100:87–99.

41. Fader DJ, Johnson TM. Medical issues and emergencies in the dermatology office. *J Am Acad Dermatol* 1998;36:1–16.

42. Freeman TM. Anaphylaxis diagnosis and treatment. *Allergy Immunol Clin North Am* 1998;25:809–817.

43. Kagy L, Blaiss MS. Anaphylaxis in children. *Pediatr Ann* 1998; 27:727–734.

44. Bedry R, Gabinski C, Paty MC. Diagnosis of scombroid poisoning by measurement of plasma histamine. *N Engl J Med* 2000; 342:520–521.

45. Naguib M, Magboul MMA. Adverse effects of neuromuscular blockers and their antagonists. *Drug Safety* 1998;18:99–116.

46. Flaherty SA. Allergic reaction to antibiotics during anesthesia: a case report. *CRNA Clin Forum Nurs Anesthetist* 1996;7: 118–125.

47. Friday GA, Fireman P. Anaphylaxis. *Ear Nose Throat J* 1996; 75:21–24.

48. Thomsen HS, Bush WH Jr. Treatment of the adverse effects of contrast media. *Acta Radiol* 1998;39:212–218.

49. Olive-Perez A. Allergy during anesthetic procedures. *Allergol Immunopathol* 1997;25:293–301.

50. Mabry RL. Management of allergic emergencies. In: Krause HF, ed. *Otolaryngic allergy and immunology.* Philadelphia: WB Saunders, 1989:297–301.

51. Frew AJ, Kay AB. Eosinophils and T-lymphocytes in late-phase allergic reactions. *J Allergy Clin Immunol* 1990;85:533–539.

52. King HC. *An otolaryngologist's guide to allergy.* New York: Thieme Medical, 1990:179.

53. Turkeltaub PC, Campbell G, Mosimann JE. Comparative safety and efficacy of short ragweed extracts differing in potency and composition in treatment of fall hay fever: use of allergenically bioequivalent doses by parallel line bioassay to evaluate comparative safety and efficacy. *Allergy* 1990;45:528–546.

54. MacIntyre D, Boyd G. Site of airflow obstruction in immediate and late reactions to bronchial challenge with *Dermatophagoides pteronyssinus. Clin Allergy* 1983;13:213–218.

55. Soto-Aguilar MC, deShazo RD, Waring NP. Anaphylaxis: why it happens and what to do about it. *Postgrad Med* 1987;82: 154–170.

56. Kniker WT. Anaphylaxis in children and adults. In: Bierman CW, Pearlman DS, eds. *Allergic diseases from infancy to adulthood.* Philadelphia: WB Saunders, 1988:667–677.

57. Fisher MM, Baldo BA. Acute anaphylactic reactions. *Med J Aust* 1988;149:34–38.

58. Schellenberg RR, Ohtaka H, Paddon HB, et al. Catecholamine responses to histamine infusion in man. *J Allergy Clin Immunol* 1991;87:499–504.

59. Dykewitz MS. Anaphylaxis and stinging insect reactions. *Comp Ther* 1996;22:579–585.

60. Brady WJ, Bright HL. Occurrence of multiphasic anaphylaxis during a transcontinental air flight. *Am J Emerg Med* 1999;17: 695–696.

61. Brazil E, MacNamara AF. "Not so immediate" hypersensitivity: the danger of biphasic anaphylactic reactions. *J Accid Emerg Med* 1998;15:252–253.

62. Paulson E. Anaphylaxis: statement on initial management in nonhospital settings. *CMAJ* 1996;154:1519–1522.

63. Patterson R, Lieberman P. Idiopathic anaphylaxis: a purely internal affair. *Hosp Pract* 1996;31:47–66.

64. Krasnick J, Patterson R, Harris KE. Idiopathic anaphylaxis: long-term follow-up, cost, and outlook. *Allergy* 1996;51: 724–731.

65. Volcheck GW, Li JTC. Exercise-induced urticaria and anaphylaxis. *Mayo Clin Proc* 1997;72:140–147.

66. Brown AFT. Therapeutic controversies in the management of acute anaphylaxis. *J Accid Emerg Med* 1998;15:89–95.

67. Toogood JH. Risk of anaphylaxis in patients receiving beta-blocker drugs. *J Allergy Clin Immunol* 1988;81:1–5.

68. Hepner MJ, Ownby DR, Anderson JA, et al. Risk of systemic reactions in patients taking beta-blocker drugs receiving allergen immunotherapy injections. *J Allergy Clin Immunol* 1990;86: 407–411.

69. Javeed N, Javeed H, Javeed S, et al. Refractory anaphylactoid shock potentiated by beta-blockers. *Cathet Cardiovasc Diagn* 1996;39:383–384.

70. Cohan RH, Leder RA, Ellis JH. Treatment of adverse reactions to radiographic contrast media in adults. *Radiol Clin North Am* 1996;34:1055–1076.

71. Cummins RO, ed. *Advanced cardiac life support 1997–1999.* Dallas: American Heart Association, 1997.

72. Hardman JG, Limbird LE, Molinoff PB, et al., eds. *Goodman and Gilman's the pharmacological basis of therapeutics,* 9th ed. New York: McGraw-Hill, 1996.

73. Seidman MD, Lewandowski CA, Sarpa JR, et al. Angioedema related to angiotensin-converting enzyme inhibitors. *Otolaryngol Head Neck Surg* 1990;102:727–731.

74. Anderson MW, deShazo RD. Studies of the mechanism of angiotensin converting enzyme (ACE) inhibitor-associated angioedema: the effect of an ACE inhibitor on cutaneous responses to bradykinin, codeine, and histamine. *J Allergy Clin Immunol* 1990;85:856–858.

75. Goldsobel AB, Rohr AS, Siegel SC, et al. Efficiency of doxepin in the treatment of chronic idiopathic urticaria. *J Allergy Clin Immunol* 1986;78:867–873.

76. Watson A. Alpha adrenergic blockers and adrenaline: a mysterious collapse. *Aust Fam Physician* 1998;27:714–715.

77. Howes L. Commentary on: alpha adrenergic blockers and adrenaline. *Aust Fam Physician* 1998;27:715.

78. Horowitz BZ, Jadallah S, Derlet RW. Fatal intracranial bleeding associated with prehospital use of epinephrine. *Ann Emerg Med* 1996;28:725–727.

79. Lundin AP, Pilkington B, Delano BG, et al. Response to inhaled beta-agonist in a patient receiving beta-adrenergic blockers. *Arch Intern Med* 1984;144:1,882–1,883.

80. Kraan J, Koeter GH, van der Mark TW, et al. Changes in bronchial hyperreactivity induced by 4 weeks of treatment with antiasthmatic drugs in patients with allergic asthma: a comparison between budesonide and terbutaline. *J Allergy Clin Immunol* 1985;76:628–636.

81. Murphy S, Kelly HW. Acute asthma in children: when first-line therapy isn't enough. *J Respir Dis* 1990;11:589.

82. Ciccolella DE, Brennan K, Kelsen SG, et al. Dose-response characteristics of nebulized albuterol in the treatment of acutely ill, hospitalized asthmatics. *J Asthma* 1999;36:539–546.

83. Heilborn H, Hjemdahl P, Daleskog M, et al. Comparison of subcutaneous injection and high-dose inhalation of epinephrine: implications for self-treatment to prevent anaphylaxis. *J Allergy Clin Immunol* 1986;78:1,174–1,179.

84. Raper RF, Fisher MM. Profound reversible myocardial depression after anaphylaxis. *Lancet* 1988;1:386–388.

85. Chrusch C, Sharma S, Unruh H, et al. Histamine H3 receptor blockade improves cardiac function in canine anaphylaxis. *Am J Respir Crit Care Med* 1999;160:1142–1149.

86. Patterson LJ, Milne B. Latex anaphylaxis causing heart block: role of ranitidine. *Can J Anaesth* 1999;46:776–778.

87. Otero E, Onufer JR, Reiss CK, et al. Anaphylaxis-induced myocardial depression treated with amrinone. *Lancet* 1991;337:682–683.

88. Bickell WH, Dice WH. Military antishock trousers in a patient with adrenergic-resistant anaphylaxis. *Ann Emerg Med* 1984;13:189–190.

89. Levi M, tenCate H. Disseminated intravascular coagulation. *N Engl J Med* 1999;341:586–592.

90. Polosa R, Phillips GD, Rajakulasingham K, et al. The effect of inhaled ipratropium bromide alone and in combination with oral terfenadine on bronchoconstriction provoked by adenosine 5′-monophosphate and histamine in asthma. *J Allergy Clin Immunol* 1991;87:939–946.

91. Beakes DE. The use of anticholinergics in asthma. *J Asthma* 1997;34:357–368.

92. Stoodley RG, Aaron SD, Dales RE. The role of ipratropium bromide in the emergency management of acute asthma exacerbation: a meta-analysis of randomized clinical trials. *Ann Emerg Med* 1999;34:8–18.

93. Zaloga GP, DeLacey W, Holmboe E, et al. Glucagon reversal of hypotension in a case of anaphylactoid shock. *Ann Intern Med* 1986;105:65–66.

94. Gavalas M, Sadana A, Metcalf S. Guidelines for the management of anaphylaxis in the emergency department. *J Accid Emerg Med* 1998;15:96–98.

95. Pollack CV. Utility of glucagon in the emergency department. *J Emerg Med* 1993;11:195–205.

96. Nannini LJ, Pedino JC, Corna RA, et al. Magnesium sulfate as a vehicle for nebulized salbutamol in acute asthma. *Am Med J* 2000;108:193–197.

97. Calhoun WJ, Bush RK. Enhanced reactive oxygen species metabolism of airspace cells and airway inflammation follow antigen challenge in human asthma. *J Allergy Clin Immunol* 1990;86:306–313.

98. Gullo A, Romano E. Naloxone and anaphylactic shock. *Lancet* 1983;1:819.

99. Chanez P, Mann C, Bosquet J, et al. Atrial natriuretic factor (ANF) is a potent bronchodilator in asthma. *J Allergy Clin Immunol* 1990;86:321–324.

100. Laviolette M, Malmstrom K, Lu S, et al. Montelukast added to inhaled beclomethasone in treatment of asthma. *Am J Respir Crit Care Med* 1999;160:1862–1868.

101. Fujimura M, Abo M, Kamio Y, et al. Effect of leukotriene and thromboxane antagonist on propranolol-induced bronchoconstriction. *Am J Respir Crit Care Med* 1999;160:2100–2103.

102. Littenberg B. Aminophylline treatment in severe, acute asthma: a meta-analysis. *JAMA* 1988;259:1678–1684.

103. Self TH, Abou-Shala N, Burns R, et al. Inhaled albuterol and oral prednisone therapy in hospitalized adult asthmatics: does aminophylline add any benefit? *Chest* 1990;98:1,317–1,321.

104. Ernst ME, Graber MA. Methylxanthine use in anaphylaxis: what does the evidence tell us? *Ann Pharmacother* 1999;33:1001–1004.

105. Davis WE, Cook PR, McKinsey JP, et al. Anaphylaxis in immunotherapy. *Otolaryngol Head Neck Surg* 1992;107:78–83.

106. Peters SP. Systemic anaphylaxis. In: Lichtenstein LM, Fauci AS, eds. *Current therapy in allergy, immunology, and rheumatology*. Philadelphia: BC Decker, 1985:75–80.

107. Weiszer I. Allergic emergencies. In: Patterson R, ed. *Allergic diseases diagnosis and management*. Philadelphia: JB Lippincott, 1985:418–439.

108. Yunginger JW, Sweeney KG, Sturner WQ, et al. Fatal food-induced anaphylaxis. *JAMA* 1988;260:1450–1452.

109. Simons FER, Roberts JR, Gu XC, et al. Epinephrine absorption in children with a history of anaphylaxis. *J Allergy Clin Immunol* 1998;101:33–37.

110. Ornato JP. High-dose epinephrine during resuscitation: a word of caution. *JAMA* 1991;265:1160–1161.

111. Clearihan L. Managing anaphylaxis in small children. *Aust Fam Physician* 1998;27:97.

112. McFadden ER Jr. Fatal and near-fatal asthma. *N Engl J Med* 1991;324:409–411.

113. Calhoun DA, Oparil S. Treatment of hypertensive crisis. *N Engl J Med* 1990;323:1177–1183.

114. Lieberman P. The use of antihistamines in the prevention and treatment of anaphylaxis and anaphylactoid reactions. *J Allergy Clin Immunol* 1990;86:684–686.

115. Sullivan TJ. Dr. Sullivan's response to Dr. Toogood's editorial. *J Allergy Clin Immunol* 1989;83:706–707.

116. Chapman KR, Verbeek PR, White JG, et al. Effect of a short course of prednisone in the prevention of early relapse after the emergency room treatment of acute asthma. *N Engl J Med* 1991;324:788–794.

117. Jantz MA, Sahn SA. Corticosteroids in acute respiratory failure. *Am J Respir Crit Care Med* 1999;160:1079–1100.

118. Bonner JR. Anaphylaxis part II: prevention and treatment. *Ala J Med Sci* 1988;25:408–411.

119. Dolowitz DA, Dougherty TF. Allergy as inflammatory reactions. *Ann Allergy* 1971;29:410–417.

120. Dolowitz DA, Dougherty TF. The use of heparin in control of allergies. *Ann Allergy* 1965;23:309–313.

121. Gang V, Gaubitz W, Gunzer U. Postheparin-diamine oxidase (histaminase) in anaphylaxis. *Klin Wochenschr* 1975;53:285–287.

122. Ferrell WJ, Jabs CM, Robb HJ, et al. Comparative study of blood clotting factors in anaphylactic and primary and secondary endotoxin shock. *Ann Clin Lab Sci* 1983;13:291–298.

123. Gervin AS. Complications of heparin therapy. *Surg Gynecol Obstet* 1975;140:789–796.

124. Dhar HL, Mukherjee B, Sanyal RK. The effect of heparin on the heart in anaphylaxis. *Am Heart J* 1967;74:489–495.

125. Boyle JP, Smart RH, Shirley JK. Heparin in the treatment of chronic obstructive bronchopulmonary disease. *Am J Cardiol* 1964;14:25–28.

126. Dougherty TF, Dolowitz DA. Physiologic actions of heparin not related to blood clotting. *Am J Cardiol* 1964;14:18–24.

127. Letourneau MA, Schuh S. Respiratory disorders. In: Barkin RM, ed. *Pediatric emergency medicine*, 2nd ed. St. Louis: Mosby 1997:1056–1126.

128. Serwonska MH, Frick OL. Anti-anaphylactic activity of glucagon in guinea pigs with beta-adrenergic blockade. *J Allergy Clin Immunol* 1988;81:238.

129. Jerrard DA. ED management of insect stings. *Am J Emerg Med* 1996;14:429–433.

130. Rolla G, Bucca C. Magnesium, beta-agonists, and asthma. *Lancet* 1988;1:989.

131. Skobeloff EM, Spivey WH, McNamara RM, et al. Intravenous magnesium sulfate for the treatment of acute asthma in the emergency department. *JAMA* 1989;262:1210–1213.

132. Bucca C, Rolla G, Oliva A, et al. Effect of vitamin C on histamine bronchial responsiveness of patients with allergic rhinitis. *Ann Allergy* 1990;65:311–314.

133. Pauling LC. *How to live longer and feel better.* New York: Avon Books, 1986:100–101.

134. Rivers JM. Safety of high-level vitamin C ingestion. *Ann NY Acad Sci* 1987;498:445–453.

# SKIN TESTING IN THE DIAGNOSIS OF INHALANT ALLERGY

## JOHN A. FORNADLEY

Skin testing is widely used as a diagnostic technique for the evaluation of inhalant allergy. Skin tests have been demonstrated to be reliable and safe indicators of antigen sensitivity and have therefore been widely accepted. The purpose of this chapter is to present the available forms of skin testing, to indicate how each is properly performed, and to review their relative advantages and disadvantages.

## HISTORY OF SKIN TESTING

Skin testing techniques have been used in the diagnosis of inhalant allergy over the past 100 years. Testing was first attempted by Blackley in 1872, who applied a grass pollen extract to excoriated skin and observed for the skin's reactivity to this extract (1). These techniques were then adapted by Noon and others, who used various techniques to assess allergic sensitivity (2,3).

In the 1930s, Hansel and Rinkel further adapted these prior techniques, using a progressive dilutional intradermal test that they argued was a superior methodology in that it offered both qualitative and quantitative assessments of allergenicity. Hansel introduced a systemic approach to serial testing of antigens using 1:10 dilutions injected in a sequential pattern intradermally (4). This technique was further refined by Rinkel, who introduced the 1:5 system of serial dilutions currently used in clinical practice (5). These techniques, among others, are reviewed in this chapter.

## SKIN TESTING TYPES

The earliest forms of allergy testing involved placing antigen onto skin that was abraded to bypass the keratin layer. A response was then assessed from the reaction of the skin to

**J. A. Fornadley:** Department of Surgery, Division of Otolaryngology, Pennsylvania State University, Hershey, Pennsylvania.

the antigen. Although critical refinements have occurred in the technique, this principle of assessing the skin's reactivity remains at the core of all skin testing. Practitioners of allergy will continue to debate which of the various "improvements" truly represents the most satisfactory testing method.

## Scratch Testing

The direct descendant of the earliest allergy testing methods is the *scratch test* technique. A 2-mm superficial skin cut is created to remove the upper layers of keratin. A drop of test antigen concentrate is placed onto this partially denuded epidermis. After a period of 10 to 20 minutes, a response is recorded based on the wheal and flare of the skin around the site. The partial removal of keratinized skin and epidermis allows a greater response than would be possible with an intact skin layer, adding sensitivity to the test. As with all later forms of skin testing, a positive and negative control test is performed in conjunction with antigen testing to ensure that the skin reaction accurately represents a response to the antigen. The positive control commonly is histamine. The negative control is saline, usually containing whatever preservative is being used in the antigen vials. If the skin is underresponsive owing to medication or chronic disease, the positive test does not elicit a reaction. On the other hand, hyperresponsiveness such as dermatographia demonstrates a positive response even with the negative control. Placement of an antigen to which the patient is not sensitive should elicit no greater response than the negative control. An antigen to which the patient has developed a significant allergy should elicit a skin response similar to the positive control.

Scratch testing has been demonstrated to present a very low likelihood of causing a serious local or systemic reaction, even if the patient is markedly allergic to the antigen (6). This wide margin of safety results from the antigen being placed on an abrasion that is very superficial. Because scratch testing enjoyed familiarity as the oldest technique, and had a satisfactory safety profile, the test continued to be used throughout most of the 20th century. Unfortunately, this technique lacks both the sensitivity and specificity to remain a viable testing alternative. An unacceptably high false-negative rate (low sensitivity) results from the superficial scratch, which allows the remaining epithelium to block a positive response. These patients therefore will be diagnosed as nonallergic when they are in fact allergic. In addition, specificity also is lost because the trauma of the scratch is sufficient to create a localized inflammatory response. This may incorrectly identify a patient as allergic when no such allergy exists (false positive).

Better techniques exist with comparable safety, and because of the poor sensitivity and specificity of scratch testing, the American Medical Association (AMA) Council on Scientific Affairs recommends against the use of this technique (7).

## Skin Prick Testing

Skin prick testing (SPT) represents a significant advance beyond scratch testing, and is one of the major testing techniques used in contemporary allergy diagnosis. It was introduced in the 1920s, and gained wide popularity in the 1970s (8). A variety of different prick testing techniques have been described in the literature. This broad, "umbrella" term has been extended to include several different techniques. An example of the technique is presented.

A drop of the test antigen concentrate is placed onto the subject's skin. A solid needle is passed through the drop into the skin, entering a known, controlled distance into the epidermis. The needle may reach the dermal–epidermal junction, but the dermis is not entered. The antigen concentrate is introduced into this puncture by the passage of the needle. This technique has been modified to include the use of multitest devices that deliver the antigen into several sites at once with equal pressure (9) (Fig. 8.1).

Prick testing is rapid and allows multiple antigens to be evaluated in a relatively short time. Results can be read and interpreted within 10 minutes of the test. Although concentrated antigen is used, the controlled depth and small quantity of antigen delivered into the skin ensures that the antigen load delivered is small enough and placed correctly to yield an acceptable level of safety. The risk of severe localized or systemic reaction is greater than with scratch testing, but remains low because the antigen does not enter the more vascular dermal layer.

The prick testing technique allows a rapid, reasonably sensitive method for evaluation of moderate to high levels of inhalant allergy. A large number of antigens (often 20 to 30 or more) can be assessed in a single session, if indicated. Patients with low levels of sensitivity may not be identified by this technique, even if the antigen is clinically significant to the symptom complex. Other methods, such as the intradermal technique discussed later, are required to detect patients with lower levels of sensitivity (10). Advantages of SPT include safety and rapidity. The means by which SPT can be used to initiate allergy immunotherapy are discussed later in this chapter.

A major disadvantage of SPT involves the possibility of missing clinically significant low-sensitivity antigens, requiring intradermal techniques to improve diagnostic efficiency. Dermatographic skin responses can create false-posi-

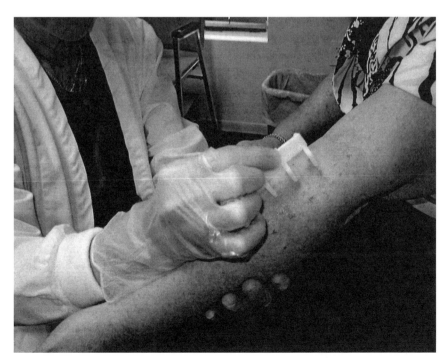

**FIG. 8.1.** Multitest device being used for multiple prick testing.

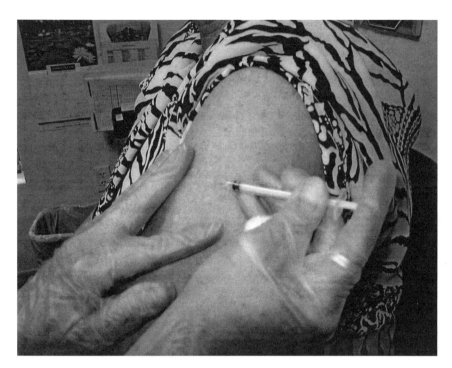

**FIG. 8.2.** Intradermal wheal being applied to the upper arm.

tive reactions or simply confound interpretation of the test. The risk of anaphylaxis is small but present. In addition, patients must be off all antihistamines for an appropriate time (7 to 10 days for long-acting antihistamines) before testing. When advantages and disadvantages are carefully considered, SPT emerges as a reasonable clinical modality in appropriate situations. Variations on this testing technique are in routine use throughout the United States.

## Intradermal Testing

Intradermal testing refers to the placement of antigen below the epidermal layer of skin (Fig. 8.2). Placing a known quantity of antigen into the dermis yields a test response that is more reproducible and provides a higher sensitivity than the more superficial skin testing techniques (11). Unfortunately, this method also has the potential to cause adverse reactions that are more frequent and of greater severity owing to the placement of antigen into the vascular dermal layer.

Intradermal testing has been extensively performed using two very different algorithms. Although both involve placement of antigen into the dermal layer, the differences in the testing situations and philosophies are great enough that these testing techniques are treated separately.

## Intradermal Testing After Skin Prick Testing

There are times when the history strongly suggests an allergy, yet the SPT result is negative. Because of this recog-

nized limitation of SPT, there is a need to identify patients with lower but still clinically important sensitivities. Intradermal testing provides a higher level of sensitivity by placing antigen into the dermal layer. Intradermal injection of concentrate is not an acceptable technique for initial testing because the risk of anaphylactic reaction from direct intradermal injection is unacceptably high. A safe initial technique, such as SPT or skin endpoint titration (SET; discussed later) must be used. These forms of testing provide an important safeguard that the patient will not react adversely to the intradermal injection, paving the way for the relatively safe use of intradermal testing. The advantage of this combination technique is that it combines the rapid screening evaluation of SPT with the much more sensitive intradermal technique.

There also are disadvantages to allergy testing with this technique. First is the reliance on the specificity of prick testing. Unless each antigen that is reported negative by SPT is subsequently tested by intradermal means, there is the potential that a significant sensitivity will be missed. Certainly, it is important to include patient history when determining allergic sensitivities, but a patient may be unaware of the relationship of a given antigen to symptoms, or the relationship could fail to be appreciated because of other, more obvious antigens. Another concern is that there are underlying vagaries of skin testing, including dermatographia, histamine release due to anxiety, and technical error that results in failure to deliver antigen to the correct level in appropriate quantities (12). All of these problems can limit the effectiveness of the sequential SPT–intradermal technique. Idiosyncratic reactions also can interfere with the testing process. In these reactions, termed a *flash responses,* the magnitude of the response to the isolated skin test suggests a far higher level of antigen sensitivity than actually exists. This may be due to cross-reactivity to a food or inhalant antigen, or it may be an idiopathic response.

## Skin Endpoint Titration

The other type of intradermal testing uses a very different algorithm, and is appropriately considered an entirely different testing system. This testing technique has been descriptively termed the *serial intradermal dilution technique,* alternatively known as *skin endpoint titration* (13). It is an approved testing modality of the AMA Council on Scientific Affairs (7). SET allows allergy tests to be safely per-

formed using only intradermal injections. This technique relies on the use of multiple dilutions of concentrate for the intradermal testing process. The margin of safety is provided by starting the testing series at an extremely dilute level of antigen, and progressing to more concentrated injections in a sequential process. By starting with an extremely dilute preparation, testing begins at a level where no anaphylactic response has been reported, even with the intradermal injection technique. If no response or a minimal response is identified after the skin has been observed for 10 minutes, a fivefold stronger dilution is placed. Sensitivity to a specific antigen is determined when the wheal of the injected antigen grows a minimum of 2 mm within the 10 minutes, and is confirmed by an additional 2 mm of growth with the next more concentrated antigen (Fig. 8.3). An *endpoint* therefore is defined as the dilution that initiates progressive

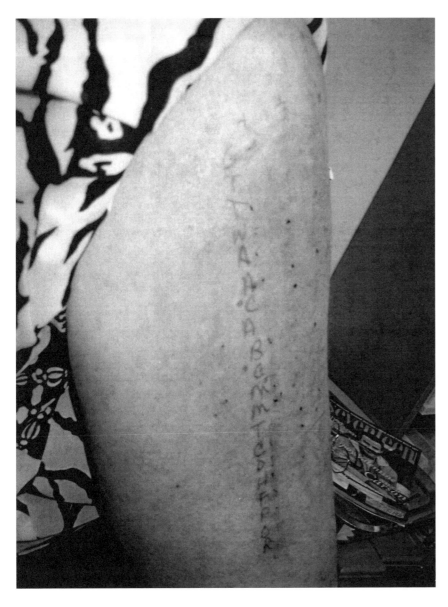

**FIG. 8.3.** Progressive whealing with skin endpoint titration.

positive whealing and is followed by confirmatory progressive whealing.

The advantage of the technique is that SET determines not only presence of an allergic response, but the patient's level of sensitivity for the test antigen. This protocol is accurate enough to allow the preparation of a desensitization regimen based on the level of sensitivity identified (14). Prospective studies have demonstrated the efficacy of immunotherapy based on SET (15).

Disadvantages of SET include the time and expense required to complete testing, given that several injections are required for each antigen tested. As with SPT, the patient must be removed from antihistamines, tricyclic antidepressants, or other medications that may limit skin response to antigen. The test can be compromised by dermatographia, but idiosyncratic or flash responses are detected by failure of the antigen to provide a normal pattern of responses with titration.

## SPECIFIC TESTING METHODOLOGIES

### Skin Prick Testing

A number of different prick test devices are commercially available. All are based on the principles discussed previously. A single generic technique is described, along with a common variation.

The patient arrives in the testing room and is positively identified. Assurance is obtained that all antihistamines or similar medications that interfere with the skin response have been stopped sufficiently in advance of the test. It also is verified that new medications have not been started that could affect the testing process. Such medications include β-blockers, which affect the safety of injection testing. The skin is clean and free of lotions, glove powder, and the like. Testing begins with a negative and positive control. One drop of saline and one drop of histamine are placed on the skin, and the planned site is marked with ink. A lancet needle is passed through this drop at a near vertical angle and is allowed to tent up the skin and enter the epidermis, and is then withdrawn. The needle is wiped between injections or, ideally, a new needle is used for each test, and the drop is then wiped away with care to avoid contact with other prick test sites. Alternatively, other devices can be used for prick testing, such as the Morrow-Brown needle (Antigen Laboratories, Liberty, MO) or the Duotip needle (Lincoln Diagnostics, Decatur, IL).

After assurance of an appropriate positive and negative response, the actual testing begins. Marks are placed on the patient's test site, usually the arms or back. One drop of the appropriate antigen diluted at 1:100 w/v is placed adjacent to each mark. A smooth, repetitive motion is developed to place the lancet through each antigen, tent the skin, withdraw the lancet, and clean it before the next prick test antigen. The antigen drops are wiped way at the end, and 10

**TABLE 8.1. GRADING SCALE FOR SKIN PRICK TESTING**

| Grade | Erythema |
|-------|----------|
| 0 | 0–10 mm |
| 1 | 11–20 mm |
| 2 | 21–30 mm |
| 3 | 31–40 mm |
| 4 | >40 mm |

minutes elapse between injection and interpretation. The test results are evaluated according the wheal-and-flare response.

One major variation that fits the definition of SPT is the use of individual antigen wells into which the needle is placed, then withdrawn, taking a tiny drop of antigen with it to the skin. Some of these devices have been adapted to perform multiple tests in one motion, such as the Multi-Test device (Lincoln Diagnostics). These variations still meet the criteria of a needle passing through a drop of concentrated antigen to enter the skin above the level of the dermis. This testing involves some additional expense for the testing devices, but may provide more reproducible results by being less technician dependent (9).

Common errors in SPT include placing the needle too deep, with subsequent bleeding and excessively deep insertion of antigen. Alternatively, insufficient penetration of the skin and superficial antigen deposition may occur. Careless wiping of the lancet can cause the antigen to contact other test areas, resulting in a skew of results. Technician variability also can occur because there is a learning curve to development of a smooth, repeatable motion for the testing process.

Skin prick testing is graded on a scale of 1 to 4 (Table 8.1).

### Translation of Skin Prick Testing to Immunotherapy

Allergy immunotherapy can be initiated using the results of SPT, but must begin at a very dilute level because the precise sensitivity of each antigen is not known. A relatively wide range of sensitivity may exist among antigens having a positive SPT, but for safety it is necessary to start all antigens at a safe dilution level. Some practitioners divide the semiquantitative results into high- and low-sensitivity groups, but in general, antigens are started uniformly at a safe, dilute level. Because antigen sensitivities vary, the more sensitive antigens reach a clinically significant level first, whereas antigens with lesser sensitivity do not provoke an immunotherapeutic response for a much longer time. As the concentration of immunotherapy is gradually increased, any antigens present with greater sensitivity may create a skin reaction before another antigen reaches an effective concentration. As immunotherapy approaches the endpoint of maximally tolerated antigen dose, or the dose of maximal symptom relief, one antigen may reach this level before the other antigens have been advanced sufficiently to provide maximal relief. This disparity may limit the efficacy of the therapy by not advancing the dose to the maximum level for all antigens. Precise dose calculation is covered in another chapter, but it can be seen that a relatively long time will elapse before the dose of immunotherapy reaches a therapeutic level for all antigens.

As an alternate technique, SPT can be used as a screening test and SET used for definitive testing before immunotherapy.

## Methodology of Skin Endpoint Titration

Before SET can be performed, the antigen must be diluted to allow safe serial titration. The method of diluting antigens from concentrate bears additional discussion.

The dilutions used to provide safe intradermal dilution testing are readily created and safely maintained on a mixing board (Fig. 8.4). Along one side, each concentrate is placed. Sequential 1:5 dilutions from concentrate are placed in succeeding rows beginning next to the concentrate.

A positive and negative control is placed, using a #3 dilution of histamine for the positive control and phenolated saline diluent for the negative control. If the hista-

mine control demonstrates positive whealing within 10 minutes, the first intradermal test is applied. Conservative SET techniques use a #6 dilution (1:312,500 w/v) of the selected antigen. A small quantity of approximately 0.05 to 1 mL is drawn into a syringe with a 26-gauge TB-type needle. The precise quantity in the syringe is not critical because the injection is not based on the quantity of fluid, but rather the size of the wheal created. The needle is placed into the dermal layer, and antigen is injected to create a 4-mm wheal (Fig. 8.5). Practice results in the creation of a smooth, round wheal without injecting too superficially or deeply, and without irregularities or "pseudopods" extending out from the wheal. After 10 minutes, the wheal is observed. If the wheal has not increased in size by at least 2 mm, the wheal is considered negative, and a second wheal of the next higher dilution is placed. If the wheal has grown more than 2 mm, but has not developed into a large (>13 mm) reaction, this is recorded, and a second wheal also is placed. If a major reaction occurs, no further wheals are placed.

The following illustrations demonstrate the possible outcomes of SET and their interpretations.

Negative titration

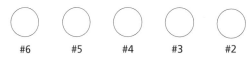

#6    #5    #4    #3    #2

The sequential injections (termed *titration*) proceed to the #2 dilution without any change of greater than 2 mm. The patient is considered not to be allergic to this antigen.

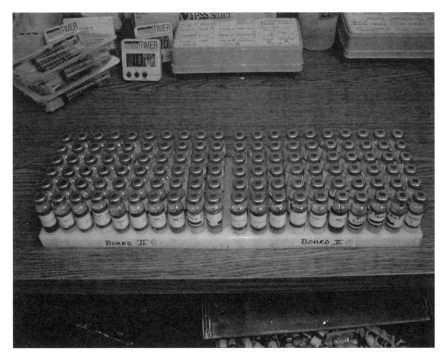

**FIG. 8.4.** Testing boards for skin endpoint titration (SET).

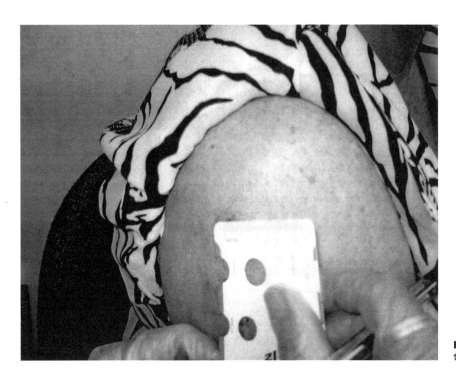

**FIG. 8.5.** A 4-mm wheal being measured on the skin.

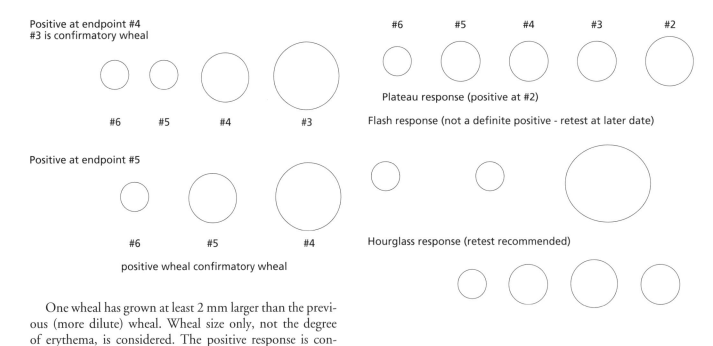

Positive at endpoint #4
#3 is confirmatory wheal

#6  #5  #4  #3

Positive at endpoint #5

#6  #5  #4

positive wheal confirmatory wheal

#6  #5  #4  #3  #2

Plateau response (positive at #2)

Flash response (not a definite positive - retest at later date)

Hourglass response (retest recommended)

One wheal has grown at least 2 mm larger than the previous (more dilute) wheal. Wheal size only, not the degree of erythema, is considered. The positive response is confirmed by the next more concentrated wheal growing by at least an additional 2 mm. The first wheal to increase by 2 mm is termed the *endpoint wheal,* whereas the second is termed the *confirmatory wheal.*

Plateau response (negative)

## Abnormal Responses

Sometimes the skin does not demonstrate one of the normal patterns. The most likely abnormal response is a *flash response,* with one dilution creating a dramatic wheal not forecast by the prior injections. This flash response does not indicate endpoint sensitivity, and should never be used in dose calculation for immunotherapy; it is not even a specific indicator of allergic disease. This antigen should be titrated again at a later date. When such a false response occurs, the likelihood of another titration yielding abnormal responses is increased. If a second abnormal titration response is identified, testing should be concluded for the day.

The *hourglass response* shows an increased size of one wheal, but the next more concentrated wheal is smaller, not larger. The larger wheal is not considered an endpoint. It is reasonable to continue the titration further to detect an endpoint. The presumption is that the abnormal response is due to spread of antigen into the dermal layers, or increased injection quantity. However, if further abnormal responses occur, testing should be concluded for the day.

The *plateau response* is another abnormal titration result. In this case, an enlarged wheal is followed by one or more wheals that continue at the same size without increasing. If a larger wheal eventually occurs, as noted in the illustration, the endpoint is defined as the final wheal to have increased by at least 2 mm before the larger confirmatory wheal.

### Shortcuts Involving Skin Endpoint Titration Testing

The term *shortcut* often carries a negative connotation by implying that a technique may "cut corners," adversely affecting patient care. This is not true of the steps discussed here. The SET method was presented in its strict, standard format for illustration purposes. If SET were performed exactly as described in the preceding section, it would be a prolonged, expensive technique with much wasted time.

### Shortcut 1

It is reasonable to titrate several different antigens at the same time, rather than completing a single antigen before proceeding to the next one. The arm is marked for identification purposes, and different antigens are simultaneously placed. By convention, the antigens are placed vertically, and the different dilutions of each antigen proceed across a horizontal line.

### Shortcut 2

A complete SET series includes an endpoint wheal and a confirmatory wheal; it should be evident that when the initial (#6) dilution is negative, it is safe to "skip" to an injection two dilutions more concentrated. If this "skip" dilution does not grow by at least 2 mm, an additional skip to two dilutions more concentrated can be accomplished. If the dilution shows growth of 2 mm, suggesting that it may be an endpoint, then the immediate next more concentrated dilution is placed. If the dilution increases by 4 mm or greater, then the wheal is suspected of being a confirmatory wheal, and the "skipped" dilution is placed.

### Advanced Shortcut 3

Because the #6 dilution is a safe starting point and rarely an endpoint, the #4 should be, at most, the confirmatory

wheal. Some have advocated shortening SET further. Carefully selected, nonasthmatic patients may be safely tested for antigens that are not currently in season by using the following technique. A #4 dilution (1:12,500 w/v) is placed, and if no response occurs in 10 minutes, a #2 (1:500 w/v) is placed. If no response is noted, the titration is completed and the patient is considered not allergic to the antigen. If a response is seen, the other dilutions are placed, and the titration read as in the traditional fashion. Certainly this technique increases the potential for adverse reactions, and therefore should be used, if at all, by experienced testers with informed, carefully selected patients.

## SCREENING FOR ALLERGIES USING SKIN TESTING

The performance of screening tests for allergic disease is a topic of some controversy. A successful screening test sacrifices a small amount of sensitivity or specificity to provide inexpensive, more rapid identification of atopic patients. Skin testing for allergy screening has been described in both SET and SPT formats. SPT allows rapid testing of a wide spectrum of antigens. SPT, as noted previously, fails to identify antigens with low sensitivity, but identifies most positives with clinical significance. The "screening" portion of SPT techniques is the actual testing, because SPT involves placing a relatively large number of antigens common to the environment or suspect based on history onto the test arm for evaluation. Follow-up testing of related antigens or intradermal testing for highly suspect antigens follows this initial screening test. Screening with SPT therefore involves performing a panel of prick tests to assess whether the patient is allergic at a moderate to high sensitivity. As noted, this protocol does not allow a quantitative view of individual allergens, but does permit rapid insight as to whether the person is atopic.

Skin endpoint titration involves a much greater time investment in testing for each antigen, and there is no convenient way dramatically to shorten the time beyond the shortcuts mentioned previously. Instead, SET screening uses relatively few antigens. These antigens are chosen as the most common representatives of pollens, epidermals, and dusts in the geographic area. The SET panel can identify even subtle atopy by screening for key antigens in each category. This method takes advantage of the phenomenon of related antigen cross-reactivity. Cross-reactivity is the tendency of closely related antigens to have similar antigen–antibody binding sites. A patient who screens negative to the most common grass, tree, weed, mold, dander, and dust antigens is very unlikely to have a significant inhalant allergy contribution to his or her symptom complex from the less common antigens in these classes. Because of this phenomenon, it is important critically to examine even very slight positive responses because these may represent cross-reactivity, and further testing of related antigens is required to ascertain which species provides the dominant allergen. Screening may include specific antigens that appear in a patient's history. Grasses, such as timothy and June, share sufficient antigenic sites that a patient who has developed an allergy to June grass may give a positive reaction to a skin test for timothy. Because of the ability of SET to identify even low-sensitivity responses, a screening test can use one or two antigens in a class. A positive response indicates a need to test further based on history and the types of antigen available in the geographic area. Cross-reactivity works well for most pollen families, particularly grasses. An example of SET screening based on cross-reactivity would include one or two grasses common to the area, two to three trees, two or more weeds, a selection of appropriate molds, one dust or dust mite, and epidermals such as cat, dog, or other appropriate animal dander. This method is an effective screening tool for allergic disease. Positive findings are evaluated by expanding the testing to determine which antigen is the most reactive. Chapter 9, *In Vitro Testing of Inhalant Allergy,* discusses the phenomenon of cross-reactivity in greater detail.

Positive findings in each category trigger follow-up SET for other suspect antigens in this group. Because SET is performed using the same algorithm for screening as for complete testing, the tests that show positive demonstrate the actual endpoint and do not need to be repeated.

## Desensitization Plan Based on Skin Testing

After skin testing, patients with appropriate indications may be considered for desensitization immunotherapy. Calculation of desensitization therapy varies based on the type of allergy testing that was selected.

If SPT is the testing performed, only the qualitative level of sensitivities of each antigen is known. In this situation, immunotherapy must begin with extremely dilute serum (to diminish the risk of an anaphylactic reaction). The qualitative responses can be categorized according to "high" and "low" sensitivity, divided by the amount of skin response noted to the testing. This semiquantitative calculation is a reasonable, acceptable technique in routine contemporary use. An argument can be made that the initiation of injections at such a dilute level may delay the efficacy of desensitization therapy, and may lack the safety of other methods. Nonetheless, the procedure is time tested and efficacious.

The other option available for patients who have been tested by SPT is to perform SET or in vitro testing to obtain more accurate knowledge of the level of antigen sensitivity, as noted later.

When allergy testing is performed using SET, the actual level of sensitivity of each antigen is known. Each antigen can be mixed into a desensitization vial according to the level of sensitivity, allowing the immunotherapy to be indi-

vidualized according to how sensitive the patient is to each antigen. This permits therapy for each antigen to be initiated individually at the level of the patient's sensitivity. This is discussed further in Chapter 12.

## SAFETY OF SKIN TESTING

Safety is a critical issue in skin testing. Fatalities have been reported with both prick and intradermal tests, and are directly related to the quantity of antigen introduced. For that reason, SPT usually is conducted before single-dilution intradermal tests are used. With SET, very dilute intradermal injections are used initially to reduce the likelihood of serious systemic reactions. Serious reactions with SET therefore are uncommon (16). Even very dilute injections of antigenic sera, however, can elicit anaphylactic reactions in susceptible people. Any office that performs skin testing therefore must be adequately equipped and prepared to treat these untoward reactions. A discussion of the treatment of systemic reactions with skin testing and immunotherapy is provided in Chapter 7.

When practiced consistently, and when following guidelines adopted by national organizations such as the American Academy of Otolaryngic Allergy, (17) skin testing is a safe and effective means of assessing a patient's reactivity to suspected antigens and of guiding the initiation of desensitization immunotherapy.

## REFERENCES

1. Blackley CH. *Experimental researches on the causes and nature of cattarrhus aestivus.* London: Balliere, Trindall, & Cox, 1873.
2. Noon L. Prophylactic inoculation against hayfever. *Lancet* 1911; 1:1572–1573.
3. Cooke RA. The treatment of hayfever by active immunization. *Laryngoscope* 1915;25:108–112.
4. Hansel FK. *Allergies of the nose and paranasal sinuses.* St. Louis: Mosby, 1936.
5. Rinkel HJ. Management of clinical allergy: II. ideologic factors in skin titration. *Arch Otolaryngol* 1963;77:42–75.
6. Gordon BR. Allergy skin tests for inhalants and foods: comparison of methods in common use. *Otolaryngol Clin North Am* 1998; 31:35–54.
7. American Medical Association Council on Scientific Affairs, Panel on Allergy. In vivo diagnostic testing and immunotherapy for allergy. *JAMA* 1987;258:1363–1367.
8. Pepys J. Skin testing. *Br J Hosp Med* 1975;10[Suppl]:1–59.
9. Kniker WT. Multi-test skin testing in allergy: a review of published findings. *Ann Allergy* 1993;71:485–491.
10. Nelson HS. Diagnostic procedures in allergy: I. allergy skin testing. *Ann Allergy* 1983;51:411–417.
11. Kniker WT, Hales SW, Lee LK. Diagnostic methods to demonstrate IgE antibodies: skin testing techniques. *Bull NY Acad Med* 1981;57:524–528.
12. Gordon BR. Allergy skin tests and immunotherapy: comparison of methods in common use. *Ear Nose Throat J* 1990;69:47–62.
13. Mabry RL, ed. *Skin endpoint titration.* New York: Thieme Medical, 1992.
14. King HC. Skin endpoint titration: still the standard? *Otolaryngol Clin North Am* 1992;25:13–26.

15. Krouse JH, Krouse HJ. Efficacy of immunotherapy based on skin endpoint titration. *Otolaryngol Head Neck Surg* 2000;123: 133–137.
16. Hurst DS, Gordon BR, Fornadley JA, et al. Safety of home-based and office allergy immunotherapy: a multicenter prospective study. *Otolaryngol Head Neck Surg* 1999;121:553–561.
17. Fornadley JA, Corey JP, Osguthorpe JD, et al. Allergic rhinitis: clinical practice guideline. Committee on Practice Standards, American Academy of Otolaryngic Allergy. *Otolaryngol Head Neck Surg* 1996;115:115–122.

## BIBLIOGRAPHY

**Goldman JL, ed.** *The principles and practice of rhinology.* New York: John Wiley & Sons, 1987.

**King HC.** *An otolaryngologist's guide to allergy.* New York: Thieme Medical, 1990.

**Krause HF, ed.** *Otolaryngic allergy and immunology.* Philadelphia: WB Saunders, 1989.

**Middleton E, Reed CE, Ellis EF, et al., eds.** *Allergy principles and practice,* 4th ed. St. Louis: Mosby, 1993.

# IN VITRO TESTING FOR ALLERGIES

## IVOR EMANUEL

This chapter discusses the current status of in vitro testing for allergen-specific immunoglobulin E (IgE) and examines various applications of this technology in routine clinical practice. The clinical benefits derived from the identification and quantitation of specific IgE, the standardization of diagnostic techniques, the interpretation of data, and the role of these measurements in diagnosis of atopic manifestations also are discussed.

The purpose of in vivo testing is to demonstrate the presence of IgE antibodies in the serum and thereby establish that sensitization to an allergen has occurred. This technique can provide the basis for an etiologic diagnosis of allergic diseases that most commonly affect the tissues of the respiratory tract, but can also involve the conjunctiva, skin, or the gastrointestinal tract. In addition, most cases of systemic anaphylaxis are precipitated through allergic mechanisms based on IgE antibodies.

## HISTORY OF IN VITRO TESTING

No description of the use of in vitro allergy testing would be complete without a brief overview of the history leading to the development of the assays in current use. In 1921, Prausnitz and Kuster first demonstrated that skin-sensitizing activity could be passively transferred from people with allergy to those without allergy. The active substance in the serum thought to be responsible for this reaginic activity was termed *reagin*. It was not until the 1960s, when new techniques for fractionation and definition of proteins were developed, that it became clear that "reagin" was an immunoglobulin. In 1966, through the efforts of the Ishizakas in the United States (1) and Johansson and Bennich in Sweden (2), this immunoglobulin ultimately was identified as representing a unique class of immunoglobulin, thereafter called *IgE*. Early in the following year, Johansson et al. developed

the first radioimmunoassay for detecting IgE, the radioallergosorbent test (RAST) (2).

The principle of the RAST involves the performance of a typical sandwich assay. The allergen preparation is chemically linked to a solid-phase support (a paper disk in the original assay). The allergen on the solid phase is then incubated with the patient's serum. If IgE antibodies are present in the serum sample, their Fab portion binds with the allergen, which in turn is chemically bound to the solid phase. After the first step of the test, the solid phase is washed to remove all the nonspecific IgE to that particular allergen. In the second step, the allergen–antibody complex thus created is incubated with a readable marker. This marker was originally a radioactive isotope I-125. After the second incubation, all the free marked anti-IgE is removed. Any IgE left on the solid phase binds with the marked anti-IgE, forming a new complex, which is then measured.

In the original RAST assay, the solid phase was a paper disk with the allergen covalently linked with cyanogen bromide, and the readable marker was a radioisotope. The results were then read on a gamma counter. In the specific IgE assays that have been developed subsequently, different solid phases have been used, such as various plastic polymers, cellulose sponge, and even a liquid preparation. In addition, various forms of enzymatic markers, read by calorimetry, immunofluorescence, and spectrophotometry, have replaced radioisotopes. Today's computerized assays are almost fully automated and hands-free. As a result, the original 2- or 3-day test has been shortened to less than 3 hours. Better technology regarding allergen binding has increased the sensitivity of the solid phase, without losing specificity and with much less nonspecific IgE binding. Therefore, most of the new assays for the measurement of specific IgE are more efficient and sensitive than the original RAST assay without any loss of specificity.

In the mid-1970s, there was only one in vitro allergy diagnostic assay, the Phadebas RAST (Pharmacia Diagnostics, Uppsala, Sweden). Investigators had reported good correlation between RAST scores and the allergy history, response to allergen challenge, and serial endpoint titration. In 1975, Kelso and colleagues (3), writing about RAST

**I. Emanuel:** Affiliate, University of California Teaching Hospitals and California Pacific Medical Center, San Francisco, California.

use in allergy management, stated " . . . the introduction of RAST has been a milestone in the transition of allergy from a practice based on definitive biochemical information derived from the clinical chemistry laboratory." Unfortunately, in the late 1970s and early 1980s, an era of controversy arose over the value of RAST. Its conservative cutoff point, which allowed for a large number of false-negative results compared with skin testing, hampered the use of the Phadebas RAST in the United States. These results led to much controversy over the assay's clinical usefulness, and the decreased sensitivity of the Phadebas RAST is still widely used as an argument by those physicians who prefer skin testing over in vitro testing. The controversy occurred because of the lower sensitivity of the Phadebas RAST.

The original RAST test had four reagenic reference standards. Standard A [50 Phadebas RAST Units (PRU)], taken from pooled serum from patients highly sensitive to birch pollen; standard B (a fivefold dilution of A); standard C (a fivefold dilution of B); and standard D (a twofold dilution of C). The original scoring system, based on the use of these reference standards and a cutoff of 1.0 PRU, was found to be poorly sensitive to clinical allergy. In 1980, as a result of these findings and in response to the assay's poor sensitivity, a new Phadebas RAST was introduced, with a new cutoff point set at 0.35 PRU (4) (Fig. 9.1). In Europe, this new cutoff point was accepted as sufficient to differentiate atopic from nonatopic patients. Unfortunately, this new cutoff level did not solve the sensitivity concerns in the United States, where the assay was still deemed to have less sensitivity than skin testing.

This lesser sensitivity led directly to the development of the Modified RAST Test (MRT) by Fadal and Nalebuff in the late 1970s (5). With procedural and interpretive changes, they effectively increased the sensitivity of the

RAST without significantly decreasing its specificity. Several changes were incorporated into the performance of the test that increased its sensitivity. First, the initial incubation period was increased from 3 to 18 hours. In addition, to guarantee that the allergen disk was kept moist through the entire incubation, the volume of the test serum was increased from 50 to 100 mL. When less test serum was used, some disks dried out during the overnight incubation. After the second incubation with labeled antihuman IgE and before counting the bound radioactivity, an extra step was added. The coated allergen disks were removed from the original polystyrene tubes and, before counting, were placed into fresh ones. This procedure was done to ensure that only radioactivity immunologically bound to the disk was measured.

Improved reproducibility of assay results between laboratories was accomplished by the use of a time-of-count control (the time used to count each disk, requiring a known 25 U/mL sample of IgE to reach 25,000 counts when tested against an anti-IgE disk and run in parallel with the atopic sera under study). When this test was initially done, the average nonspecific binding in the MRT system averaged 500 counts, or 2% of that obtained by the 25 U/mL IgE time control. In the original MRT system, the lower limit of detectable levels of allergen-specific IgE was either human cord serum, serum from nonatopic patients, or serum from highly atopic patients tested against an inappropriate allergen. With an enzymatic tracer, the nonspecific binding was somewhat higher, at 375 counts. With the enzymatic markers, the cutoff point was 750 counts, or 3% of the time control. Scores above 750 counts were divided into distinct classes, each representing approximately a fivefold increase in the amount of specific IgE antibody present in the sample. The MRT (Pharmacia-Ventrex, Kallestad, Sweden) be-

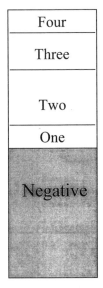
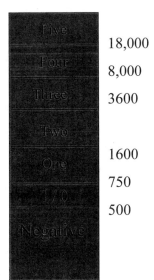

| | |
|---|---|
| Five | 18,000 |
| Four | 8,000 |
| Three | 3600 |
| Two | |
| One | 1600 |
| 1/0 | 750 |
| Negative | 500 |

**FIG. 9.1.** Original versus modified radioallergosorbent test.

came the most widely used in vitro allergy diagnostic assay in the United States and was considered by many to be the gold standard against which all such assays were compared. The original MRT is still available today, but has been somewhat automated (HY.TEC; Hycor Corporation, Irvine, CA).

Throughout the 1980s, various other in vitro assays were introduced into the U.S. market (6). One of the first such methods was the fluorescent allergosorbent test (FAST), which used individual plastic polymer wells bound with antigen as the solid phase. It also was read using a fluorescent marker. Unfortunately, even though the assay underwent multiple technical changes to improve its efficiency, the results were inconsistent from allergen to allergen, and the assay finally was withdrawn from the marketplace. Another in vitro assay for allergy diagnosis, developed around the same time, was the modified allergosorbent test (MAST) (MAST ImmunoSystems, Mountain View, CA). This assay remains available today. Numerous studies performed in the mid- to late 1980s showed this assay's results to be closer to those of the Phadebas RAST assay than the MRT. In other words, although the assay had excellent specificity, it had a significantly lower sensitivity.

The late 1980s and early 1990s saw another proliferation of new in vitro IgE assays. The Matrix (Abbott Laboratories, Abbott Park, IL) and the Magic-Lite (Corning, Corning, NY) assays were short-lived and never brought to market. The AlaStat assay (DPC, Los Angeles, CA) also was introduced during this period. This assay used a liquid instead of a solid phase, which allowed the assay to be significantly automated. Studies done at that time showed an inconsistency from allergen to allergen. This assay, with some technological changes, is still in use today.

This era also gave rise to a new, technologically advanced assay, the Pharmacia CAP System (Pharmacia Diagnostics) (7), which assay uses a flexible hydrophilic carrier polymer encased in a capsule (ImmunoCAP). This solid phase binds at least three times more protein than the original paper disk. Specific combinations of monoclonal and polyclonal anti-IgE antibodies labeled with a fluorescent enzyme reagent, β-galactoside, are used to determine the allergen-bound specific antibody. After washing and addition of the substrate, the quantity of bound IgE is measured by the amount of fluorescence detected in a fluorometer. There are two scoring methods available for this assay. In one, the assay results are expressed quantitatively in kilounits (kU)/L, with the positive–negative cutoff at 0.35 kU/L. In the other method, the alternate scoring method (ASM), used only in the United States, the ratio of the sample measurement to that of the 0.35 IU/mL calibrator, expressed as a percentage, is reported.

## QUALITY OF IN VITRO ASSAYS

To fulfill criteria for accurate measurements, all components in a test system have to be standardized both separately and in a combination battery. An assay for IgE antibody should be sensitive, specific, accurate, and reproducible and not produce elevated values in the presence of high total serum IgE. The detecting antibodies should be absolutely IgE specific without cross-reactivity with IgG, and give the same result when repeated over a period of time. To give results in true quantitative terms, assays should be related to a reference curve and calibrated against an international standard, preferably the World Health Organization standard for IgE. Allergen extracts used for preparation of the solid phase should contain all the important components in sufficient quantities so that the results are not spuriously elevated by the presence of high total IgE or IgG antibody levels. The test system should use allergen sources that do not contain contaminating allergens from other sources. A positive value should be reproducibly positive and a negative value must be reproducibly negative.

A large number of comparative studies in Europe, Japan, and the United States have shown the CAP assay to be far more sensitive than the Phadebas RAST, yet with the same specificity. The CAP method also has shown an excellent correlation with skin testing. With the ASM scoring method, the assay has shown good concordance with the MRT, but with better specificity. The CAP assay is totally automated and is fully completed in 3 hours. There are various models available, depending on the test volume of the user. A fully integrated desktop unit, the UniCap, is available for the physician's office or a small laboratory, where a smaller volume of testing occurs. At this time, the Pharmacia CAP System is the most widely used assay for determining specific IgE in the world.

## DIAGNOSIS OF ALLERGIC DISEASE

Demonstration of the presence of specific IgE antibodies is an essential part of the diagnosis in cases of allergic disease related to aeroallergens, insect venom, latex, foods, occupational allergens, and drugs. Knowledge of the specific cause of an allergic disease allows detailed education of patients, rational avoidance measures, and the design of therapeutic regimens.

Allergic disease is initiated by the exposure of susceptible individuals to proteins or glycoproteins in the environment (i.e., allergens) that can stimulate the production of specific IgE antibodies. This process is termed *sensitization.* Repeated exposure to these allergens can lead to further increases in sensitization and also to mediator release from mast cells, which plays a major role in clinical disease. The medical history and physical examination are used first to identify whether the patient's symptoms are compatible with those of an allergic disease. Clinical assessment may be sufficient to identify causes, make judgments of severity, and formulate preliminary treatment plans.

The diagnosis of allergy can be a difficult process because

(a) the history is often complex, (b) allergens from a number of different sources may be involved, and (c) other pathologic processes can induce similar symptoms. A clinical history usually can distinguish between seasonal symptoms as a result of pollen exposure and perennial symptoms related most often to indoor allergens. The history cannot provide accurate identification of the specific sensitivity, which is essential either for immunotherapy or allergen avoidance, a major part of the treatment of perennial allergic disease.

The methods used to establish the presence of allergic disease and to define the causal factors are of two types: clinical tests to investigate whether exposure contributes to the symptoms, and tests for sensitization. Tests for symptoms include direct challenges with the allergen believed to be causal, avoidance trials to test whether symptoms abate, and medication trials that support an allergic etiology of the symptoms (e.g., with antihistamines or local steroids). Tests for sensitization include skin tests and in vitro measurements of allergen-specific IgE. The tests for sensitization are inherently less direct than challenge, but their correlation with clinical symptoms is high.

The amount of specific IgE antibody detected in vitro usually is reported in class ranges of 0 to 6. Alternatively, quantitative measurements can be made in mass units (units per milliliter) or in relation to a standard value (percentage of a control value). Often, a single value is reported as the threshold for regarding a test as positive or negative, and for increasing degrees of sensitivity, regardless of the allergen or clinical situation. It often is difficult to define a single threshold level that produces clinical symptoms. An advantage, however, of the in vitro systems is that the technical detection limit can be quantitated.

## IN VITRO AND SKIN TESTING

Evidence for specific sensitization can be obtained by tests for IgE antibody in vitro and skin testing in vivo. In the evaluation and interpretation of in vitro results, compared with skin tests on the same patients, the clinician must consider that different environmental factors and pharmaceutical therapies may have different effects on in vivo compared with the in vitro parameters. For example, antihistamines, hormonal factors, age, and the site on the body can all selectively influence skin test responses. Even if the two tests are performed with the highest possible standards, using well defined allergens, there may be a substantial difference between the results. The specific IgE antibody level may be 100-fold different in various individuals where the skin tests results are very similar. In addition, serum IgE antibodies (and skin test results) may change over time in response to increased or decreased exposure to antigen. Effects are more marked for nasal, bronchial, or conjunctival challenge than they are for skin tests.

Neurogenic and other nonspecific components of hyper-

responsiveness can all influence the response to in vivo challenge. Variation in the relative concentrations of allergens in the skin test solutions can change the results from more specific and less sensitive to more sensitive and less specific. Similar exercises can be undertaken with in vitro tests. With some less common allergens, the constituents of the extracts are not well defined, and consequently it is difficult to define the extract used either for in vitro tests or for skin test reagents.

## ABSOLUTE INDICATIONS FOR IN VITRO TESTING

There are special situations where in vitro testing may be specifically indicated. These include both patient-related issues and problems with certain antigens. Skin testing may be impossible if the patient is unable to discontinue antihistamines or tricyclic antidepressants. It often is difficult to skin test patients with generalized skin disease (e.g., atopic dermatitis, dermatographism, or urticaria). Most physicians avoid skin testing during pregnancy. There also are allergens foe which skin testing requires specific precautions or titration of the allergen (e.g., venom or latex), and in vitro testing therefore is safer. There also are patients who have had life-threatening anaphylactic reactions to a food or drug, for whom in vitro testing has no risk of anaphylaxis and may be clinically preferable.

## TOTAL SERUM IMMUNOGLOBULIN E

Should a total serum IgE be part of an in vitro allergy evaluation? When performed alone, total serum IgE may be useful only when the test result is elevated, because in many instances the patient may have a normal total IgE level with an elevated specific IgE result to one or more allergens. Some have argued that knowledge of total serum IgE and the absolute and relative amounts of specific IgE antibodies helps to identify relevant aeroallergens or warns that important allergens may have been missed. For example, when a patient with rhinitis or asthma is found to have a total serum IgE of 600 IU/mL but no positive tests for specific inhalant allergens, it is useful to consider testing for a wider range of allergens, such as foods, other molds, or dermatophytes.

## IN VITRO ASSAYS IN CHILDHOOD

In vitro assays also can be used to follow the development of sensitization in childhood (8). The clinician's awareness of sensitization to foods can be clinically helpful in recommending allergen avoidance measures (9). In addition, studies have shown that the risk of clinical disease, especially asthma, can be predicted in patients who have an elevated

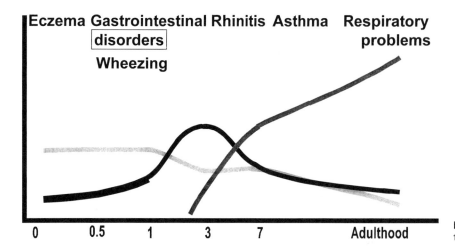

**FIG. 9.2.** Age and atopic allergy manifestations.

IgE to certain foods and aeroallergens, but who have no active allergic disease (10). Therefore, in children with a strong family history of atopic allergy, especially asthma, it may be prudent to test them in infancy or as toddlers (11, 12).

A striking temporal pattern of specific IgE antibodies and related symptoms has been identified in small children (7). Clinical symptoms frequently present in the order of eczema, then gastrointestinal problems, and, finally, rhinitis and asthma. This temporal sequence has been labeled *the allergy march* (13) (Fig. 9.2). In keeping with this model, the pattern of IgE antibody production usually starts with

food-specific IgE antibodies, often to egg white. These IgE antibodies have been shown to be predictive of the later appearance of IgE antibodies to inhalants like dust mite and pollen. Equally important, the IgE antibodies and skin test results may be detectable before any symptoms occur. Furthermore, this evidence of sensitization to egg proteins has been reported to be predictive of subsequent development of asthma and respiratory symptoms (Fig. 9.3). The reproducible and quantitative features of in vitro systems make it easier to interpret this kind of predictive information.

Further studies are needed to confirm whether repeated assays of IgE antibody should be recommended as part of

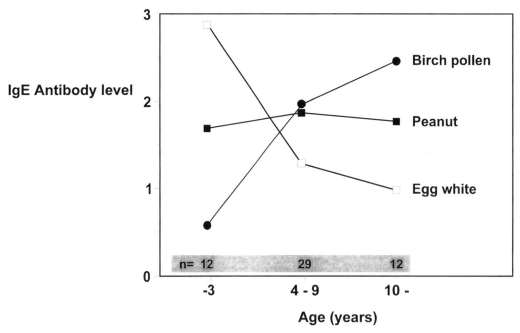

**FIG. 9.3.** Age and IgE sensitization changes.

routine practice (14). Monitoring the levels of specific IgE antibodies before and after major alterations in allergen exposures and relating this value to measures of disease severity has been done in relation to mite and pollen exposure. Results of this kind could lead to the use of in vitro testing results as predictors of clinical disease and as an index of disease severity.

## ALLERGY SCREENING

The concept of using an allergen screen for in vitro allergy diagnosis was developed primarily because of the concern about the widespread use, abuse, and cost of performing in vitro assays. It has been clearly shown in most cases that there is no need to perform a large initial battery of tests, which can only raise the overall costs of the assay to an unnecessary level. Screening for allergens is based on prevalence of the allergen, both in the general population and the specific geographic region. The cross-reactivity of allergens (e.g., grass pollen) also should be taken into account. The use of an allergen screen, consisting of at least one highly prevalent representative of each major inhalant allergen group (e.g., pollen, dust mite, mold, and animal dander) has been shown to detect 95% of atopic patients with allergy (15–18).

Another screening assay developed involves a mixture of allergens from different allergen groups on a single solid phase (e.g., Phadiatop; Pharmacia Diagnostics). An additional type of screen is the "miniscreen," in which quantitative determinations of a small number of different individual allergens, grouped by prevalence, are performed. These groups of selected antigens usually differ from each other depending on the different pollen species in a geographic area. The miniscreen therefore could contain from 6 to 15 inhalant allergens, depending on the patient's age, symptoms, and geographic location. An appropriately chosen battery of 8 to 12 allergens is 96% efficient and 94% sensitive in detecting patients who have class 2 or higher responses on a full test battery. These initial screening batteries normally contain two to three trees, grasses and weeds, a small number of molds, dust mites, and one or two animals. In infants and children, common foods such as milk, egg, soybean, wheat, peanuts, and corn should be used in the screen in place of most of the pollens (Fig. 9.4). Only if these allergen screens are positive and the patient is sick enough to warrant immunotherapy should any additional in vitro allergy testing be performed. The choice of additional tests to be performed depends on the results of the miniscreen. Using any of these screening procedures in the initial diagnostic evaluation spares nonallergic patients from further unnecessary allergy testing, thereby significantly reducing the cost of allergy care (19).

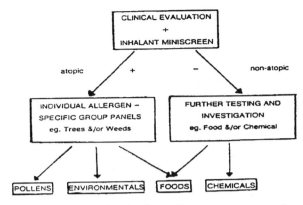

**FIG. 9.4.** In vitro testing in allergy diagnoses: summary of use.

## THE GOLD STANDARD FOR DETECTION OF ALLERGEN-SPECIFIC IMMUNOGLOBULIN E

The premises that underlie a diagnosis of IgE-mediated allergic disease are that the patient's history supports the diagnosis, that specific IgE antibodies are present, and that allergen exposure has occurred sufficiently to cause sensitization and produce disease. The reliance on clinical data as the gold standard is not appropriate because histories can be highly subjective. No gold standard for assessing the sensitivity and specificity of skin tests and in vitro testing for allergen-specific IgE has been found (20,21). Part of the reason for this may be the confusion that arises when these tests are considered tests for clinical diagnosis rather than tests for detection of specific IgE antibodies. Most clinicians consider skin testing to be the gold standard for detecting specific IgE, and thus any other test should be compared with skin testing (22).

There are many reasons for discrepancies in comparing results between skin tests and in vitro tests. It is legitimate to ask whether either test modality has achieved optimal standardization. For example, several reports have found there are significant variations in the quality of skin testing and in vitro testing over time; therefore, the test to be used needs to be selected carefully. It is easier to investigate the specificity of the IgE antibodies measured with an in vitro test than a skin test.

## IMMUNOTHERAPY

Immunotherapy is effective only in IgE-mediated disease, and the patient's symptom relief is only for those allergens treated, providing the dose of allergenically active material is of significant size to produce immunologic change. Studies have shown that by incorporating the direct measurement of specific IgE into the decision-making process, allergen immunotherapy treatment is limited to those patients with detectable levels of serum specific IgE antibody, and fewer patients therefore are started on immunotherapy. The first immunotherapy protocol based on in vitro assay results was developed using the MRT in 1977 by Fadal and Nalebuff. This technique was known as *RAST-based immunotherapy*. Using the RAST class scoring system as the guide to the initial tolerated immunotherapy dose, safe treatment sets were developed. Also, fewer but still appropriate allergens are selected for immunotherapy. In addition, it has been demonstrated that initial treatment doses for allergens associated with low scores can be administrated at a much higher level than was previously considered possible. With extremely high scores, the physician also is alerted to the fact that the patient is at risk for having an adverse reaction, and therefore a lower concentration of allergen can be used initially in the patient's buildup phase, which should be slow and careful in those patients with a high serum concentration of specific IgE.

## ADVANTAGES OF IN VITRO TESTING

There are some significant advantages to the use of in vitro assays. In vitro testing is convenient for patients in that it is quick and easy to do, especially in children. It can allay apprehension in both children and parents. It is safe, and does not have the risk of anaphylaxis that is possible with skin testing. The use of medications does not affect the assay and it is the most effective and safe allergy test for patients with dermatographia or dermatitis and those with a history of anaphylaxis. An appropriate in vitro assay also is accurate and very specific, with few false-positive results (23). The latter is a major advantage over skin testing, where false-positive results can easily occur, thus leading to inappropriate therapy, whether it be pharmacologic treatment or immunotherapy. This unnecessary treatment significantly increases the cost of the illness by much more than the cost of the in vitro test itself, because the cost of the diagnostic portion of allergy management is small compared with treatment.

## SUMMARY

In vitro assays in general are scientific, accurate, and reproducible in determining and quantifying the presence of specific IgE in the serum, and therefore identifying those patients with true atopic or IgE-mediated allergy. In vitro assays therefore should be part of every physician's armamentarium for establishing true IgE sensitization. Physicians using these assays should understand the differences in efficiency, reproducibility, and accuracy of the many in vitro methodologies available today, and they should be informed in the choice of appropriate screening panels for their region of practice. Only after an accurate diagnosis is made can the effective management of an allergic patient begin.

## REFERENCES

1. Ishizaka K, Ishizaka T, Hornbrook MH. Physicochemical properties of reaginic antibody: V. correlation of reaginic activity with the E-globulin antibody. *J Immunol* 1966;97:840.
2. Johansson SGO, Bennich HH. The clinical impact of the discovery of IgE. *Ann Allergy* 1982;48:325.
3. Kelso JM, Sodhi N, Gosselin VA, et al. Diagnostic performance characteristics of the standard Phadebas RAST, modified RAST, and Pharmacia CAP System versus skin testing. *Ann Allergy* 1991; 67:511–514.
4. De Filipi I, Yman L. Clinical accuracy of updated version of the Phadebas RAST test. *Ann Allergy* 1981;46:249.
5. Nalebuff DJ. An enthusiastic view of the use of RAST in clinical allergy. *Immunol Allergy Pract* 1981;3:18.
6. Perelmutter L, Emanuel I. Assessment of in vitro IgE testing to diagnose allergic disease. *Ann Allergy* 1985;55:762.
7. Ahlstedt S. Mediators in allergy. *Clin Trends ACI Int* 1998;1012: 37–41.
8. Nickel R, Kulig M, Forster J, et al. Sensitization to hen's egg at the age of twelve months is predictive for allergen sensitization to common indoor and outdoor allergens at the age of three years. *J Allergy Clin Immunol* 1997;99:613–617.
9. Hattevig G, Kjellman B, Bjorksten B. Appearance of IgE antibodies to ingested and inhaled allergens during the first 12 years of life in atopic and non-atopic children. *Paediatr Allergy Immunol* 1993;4:182–186.
10. Sampson HA, Ho DG. Relationship between food-specific IgE concentrations and the risk of positive food challenges in children and adolescents. *J Allergy Clin Immunol* 1997;100: 444–451.
11. Sasai K, Furukawa S, Muto T. Early detection of specific IgE antibody against house dust mite in children at risk of allergic disease. *J Pediatr* 1996;128:834–840.
12. Sigurs N, Hattevig G, Kjellman. Appearance of atopic disease in relation to serum IgE antibodies in children followed up from birth for 4 to 15 years. *J Allergy Clin Immunol* 1994;94:757–763.
13. Bergmann RL, Wahn U, Bergmann KE. The allergy march: from food to pollen. *Environ Toxicol Pharmacol* 1997;4:79–83.
14. Wahn U, Bergmann R, Kulig M. The natural course of sensitization and atopic disease in infancy and childhood. *Pediatr Allergy Immunol* 1997;8[Suppl 10]:16–20.
15. Eriksson NE. Allergy screening with Phadiatop and CAP Phadiatop in combination with a questionnaire in adults with asthma and rhinitis. *Allergy* 1990; 45:285–292.
16. Hamburger R. The value of laboratory screening tests for allergy to the general practitioner in an HMO to assist in diagnosis and referral. Presented at: Annual Meeting of the American Academy of Pediatrics, Boston, October 27, 1996.
17. King WP. Efficacy of a screening radioallergosorbent test. *Arch Otolaryngol* 1982;108:81.
18. Nalebuff DJ. Use of RAST screening in clinical allergy: a cost effective approach to patient care. *Ear Nose Throat J* 1985;107.
19. Poon AW, Goodman CS, Rubin RJ. In vitro and skin testing for allergy: comparable clinical utility and costs. *Am J Managed Care* 1998;4:969–985.
20. Emanuel IA. Comparison of in vitro allergy diagnostic methods. *Immunol Allergy Pract* 1985;7:10–83.
21. Emanuel IA. Comparison in vitro allergy diagnostic assays. *Ear Nose Throat J* 1990;69:27–41.
22. Williams PB, Dolen WK, Koepke JW, et al. Comparison of skin testing and three in vitro assays for specific IgE in the clinical evaluation of immediate hypersensitivity. *Ann Allergy* 1992;68: 35–45.
23. Nelson HS. Variables in allergy skin testing. *Allergy Proc* 1994; 15:265–268.

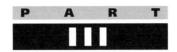

# MANAGEMENT SYSTEMS FOR ALLERGIC DISEASE

# 10

# ENVIRONMENTAL MANAGEMENT

## ANIL GUNGOR
## BERRYLIN J. FERGUSON

Avoidance of allergen is the safest and most effective method of managing allergic rhinitis. It is not always possible or practical for the patient to avoid all allergens; hence, other management, including pharmacotherapy and immunotherapy, often is used. The efficacy of these other therapeutic modalities is enhanced with the implementation of environmental controls (1).

This article explores environmental controls as a means of preventing allergies, provides practical guidelines in instructing the patient in the implementation of allergen reduction strategies, and critically evaluates various allergy control measures such as air filters, vacuums, and acaricides.

## APPROACH TO THE PATIENT WITH ENVIRONMENTAL ALLERGENS

The first step in the approach to the patient with allergies is a careful history. The history may be sufficient to advise patients regarding pertinent environmental controls. For example, if allergy symptoms worsen on exposure to cats, then the person almost certainly is allergic to cat. Patients with pollen allergies usually suffer seasonal bouts of sneezing, rhinorrhea, and itchy eyes. In the more northern climates, distinct seasons with distinct pollen counts allow us to assume that patients with more symptoms in the spring are allergic to tree pollen, those with mainly summer symptoms have classic "hay fever" and are allergic to grass pollen, and those with symptoms in the late summer that persist to the first frost have weed allergy.

Environmental controls of these exposures are avoidance of the outdoors when these pollen counts are high and the institution of vehicle and housing behaviors that minimize exposure to the outdoors. Environmental controls for seasonal hay fever–like symptoms restrict freedom and frequently are difficult to implement.

Patients with chronic symptoms frequently are unable to pinpoint triggers. Often these patients have perennial allergens, such as dust mite and mold. Common symptoms of perennial allergic rhinitis are fatigue and chronic nasal congestion, frequently worse in the winter. In contradiction to pollen avoidance, environmental controls to reduce exposure to dust mite and mold often can be highly effective without significantly reducing freedoms or altering lifestyle. Implementation of methods to reduce dust mite (i.e., mattress covers and hot water washes of bedding) and mold (i.e., dehumidification of the basement) should be explored with the patient. Because molds can be present both indoors and outdoors, complete elimination of mold often is impossible.

A complete history ascertains the presence of cigarette smoke (either primary or secondhand), pets (whether indoor or outdoor or in the bedroom), type of heating or air conditioning, and the setting of the house (either urban, suburban, or rural).

In children with allergies, one of the most common and preventable causes of persisting symptoms is exposure to environmental tobacco smoke. If the patient or members of the household are smoking, clear and firm instructions regarding its ill effects must be given, accompanied by advice on methods to stop smoking. The patient's commitment to the implementation of environmental controls can be determined during the interview, and the simplest, most effective measures should be targeted initially. If the implementation of simple primary measures is ineffective, then more extensive instruction and recommendations can be pursued. Allergic rhinitis without asthma is not a life-threatening condition. Thus, the nuisance or bother of implementing environmental controls must be balanced against nuisance and bother of the symptoms of allergic rhinitis. Occasionally, the patient would rather suffer with his or her allergic rhinitis than give up the presence of a pet on the bed, for example. The patient must be apprised of the effect of continued allergens on other members of the household who have allergies, and instructions regarding environmental control measures and their implementation must be more emphatic if the patient and other members of the

**A. Gungor:** Department of Pediatric Otolaryngology, Children's Hospital of Pittsburgh, Pittsburgh, Pennsylvania.

**B. J. Ferguson:** Department of Otolaryngology, University of Pittsburgh School of Medicine, Pittsburgh, Pennsylvania.

household experience the more life-threatening or costly complications of allergy, including recurrent or chronic rhinosinusitis and asthma.

The patient directly controls environmental management. Once the history or allergy testing strongly suggests the causative allergen, the physician must convey the importance of environmental management to the success of allergy control. Families vary widely in their commitment to the implementation of environmental controls, their personal financial resources, energy level, demands on time, and other factors that are critical to the success of avoidance treatment. The patient's allergist can advise and support, but the difficulties of compliance, with the limiting and sometimes expensive implementation of environmental controls, must be considered individually.

## PREVENTION OF ALLERGY

Allergic symptoms do not occur with primary exposure. Immunoglobulin E (IgE) to the allergen is not generated until after one or many exposures to the allergen. Only when sufficient IgE has been produced to occupy mast cells can the patient manifest allergic symptoms, which occur when the allergen cross-links the IgE molecules present on the mast cell, causing degranulation. In the child who is at high risk for development of allergy because of the presence of allergies in both parents, environmental controls should be instituted, ideally before the birth of the child. Hide et al. in a randomized, controlled trial showed that environmental controls for dust mites during the first 12 months of life in high-risk children prevented the development of allergic rhinitis at 12 months and at 24 months, compared with control subjects. The children treated with strict environmental controls had a significant decrease in positive skin prick reaction compared with the children in homes without environmental controls in place (2).

Allergen sensitivity may be increased with exposure to multiple factors independent of the allergen, especially concomitant exposure to environmental tobacco smoke. Lindfors et al. in a prospective study of 189 asthmatic children showed that the risk of sensitization to cat is low (9%) if there is no household cat, whereas the incidence of cat sensitization increases proportional to cat exposure but is dramatically increased if, in addition to the cat, there is house dampness and environmental tobacco smoke, with 80% of these children showing IgE sensitivity to cat (3).

The other area where prevention of allergy should be strongly considered is in patients involved with laboratory animals, such as mice, rodents, and rabbits. These animals are highly allergic, and the incidence of sensitization in patients who fail to prevent sensitization through the use of gloves and masks is as high as 46%, substantially greater than the 20% incidence of allergies in the general popula-

tion (4). It is far easier to prevent sensitization than it is to deal subsequently with the results of sensitization.

## ENVIRONMENTAL CONTROLS IN SENSITIZED PATIENTS

The first focus of environmental management should be on the bedroom because this usually is the area of the house where inhabitants spend the most time. This approach also ensures the achievement of highest yield from effort and money spent for environmental control.

Three basic control principles apply for all inhalant allergens:

1. Remove the source of the allergen if possible
2. Remove accumulated allergen
3. Prevent the return of the allergen

With indoor allergens, management consists of decreasing the presence of the allergen. With outdoor allergens, management principles emphasize "cocooning" the patient to avoid exposure. The following sections deal with pollen, mold, dust mite, pet (cat and dog), rodents, cockroach, and tobacco smoke individually.

## POLLEN

Allergenic pollens range from 15 to 50 $\mu$m in size (e.g., ragweed, 23 $\mu$m diameter). Indoor pollen exposure is reduced by keeping windows closed during times of high pollen counts, by the use of air conditioning to filter air, and the avoidance of inward-directed window fans. More aggressive measures include removing allergenic plants and trees that are immediately adjacent to the dwelling, and the use of room or house air filtration devices. Wilson et al. showed that particles more than 10 $\mu$m in diameter are too large to reach the lower airways and are primarily responsible for upper airway disease (i.e., allergic rhinitis) (5). It still is possible for fragments of pollen (approximately 7 $\mu$m) to reach the lower airway and cause asthma symptoms (6).

Although staying indoors during specific pollen seasons may provide considerable relief, it also is socially restrictive and becomes an increasing hardship if the patient is allergic not only to trees, for example, but also to grasses, molds, and weeds. This would essentially restrict the patient to the indoors for at least 6 months of the year in northern climates and year round in the more southern areas of the United States.

Pollens are most prevalent in the air in the morning as the sun rises and the air warms. Staying indoors at this time reduces pollen exposure at the most critical period of the day. Regional pollen counts are published in major newspapers and provided by television weather forecasters in the area. When pollen levels are exceptionally high, the pollen-allergic patient should plan on spending more time indoors. When it is necessary to go outside, patients should choose calm days when the air is still, or within 2 hours of a rain. Most pollen is washed from the air during a rain. Wearing a hat, glasses, and a mask limits outdoor exposure to pollen. After outdoor activities, patients should remove clothing immediately and shower and shampoo to remove pollen from their skin and hair. Control of exposure to seasonal pollen can be relatively simple but not practical in most situations.

## Seasonal Variation in Pollen Counts

Peak pollination, unfortunately, occurs when people most want to be outside. In temperate climates, tree pollen is the earliest pollen of the year. Trees primarily pollinate in the spring, starting as early as February in some parts of the country. One species of tree may pollinate for a few weeks, followed by pollination by other species. There is considerable overlap in tree pollination and the season may last until June, depending on the geographic area, temperature, and rainfall. Summer is the peak pollination season for grasses, but it frequently overlaps the tree pollination season to some degree as well as extending into the fall weed pollination season. In some areas, grasses pollinate throughout the year. Fall is primarily weed pollination season, starting in August and continuing until the first frost, although timing and duration vary geographically. In addition, widespread distribution of pollen through high winds over great distances is possible (7).

Patients often are unaware of the appearance of the tree, grass, or mold that is causing their symptoms and may mistakenly attribute their symptoms to a pollen they can readily see, such as pine, which is much less allergenic than the more buoyant pollens that are less apt to coat the ground. In extreme situations, removal of the shrub or plant from close proximity to the house can be undertaken. Keeping the grass cut short can minimize pollination from grass. Nevertheless, pollen can still be blown great distances and the pursuit to remove allergenic pollinating plants from the environment must be tempered with this knowledge. Mary Jelks has written an excellent, well illustrated short book on allergy plants that cause sneezing and wheezing. It is a valuable tool for the education of patients (7).

## MOLD

Mold is present year round. Outdoor mold counts are highest during the warmer months and usually lower after first frost. Mold spores range from 5 to 50 μm but in general are larger than most pollen grains. The same strategies for avoiding outdoor mold exposure as for the pollens can be pursued. The reduction of exposure to indoor mold should be pursued vigorously.

The most commonly identified indoor molds are *Aspergillus, Penicillium,* and *Rhizopus.* This is in contradistinction to the high outdoor mold counts, in which *Alternaria, Cladosporium,* and *Helminthosporium* predominate. Regardless of the species present, environmental control measures are the same because all molds grow better in damp areas.

Outdoor molds peak in the evening hours when the temperature drops at sunset. An avoidable common exposure to molds is lawn work. Patients who complain of severe allergies when mowing the lawn frequently are not allergic to grass because lawn grasses do not pollinate when kept closely mowed. Rather, they are reacting to the molds and smut that are present in the grass roots and become airborne when the grass is mowed. Mold-allergic patients should either avoid lawn work or wear a facemask. The same goes for raking leaves or piles of cut grass. Rain usually clears the air of pollen, but mold spores are be released and frequently peak approximately 2 hours after the rain. During this time, mold-allergic patients should stay indoors.

An occupational hazard for farmers is mold exposure from molds and smuts growing on grain. Stables and barns frequently are moldy, with mold growing on animal droppings, litter, hay, and feed. Decaying vegetation promotes heavy mold growth, and the compost pile should not be close to the house.

Indoor mold exposure occurs on indoor plants, shower curtains, and in areas of dampness in basements and garages, drip pans beneath refrigerators and freezers, and around condensers. Old books, bird droppings, firewood, and piled newspapers frequently are moldy. Christmas tree allergies frequently are not a tree allergy but a mold allergy because the trees have been cut and packed in the presence of snow and frost that, with warming, provide the humidity that allows prolific mold growth.

The best method of environmental management of indoor mold is to keep humidity low and prevent wet areas on walls and carpets. Maintaining the humidity below 50% reduces the growth and germination of mold significantly. A humidity gauge can be used to assess humidity levels.

Chemical fungicides include chlorine bleach and specific mold-inhibiting preparations. Soap and water also can reduce mold and mildew for a short time. Irritating, harsh chemicals should be avoided. A dehumidifier should be placed in the basement. Carpeting should be avoided in the basement. If a basement smells like a basement, it almost certainly has mold growing in it.

## DUST AND DUST MITES

House dust is a combination of over two dozen identified or suspected allergens. The potency of the allergen depends largely on the age of the dust. Older dust is more allergenic. House dust is generated in any living environment and includes degenerating residues of upholstery, carpets, mattresses, bedding, an assortment of molds, insect parts, food particles, mites, pollens, and hair from pets and vermin (8). Winter is the worst dust allergy season, when low temperatures result in tightly closed houses. Complete removal of dust is not practical.

Various dust mites also are present in house dust but can be considered independently of house dust because they are found primarily in the bedroom and specifically on the bed.

The dust mite is a microscopic creature with a worldwide distribution, but is absent at high altitudes. Dust mites are sightless arachnids up to 0.3 mm long and related to tics and scabies mites in the order Acaridae. In North America, *Dermatophagoides farinae, Dermatophagoides pteronyssinus,* and *Euroglyphus maynei* are the most common species. *D. farinae* tends to predominate in areas in which there are 3 or more months of dry weather, whereas *D. pteronyssinus* predominates in more humid areas such as Atlanta and the Pacific Northwest (9). Storage mites, including *Blomia,* are found in stored foods and grains and may be important allergens (10). Dust mites rarely grow at elevations of over 5,000 feet.

Dust mites and their feces are powerful antigens. Major allergens of two distinct house dust mites have been identified and standardized as Der p1 and Der f 1, representing *D. pteronyssinus* and *D. farinae,* respectively (11). Mite particles can vary from 5 to 20 μm in diameter. The allergens are similar in size to grass pollen grains (10 to 14 μm).

This relatively large particle is not readily airborne unless disturbed with bed making or vacuuming. Dust mites resettle quickly, within 1 to 2 hours (12). Dust mites feed on human skin scales, and the highest concentration of dust mites is found in the bedroom (11).

In colder climates, infestation and proliferation depend primarily on factors determining indoor microclimate and humidity, such as ventilation, insulation, and dampness. Relative humidity of 70% to 80% increases the dust mite population (9). Lowering the humidity below 50% helps to slow dust mite growth and diminish their byproducts. Dust mite–allergic patients should be cautioned not to introduce humidifiers into the bedroom.

Sensitization to dust mites seems to be dose dependent among susceptible people. Exposure to more than 2 μg of Der p1 increases the risk of mite sensitization. Levels greater than 10 μg/g of Der p 1 is a risk factor for wheezing in asthmatic patients (11).

## Methods Used to Estimate Exposure to Dust Mites

Methods used to estimate exposure to dust mites are mite counts, assays of mite allergens, and measurements of guanine.

Mite counts permit identification of live and dead mites, require expertise, are time consuming, and do not assess allergens and fecal pellets.

Direct measurement of mite allergens and dust samples is possible with enzyme-linked immunosorbent assay (ELISA). Although basically used as a research technique at present, the ELISA-based technique is available for routine monitoring.

Guanine, which is an end product of purine digestion/extraction that is excreted in mite feces, also can be measured to estimate exposure. Acarex is a semiquantitative assay for guanine and may be a useful test to improve patient compliance with mite reduction measures.

## Measures to Reduce Dust Mite Exposure

Covering bedding pillows or mattresses with a special tightly woven or plastic cover under regular bedding prevents exposure to dust mites. A number of such products are available, and the texture has been improved to prevent the feeling of sleeping on plastic. Pillow and mattress covers impermeable to dust mites are available from commercial allergy supply houses. These covers must be cleaned regularly by washing them in hot water, but less frequently than sheets and pillow case covers. Laundry detergents do not augment the efficacy, but regular washing of bedding in water above 130°F destroys the mite population. Even cold-water washes remove the allergen, although they do not kill dust mites. Standard dry cleaning kills dust mites but does not effectively remove the allergen. Tumbling pillows or duvets for 1 hour in a dryer set to high (59°C) effectively kills the dust mite but does not remove it from the bedding (13).

Avoidance of dust catchers, especially in the allergic person's bedroom, is another cost-effective way to reduce dust mites. Books on open shelves tend to accumulate larger amounts of dust and mold. Removal of draperies and curtains is recommended. Closet shelves and their contents should be cleaned regularly, preferably with a damp sponge or cloth. The tops of window frames and doorframes are typically major accumulators of dust but, if undisturbed, rarely exacerbate allergy symptoms. Ceiling fans not only stir up dust from the room, they collect large amounts of dust on the fan lids unless cleaned frequently. Items to avoid include horizontal blinds, stuffed animals, and multiple shelves. Carpeting and upholstered furniture should be minimized. Periodic airing and exposure for just 10 minutes of rugs, drapes, and upholstered furniture to sunlight kills the dust mites present in these furnishings. A 3-hour exposure of mite-infested carpet to sunlight at temperatures of 80°F to 90°F results in a complete killing of all dust mites present. The mites are killed mainly by dehydration (14). Small area rugs that can be washed regularly are preferable to wall-to-wall carpeting. In areas where the winter is dry, a carpet may be put down in November and removed in May. For the rest of the house, removing carpets and replacing old furniture helps, but often is impractical.

In children, dust mite sensitivity usually is the first to appear. Dust mite proofing children's rooms includes measures already reviewed, but especially important are covering the child's bed mattress with dust-proof material and replacing stuffed animals with one or two toys made of washable foam and terry cloth, which are then washed weekly.

Chemical acaricides are effective in killing dust mites and reducing their population; however, they often are more effective if applied for longer than manufacturers' recommendations. An application every 3 months is necessary to maintain low dust mite antigen levels because the mite population will be replenished. Long-term effectiveness of acaricides has been questioned.

Benzyl benzoate kills dust mites but does not denature their antigenic protein (15). When patients use benzyl benzoate powder according to the manufacturer's direction, they found it was no different from baking soda in reducing dust mites (16). Other investigators have shown that benzyl benzoate is effective only when left on carpets a minimum of 12 hours, brushed in twice, and when used on ventilated carpets on wood floors, but not on carpets on concrete slabs. Benzyl benzoate is effective for up to 3 months but is not still effective at 6 months despite the manufacturer's recommendation. Except for sunlight, all commercially available acaricides are costly, must be repeated several times a year, and may be unpleasant to use because of odor (17). Acarosan (Searle, Peapack, NJ) is a benzyl benzoate–based acaricide, produced as an aerosol foam for furniture and beds and a moist powder for carpets. These products are not currently commercially available. Benzyl benzoate reduces allergic symptoms if combined with effective cleaning (18).

Paragerm (Laboratoire Paragerm, Carros, France) is a nontoxic acaricide that has been used for over 40 years in Europe. It contains ten components, including various antiseptics. It acts promptly, is easy to use, and lasts at least 2 months. Unfortunately, it has an offensive odor (19).

Some commercially available compounds contain tannic acid, which denatures dust mite allergens but does not kill mites (20). Tannic acid denatures protein, and a 4-hour treatment of carpeting can significantly reduce mite allergen levels as well as lower concentrations of cat allergen. Because tannic acid does not kill mites, the application must be repeated every 6 to 8 weeks (21). High levels of cat allergen block the effect of tannic acid.

Effective control of dust and mold requires cleaning air ducts to remove accumulated allergens. Duct cleaning services typically are expensive and should be investigated before use to be certain the contractor does not introduce chemicals into the duct system that may provoke a serious reaction of their own.

## CATS AND DOGS

Two percent of the population in the United States is allergic to cats, and cat exposure is a significant risk factor for emergency department visits for asthma flares. Fel d 1, the major cat allergen, remains airborne in undisturbed conditions because a significant proportion is associated with particles less than 2.5 $\mu$m in diameter (22). It is among the most widely studied antigen in terms of dosage necessary for disease provocation, incidence of allergy, and biochemical structure. Cat antigen provokes symptoms in quantities as small as 8 $\mu$g/g of dust. Unfortunately, quantities this small persist for 4 months or more after the removal of the cat from the house. This extraordinary persistence occurs because cat dander is difficult to remove with vacuuming, adheres to clothing, and can be carried into the house from external sources (23). Control of cat antigen is important because of the severity of symptoms it causes with small dosages.

Fel d 1 is produced from the pelt and saliva, although less than 10% of Fel d 1 comes from cat saliva and the cat breathing. The major source of Fel d 1 is the pelt (24), which suggests that regularly washing the cat could reduce the source. Unfortunately, this may not always be the case. Glinert et al. demonstrated that a cat washed at monthly intervals over 7 months had significantly reduced cat allergen (25). This study was limited to just a few cats, however, and in a much larger study, Klucka et al. showed that washing was ineffective (26). Removing the cat from the bedroom, maintaining hard, polished floors that are cleaned weekly, reducing the amount of upholstered furniture, and good air filtration are measures that help control cat antigen. The effectiveness of weekly washing of the cat diminishes with low ventilation rates and upholstered furnishings (24). Although it may take 16 to 24 weeks for the level of antigen to fall to precat exposure levels, this reduction can be improved with vigorous high-efficiency particulate arrestor (HEPA) cleaning and removal of upholstered furniture and carpet. De Blay et al. showed that HEPA filtration for 3 hours reduced airborne Fel d 1 by 50%, and if a HEPA vacuum cleaner was used first, the airborne allergen decreased by 98% (24).

Despite the best attempts to provide an animal dander–free environment, the patient may continue to be exposed unknowingly. In a report from Sweden, cat allergen was found to be higher in classrooms than in some houses with a cat (23). Children with cats carry cat allergen to school on their clothes. Fel d 1 has been detected in carpet dust of houses where cats have never been present (27).

Dog allergens have been found in 60% of homes in the Baltimore area (28). Dog saliva and dog dander appear to be the main sources of dog allergen Can f 1. The recent development of a Can f 1 ELISA may help measure dog allergen exposure levels in homes and public places. Dog allergen, like cat allergen, can be detected in public places, including schools (29).

Whether certain dogs are less allergenic than others cannot be answered definitively because available species-specific dog antigens do not correlate with symptoms related to specific dog breeds. We know that many dog-allergic patients tend to react only to some dogs and not to others. But no data exist to recommend one breed over another at this time (30).

Patients who are not allergic to dogs may experience exacerbation of other allergies if pollens or molds cling to the dog's coat and are then brought into the house.

Allergic owners should be encouraged to ban the offending pet from the bedroom and certainly to ban it from sleeping on the bed. Sometimes it is necessary to banish the pet from the house; however, quite a few pet owners are more likely to get rid of their allergist before they get rid of their pets. Fortunately, frequent vacuuming with a HEPA vacuum cleaner and good air filtration combined with pet management usually help keep animal danders under control. HEPA air cleaners are particularly effective (31).

## Environmental Control Devices

Although several products are marketed to reduce animal dander, it has not been shown that products in addition to water improve the reduction of animal allergen. In studies showing marked decreases in Fel d 1 in frequently bathed cats, only distilled water was used. Products used to decrease nonseasonal hair shedding and improve skin condition in dogs and cats may decrease airborne allergens, but this method has not been investigated. In a controlled trial involving dogs and cats, 80% of pet owners indicated that the daily application to the pet of a preparation of essential nutrients (LoShed; Immunovet, Tampa, FL) reduced shedding by over 50%, whereas 90% of control animal owners reported no change in animal shedding. Whether this improves allergy symptoms was not studied.

## RODENTS

Animal handlers, laboratory workers, scientists, and people living in poor sanitary conditions are exposed to rodents on a regular basis. Rodents have permanent proteinuria and often aerosolize their urine by spraying. Humans then inhale these urinary proteins and hypersensitivity develops. Rodents should not be introduced as pets if the family is at high risk for development of allergies. Rodent infestation must be eliminated. Occupational exposure to rodents should be limited by wearing gloves and a mask to decrease the development of hypersensitivity (32). Birds, cows, and horses have been reported as significant sources of allergen for atopic people exposed to these allergens (33).

## COCKROACHES

The cockroach was first recognized as a source of indoor allergen in the 1960s, and since then has been associated with respiratory allergy, particularly asthma, in inner city children (34,35). Cockroaches are important sources of indoor allergens in semitropical southern climates and overcrowded, older buildings in the inner city. Socioeconomic status and race are independent risk factors for cockroach allergen exposure, both in home and school settings (36, 37). There is a clear dose–response relationship between cockroach allergen exposure and sensitization in children with asthma (38). In some parts of the United States, cockroaches are present in every house regardless of its cleanliness or the socioeconomic status of its owners. In these houses, cockroach may be the dominant foreign protein in dust (39). Twenty percent of homes with no visual evidence of cockroach infestation have been found to have significant levels of cockroach allergen. Most studies on cockroach allergens focus on American and German cockroaches, and several major allergens have been identified (35). The actual allergen source is still unclear, but it may be a substance secreted by the insect that is deposited on their body and wings. Of the seven or eight indoor species, the American cockroach *(Periplanata americana)* and the German cockroach *(Blatta germanica)* predominate in the United States. The oriental cockroach *(Blatta orientalis)* is more common in the United Kingdom. Water and food sources are the key to population growth.

Two methods can be used to help estimate exposure to cockroach allergen: traps or visual evidence of infestation and assays of cockroach allergen. Cockroach traps permit the identification of the type of species but do not assess allergens in fecal pellets. Allergens derived mainly from fecal pellets and body parts include Bla g 1 and Bla g 2, the major allergens of German cockroaches. Direct measurements of Bla g 1 and Bla g 2 allergens and dust samples are possible with an ELISA technique (35).

The highest concentration of cockroach allergen is usually from the kitchen and dust from the bedroom (37,38). Cockroach allergens are similar in size to dust mite allergens. They are greater than 10 μm, can be detected only in disturbed air, and settle down again and fall within 10 minutes (40). The sampling of settled dust from reservoirs is a widely used method of detecting cockroach allergen. Ridding the house of cockroaches is a difficult task, and an entire industry is focusing on this problem.

## TOBACCO SMOKE

Surveys indicate that up to 76% of United States children live in a home in which there is at least one smoker. It is estimated that up to 12.4 million children younger than 5 years of age are exposed to cigarette smoke at home (41). Environmental tobacco smoke is composed of more than 3,800 different chemical compounds. Cigarette smoking is a key factor that determines the level of suspended particulate matter (particulates <2.5 μm) and respirable sulfates and particles in indoor air. Concentrations of respirable suspended particulate matter can be two to three times higher in homes in which smokers reside than in homes with no smokers. Passive smoking is associated with children having higher rates of lower respiratory illness in the first year of life, decrements in pulmonary function tests, higher rates of middle ear effusion, and sudden infant death syndrome. In addition, children with asthma, whose parents smoke, have more severe symptoms and more frequent exacerbations (42,43). Although tobacco smoke is not in itself an allergic trigger, it increases sensitivity in the airways to allergens.

## FILTERS

Over $350 million was spent in 1999 in the United States on portable air cleaners, triple the amount spent in the early 1990s (44).

To date, there are very few studies demonstrating reduction in symptoms, despite a measurable decrease in airborne allergens such as cat dander (31,44,45). Van der Heide et al. were the first to show that a physical symptom is improved with the use of an air cleaner (in this case, a HEPA filter placed in the living room and bedroom of allergic children with asthma and a cat or dog). The children had a significant decrease in airway responsiveness compared with children in the placebo group (31).

Although several studies are ongoing to validate claims of the air cleaning business, it is important to be wary of past and current testimonials until further studies are completed. In particular, ozone-generating devices actually can be dangerous. In January of 2000, *Consumer Reports* tested a "personal" air cleaner that hangs around the neck. After 1 hour in a test chamber, the particle concentration in the surrounding air was "barely reduced." Around-the-neck models often use ionization, which emits small levels of ozone. Ozone cleaners usually are ineffective because the ozone levels required to remove most contaminants would be unsafe. The Federal Trade Commission (FTC) won a suit against Alpine Industries (Greenville, TN) in November of 1999 charging that the claims of removing allergens and killing mold, bacteria, and viruses were exaggerated. FTC experts also testified that the machine (Living Air ozone cleaner) produced up to five times as much ozone as is permitted under U.S. Food and Drug Administration (FDA) rules (44).

In recommending filters to patients, clinicians must keep in mind that high cost does not necessarily correspond to high efficacy. Many patients will probably be better off with an appropriate-size bedroom air cleaner. Filters that replace the heating system's existing filter do slow airflow and increase energy bills because the system has to run longer to heat or cool the house. Allergenic pollens range from 15 to 50 μm in size. The standard fiberglass filter that comes with most air conditioners usually does not filter these out. For allergic patients, there are three basic types of filters that need to be considered, although there are many variants. These are HEPA filters, electronic precipitation, and electrostatic filters. Each is discussed separately in the next sections, along with ozone generators.

## High-efficiency Particulate Arrestor Filters

High-efficiency particulate arrestor filters are the most efficient type of filter available. HEPA filters were developed by the atomic energy commission to remove radioactive dusts from plant exhausts. The filter is composed of a paperlike material made of very thin glass fibers that is pleated to increase surface area and is interposed between the air intake and output. Most HEPA filters capture particles down to 0.3 μm in diameter. This is a pore size that effectively filters out pollen grains, dust mites, mold spores, and animal danders. To qualify as a HEPA filter, the filtered air must be cleaned to 99.97% at the 0.3-μm level. The HEPA filter actually is more efficient above and below the 0.3-μm particle size and becomes more efficient with use. It is a long-lasting filter (2 to 5 years) and is virtually maintenance free. The replacement filters cost an average of $22 to $140 a year, depending on how often a filter change is recommended. Most HEPA filters are combined with a prefilter, which removes larger particles. A carbon filter also may be added to remove odors (1).

For a patient who can afford a central HEPA filtration system, access to the filter and simplicity of changing the filter are important factors to be considered for the periodic cleaning required. For patients who are not able or not willing to invest in the central HEPA filtering system, portable HEPA filtration systems can be considered. These portable room air cleaners are kept with both a HEPA filter and a charcoal prefilter incorporating a blower system that draws air through the filters and circulates it. These air cleaners are available in several sizes and should be matched to the room size accordingly.

## Electronic Precipitator

An electronic precipitator is a filtering system designed to remove allergens from indoor air. Indoor air passes over a series of electronically charged plates that attract the passing air particles. The charged particles deposit on the plates, which removes them from the air. If the precipitator is integrated into a household air conditioning system, ambient air access to the filter and frequent cleaning are essential for optimal functioning. If the electronic precipitator is not cleaned frequently, particulate deposits build up on the plates and, in time, a passage is developed through the filter that allows particles in the ambient air to escape back into the living space. If the charged particles are not removed from the air onto the plates, they adhere to the ceiling, walls, and upholstery of the living area, resulting in accumulation of dark, greasy deposits. Low levels of ozone also may be produced. Regular cleaning of the plates is important. Secondhand smoke can remove the charge from the filter and decrease filtering capacity (1).

## Electrostatic Filters

Electrostatic filters are somewhat less effective in removing particulate matter from the air than the HEPA filters or electronic precipitators, but they are simple to install. An electrostatic filter requires no special ductwork and no electrical connections. It can be tailored to fit in the same space as a fiberglass filter and removes particular materials from the air by electrostatic attraction. It is necessary to clean the electrostatic filter at frequent intervals or the efficiency of filtration will suffer. Huang (46) showed that a bedroom electrostatic air filter resulted in a significant improvement in allergic symptoms in allergic children, as well as fewer missed work days by the parents and fewer school days lost by the patients.

## Ozone Generators

Ozone generators convert oxygen to ozone by a high-voltage electric charge. Ozone is a powerful oxidant that can destroy microorganisms such as dust mites and molds, as well as gas molecules. Dust particulates are not affected. The FDA limit for ozone from electronic air cleaners is 50 parts per billion. If that limit is exceeded, ozone can be quite toxic. Ozone is used to clear smoke smells from burned areas. During the treatment, the area is sealed because exposure to these high levels of ozone would be lethal (1,44).

## Vacuum Cleaners

Super-filtering vacuum cleaners are most effective in removing dust mites, and prevent their disbursement back into the air during vacuuming. Single-layer vacuum cleaner bags usually perform poorly compared with most of the two- and three-layer microfiltration bags. Vacuum cleaners designed for allergic patients leak lower amounts of allergens. HEPA vacuum cleaners are regularly available for prices of $100 up to $1,000. For the allergic patient, low emissions are critical to the success of an environmental control program because vacuum cleaners that emit allergens in their exhaust move the allergens during vacuuming but do not remove them from the environment being vacuumed. Vacuum cleaners with 97% efficiency are marketed as HEPA-like vacuum cleaners or "allergy vacuums." The criterion for a true HEPA vacuum cleaner actually is 99.97% efficiency. Water-filtered vacuum cleaners generally are less effective. They also create aerosolized water particles that may make

humidity control more difficult and actually increase the number of allergens in the environment (1).

## CONCLUSION

Environmental controls usually are most effective for indoor allergens. The bedroom should be targeted first. Reduction of exposure to outdoor allergens such as pollen usually results in limitation of the allergy sufferer's outdoor activities. This chapter reviews environmental controls in terms of efficacy and expense. The approach to the patient is critical and reviewed in detail. Environmental controls require patient compliance and implementation to be effective.

## REFERENCES

1. Ferguson BJ. Environmental controls in allergy. *Curr Opin Otolaryngol* 1995;3:44–49.
2. Hide DW, Matthews S, Matthews L, et al. Effect of allergen avoidance in infancy on allergic manifestations at age two years. *J Allergy Clin Immunol* 1994;93:842–846.
3. Lindfors A, van Hage-Hamsten M, et al. Influence of interaction of environmental risk factors and sensitization in young asthmatic children. *J Allergy Clin Immunol* 1999;104:755–762.
4. Reeb-Whitaker CK, Harrison DJ, et al. Control strategies for aeroallergens in an animal facility. *J Allergy Clin Immunol* 1999;103:139–146.
5. Wilson AF, Novey HS, Berke RA, et al. Deposition of inhaled pollen and pollen extract in human airways. *N Engl J Med* 1973;288:1056–1058.
6. Rosenberg GL, Rosenthal RR, Normal PS. Inhalation challenge with ragweed pollen in ragweed sensitive asthmatic. *J Allergy Clin Immunol* 1975;55:126(abstr).
7. Jelks M. *Allergy plants.* Tampa, FL: World Wide Printing, 1987.
8. National Institute of Allergy and Infectious Diseases. *Dust allergy.* NIH publication no. 83-490. Bethesda, MD: National Institutes of Health, revised November, 1982.
9. Platts-Mills TAE, Chapman MD. Dust mites: immunology, allergic disease, and environmental control. *J Allergy Clin Immunol* 1987;80:755–774.
10. Scinto JD, Bernstein DI. Immunotherapy with dust mite allergens. *Immunol Allergy Clin North Am* 1992;12:53–67.
11. Platts-Mills TAE, Vervloet D, Thomas WR, et al. Indoor allergens and asthma: report of the Third International Workshop. *J Allergy Clin Immunol* 1997;100[6-1]:S2–24.
12. Wood RA, Eggleston PA. Management of allergy to animal danders. *Immunol Allergy Clin North Am* 1992;12:69–84.
13. Mason K, Riley G, et al. Hot tumble drying and mite survival in duvets. *J Allergy Clin Immunol* 1999;104:499–500.
14. Tovey ER, Woolcock AJ. Direct exposure of carpets to sunlight can kill all mites. *J Allergy Clin Immunol* 1994;93:1072–1074.
15. Lau-Schadendorf S, Ruxhe AF, Weber AK, et al. Short-term efficacy of benzyl benzoate on mite allergen concentration in house dust. *J Allergy Clin Immunol* 1989;83:263(abst.)
16. Huss RW, Huss K, Squire EN, et al. Mite allergen control when acaricide fails. *J Allergy Clin Immunol* 1994;94:27–32.
17. Platts-Mills TAE. Aerobiology and inhalant allergens. In: Middleton E Jr, Reed CE, Ellis EF, et al., eds. *Allergy principles and practice,* 4th ed, vol 1. St. Louis: Mosby, 1993:523–525.
18. Kniest M, Young E, Van Praag MCG, et al. Clinical evaluation

of a double-blind dust mite avoidance trial with mite-allergic rhinitis patients. *Ann Allergy* 1991;67:25–31.

19. Massey DG, Fournier-Massey G, James RH. Minimizing acaricides and house dust in the tropics. *Ann Allergy* 1993;71:439–444.

20. Green WF. Abolition of allergens by tannic acid. *Lancet* 1984;88:77–82.

21. Woodfolk JA, Hayden ML, Miller JD, et al. Chemical treatment of carpets to reduce allergen: a detailed study of the effects of tannic acid on indoor allergens. *J Allergy Clin Immunol* 1994;94:19–26.

22. Luczynska CM, Li Y, Chapman MD, et al. Airborne concentrations and particle size distribution of allergen derived from domestic cats. *Am Rev Respir Dis* 1990;141:361–367.

23. Munir AKM, Einarson R, Shou C, et al. Allergens in school dust: the amount of the major cat (Fel d 1) and dog (Can f 1) allergens in dust from Swedish schools is high enough to probably cause perennial symptoms in most children with asthma who are sensitized to cat and dog. *J Allergy Clin Immunol* 1993;91:1067–1074.

24. De Blay F, Chapman MD, Platts-Mills TAE. Airborne cat allergen (Fel d 1): environmental control with the cat in situ. *Am Rev Respir Dis* 1991;143:1334–1339.

25. Glinert R, Wilson P, Wedner HF. Fel d is markedly reduced following sequential washing of cats. *J Allergy Clin Immunol* 1990;85:327(abstr).

26. Klucka CV, Ownby DR, Green J, et al. Cat shedding of Fel d 1 is not reduced by washings, Allerpet-c sprays or acepromazine. *J Allergy Clin Immunol* 1995;95:1164–1171.

27. Bollinger ME, Eggleston PA, Flanagan E, et al. Cat antigen in homes with and without cats may induce allergic symptoms. *J Allergy Clin Immunol* 1996;97:907–914.

28. Wood RA, Chapman M, Adkinson N, et al. The effect of cat removal on allergen content in household dust samples. *J Allergy Clin Immunol* 1989;83:730–734.

29. Schou C, Hansen G, Linter T, et al. Assay for the major dog allergen Can f 1: investigation of house dust samples and commercial dog extracts. *J Allergy Clin Immunol* 1991;88:847–853.

30. Lindgren S, Belin L, Dreborg S, et al. Breed specific dog dandruff allergens. *J Allergy Clin Immunol* 1988;82:196–204.

31. Van der Heide S, van Aalderen WMC, et al. Clinical effects of air cleaners in homes of asthmatic children sensitized to pet allergens. *J Allergy Clin Immunol* 1999;104:447–451.

32. Ipsen H, Klysner SS, Larsen JN, et al. Allergenic extracts. In: Middleton E Jr, Reed CE, Ellis EF, et al., eds. *Allergy principles and practice,* 4th ed, vol 1. St. Louis: Mosby, 1993:535–537.

33. Sarpong SB, Corey JP. Assessment of the indoor environment in respiratory allergy. *Ear Nose Throat J* 1988;77:960–964.

34. Kang B. Study on cockroach antigen as a probable causative agent in bronchial asthma. *J Allergy Clin Immunol 1976;58:357–365.*

35. Pollart S, Smith TF, Morris EC, et al. Environmental exposure to cockroach allergens: analysis with monoclonal antibody-based enzyme immunoassays. *J Allergy Clin Immunol* 1991;87:505–510.

36. Sarpong SB, Wood RA, Karrison T, et al. Cockroach antigen (Bla g 1) in school dust. *J Allergy Clin Immunol* 1997;99:486–492.

37. Sarpong SB, Hamilton RG, Eggleston PA, et al. Socioeconomic status and race as risk factors for cockroach allergen exposure and sensitization in children with asthma. *J Allergy Clin Immunol* 1996;97:1393–1401.

38. Eggleston PA, Rosenstreich D, Lynn H, et al. Relationship of indoor allergen exposure to skin test sensitivity in inner city children with asthma. *J Allergy Clin Immunol* 1998;102:563–570.

39. Pollart SM, Platts-Mills TAE, Chapman MD. Identification, quantitation, and purification of cockroach (CR) using monoclonal antibodies (mAb) (abstract). *J Allergy Clin Immunol* 1989;83:293.

40. Sarpong SB, Wood RA, Eggleston PA. Aerodynamic properties of cockroach allergens. *J Allergy Clin Immunol* 1995;95:262(abstr).

41. Agudo A, Bardagi S, Romero PV, et al. Exercise-induced airways narrowing and exposure to environmental tobacco smoke in school children. *Am J Epidemiol* 1994;140:409–417.

42. Frischer T, Kuehr J, Meinert R, et al. Maternal smoking in early childhood: a risk factor for bronchial hyperresponsiveness to exercises in primary school children. *J Pediatr* 1992;121:17–22.

43. Jindal SK, Gupta D, Singh A. Indices of morbidity and control of asthma in adult patients exposed to environmental tobacco smoke. *Chest* 1994;106:746–749.

44. Parker-Pope T. Popular air cleaners pull in consumers but do they work? *Wall Street Journal* April 7, 2000:B1.

45. Wood RA, Johnson EF, Van Natta ML, et al. A placebo-controlled trial of a HEPA air cleaner in the treatment of cat allergy. *Am J Respir Crit Care Med* 1998;158:115–120.

46. Huang SW. The effects of an air cleaner in the homes of children with perennial allergic rhinitis. *Pediatr Asthma Allergy Immunol* 1993;7:111–117.

# 11

# PHARMACOTHERAPY OF OTOLARYNGIC ALLERGY

## HELEN FOX KRAUSE

The incidence of allergy has increased in recent years, especially in the industrial world. The pharmaceutical industry has responded by producing newer therapeutic agents with good efficacy and fewer adverse and side effects. The options for pharmacotherapy continue to expand.

In otolaryngic allergy, we are concerned primarily with allergic rhinitis and conjunctivitis, although at times we also may see patients with food allergy, eczema, and urticaria. In selection of pharmacotherapy for these patients, certain variables must be taken into consideration. Patient age is important. Children and the elderly may have adverse responses to agents safe for adults. If a patient has other medical problems, such as glaucoma, prostatic hypertrophy, or cardiac disease, certain drugs may be contraindicated or there may be possible drug interactions with other essential medications.

Understanding the pathophysiology of the early and late allergic responses helps determine which medications are selected for a particular patient. In the early phase, there may be sneezing and itching of the nose, eyes, ears, and throat that is neurogenically induced. There may be an increase in secretions from the nose, increased tearing, and mild nasal congestion. These symptoms are triggered by the release of histamine, tryptase, cytokines, and products of arachidonic acid metabolism. Cells of the immune system also become involved, including T cells, eosinophils, and basophils. More chemical mediators are released, especially the interleukins, producing an inflammatory reaction at times more severe than the earlier response. Other chemicals, including histamine, also are released (1). The patient becomes markedly congested and may continue to experience the earlier symptoms. Seasonal and perennial rhinitis may have similar symptoms, although the secretions in the latter may be more tenacious and the patient may complain of more postnasal drainage.

Pharmacotherapy for allergic disease may control symptoms once they have started or may prevent them by acting on the immunologic mechanisms involved. Some available medications are effective for the early response only, others for the late response. Newer medications may alter both responses, early and late. It is important to recognize which symptom complex is active. For example, antihistamines do little to control congestion, whereas decongestants do not help the sneezing, itching, and rhinorrhea.

Available pharmacotherapeutic agents include antihistamines, nasal steroids, decongestants, mast cell stabilizers, leukotriene modifiers, and others, which include mucolytics and anticholinergics to help relieve some symptoms. Additional classes of drugs are being investigated. New drugs may be developed with fewer side effects or designed to act against a specific chemical mediator.

## ANTIHISTAMINES

For many years the most commonly used drugs to control or prevent the symptoms of allergy have been antihistamines. Antihistamines were developed to antagonize histamine, one of the major mediators of the early-phase allergic reaction. Many of the six classes of older classic antihistamines (Table 11.1) are now available as over-the-counter (OTC) drugs. The primary mechanism of all antihistamines is competitive, dose-related binding to type 1 histamine ($H_1$) receptors on the target organ. They relieve sneezing and itching and reduce the rhinorrhea and tearing of the allergic reaction. Some of the newer compounds also may have mast cell–stabilizing and antiinflammatory activity.

The classic antihistamines are effective drugs, quickly absorbed with a rapid onset of $H_1$ receptor antagonism. Because they have a short duration of activity, long-acting formulations have been developed. These drugs are lipophilic and easily cross the blood–brain barrier, producing sedation (2), variable degrees of anticholinergic activity, and at times gastrointestinal and cardiac effects. They should not be used by patients with diabetes, glaucoma, prostatic hypertrophy, or cardiac disease. They may have prolonged

**H. F. Krause:** Department of Otolaryngology, University of Pittsburgh, Pittsburgh, Pennsylvania.

## TABLE 11.1. ANTIHISTAMINES: CLASSIC

| Classification | Generic Name | Trade Name |
|---|---|---|
| Ethanolamines | Diphenhydramine | Benadryl |
| | Clemestine | Tavist |
| Ethylenediamines | Tripelennamine | Pyribenzamine |
| Alkylamines | Chlorpheniramine | Chlor-Trimeton |
| | Brompheniramine | Dimetane |
| Piperazines | Hydroxyzine | Atarax |
| | Meclizine | Antivert |
| Phenothiazines | Promethazine | Phenergan |
| | Trimeprazine | Temaril |
| Piperidines | Cyproheptadine | Periactin |

ity. For the most part they are lipophobic, not passing easily through the blood–brain barrier, have little affinity for central $H_1$ receptors, and therefore are nonsedating or less sedating then the classic antihistamines. They are easily absorbed and have little anticholinergic effect. These second-generation drugs are metabolized in the liver and excreted fecally or renally. Some are metabolites of previously developed drugs. The newer antihistamines have a rapid onset of action and their half-lives are relatively long, so they may be administered once or twice a day. They do not have the same drug interactions as the classic antihistamines and may be used safely for those patients with glaucoma, diabetes, prostatic hypertrophy, and cardiac and thyroid disease. The effectiveness of their $H_1$ antagonism is similar to that of the older antihistamines, perhaps slightly better, and there may be other actions such as cell membrane stabilization or some degree of antiinflammatory effect by decreasing the migration of inflammatory cells to the target organ (1).

The first of the second-generation antihistamines to be developed were terfenadine (1985) and astemizole (1988). These are efficacious antihistamines but were found to have drug interactions with other products using the same cytochrome p450 enzymes for metabolism, such as the macrolides and antifungal drugs. If liver function is decreased, these agents can be dangerous. The effects of increased levels of these agents produced cardiac changes resulting in torsades de pointes, a life-threatening arrhythmia (2–5). Both have been withdrawn from the market in the United States.

psychomotor effects, which can be dangerous. Also, this group of drugs may adversely interact with other drugs, especially central nervous system depressants such as monoamine oxidase inhibitors, tricyclic antidepressants, narcotics, alcohol, barbiturates, anti-Parkinson agents, and other sedatives. They may decrease the effect of oral contraceptives, progesterone, reserpine, and thiazide diuretics and may inhibit the action of anticoagulants. Some of these drugs may have paradoxical activity, producing stimulation in both the cardiac and central nervous systems.

Newer antihistamines have been developed to offset the adverse effects and drug interactions of the classic antihistamines (Table 11.2). Some have additional antiallergic activ-

## TABLE 11.2. SECOND-GENERATION ANTIHISTAMINES

| Classification | Generic Name | Brand Name | Dosage |
|---|---|---|---|
| Alkylamines | Acrivastine (with 60 mg of pseudoephedrine) | Semprex-D | 8 mg qd to qid |
| Piperizine | Ceterizine | Zyrtec | 10 mg qd |
| Piperidine | Astemizole[a] | Hismanal | 10 mg qd |
| | Ketotifen | | |
| | Ophthalmic | Zaditor | 1 qtt (0:025%) q8–12h |
| | Oral[a] | Zaditen | 2 mg bid |
| | Loratadine | Claritin | 10 mg qd |
| | Terfenadine[a] | Seldane | 60 mg bid |
| | Ebastine[b] | Cedex | 10 mg qd |
| | Epinastine[b] | | 10 mg qd |
| Miscellaneous | Azelastine | Astelin | |
| | Oral[a] | | 2 mg qd |
| | Nasal | | 2 sprays (0.1%) qd or bid |
| | Levocabastine | | |
| | Ophthalmic | Livostin | 1 qtt (0.5 g/L) qid |
| | Nasal[a] | | |
| | Olapatidine | Patanol | 1 or 2 qtt (0.1%) bid |
| | Emedastine | Emadine | 1 qtt qd to qid |

[a]No longer available in the United States.
[b]Not available in the United States.

The next drug to be developed was loratadine (1993). Although it uses the same cytochrome p450 enzyme system for metabolism, it does not block the delayed potassium rectifier system that produces the Q-wave prolongation of torsades de pointes (5). Loratadine was developed from the classic drug azatadine but does not have the sedating and other classic side effects. It preferentially blocks peripheral $H_1$ receptors and binds poorly to α-adrenergic receptors. The half-life is biphasic, initially 7.8 to 11 hours, and the active metabolite has a serum half-life of 17 to 24 hours, allowing a 10-mg dose to be effective for 24 hours (6). It is available in several forms: alone in two forms and with pseudoephedrine in 12- and 24-hour preparations. A pediatric form also is now available. It has been approved for use by military pilots and is in the U.S. Food and Drug Administration (FDA) pregnancy category B (7,8).

Acrivastine is another second-generation drug with a short half-life of 1.5 hours and therefore a short duration of action. However, it is effective very rapidly and produces little sedation or antimuscarinic activity. It is secreted renally. Its dosage regimen is 8 mg four times a day or, when combined with 60 mg of pseudoephedrine, three times a day. A delayed-release formulation of acrivastine 12 mg with 60 mg of pseudoephedrine has been developed for twice-a-day use (9). Only the twice-a-day preparation is available in the United States.

Cetirizine is a metabolite of the classic antihistamine, hydroxyzine. It has excellent antiallergenic activities for respiratory and dermatologic allergies (1). It is classified as a sedating antihistamine, although its degree of sedation is dose related. For seasonal and perennial allergic rhinitis, a 10-mg dose once daily is the usual for adults, with 5 to 10 mg in a suspension form used for children (10–13). Cetirizine is excreted primarily renally, so kidney function is very important. No drug interactions or anticholinergic effects have been reported, and no cardiovascular changes associated with its use have been found (14). An important additional action of this drug is its ability to block the migration of inflammatory cells, primarily eosinophils, to target organs (15). It also may have an effect on T-cell activity. It improves allergic status asthmaticus and is very effective in urticaria.

Fexofenadine is the active metabolite of terfenadine with comparable antihistamine benefits without the adverse cardiac effects (13–15). Studies demonstrate that it also has antiinflammatory activity. Other studies have shown no effect on driving or other psychomotor performance (16). The doses now available are 60 mg with and without pseudoephedrine in 12-hour doses, so an evening dose without decongestant stimulation can be avoided (17). A 180-mg dose once a day as well as a 30-mg pediatric dose became available in 2000 in the United States. A 120-mg daily dose is available in other countries (18). This drug has been studied at levels up to 480 mg without adverse effects. Fexofenadine has been approved for military pilots after a 2-week

ground trial. It is FDA pregnancy category C according to the package insert, but the American Academy of Obstetricians and Gynecologists and the American College of Allergy, Asthma and Immunology have stated that it may be used after the first trimester, just as loratadine may be used (8).

Philpot has compared the safety of these second-generation antihistamines (19). All are effective in allergic rhinitis and all are safe, although cetirizine may be somewhat sedating for some patients. He states that all three are safe for pediatric use and in the elderly as long as kidney function is adequate.

Some new antihistamines now available are effective as topical preparations.

Azelastine has activity in both early and late allergic reactions as a nasal spray in seasonal and perennial allergic rhinitis (20–23). It inhibits the production or release of mediators in in vitro studies, including histamine, leukotrienes, serotonin, kinins, and superoxide free radicals. Onset of action is within 1 hour with the dosage of two sprays (0.1% = 0.137 mg/spray) per nostril once or twice a day. It is nonsedating in the nasal form available in the United States, but more sedating in the oral form available in Europe, where it is used as an antiasthma drug. Some studies suggest improvement in congestion. The only adverse effects reported are dysgeusia, a bitter metallic taste, from both forms and a slight increase in headaches (23). There is both fecal and urinary excretion.

There are a number of allergic eye disorders (see Chapter 21), the most common of which are seasonal and perennial allergic conjunctivitis. There are several therapeutic options now available (24). Levocabastine is available in the United States as a topical antihistamine eye solution that is very effective for allergic conjunctivitis (8,24). The dosage is 1 drop (0.5 g/L) four times a day or as needed. The eye preparation is very effective, does not cause sedation, and has no adverse side effects except mild initial stinging. It is minimally absorbed, undergoes slight hepatic metabolism, and is excreted primarily by the kidneys. There is a nasal spray available elsewhere, but not in the United States.

Emedastine is an eye solution that is a potent topical antihistamine. It is safe and long lasting but not yet available in the United States. It has flexible dosing of one to four times a day and is safe for children as young as 3 years of age (24–26).

Olopatadine is a topical ophthalmic preparation (0.1% solution) that has antihistamine and mast cell–stabilizing benefits (24–27). No adverse effects have been reported except occasional headaches and a possible stinging sensation. It provides 8 hours of relief from itching and tearing with one or two drops in each eye when used twice a day. It may be used in children as young as 3 years of age. It has no α-adrenergic effects, and no effects on dopamine, muscarinic, or serotonin receptors. It does contain benzalkonium chloride as a preservative. It is listed as an FDA pregnancy category C drug and should not be used by nursing mothers.

Released in 1999 in the United States, ketotifen fumarate, another ophthalmic preparation (0.025% solution), has both antihistaminic and mast cell–stabilizing properties. In addition, it inhibits mediator release from basophils and neutrophils, inhibits chemotaxis and degranulation of eosinophils, and demonstrates antileukotriene activity. It also antagonizes platelet-activating factor (28–31). It has been available since 1991 in Japan, as well as more recently in some Central and South American countries. Adverse effects are rare, consisting primarily of conjunctival injection and headaches. The dosage is one drop in each affected eye every 8 to 12 hours. It is in pregnancy category C and should not be used by nursing mothers (32). It may be used by children as young as 3 years of age.

Oral ketotifen has been available since 1976 in Japan and Europe for the treatment of allergies, especially asthma. It is somewhat sedating when taken orally.

There are a number of other antihistamines that are available elsewhere in the world but not in the United States, or are in the research stage.

Ebastine is available in some European countries. It is metabolized to two major metabolites. The dose is 10 mg once daily, although the 20-mg dose may reduce the time for maximal efficacy in severe allergy (8,33,34). Although no actual cardiac events have been reported, there has been some question about such effects with the parent compound, but not with the active metabolite, carebastine.

Epinastine is available in South America. It suppresses interleukin-8, a cytokine that promotes eosinophil migration in the inflammatory late allergic reaction. It also may inhibit the formation and release of leukotriene C4. It has been found effective in 10- and 20-mg doses. There have been no adverse cardiac events (35).

Mizolastine is an extensively studied, nonsedating antihistamine. There is a significant prophylactic effect in its ability to delay the onset of seasonal allergic rhinitis (7,36, 37). Compared with loratadine in perennial allergic rhinitis, there is 69.8% improvement with the mizolastine and 64.8% with loratadine. Mizolastine has shown no cholinergic effects. Its dosage is 10 mg/day for adults. It is available in the United Kingdom, Switzerland, Denmark, the Netherlands, and Canada for seasonal allergic rhinitis and chronic idiopathic urticaria, but it is not currently available in the United States. It is being studied for use in asthma (38).

A number of antihistamines are still in the research stage. Norastemizole is one of the metabolites of astemizole that has effective $H_1$ antagonism and inhibits formation and release of inflammatory mediators from mast cells. It appears to have the same benefits as its parent compound without the adverse cardiac effects. It will have 13 to 16 times the antihistamine effect of astemizole. The onset effect may be as rapid as 29 minutes. It will not have astemizole's

prolonged antihistamine effects, however, lasting only 24 hours after one dose (34,39).

The active metabolite of loratadine, descarboethoxyloratadine (desloratadine), was submitted to the FDA for approval in early 2000. It has a wide margin of safety and a more rapid onset of action than its parent. It is highly selective for $H_1$-receptors and has no anticholinergic effects.

Levocetirizine is one of the two active metabolites of cetirizine. It has the same or more activity than its parent with less sedation. A number of further studies will be necessary before it is ready for release (39).

Carebastine has all the beneficial activity of its parent compound, ebastine, but with no QT segment prolongation, and may replace ebastine.

Rupatadine is a new agent with two actions. It has shown antagonism against histamine and platelet-activating factor in animal studies. It may prove useful in treatment of allergic and other inflammatory diseases.

## DECONGESTANTS

No new decongestants have been developed in recent years. Their action is to decrease nasal edema in the late allergic reaction. They stimulate adrenergic receptors and are sympathomimetic (49,41). They are available as oral or topical drugs (Table 11.3). The oral drugs often are combined with antihistamines, guaifenesin, dextromethorphan, or other drugs. Those most common in oral use are pseudoephedrine, phenylpropanolamine, and phenylephrine. The latter is the least effective orally (41). The topical nasal drugs usually are available OTC, except for cocaine and epinephrine. Phenylpropanolamine preparations were withdrawn from the market on order of the FDA because they were shown to promote an increased incidence of hemorrhagic stroke in certain patients.

Overuse of the topical preparations produces a rebound

**TABLE 11.3. DECONGESTANTS**

| Generic Name | Trade Name |
|---|---|
| Pseudoephedrine (oral) | Sudafed |
| Phenylpropanolamine (oral) with guaifenesin | Entex LA |
| Phenylephrine (oral/topical) | Entex capsules/ Neo-Synephrine |
| Ephedrine (oral/topical) | Ephedrine |
| Oxymetazoline (topical) | Dristan |
| Tetrahydrozoline (topical) | Tyzine |
| Naphazoline (topical) | Privine |
| Xylometazoline (topical) | Otrivine |
| Epinephrine (systemic/topical) | Adrenaline Primatene |
| Cocaine (topical) | Cocaine |

effect known as *rhinitis medicamentosa* or *chemical rhinitis.* Overuse of both the oral and topical forms may produce dangerous systemic effects (1,40,41). They must be used with great care and should not be used in patients with heart disease, arrhythmias, diabetes, glaucoma, prostate hypertrophy, ulcers, or hyperthyroidism.

Although hypertension usually is a contraindication to the use of decongestants, some studies have indicated that in selected patients with well controlled blood pressure levels, pseudoephedrine may be used. The patient must monitor his or her blood pressure to be sure it stays at an acceptable level (42).

Oral decongestants do not cause topical rebound but may have a variable effect on nasal congestion. There may be significant drug interactions with any decongestant, and they should not be used with monoamine oxidase inhibitors, β-adrenergic blockers, methyldopa, indomethacin, digitalis, and possibly theophylline. They should not be used with general anesthetics, or very cautiously, as in nasal surgery. If cocaine is chosen for use in nasal surgery, absorption may be decreased by prior use of a topical decongestant with less potential cardiovascular effects such as oxymetazoline or xylometazoline. These agents do not decrease the local anesthetic or prolonged decongestant effects of topical cocaine (43).

Exercise may improve nasal congestion by decreasing the sympathetic tone of the nasal circulation (41). Trade-name decongestants and generic forms may not be bioequivalent because the release properties often are different.

## CORTICOSTEROIDS

Corticosteroids are antiinflammatory drugs available for use in allergic rhinitis intranasally or systemically by oral, intramuscular, or intravenous routes. Their effect is primarily on the late-phase allergic reaction, although Mygind and Naclerio report that an effect may be present with the early-phase reaction as well (44).

Systemic steroids are used for the most difficult cases. Systemic administration may be necessary with severe allergic problems such as with rhinitis medicamentosa, in aspirin sensitivity, and during and after surgery in patients with asthma or severe allergic reactions (45). Oral high-dose therapy may be instituted with prednisone or methylprednisolone in tapered doses (45,46).

Steroids may be injected into the edematous anterior tips of the inferior turbinates only with extreme care and caution because of the danger of blindness that may result from embolism of the steroid or spasm of the ophthalmic artery. It is not recommended unless the physician is an experienced nasal surgeon and an explicit protocol is carefully followed (46).

Intranasal steroids diffuse across cell membranes, resulting in a series of chemical events that may take 2 or 3 days to begin to have effects. Intranasal steroids have significantly fewer side effects than systemic forms, but maintain excellent efficacy (47).

There are a number of topical nasal preparations available, all still by prescription in the United States, but many available as OTC agents in other countries (Table 11.4). The formulations dexamethasone and betamethasone are not currently available in the United States because their systemic absorption is high and there may be alteration of the hypothalamic–adrenal–pituitary axis. The other preparations have variable bioavailability and include beclomethasone dipropionate, flunisolide, fluticasone propionate, triamcinolone acetonide, budesonide, and monomethasone. Fluocortin butylesterase is a powder preparation requiring a special device not available in the United States. These drugs are absorbed from the mucosa of the nose but undergo rapid hepatic metabolism and have a very short plasma half-life, so systemic effects are minimal or absent. Betamethasone, which is not available in the United States, does produce some systemic effect (43,44,46).

Adverse effects such as atrophic rhinitis, epistaxis, and septal perforations may be avoided if the patient is taught the proper technique for application. It is important that the patient be instructed to angle the applicator in the direction of the medial canthus, never toward the septum. There is less danger of nasal damage with the aqueous formulations. The efficacy of the various preparations appears to be comparable in a number of drug comparison studies (44, 48). The risk of systemic effects due to the absorption of the intranasal steroids is minimal even with long-term use. There was a question of posterior subcapsular cataracts developing from intranasal steroids, but this effect has not been proven. There has been concern about potential growth inhibition when inhaled steroids are used in children. This concern has been based on studies of inhaled steroids used for asthmatic patients. Studies on budesonide suggest that this is not a problem (49,50). The other formulations either have not been evaluated, or studies are underway. There also has been some question regarding the chronic use of intranasal steroids causing osteoporosis in postmenopausal women; this issue remains unclear (44).

The first preparation, flunisolide, produced local stinging because it contained irritating levels of propylene glycol. This stinging has been reduced in the second formulation, which contains an increased concentration of polyethylene glycol, although some patients still complain of burning. Some preparations have a floral scent because of the preservative; others are odorless.

The frequency of use of the various preparations is once or twice a day, but all authorities suggest gradually reducing the dosage to the lowest that is therapeutically necessary (44,49,51). The original delivery system of some intranasal steroids required the use of chlorofluorocarbon propellants or Freon in self-pressurized aerosols. The use of these addi-

**TABLE 11.4. INTRANASAL STEROID PREPARATIONS**

| Preparations | Delivery System | Dosage Each Nostril | Benzalkonium Chloride |
|---|---|---|---|
| Dexamethasone[a] | FHP | 2 sprays bid | Yes |
| Flunisolide | Pump | 2 sprays bid | No |
| Beclomethasone | FHP | 2 sprays bid | Yes |
| Double strength | FHP | 2 sprays qd | Yes |
| AQ | Pump | 2 sprays qd | Yes |
| Triamcinolone | FHP | 2 sprays qd | Yes |
| AQ | Pump | 2 sprays qd | Yes |
| Fluticasone | Pump | 2 sprays qd | Yes |
| Budesonide | FHP | 2 sprays bid or 4 sprays qd | Yes |
| AQ | Pump | 1 spray qd | No |
| Powder[b] | Pump | 1 spray qd | |
| Mometasone | Pump | 2 sprays qd | Yes |

[a]No longer recommended because of adrenal–pituitary axis alterations.
[b]Not available in the United States.

tives has been questioned, and they are now being phased out of use at the request of the FDA. The aqueous preparations give a better distribution onto the nasal mucosa (44). More recently, the use of the preservative benzalkonium chloride has been questioned. This additive inhibits ciliary function and may be associated with epithelial metaplasia and cell death and inhibition of neutrophil function, so its exclusion is recommended by some researchers (44,52).

## MAST CELL STABILIZERS

Mast cell stabilizers are available as nasal, ophthalmic, pulmonary, and oral preparations. The oral preparation has been approved in the United States only for mastocytosis. In other countries, the oral form also is used for treating food allergies.

The first drug in this class to be developed was cromolyn sodium (sodium cromoglycate). Its mechanism of action has not been fully described, but it is known that the mast cell membrane is stabilized, preventing release of the chemical mediators. It appears that calcium flow into the cell is inhibited, thereby preventing degranulation (45). There are other mechanisms that may prevent the late allergic reaction. Mast cell stabilizers increase phosphorylation of the 78-kd protein that terminates allergic responses or bind to sodium cromoglycate–type cell surface receptor with inhibition of protein kinase. These drugs also inhibit the inflammatory effect of neutrophils and eosinophils that produce the late-phase allergic reaction (53). This drug is effective for allergic rhinitis when used before the patient is subjected to the allergen. Originally, the recommended dosage was five to six times a day as a nasal spray, with gradual reduction to the lowest effective dose. It is now a nonprescription

drug in the United States, recommended to be used four times a day.

Nedocromil is a newer mast cell stabilizer with approximately ten times the strength of its predecessor. It is available in this country as an asthma preventative and elsewhere in the world as a nasal preparation as well. As well as being more potent, it is needed only two to four times a day, enhancing compliance. The ophthalmic preparation (2%) was released in 2000 in the United States.

Ketotifen is now available as an antihistamine–mast cell drug for allergic eye disease, as described earlier. It is nonsedating in this instance. When used orally in Europe for asthma, allergic dermatitis, and anaphylaxis, it is somewhat sedating (31).

Lodoxamide has been shown to reduce tryptase levels in allergic inflammation. In the eye, its effect is to reduce the inflammatory cells in tears after allergen challenge by inhibiting eosinophil chemotaxis. It is more potent than cromolyn (24,25).

Pemirolast potassium was approved as an ophthalmic mast cell stabilizer in 1999 for allergic conjunctivitis, but the recommendations for its use were not available as of this publication (32).

Other mast cell stabilizers are being studied and may become available in other countries. Isospaglumic acid, when used as a nasal spray, appears to have protective effects. Oxatomide is still being studied and may eventually be a useful preventive therapy (43).

## ANTILEUKOTRIENES

Cysteinyl leukotrienes ($LTC_4$, $LTD_4$, and $LTE_4$) are produced during inflammatory reactions from arachidonic acid metabolism. Receptor antagonists against these leukotrienes have been used predominantly in asthma care. Because allergic rhinitis and asthma are both inflammatory diseases with involvement of leukotrienes, a drug effective for one might be expected to be effective treatment for the other. Meltzer reviewed the literature on the drugs classified as cysteinyl leukotriene receptor antagonists (54). The oral drugs he reviewed were zafirlukast and montelukast. Since then, zileuton also has been approved. These oral medications vary slightly in effectiveness and side effects. Zafirlukast is used twice a day for patients 12 years of age and older (55); montelukast is used once a day for patients starting at 6 years of age (56). These drugs do not fully relieve the symptoms but appear to make other drugs, such as corticosteroids and antihistamines, more effective.

Very little has been published with reference to this class of drugs and nasal symptomatology. However, based on Meltzer's work (54) and that of Simon (57) and Ulualp and colleagues (58), the additive effect of these drugs should enhance the use of antihistamines and intranasal steroids.

Pranlukast is not yet available in this country. It was effective in over half the cases of moderate to severe asthma in a study in Japan (59). It may have potential for the treatment of allergic rhinitis.

## ANTICHOLINERGICS

Drugs such as ipratropium bromide and atropine, when used as nasal sprays, help suppress the thin nasal secretions that are stimulated during the early-phase reaction of allergic rhinitis. They also improve this symptom during cold exposure, in patients with vasomotor rhinitis, and in those exposed to rapid temperatures changes such as loading dock workers and butchers. There is no rebound effect. Ipratropium bromide is available in two strengths, 0.03% and 0.06% by prescription. In most cases, the lower dose is sufficient for chronic symptoms of allergy and for vasomotor rhinitis in the elderly patient. In a 1999 study, ipratropium bromide was found to be effective for rhinorrhea and had some effect on congestion in children, whereas beclomethasone improved sneezing better in a comparison study (60). In another study, the use of both drugs together enhanced the benefits for some patients (61). An OTC preparation in a lower dose is now available.

## MUCOLYTICS

Mucolytics are not antiallergy drugs but act to thin thickened secretions. Frequently, drugs such as guaifenesin are combined with other agents for symptomatic relief. The therapeutic dosage of guaifenesin is 2,400 mg/day, usually administered in divided doses.

Nasal saline thins secretions and aids in washing antigens from the nose. Nasal saline or Alkalol irrigations are especially effective if the secretions are thick and difficult to clear. Warmed, moist air and pressurized air devices also are available that may also give relief by improving the patient's nasal hygiene (43).

## MONOCLONAL ANTIBODIES

A new approach to the treatment of allergic diseases, including rhinitis and asthma, involves the use of monoclonal anti-immunoglobulin E (IgE) antibodies. These antibodies inhibit the initial expression of allergic symptoms by preventing the IgE-mediated triggering of the allergic reaction. A recombinant anti-IgE has been developed and is in clinical trials to demonstrate its safety and efficacy. The antibody represents a humanized molecule developed through a murine model, rhuMAb-E25. It has been investigated in the treatment of asthma, and has been shown to reduce the degree of allergic reactivity in atopic patients and to reduce the need for steroids and rescue medications in patients with asthma (62).

Another monoclonal antibody has been developed to antagonize the effects of the proinflammatory cytokine interleukin-5. By blocking the effect of this cytokine, which is directly associated with the symptomatic expression of allergic disease, clinicians may be able to decrease the severity of symptoms in patients with rhinitis and asthma (63).

## MISCELLANEOUS

There are other drugs on the horizon that may prove to be of value in treating allergic rhinitis. Misoprostol is such a drug. It is a synthetic prostaglandin $E_1$ analogue that appears to modulate aspects of inflammation. It may be useful in allergic rhinitis, and further research is indicated (64).

## SUMMARY

Therapy for each patient must be designed individually and determined by the symptoms and the patient's response. Some patients respond better to one class of drugs than to another type. The antihistamines were the first available agents specifically prescribed for patients with allergy. Decongestants help alleviate the congestion and stuffiness of allergic rhinitis. Intranasal steroids are very effective for both early-phase and late-phase allergic reactions. Mast cell stabilizers prevent degranulation and the cascade of mediator release, and are most effective when used prophylactically. Antileukotriene receptor antagonists have yet to be proven effective for allergic rhinitis, but appear to have great potential. Specific monoclonal antibodies also may have potential for future treatment of allergic diseases. There are other drugs and devices effective for symptomatic relief, and the future promises even more specific preparations as the pathophysiologic process of allergy is further elucidated.

## REFERENCES

1. Krause HF. Therapeutic advances in the management of allergic rhinitis and urticaria. *Otolaryngol Head Neck Surg* 1994;111: 348–354.
2. Simons FER. H$_1$-receptor antagonists: safety issues. *Ann Allergy Asthma Immunol* 1999;83:481–488.
3. Monahan BP, Ferguson CL, Killeavy ES, et al. Torsades de points occurring in association with terfenadine use. *JAMA* 1990;264: 2788–2790.
4. Smith SJ. Cardiovascular toxicity of antihistamines. *Otolaryngol Head Neck Surg* 1994;111:348–354.
5. Woosley R, Darrow WR. Analysis of potential adverse drug reactions: a case of mistaken identity [Letter]. *Am J Cardiol* 1994; 74:208–209.
6. Simons FER, Simons KJ. Second generation H$_1$-receptor antagonists. *Ann Allergy Asthma Immunol* 1991;66:5–17.
7. Simons FER. Antihistamines. In: Naclario RM, Durham SR, Mygind N, eds. *Rhinitis: mechanisms and management.* New York: Marcel Decker, 1999:267–290.
8. Position Statement. The use of newer allergy medications during pregnancy. American Academy of Allergy, Asthma, and Immunology. *Ann Allergy Asthma Immunol* 2000;84:475–480.
9. Brogden RN, McTavish D. Acrivastine: a review of its pharmacological properties and clinical potential in allergic rhinitis, pollen-induced asthma, and chronic urticaria. *Drugs* 1991;44:922–940.
10. Simons FER, McMillan JL, Simons KJ. A double blind, single dose, crossover comparison of cetirizine, terfenadine, loratadine, astemizole, and chlorpheniramine versus placebo: suppressive effect on wheal and flare during 24 hours in normal subjects. *J Allergy Clin Immunol* 1990;86:540–547.
11. Lockey RF, Findley S, Mitchell DQ, et al. Effects of cetirizine versus terfenadine in seasonal allergic rhinitis. *Ann Allergy Asthma Immunol* 1993;7:311–315.
12. Mansmann HC, Altman RA, Berman BA, et al. Efficacy and safety of cetirizine therapy in perennial allergic rhinitis. *Ann Allergy Asthma Immunol* 1992;58:348–353.
13. Breneman D, Bronsky EA, Bruce S, et al. Cetirizine and astemizole therapy for chronic idiopathic urticaria: a double blind, placebo controlled, comparative trial. *J Am Acad Dermatol* 1995; 22:192–198.
14. Pratt C, Brown AM, Rumpe D, et al. Cardiovascular safety of fexofenadine HCL. *Clin Exp Allergy* 1999;29[Suppl 3]:212–216.
15. Yownley RG. Cetirizine: a new H$_1$ antagonist with anti-eosinophilic activity in chronic urticaria. *J Am Acad Dermatol* 1991; 25:688–674.
16. Hinemarch I, Shamsi Z. Antihistamines: models to assess sedative properties, assessment of sedation, safety, and other side-effects. *Clin Exp Allergy* 1999;29[Suppl 3]:133–142.
17. Sussman GL, Mason J, Compton D, et al. The efficacy and safety of fexofenadine HCL and pseudoephedrine, alone and in combination, in seasonal allergic rhinitis. *J Allergy Clin Immunol* 1999;104:100–106.
18. Casale TB, Andrade C, Qu R. Safety and efficacy of once daily fexofenadine in the treatment of seasonal allergic rhinitis. *Allergy Asthma Proc* 1999;20:193–198.
19. Philpot EE. Safety of second generation antihistamines. *Asthma Allergy Proc* 2000;21:15–20.
20. Storms WW, Pearlman DS, Chervinski P, et al. Effectiveness of azelastine nasal solution in seasonal allergic rhinitis. *Ear Nose Throat J* 1944;73:382–394.
21. Meltzer EO, Weiler JM, Dockhorn RJ, et al. Azelastine nasal spray in management of seasonal allergic rhinitis. *Ann Allergy Asthma Immunol* 1994;74:354–359.
22. Grossman J, Halverson PC, Meltzer EO. Double-blind assessment of azelastine in the treatment of perennial allergic rhinitis. *Ann Allergy Asthma Immunol* 1999;73:141–146.
23. Storms WW. Azelastine nasal spray: treatment for symptoms of seasonal allergic rhinitis: pharmacological and clinical relevance. *Allergy Asthma Proc* 1999;20:200(abstr).
24. Abelson MB, Bielory L. *Contemporary approaches to ocular allergy management: therapeutic reference summary* [Monograph]. Milwaukee: American College of Allergy, Asthma and Immunology, 1997.
25. Abelson MB, Bielory L. *Contemporary approaches to ocular allergy.* Milwaukee: American College of Allergy, Asthma and Immunology, 1998.
26. Yanni JM, Miller ST, Gamache DA. Comparative effects of topical ocular anti-allergy drugs on human conjunctival mast cells. *Ann Allergy Asthma Immunol* 1997;79:541–545.
27. Abelson MB. Evaluation of olopatadine, a new ophthalmic anti-allergic agent with dual activity, using the conjunctival allergy challenge model. *Ann Allergy Asthma Immunol* 1998;81: 211–218.
28. Raizman MB, Abelson MB, Bielry L, et al. *New development in ocular allergies* [Monograph]. Milwaukee: The Willow Group, Inc., 1999:1–12.
29. Craps LP, Ney UM. Ketotifen: current views on its mechanism of action and their therapeutic implications. *Respiration* 1984; 45:411–421.
30. Greenwood CMB. The pharmacology of ketotifen. *Chest* 1982; 82[Suppl]:451–481.
31. Grant SM, Goa KL, Fitton A, et al. Ketotifen: a review of its pharmacological and pharmacokinetic properties, and therapeutic use in asthma and allergic disorders. *Drugs* 1990;40:412–440.
32. Fields L, Freedy T. New approvals by the FDA in 1999. *Bull Allegheny County Med Soc* 2000;89:244–247.
33. Gehanno P, Bremard-Oury C, Zeisser P. Comparison of ebastine to cetirizine in seasonal allergic rhinitis in adults. *Ann Allergy Asthma Immunol* 1996;76:507–512.
34. Murris-Espin M, Melac M, Charpennnntier J-C. Comparison of efficacy and safety of cetirizine and ebastine in patients with perennial allergic rhinitis. *Ann Allergy Asthma Immunol* 1998;80: 399–403.
35. Product insert, Flurinol (ebinastine). Boehringer Ingelheim, Ingelheim am Rhein, Germany.
36. Sabbah A, Dalle J, Wade AG, et al. Comparison of the efficacy, safety, and onset of action of mizolastine, cetirizine, and placebo in seasonal allergic rhinoconjunctivitis. *Ann Allergy Asthma Immunol* 1999;83:319–325.
37. Simons FER. H$_1$-receptor antagonists: clinical pharmacology and therapeutics. *J Allergy Clin Immunol* 1988;84:845–861.
38. Mizolastine. *Drug Information Line* 412-369-4600.
39. Handley D. *Clinical advances in stereoisomers and active metabolites: new developments for allergy and asthma therapy. Symposium highlights.* American College of Allergy Asthma Immunol 1999: 17–19.
40. Krause HF. Pharmacotherapy for allergic nasal disease. *Curr Opin Otolaryngol Head Neck Surg* 1994;2:147–153.
41. Eccles R. Nasal airflow and decongestants. In: Naclario RM, Durham SR, Mygind N, eds. *Rhinitis: mechanisms and management.* New York: Marcel Dekker, 1999:291–312.
42. Beck RA, Mercado DL, Segun SM, et al. Cardiovascular effects of pseudoephedrine in medically controlled hypertensive patients. *Arch Intern Med* 1992;152:1242–1245.
43. Krause HF. Pharmacotherapy of perennial and seasonal allergic rhinitis. *Clin Immunother* 1995;3:308–324.

44. Mygind N, Naclerio RM. Intranasal corticosteroids. In: Naclerio RM, Mygind N, Durham SR, et al., eds. *Rhinitis: mechanisms and management.* New York: Marcel Dekker, 1999:221–256.

45. Krause HF. Surgery in the allergic patient. In: Krause HF, ed. *Otolaryngic Allergy and Immunology.* Philadelphia: WB Saunders, 1989:279–288.

46. Mabry RL. Corticosteroids in rhinology. *Otolaryngol Head Neck Surg* 1993;108:768–770.

47. *Corticosteroids (nasal)* [monograph]. Rockville, MD: United States Pharmacopeia, 1994.

48. Ledford DK, Lockey RF. Allergic rhinitis: offering relief this season. *J Respir Dis* 1998;19:647–666.

49. Creticos P, Fireman P, Settipane GA. Intranasal budesonide aqueous pump spray (Rhinocort Aqua) for the treatment of seasonal allergic rhinitis. *Allergy Asthma Proc* 1998;19:285–294.

50. Meltzer EO. Clinical and anti-inflammatory effects of intranasal budesonide aqueous pump spray in the treatment of perennial allergic rhinitis. *Ann Allergy Asthma Immunol* 1998;81:128–134.

51. Nayak AS, Banov C, Corren, et al. Once daily mometasone furoate dry powder in the treatment of patients with persistent asthma. *Ann Allergy Asthma Immunol* 2000;84:417–424.

52. Steinsvag SK. *Benzalkonium chloride: the adverse effects of excipient preservatives in nasal corticosteroids* [monograph]. Med Learning Center Inc. and Dannemiller Memorial Educational Foundation, San Antonio, TX, 1999.

53. Frieri M. Antigen-specific anti-allergic inflammatory effects of sodium cromoglycate: is there a new cellular mechanism? [Editorial]. *Ann Allergy Asthma Immunol* 1999;83:493–494.

54. Meltzer EO. Role for cysteinyl leukotriene receptor antagonist therapy in asthma and their potential role in allergic rhinitis based on the concept of "one linked airway disease." *Ann Allergy Asthma Immunol* 2000;84:176–187.

55. Grossman J, Smith LJ, Wilson AM, et al. Long-term safety and efficacy of zafirlukast in the treatment of asthma: interim results of an open-label extension trail. *Ann Allergy Asthma Immunol* 1999;82;361–369.

56. Noonan M, Knorr B, Noonan G, et al. Evaluation of the safety profile of montelukast (MK-0476) in adult and pediatric patients (ages 6 to 14 years). *Asthma Allergy Proc* 1999;20:200(abstr).

57. Simon RA. The role of leukotrienes and anti-leukotriene agents in the pathogenesis and treatment of allergic rhinitis. *Clin Rev Allergy Immunol* 1999;17:271–275.

58. Ulualp SO, Sterman BM, Toohill RJ. Anti-leukotriene therapy for the relief of sinus symptoms in aspirin triad disease. *Ear Nose Throat J* 1999;78:604–606.

59. Kohrogi H, Iwagoe H, Fujii K, et al. The role of cysteinyl leukotrienes in the pathogenesis of asthma: clinical study of leukotriene antagonist pranlukast for 1 year in moderate and severe asthma. *Respirology* 1999;4:319–323.

60. Milgrom H, Biondi R, Georgitis JW, et al. Comparison of ipratropium bromide 0.03% with beclomethasone dipropionate in the treatment of perennial rhinitis in children. *Ann Allergy Asthma Immunol* 1999;83:105–111.

61. Dockhorn R, Aaronson D, Bronsky E, et al. Ipratropium bromide nasal spray 0.03% and beclomethasone nasal spray alone and in combination for the treatment of rhinorrhea in perennial rhinitis. *Ann Allergy Asthma Immunol* 1999;82:349–359.

62. Barnes PJ. Anti-IgE therapy in asthma: rationale and therapeutic potential. *Int Arch Allergy Immunol* 2000;123:196–204.

63. Lotvall J, Pullerits T. Treating asthma with anti-IgE and anti-IL5. *Curr Pharm Des* 1999;5:757–770.

64. Babakhin AA, Nolte H, DuBuske LM Effect of misoprostol on the secretion of histamine from basophils of whole blood. *Ann Allergy Asthma Immunol* 2000;3:361–365.

# AEROALLERGEN IMMUNOTHERAPY

**RICHARD C. HAYDON III**
**BRUCE R. GORDON**

We cannot precisely control the effects of all stimulation coming from our external environment. However, through adaptation, our body has the ability to inhibit the effects of certain types of stimulation, if the stimulation schedule is regular, smooth, and without abrupt changes in stimulus intensity. Such is the approach to aeroallergen immunotherapy, where the body is regularly exposed to an antigenic stimulus. Immunotherapy is a method of modulating the body's immune system to enable it to tolerate the effects of environmental allergenic stimulation that cannot otherwise be controlled. Immunotherapy treats immunoglobulin E (IgE)-mediated allergic symptoms by intentional exposure to regular, progressive doses of the same specific aeroallergens that are responsible for producing symptoms. When successful, immunotherapy eventually results in downregulation of the immunologic response, and control of symptoms associated with usual levels of environmental exposure to the treated aeroallergens.

## ORIGINS OF IMMUNOTHERAPY

It was the successful use of the passive transfer of antibodies against toxins, demonstrated by Pasteur, Von Behring, and Kitasato (1), that gave birth to the concept of aeroallergen immunotherapy. Pollen-induced illness was believed to be caused by toxins, leading to early attempts at pollen immunization (2,3). For example, Curtis (4) used whole-weed extracts with success in alleviating symptoms. In the hands of others, anaphylaxis ensued (2), but animal studies carried out by Besredka and Steinhardt in 1907 indicated that technical details of the doses and immunization schedule were responsible for the anaphylactic problems, rather than properties of the antigen extracts (5). Leonard Noon then introduced the concept of quantitation into pollen treatment, by

choosing treatment doses based on measurement of pollen sensitivity in each individual, through conjunctival titration challenges (3). Using a measurably safe, progressive, and reproducible escalation of doses, Noon and Koessler (2,3) were able to demonstrate resistance to pollen challenge in pollen-sensitive patients who had been treated with immunotherapy. The benefits of immunotherapy were shown to last for at least a year, after 1 or 2 years of therapy (3,6). By 1915, Cooke had introduced immunotherapy into the United States (7,8).

## EFFICACY AND MECHANISM OF ACTION OF IMMUNOTHERAPY

Immunotherapy is the third useful treatment modality for allergy, in addition to avoidance therapy and pharmacotherapy. Immunotherapy has been shown to be an effective treatment for allergic rhinitis, asthma, and insect sting allergy (9–18). In many cases, aeroallergens cannot be completely avoided, especially in patients who are allergic to multiple allergens or who are among the estimated 61% of U.S. households with pets (19,20). Fortunately, immunotherapy increases tolerance to allergens, so it can supplement avoidance and pharmacotherapy efforts (19) without fear of adverse interaction with these other modalities. Also, although modern allergy pharmacotherapy is very free of immediate side effects, the long-term effects of these medications, when used over an entire life, are unknown (21). Immunotherapy, on the other hand, enjoys the unique advantage of effecting a specific, durable modulation of the immune system (19,21), using antigens to which patients are normally exposed. Also, immunotherapy has been in use for several generations, and has not been shown to be responsible for systemic adverse effects other than those due to accidental production of anaphylaxis. Furthermore, with current consumer emphasis on wellness and self-direction of medical care, any treatment that treats the cause rather than the symptoms is easily embraced (21). Finally, immunotherapy treatment costs are moderate (22), yet successful immunotherapy favorably affects quality of life and reduces

**R. C. Haydon III:** Department of Surgery, Division of Otolaryngology, University of Kentucky College of Medicine, Lexington, Kentucky.
**B. R. Gordon:** Department of Otology and Laryngology, Harvard University, Cambridge; Associate Surgeon, Massachusetts Eye and Ear Infirmary, Boston; Chief of Otolaryngology, Cape Cod Hospital, Hyannis, Massachusetts.

costs from pharmacotherapy, sick days, and reduced productivity (23).

A large body of literature demonstrates the efficacy of immunotherapy. In studies that predominantly used symptom and medication scores, patients receiving immunotherapy for allergies to grass pollen (10,24–35), mountain cedar pollen (35,36), birch pollen (37–39), ragweed, dust mite, cat, and *Alternaria* enjoyed relief (10,18,24–36,40–46). Symptom–medication scores improve even in patients who have been previously poorly controlled with pharmacotherapy (34). Objective clinical testing also has been used to demonstrate immunotherapy efficacy in patients with asthma sensitive to ragweed (47). In addition, improvement in the endoscopic appearance of nasal mucosa and in quality of life of patients with rhinitis occurs when immunotherapy is based on quantitative testing by skin endpoint titration (SET) (48).

In addition to direct clinical improvements, immunotherapy causes measurable changes in many immunologic parameters. T lymphocytes play a major role in the cascade of events during the allergic inflammatory response (49). They regulate IgE production, maturation of some mast cell populations, macrophage activation, and granulocyte mediator release (50). During effective immunotherapy, there are increases in allergen-specific suppressor T cells (51, 52). Some of these inhibit the synthesis of allergen-specific IgE (50,52), and others cause a decrease in production of proallergic cytokines by allergic immune response cells (52–54). Finally, T helper cells stimulate production of allergen-specific IgG.

During dose escalation, there is a gradual increase in allergen-specific IgG1 and IgG4 antibodies (25,27,29,30, 36,41,55,56) to a plateau well above pretreatment levels (19,57,58). These antibodies have been termed *blocking* antibodies because they compete with IgE for allergen binding (58–60) and have been shown to provide passive protection from experimental anaphylaxis (2,3,60,61). Although increases in IgG1 predominate early in treatment, IgG4 rises later, as optimal immunotherapy doses are reached. IgG4 elevation also is temporally related to symptom improvement (62), and so is more strongly correlated with clinical change, as measured by symptom–medication scores, than are all other measured immunologic parameters (19, 63–66). With discontinuance of immunotherapy, allergen-specific IgG4 is degraded, and its level falls (67).

During the first 2 to 3 months of immunotherapy, allergen-specific IgE rises above pretreatment levels, usually by twofold or more (19,41,42,68,69). Then, during the next 18 to 24 months, IgE levels gradually decline to below pretreatment levels (19,41,42,69–71). This inhibition of IgE synthesis is believed to be caused by the generation of allergen-specific suppressor T cells (50,51). Unlike levels of IgG blocking antibody, these declines in IgE do not directly parallel, and thus do not correlate with, clinical improvement (58). The drop in IgE does, however, inversely corre-

late with the onset of the rise in IgG blocking antibody, a relationship known as the *scissors pattern* of antibody response (72). A reduction in specific IgE levels does imply a reduction in allergen sensitivity because the degree of sensitivity is in general proportional to specific IgE levels (22). Similar to the rises in IgE that are seen during the early stages of immunotherapy with aeroallergens, allergen-specific IgE also typically rises in nonimmunized allergic patients after natural seasonal exposure to allergens to which those patients are allergic. In patients who are effectively treated by immunotherapy, this typical postseasonal IgE rise is substantially decreased (36,51,71,73). Synthesis of other immunoglobulin classes also is affected because allergen-specific B lymphocytes that produce both IgA and IgM increase during immunotherapy. This has potential beneficial effects on mucosal immune barrier function, and may help limit antigen penetration into the body (74). For example, ragweed-specific IgA and IgG are both increased in nasal secretions during immunotherapy (57).

Studies of antigen-induced histamine release indicate that basophil reactivity and sensitivity also are downregulated during immunotherapy. There is a decrease in the total amount of histamine release (75–77), a reduced response during pollen seasons (78), and an elevation in the threshold for histamine release (75–77). Decreased production of histamine-releasing factors from monocytes during grass pollen challenge in patients on immunotherapy (31) suggests that these changes may be due to decreased release of proinflammatory cytokines. Patients on immunotherapy show both an improvement in histamine challenge tolerance (73) and an increase in the threshold to a variety of other mediators, including prostaglandin $D_2$, TAME(N-alpha-tosyl-L-arginine methyl ester)-esterase, leukotrienes, and kinins (79, 80). The reduction in histamine release from immunotherapy treatment precedes any decrease in IgE or increase in IgG (81), and may explain the reductions in skin and nasal reactivity that also precede these antibody changes (68,80).

Clinical changes also accompany successful immunotherapy. As increasing doses of antigen extracts are injected, tolerance develops both to the extracts and to natural allergen exposures (19). Responsiveness to nasal or bronchial challenge decreases, skin reactivity lessens, and symptoms diminish (82,83). Fewer medications, office or emergency department visits, and hospitalizations are necessary (84). Although immunotherapy elevates the provocation threshold for symptoms, it does not abolish symptom provocation. In fact, experimental challenges with purposefully high doses can produce symptoms equal to those produced before beginning immunotherapy (19).

Lessened skin reactivity during and after immunotherapy has been observed through suppression of the immediate response to intradermal tests (29,30,32). Significant decreases in symptoms, medication scores, and intensities of prick test results are seen after immunotherapy against dust mite *(Dermatophagoides pteronyssinus)* (18,41–43), *Al-*

*ternaria* extract (56), and birch pollen (38). Suppression of the late-phase response to intradermal tests also has been documented (32,36,80), and likely is due to a decrease in mast cell and basophil chemoattractants (85) because the late phase depends on the recruitment of these cells (86). Suppression of eosinophil migration into skin and nasal mucosa during the late-phase response (32,87), as well as reduction of eosinophil chemotactic factor (38,39) and eosinophil cationic protein levels (38), also have been observed. Also, decreases in infiltrating CD3 and CD4 T lymphocytes in the late-phase skin response have been documented (32).

Finally, challenge tests also are affected by immunotherapy. Reduced immediate-phase mucosal reactivity was demonstrated during conjunctival (32) and nasal challenge tests (30,41,43). Significant decreases in nasal challenge test sensitivity have been shown after immunotherapy for dust mite (18,41–43), *Alternaria* (56), and birch (38). Suppression of the late-phase response to nasal challenge tests also has been documented by measuring significant reductions of inflammatory mediators in late-phase nasal secretions (79).

## CLINICAL ASSESSMENT OF IMMUNOTHERAPY CANDIDATES

### Indications for Immunotherapy

The only patients for whom allergen immunotherapy is absolutely indicated are those who have severe IgE-mediated anaphylactic reactions to *Hymenoptera* venom (88). Left untreated, such patients are at risk of anaphylaxis and death from future stings (19). In most other situations, immunotherapy is used for non–life-threatening conditions (88), and yet immunotherapy is potentially life threatening (89). Therefore, immunotherapy intervention "should not be undertaken lightly, haphazardly, or arbitrarily" (51). Three prerequisites should be satisfied in candidates being considered for immunotherapy. First, the candidate should have proven IgE-mediated allergic disease (15,69,90) such as allergic rhinoconjunctivitis, asthma (19), or insect sting anaphylaxis (9,15). Allergen immunotherapy has not been proven, by rigorous studies, to be effective for patients with non–IgE-mediated rhinitis or asthma, chronic bronchitis, or emphysema. Immunotherapy also is still unproven for urticaria, atopic dermatitis, food allergy, headache, and drug reactions, even though these conditions are sometimes IgE mediated and clinically often do improve with immunotherapy. In such cases, a careful informed consent discussion is useful to clarify both the potential benefits, as well as possible drawbacks, of immunotherapy. Second, allergic symptoms should directly correlate (9) with natural exposures to specific allergens that have tested positive, using intradermal or in vitro techniques that quantitate IgE-mediated hypersensitivity (19,22,91–96). Mere presence of positive skin or in vitro tests, without correlated symptoms, is not a good

reason to embark on immunotherapy (9,91–94). Because there is not always concordance between the level of allergen reactivity from diagnostic testing and its importance in causing symptoms, the two must be plausibly related to consider immunotherapy. This admonition is especially important in the patient who tests weakly positive. Third, the degree of improvement from appropriate pharmacotherapy and environmental avoidance should be insufficient, or these treatment methods must be inapplicable or unfeasible. Side effects (19,49), inconvenience, or cost can hamper medication use. Rarely, contraindications or the fear of potential side effects prevents pharmacotherapy (21). All of these factors can cause noncompliance and poor efficacy (49). Satisfactory environmental avoidance frequently is even more difficult to achieve (19). Although some physicians believe that formal IgE testing should not be carried out unless immunotherapy is contemplated (51), testing often is helpful in teaching avoidance measures, and should be used whenever knowledge of sensitivities might improve environmental control. Despite such help, the patient who reacts to many seasonal pollens, or to molds, dust mites, or pets, often is unable to minimize exposure without difficult, often expensive, lifestyle changes.

Duration and severity of symptoms also exert a major influence on indications for immunotherapy because "immunotherapy is not appropriate for treatment of trivial, equivocal, or evanescent symptoms" (22). Short exposure periods resulting in symptoms lasting only several weeks per year may not be significant enough to warrant immunotherapy. However, if symptoms span two or more seasons each year (9,69), or more than one season, totaling 6 months or more (21), or become perennial, then the risk of complications, such as development of reactive lower airway disease, increases. Like rhinitis, asthma may benefit from the long-term antiinflammatory therapy that immunotherapy offers. Even if the anticipated symptom duration each year spans one season only, it still may be appropriate to consider immunotherapy if the symptoms are severe (21), if symptoms are becoming progressively worse each year (69), or if the patient and physician agree that this is the best approach. One other strong factor favoring immunotherapy is in severe allergic conditions that require regular use of corticosteroids (96,97), where immunotherapy can serve as a corticosteroid-sparing treatment (22).

Frequently, the compliant behavior that is necessary for successful immunotherapy is easier for patients to maintain than the behavior changes required for environmental avoidance or chronic pharmacotherapy. However, when immunotherapy compliance is not satisfactory, the consequences are significant because successful immunotherapy depends on regular treatment to effect desired immunologic change. Therefore, immunotherapy should not be undertaken without a minimum 1-year compliance agreement between physician and patient. In addition, immunotherapy candidates should be carefully informed of the 3- to 5-

year time frame needed to complete immunologic changes. The clinician should beware of patients who have a history of many broken appointments because they are not likely to benefit from immunotherapy (22).

Age is another factor to consider. Although very young and very old patients may be good immunotherapy candidates (9), most of the controlled studies showing immunotherapy benefit have been carried out on patients ranging from 6 to no more than 50 years of age (98). Significant inhalant allergy is uncommon before 2 years of age (21), and symptomatic pollen sensitivity rarely occurs before the age of 5 years (21). But when inhalant allergy does begin early, it usually involves cat, dust, and mold sensitivity, and may be amenable to environmental modification. In some cases, young children who might benefit from immunotherapy may not accept injections. In these cases, sublingual immunotherapy can be considered. With aging, acute symptoms of inhalant allergies often become less severe, but chronically damaged mucosa from either long-standing rhinosinusitis or asthma is common. Limited studies in patients older than 60 years of age have shown immunotherapy to be effective for rhinitis, asthma, conjunctivitis, and insect sting allergy. Immunotherapy should not be expected to reverse the fixed, irreversible obstructive component of asthma (9), or heal long-standing chronic sinusitis with irreversibly injured mucosa. However, immunotherapy may still benefit these patients by preventing the allergic inflammation from continuing to worsen.

## Contraindications to Immunotherapy

The only absolute contraindication to immunotherapy is failure to prove that a relevant allergy exists (21,22). However, there are a number of conditions during which immunotherapy is either relatively contraindicated or should be carried out only with extra caution. At the top of the list of relative contraindications to beginning immunotherapy is the asthmatic patient who is less than optimally controlled. There is always a higher risk of serious anaphylactic reactions during immunotherapy in asthmatic patients, especially those who are highly sensitive or who have a history of many emergency department visits. Most fatalities from immunotherapy have occurred in asthmatic patients, particularly when significant asthma symptoms immediately preceded allergen administration (9,52,99,100). Although many patients with asthma might benefit from immunotherapy, institution of effective medical therapy and environmental controls normally should precede attempts at immunotherapy (22). If obstructive symptoms have recently worsened significantly, especially if pulmonary function tests show less than 70% of predicted normal values (101), then initiation or escalation of immunotherapy should be carried out with extreme caution (9).

A second relative contraindication is treatment with β-adrenergic blocker drugs. If these patients undergo anaphy-

laxis, the reaction may be both more severe (102) and more refractory to emergency treatment with adrenergic agents such as epinephrine (9,21,103). β-Adrenergic blockade causes increased production of inflammatory mediators during an allergic reaction, and also increases the severity of allergic symptoms by blocking smooth muscle relaxation in the airway (21,103). Thus, in a patient with asthma, the risks of β-blockade are even greater (9). Use of a cardioselective β-blocker only reduces the risk of asthma exacerbation during a reaction; it does not decrease the severity of other allergic symptoms. Cardioselective β-blockers also do not improve the treatment of anaphylaxis, including the unopposed α-adrenergic stimulation that may occur with the use of epinephrine, which can lead to a possible hypertensive crisis (21,104). Therefore, it is wise to try to switch immunotherapy candidates who are on β-blockers to alternate drugs. In patients who must remain on β-blockers, the benefits of immunotherapy must be carefully weighed against the increased risks of an anaphylactic emergency (22). An informed consent discussion is advisable with patients who cannot be weaned from their β-blocker.

Immunotherapy during pregnancy also deserves special attention. Although immunotherapy itself is not injurious to either mother or fetus, anaphylaxis from immunotherapy is potentially injurious (105). The greatest risks for anaphylaxis usually are present either during early escalation of immunotherapy (21,106) or at very high doses, at or above the maximally tolerated dose (MTD). Therefore, it usually is not prudent to initiate immunotherapy during pregnancy (107), or to escalate doses in patients who are already on treatment (21). Also, dose levels for immunotherapy already in progress may need to be decreased (9). It is recommended that the patient's obstetrician be consulted about the decision to continue immunotherapy during pregnancy (21,22). After parturition, it is possible to resume normal escalation immunotherapy, even if the patient is breast feeding (9).

Patients who have established immune dysregulation also deserve special attention. It has been reported that autoimmune disease can develop in patients who are undergoing immunotherapy (108). However, there are no prospective studies indicating that immunotherapy either causes or aggravates immune complex disease (109), vasculitis, or autoimmune disease (110). Similarly, there are no published studies of immunotherapy efficacy in congenital or acquired immunodeficiency states such as Wiskott-Aldrich syndrome and acquired immunodeficiency syndrome (9), both of which can be associated with IgE dysregulation (111). Prudent judgment would avoid immunomodulatory therapy in patients who already have established evidence of immune dysregulation because the potential risks of immunotherapy in these conditions may outweigh the potential benefits (9). Exceptions may be appropriate when allergy symptoms are severe, or in patients who require long-term systemic corticosteroids for their IgE-mediated allergies (21,112). In such cases, obtaining informed consent is recommended (22).

Specific immunotherapy also is not currently recommended for allergic bronchopulmonary aspergillosis or for hypersensitivity pneumonitis, although both diseases are associated with IgE elevations. Whenever the causative allergen cannot be avoided, immunotherapy may not result in improvement, and can potentially exacerbate the condition (9). However, in the closely similar condition of allergic fungal sinusitis, specific immunotherapy can be administered after complete removal of fungal contents from the affected sinuses, and appears to be of substantial benefit (113,114).

## ALLERGY TESTING AND INTERPRETATION

Potential candidates for immunotherapy must undergo IgE testing for appropriate allergens and results should be documented. Selection of the appropriate test to use to determine allergic sensitivity is very important because immunotherapy is based on the interpretation of the results. In the modern era, there are essentially four testing options. There are two types of in vivo tests, either combined prick and intradermal skin tests, or SET. The other two types of useful tests to determine allergic sensitivity are the radioallergosorbent test (RAST) (115) and the many variants of enzyme-linked immunosorbent assays (ELISA) (116). All four testing methods are sensitive and safe (22). Three of these test methods are quantitative, allowing estimation of the patient's degree of sensitivity to each tested antigen. Measuring quantitative antigen reactivity is advantageous because not all antigens that test positive are identified at equal concentrations. An appreciation of these quantitative differences forms the basis for differential immunotherapy dosing for each individual antigen according to the patient's sensitivity. It also allows for use of an aggressive, but confidently safe, immunotherapy starting dose (117,118). In practical terms, this means that it is not necessary to start immunotherapy for every antigen, on every patient, at the same very weak dose. This approach decreases the time to attain maintenance, and speeds the onset of symptomatic improvement. Knowledge of the individual antigen sensitivities allows the starting concentrations for each antigen to be independently regulated, even though they are in the same treatment vial. Knowledge of these individual sensitivities also allows for the escalation schedules for antigens of like sensitivity to be regulated independently of other allergens. For instance, less sensitive allergens can be combined into one treatment vial and started at a high initial dose, whereas highly sensitive antigens are combined in another treatment vial and started at a very weak initial dose. Such separation of antigens with different degrees of sensitivity helps prevent reactions during escalation. To be able to escalate doses of like-sensitivity antigens together, so that maintenance levels are all reached at close to the same time, allows escalation to progress more efficiently than if the relative sensitivities were unquanti-

tated and thus not known (22). Furthermore, knowing the degree of sensitivity also permits safe coseasonal immunotherapy treatment (117,119).

Interpretation of positive allergy test results requires the experience and judgment of a knowledgeable physician (51). Overinterpretation of skin tests that are not correlated with symptom production may have led to more diagnostic errors and immunotherapy failures in the management of allergic disease than any other factor (120). The clinician should strive to treat only those allergens for which there is clinical evidence of relevance (19). Including clinically irrelevant allergens in immunotherapy treatment is wasteful and may sensitize to allergens that were previously unimportant (19,121). Careful attention to control tests also is critical because drugs with type 1 ($H_1$) antihistamine properties block whealing, and can prevent positive skin tests from forming. This effect can be detected by comparison with appropriate positive controls, such as dilutions of histamine. Nonspecific false-positive whealing also can occur, especially due to concentrated solutions of the glycerin preservative that is commonly used in aqueous allergen extracts. False-positive results are a problem primarily when testing concentrated allergen dilutions, particularly dilutions #1 [1:100 weight/volume (w/v)] and #2 (1:500 w/v), but can be detected by comparison with negative controls containing glycerin concentrations identical to that present in antigen-containing dilutions. Rarely, nonspecific whealing occurs with even more dilute glycerin solutions, so that skin testing is unreliable and in vitro testing must be used. Failure to use proper controls can result in either the spurious detection of allergies that do not exist, or in the failure to detect allergies that do exist.

## PREIMMUNOTHERAPY COUNSELING AND CONSENT

Once a candidate has met the necessary indications and has been tested, a counseling session is recommended before making a final decision to treat. This meeting should provide an explanation of (a) the immunotherapy concept; (b) the basic differences between immunotherapy, pharmacotherapy, and environmental avoidance; (c) the indications (including a dissatisfaction with outcomes obtained from appropriate pharmacotherapy and environmental avoidance); (d) special risks or circumstances requiring special precautions; (e) the proposed length of treatment; and (f) the potential for allergy injection reactions. Immunotherapy candidates should be told that months of treatment will be needed to produce some symptom relief, and that years of treatment will be required to obtain lasting relief (22). They need to understand that failure to have regular treatments over long periods defeats the whole purpose of the program. They also need to know that immunotherapy may not result in permanent cure. Discontinuance of treatment, even after faithful compliance for several years, may result in return of symptoms (69,122) and necessitate reinstitution of therapy (22). Allergy reactions that may occur during immunotherapy also should be discussed with candidates. Patients should be clearly informed that although systemic reactions are not expected, reactions can and may occur, and can rarely result in death. Candidates also should be told that, unlike systemic reactions, local reactions are expected, and normally help to define the MTD. It is good practice to have immunotherapy patients sign an informed consent form, just as they should before any invasive procedure. And finally, when immunotherapy is scheduled to begin, candidates should be given a prescription and instructed in the use of a self-administered epinephrine kit that can be used in case a significant reaction occurs after an office or home immunotherapy treatment. Follow-up treatment assessment meetings between patient and physician, at least two to three times a year initially, and approximately every 6 to 12 months thereafter, are recommended.

## INITIAL IMMUNOTHERAPY DOSE

During the initial phase of escalation immunotherapy, IgE antibodies begin to rise while there has not yet been an increase in protective IgG blocking antibodies. It should be no surprise that this initial escalation is associated with higher risk for anaphylaxis (106). The simplest approach to reduce this risk is to give all patients very weak starting doses. In fact, this was the standard approach early in the 20th century. Given the crude understanding of anaphylaxis mechanisms and poor quantification techniques at that time, conservative immunotherapy initiation was appropriate. Many allergists who base immunotherapy on prick testing continue to initiate therapy at arbitrary low doses that they believe are low enough to minimize the risk of anaphylaxis (19,58,123). However, the actual initiating dose varies greatly among physicians (82,95,96,124–127), from as dilute as 1:1,000,000,000 w/v to as concentrated as 1:5,000 w/v (51,126–128). Table 12.1 illustrates starting doses based on prick testing or tenfold intradermal testing, as reported by several general allergists (129–132), and shows comparable starting doses based on quantitative testing by in vitro techniques or SET, using a fivefold dilution system. For sensitive patients, an initial starting dose, based on SET or in vitro testing, of 0.05 mL of dilution #6, is as conservative, or more conservative, than all but Bierman's recommendation. And, for average patients, the wide range of starting doses used by general allergists indicates uncertainty over what constitutes a safe starting dose when a quantitative method of testing has not been used.

## Quantitation-based Initial Dose

An inherent disadvantage of these starting dose techniques is that prick tests and single-dilution intradermal tests used

**TABLE 12.1. COMPARISON OF IMMUNOTHERAPY STARTING DOSES BASED ON PRICK TESTS OR TEN-FOLD DILUTION INTRADERMAL TESTS, AND STARTING DOSES BASED ON SET OR IN VITRO TESTS**

| Patient Type and Authors | Starting Antigen Concentration (w/v) | Starting Injection Volume (mL) | SET/In Vitro Equivalent Concentratio (w/v) | SET/In Vitro Equivalent Volume (mL) |
|---|---|---|---|---|
| **Sensitive patients** | | | | |
| Bierman et al. (126) | 1:1,000,000 | 0.05 | 1:312,500 dilution #6 | 0.02 |
| Van Metre and Adkinson (19) Creticos (122) | 1:200,00 | 0.10 | 1:312,500 dilution #6 | 0.16 |
| Galant (132) | 1:100,000 | 0.05 | 1:312,500 dilution #6 | 0.16 |
| Patterson et al. (128) | 1:50,000 | 0.05 | 1:62,500 dilution #5 | 0.06 |
| **Average patients** | | | | |
| Nelson et al. (129) | 1:100,000 | 0.05 | 1:62,500 dilution #5 | 0.03 |
| Bernstein and Bernstein (130) | 1:100,000 | 0.10 | 1:62,500 dilution #5 | 0.06 |
| Ledford and Lockey (9) Grammer (131) | 1:10,000 | 0.05 | 1:12,500 dilution #4 | 0.06 |
| Patterson et al. (128) | 1:5,000 | 0.05 | 1:2,500 dilution #3 | 0.03 |

SET, skin endpoint titration.

to confirm allergy are only qualitative tests. Single-dilution skin tests do not accurately quantify individual allergen sensitivities (54,133–137), and thus the safe application of relatively high antigen doses at the beginning of immunotherapy has not been predictably achievable with prick-based methods. Therefore, when nonquantitative tests are used, the starting dose chosen often is the same very weak dilution used for sensitive patients. On the other hand, quantitative testing with either SET or in vitro techniques determines the individual sensitivities to each allergen, so that a safe starting dose can be chosen for each allergen and for each patient (9). Experience has shown that immunotherapy, for each antigen, can be safely started at doses 5 to 20 times stronger than the dilution that causes an endpoint wheal to form (14,118). Quantitative measurements of skin reactivity therefore can be used to predict starting doses that are high enough to achieve immunotherapy goals more rapidly, and with safety. Fadal has found that most allergens tested using RAST have low sensitivity scores (85% are classes 1 through 3) (51), and similar observations have been made using SET. Therefore, most immunotherapy starting doses derived from quantification tests allow injections to be given from relatively concentrated allergen solutions, closer to final maintenance levels than those that are based on prick tests (14,138,139). When higher doses are possible, it can greatly shorten the time needed to reach maintenance treatment levels (140). Immunotherapy based on quantification tests permits safe and aggressive initial dosing when sensitization is low and high doses are desirable, but alerts the therapist in advance to those allergens to which the patient is highly sensitive, so that in these cases initial dosing may be more dilute (95,141,142).

Although qualitative and quantitative testing methods do demonstrate differences in generic techniques, many of those who use prick-based immunotherapy do, in fact, adjust the starting dose based on clinical experience (22). For example, Creticos has recommended tailoring the initial dose based on a quantitative vial test (49). Van Metre et al. (58) also showed that patients normally could tolerate 0.10 mL of the endpoint dilution that induces a skin reaction. Finally, Ledford and Lockey suggested that starting doses can be adjusted "depending on clinical judgment" (9).

The use of quantification tests to calculate an immunotherapy starting dose is not new. Hansel (143) in 1936 and Furstenberg and Gay (144) in 1937 based their starting treatment doses on tenfold dilutional SET. In 1939, Greene reported basing the starting treatment dose on serial dilution scratch testing (145), and serial dilution prick tests also have been described. The modern SET quantification technique was described by Rinkel in 1962, and is based on a titrated skin endpoint derived from a fivefold series of allergen dilutions (146,147). SET titrations clearly illustrate the fact that patients vary in sensitivity to individual antigens and therefore in tolerance to initial antigen doses. SET-based starting doses are derived from a quantified response, which enables the clinician to choose a high and yet safe starting dose.

The usual starting dose of 0.05 mL volume from a multidose vial that is prepared from SET or RAST testing results is not arbitrary. This first dose contains a fivefold greater amount of each antigen than the endpoint amounts that initiated progressive positive whealing during SET testing. This initial treatment dose actually is the same dose that was already given during SET testing to produce the larger confirmatory wheal necessary for the establishment of each endpoint (21). In practice, starting doses ranging from 5 to 10 (69,148–151) to 20 times greater than the endpoint doses for each antigen have been reported to be acceptably safe (3,126,151,152). The 0.05-mL starting dose, then, has been experimentally verified, and quantitative testing allows the clinician to predict that the starting dose will be strong enough to be at or just above the threshold of provoking skin reactions. It also is a dose that has been determined to be weak enough not to cause unwanted reactions. To be able confidently to begin therapy at a level that is neither too strong nor too weak has great advantages.

## Initial In Vitro–based Immunotherapy Dose

There may be more physicians currently using in vitro allergy diagnosis than there are allergists using skin testing methods (51). Like SET tests, the in vitro RAST and ELISA allergy tests accurately quantify responses and have been shown to correlate reliably with allergic disease history, mucosal provocation tests, and titration skin tests. Because the concept of RAST-based immunotherapy was derived from the concept of SET-based immunotherapy, in vivo tests also can accurately identify safe initial immunotherapy doses (55,153–159). Since 1977 (158), starting doses based solely on in vitro modified RAST techniques have been in use (95,141,142,160,161). Endpoints based on SET and in vitro class scores based on modified RAST or ELISA correlate exactly (Table 12.2). The only potential confusion lies in the fact that the numeric assignments for the in vitro classes correlate with the SET endpoint dilution number that is one fivefold dilution higher (weaker), often referred to as the *RAST minus one* relationship. As an example, a patient with ragweed allergy who has an in vitro score of class 3, if simultaneously skin tested, would typically reach endpoint on a #4 dilution. The immunotherapy starting dose derived from in vitro results would, therefore, be calculated based on the expected SET endpoint (Table 12.2).

## Low-sensitivity Positive Test Results

The in vitro class 0/1 is an equivocal class, where the level of detectable IgE is just slightly above the background level of the assay, and correlates with an endpoint of dilution #1, or 1: 100 w/v in SET testing. Controversy exists about whether these low-sensitivity inhalant test results have meaning in allergy diagnosis and treatment. However, many otolaryngology patients with chronic symptoms exhibit such low-level positive test results. So, when patient symp-

**TABLE 12.2. MIXING A 5-mL MULTIANTIGEN, TEN-DOSE TREATMENT VIAL FROM NONSTANDARDIZED ALLERGEN EXTRACTS, BASED ON QUANTIFICATION ALLERGY TESTS (SET OR IN VITRO)**

| *In Vitro* Class | SET Endpoint | Antigen Concentration (w/v) to Add to Vial | Volume (mL) to Add to Vial | Final Antigen Concentration (w/v) in Vial |
|---|---|---|---|---|
| 5 | 6 | 1:12,500 w/v (dilution #4) | 0.20 mL | 1:312,500 w/v |
| 4 | 5 | 1:2,500 w/v (dilution #3) | 0.20 mL | 1.62,500 w/v |
| 3 | 4 | 1:500 w/v (dilution #2) | 0.20 mL | 1:12,500 w/v |
| 2 | 3 | 1:100 w/v (dilution #1) | 0.20 mL | 1:2,500 w/v |
| 1 | 2 | 1:20 w/v (concentrate) | 0.20 mL | 1:500 w/v |
| 0/1[a] | 1[a] | 1:20 w/v (concentrate) | 0.20 mL[b] or 1.00 mL[c] | 1:500 w/v[b] or 1:100 w/v[c] |

SET, skin endpoint titration.
[a]Low-sensitivity positive.
[b]Optimum-dose therapy.
[c]Maximum tolerated dose therapy.

toms correlate with positive tests in this range, some physicians include these low-sensitivity allergens in the immunotherapy treatment mixture. Other physicians treat only for higher-strength positive results. If facilities are available for nasal or bronchial allergen challenges, these would be appropriate methods to resolve the clinical relevance of these low-sensitivity results (124,125).

## Mixing Inhalant Immunotherapy Vials

Once the decision is made to treat, and the relevant positive tests are evaluated, one or more treatment vials are mixed. During escalation, 5-mL multiantigen, multidose vials usually are prepared, each of which contains ten doses of 0.5-mL volume. For some patients, small dose volumes or less frequent injections may permit 2.5-mL vials to be prepared, with significant antigen cost savings. For example, if a maintenance dose is 0.2 mL, a 2.5-mL vial would contain 12 doses, enough for 3 months of weekly treatment. Similarly, at a maintenance dose of 0.4 mL, a 2.5-mL vial would provide 3 months of biweekly treatment. Some physicians prefer to dispense multiantigen, single-dose vials, particularly for patients on home immunotherapy. When single-dose vials are used, a multidose vial is prepared first, and then the appropriate doses are measured into prelabeled, 2-mL single-dose vials and diluent added to bring each vial to the same volume. Patients are then instructed to withdraw and inject the entire contents of the appropriately numbered vial for each week.

An example of vial mixing is shown in Table 12.3. The hypothetical patient is a young adult with rhinoconjunctivitis and mild asthma who has perennial symptoms with distinct worsening in the summer and also in late fall and early winter. In this case, testing produced 24 positive tests, ranging from an endpoint of #1, not very sensitive, to #7, exquisitely sensitive. Testing was completed in the Northeast, in early May. Summer symptoms often indicate grass

sensitivity, and testing shows very strong reactions to all three grass families. Because grass will be in season before doses can be substantially advanced, grass should be placed in a special, separate treatment vial until the grass season is past. Trees do not require special treatment because only oak and pine are still in bloom in May, and both are relatively low sensitivity. Safe coseasonal treatment for trees may be initiated based on the recently completed RAST or SET results. Dermatophytes also normally are treated separately because most people cannot tolerate advancement much beyond endpoint doses. All other allergens are divided into either high- or low-reactor vials, based on endpoints. A decision also has to be made about whether to treat the antigens reaching endpoint on the #1 dilution. These are all molds, and the patient has increased symptoms during the primary mold season of late fall and early winter, so a decision is made to treat these antigens.

Recall that the 7-mm endpoint wheal for each antigen was produced from injection of 0.01 mL of that dilution. The initial treatment vial begins at a treatment dose for each antigen equal to 0.05 mL of the endpoint dilution, and escalates to a maximum dose of 0.5 mL. To treat 24 antigens would require from a 1.2- to 12-mL injection from the endpoint dilutions, clearly not a reasonable injection volume. Therefore, volume reduction is accomplished by using dilutions that are 25-fold more concentrated than the endpoint, commonly referred to as *two dilutions to the right*. To prepare ten doses would require 10 × 0.5, or 5 mL of the endpoint dilution for the maximum dose for each antigen. This is equal to 1 mL of the next more concentrated dilution, or 0.2 mL from the solution that is two dilutions more concentrated. A vial therefore is prepared by adding 0.2 mL for each antigen, taken from a dilution that is 25-fold more concentrated than the endpoint dilution, and the total volume is adjusted to equal 5 mL by adding appropriate amounts of glycerin and phenol saline diluent (Table 12.3). A 2.5-mL vial is similarly prepared, but uses only a 0.1-mL volume of each antigen.

**TABLE 12.3. EXAMPLE OF INITIAL INHALANT TREATMENT VIAL PREPARATION. 5-mL MULTIANTIGEN, 10-DOSE VIALS. 24 ALLERGENS POSITIVE BY HISTORY AND TESTING**

| Inhalant | Endpoint Dilution | Volume to Add (mL), Two Dilutions Stronger | |
|---|---|---|---|
| **High-reactor vial**[a] | | | |
| Mite mix | #5 | 0.20 | #3 |
| Cat | #4 | 0.20 | #2 |
| Cockroach, American | #5 | 0.20 | #3 |
| Red cedar | #4 | 0.20 | #2 |
| Box elder | #6 | 0.20 | #4 |
| White oak | #4 | 0.20 | #2 |
| Short ragweed | #5 | 0.20 | #3 |
| *Alternaria tenuis* | #5 | 0.20 | #3 |
| *Ustilago maydis* | #4 | 0.20 | #2 |
| **Antigen volume** | | **1.80** | |
| 50% Glycerin[b] | | 1.00 | |
| Phenol saline | | 2.20 | |
| **10-Dose vial** | | **5.00** | |
| | | | |
| **Low-reactor vial**[a] | | | |
| Dog | #2 | 0.20 | concentrate |
| Paper birch | #2 | 0.20 | concentrate |
| White pine | #2 | 0.20 | concentrate |
| Lambs quarters | #2 | 0.20 | concentrate |
| Common mugwort | #3 | 0.20 | #1 |
| *Aspergillus* mix | #3 | 0.20 | #1 |
| *Cladosporium cladosporoides* | #3 | 0.20 | #1 |
| *Epicoccum purpurascens* | #2 | 0.20 | concentrate |
| *Fusarium oxysporium* | #1 | 1.00 | concentrate |
| *Helminthosporium solani* | #2 | 0.20 | concentrate |
| *Penicillium* mix | #1 | 1.00 | concentrate |
| **Antigen volume** | | **3.80** | |
| 50% Glycerin[b] | | 0 | |
| Phenol saline | | 1.20 | |
| **10-Dose vial** | | **5.00** | |
| | | | |
| **Special treatment vial**[c] | | | |
| *Candida albicans* | #3 | 0.20 | #1 |
| **Antigen volume** | | **0.20** | |
| 50% Glycerin[b] | | 1.00 | |
| Phenol saline | | 3.80 | |
| **10-Dose vial** | | **5.00** | |
| | | | |
| **Special treatment vial**[c] | | | |
| Bahia grass | #6 | 0.20 | #4 |
| Bermuda grass | #5 | 0.20 | #3 |
| Timothy grass | #7 | 0.20 | #5 |
| **Antigen volume** | | **0.60** | |
| 50% Glycerin[b] | | 1.00 | |
| Phenol saline | | 3.40 | |
| **10-Dose vial** | | **5.00** | |

[a]Combining antigens of like sensitivity.
[b]Preserves antigen potency.
[c]To prevent allergen overload.

## Safety Vial Test

Beginning immunotherapy at levels that are close to maintenance is intended to achieve therapeutic goals more quickly. But because these are potent initial doses, before administering the first injection, and especially if this dose has been derived from an in vitro test, an intradermal safety vial test is recommended (22,69,84,92–94,141,142,156,160,161). A vial test is mandatory before beginning treatment based on in vitro diagnosis, and is strongly suggested before beginning any immunotherapy treatment. The vial test allows the clinician who wishes to initiate therapy at a high dose to test the water before jumping in. A vial test accomplishes this by injecting 0.01 mL of the treatment vial mix intradermally, where the reaction can be easily assessed. Thus, it is a biologic indicator of tolerance to the prescribed injection, and poses a lower level of risk than if a larger dose were given subcutaneously (51).

A significant reaction to the first subcutaneous injection may result from a host of reasons. For example, because of human error, the treatment vial contents may be improperly calculated or mixed (22). Many other variables also have been found to affect the risk of reaction (162) and, in fact, receiving the first injection from a new vial is one of the most important risks. Therefore, any patient who is about to start injections with previously untreated antigens, or receive an injection from a newly mixed treatment vial, is best served if an intradermal vial test is performed first. When the treatment vial is based on an in vitro test (69), there should be no exceptions to performing an initial vial test. The in vitro–based immunotherapy patient has never been skin tested to the actual antigens that will be used in therapy. And, unlike the patient who has undergone skin tests, the in vitro patient also has not necessarily been tested with exactly the same extracts that will be used in immunotherapy (21). Thus, patients who have been tested with in vitro methods have a higher chance of discrepancies between the level of reactivity determined by the in vitro tests and the actual reactivity to the extracts mixed from the clinician's treatment concentrates.

The vial test is performed by injecting intradermally the smallest easily measurable dose, 0.01 mL, of the treatment vial contents (162), producing a 4- to 5-mm, sharply demarcated skin wheal identical to the test wheal used in SET testing (51). The resulting skin reaction is then read in 10 (21,69,162) to 15 (51) minutes. A positive whealing response is expected, and proves a biologically active allergen treatment dose (50). Most test wheals are in the range of 9 to 13 mm and indicate tolerance to the initial dose (50). If the wheal grows no larger than 11 mm, then the first subcutaneous injection of 0.05 mL may be given during that same visit. If it enlarges to 12 to 13 mm, then the first injection should be given at the next visit, 3 to 7 days later. However, if the wheal enlarges to 14 mm or more—and it is this circumstance that is safely identified by the vial test—then the treatment vial is too strong. When this oc-

curs, the vial may either be diluted 1:5 and retested (21), or the original undiluted vial may be retested during the next visit (69). If the vial test wheal enlarges to greater than 15 mm, then the vial should be diluted. A 1:5 dilution is created by taking 1 mL from the treatment vial and mixing it with 4 mL of diluent. This produces a new 5-mL treatment vial that is effectively a #1 dilution from the original vial. This more dilute vial usually gives a skin test in the range of 13 mm or less, so that escalation may then proceed with the diluted vial. If the diluted vial test wheal is still too large, then further dilutions may be carried out until a vial test resulting in acceptable wheal size is found. If multiple vial dilutions are required, the clinician should consider whether there has been an error in vial manufacture, or if an important allergen has come into season. In either case, it may be wise to recheck the skin endpoints by partially retesting that patient.

## Vial Testing Subsequent Treatment Vials

Vial testing may not be necessary before giving the first injection from vials subsequent to the first treatment vial, provided that antigens to which the patient has not yet been subcutaneously exposed have not been added. Although omitting subsequent vial tests does not guard against mixing errors, some believe that vial tests done during the early phases of escalation may be misleading, and can lead to inappropriate slowing of the escalation (21). During the early phases of escalation, skin reactivity is unlikely to have been reduced significantly, whereas the skin wheal produced by a vial test from a vial that is five times stronger than the previous vial may be large enough to induce excessive caution. As an alternative to testing subsequent vials, many clinicians decrease the first dose from a new vial to one half of the last dose given from the old vial. For example, if the last injection was 0.5 mL from the previous vial, then the first injection from the new, fivefold stronger vial would be 0.05 mL, rather than 0.10 mL (21,163). Other clinicians do normally use a vial test before giving any initial injection from any new vial. At high immunotherapy doses, an intradermal vial test injection may be painful, or may produce a large, visible, lingering reaction. If this occurs, subsequent 0.01 mL safety tests may be given subcutaneously, and patients are observed for systemic symptoms rather than evaluating the skin reaction. Alternately, at these high antigen doses, some physicians elect to omit the vial test, instead reducing the initial dose from every new vial.

## IMMUNOTHERAPY ESCALATION

## Immunotherapy Escalation Schedules

Successful immunotherapy is predicated on many factors. One critical factor is the achievement of high treatment doses that are close to levels that can produce large local or systemic reactions, administered for long periods (19). To

**TABLE 12.4. IMMUNOTHERAPY DOSE ESCALATION EXAMPLE USING 1:5 DILUTIONS, AVERAGE PATIENT, SINGLE ANTIGEN VIAL. POSITIVE TEST ON SKIN ENDPOINT TITRATION ENDPOINT #4 (IN VITRO CLASS 3)**

| Office Visit No. | Antigen Added to 5-mL, 10-Dose Treatment Vial (w/v) | Vial Final Antigen Concentration (w/v) | Injection Volume (mL) | Comment |
|---|---|---|---|---|
| **First treatment vial** | | | | |
| 1 | 0.2 mL of 1:500 (dilution #2) | 1:12,500 | 0.01 ID[a] | ⇐ Vial safety test |
| 1 or 2 | | | 0.05 | |
| 3 | | | 0.10 | Slow initial escalation |
| 4 | | | 0.15 | |
| 5 | | | 0.20 | |
| 6 | | | 0.25 | |
| 7 | | | 0.30 | |
| 8 | | | 0.35 | |
| 9 | | | 0.40 | |
| 10 | | | 0.45 | |
| 11 | | | 0.50 | |
| **Second treatment vial** | | | | |
| 12 | 0.2 mL of 1:100 (dilution #1) | 1:2,500 | 0.01 ID[a] | ⇐ Vial safety test |
| 12 or 13 | | | 0.05 | ⇐ Reduced dose |
| 14 | | | 0.10 | |
| 15 | | | 0.20 | More rapid |
| 16 | | | 0.30 | escalation |
| 17 | | | 0.40 | |
| 18 | | | 0.50 | |
| **Third treatment vial** | | | | |
| 19 | 0.2 mL of 1:20 concentrate[b] | 1:500 | 0.01 ID/SC[a] | ⇐ Vial safety test |
| 19 or 20 | | | 0.05 | ⇐ Reduced dose |
| 21 | | | 0.10 | |
| 22 | | | 0.20 | Rapid escalation until |
| 23 | | | 0.30 | symptoms occur, |
| 24 | | | 0.40 | then slower |
| 25 | | | 0.45 | |
| 26 | | | 0.50 | |
| **Fourth treatment vial** | | | | |
| 27 | 1.0 mL of 1:20 concentrate[c] | 1:100 | 0.01 SC[a] | ⇐ Vial safety test |
| 27 or 28 | | | 0.05 | ⇐ Reduced dose |
| 29 | | | 0.10 | |
| 30 | | | 0.15 | |
| 31 | | | 0.20 | Slow escalation near |
| 32 | | | 0.25 | maximum |
| 33 | | | 0.30 | tolerated dose |
| 34 | | | 0.35 | |
| 35 | | | 0.40 | |
| 36 | | | 0.45 | |
| 37 | | | 0.50 | |

ID, intradermal; SC, subcutaneous.
[a]Vial test.
[b]Optimum-dose therapy.
[c]Maximum tolerated dose therapy.

achieve this goal, the patient must acquire immunologic tolerance to these high doses by being subjected to a series of regular antigen exposures of progressively increasing intensity. Contemporary escalation schedules are more similar than different, and reflect the judgment, experience, and risk tolerance of the clinician. Table 12.4 illustrates a conservative escalation schedule suggested for use with in vitro– or SET-based immunotherapy. If the vial test indicates the treatment vial is satisfactory, then immunotherapy injections are given at weekly or twice-weekly intervals (21),

escalating the dose until satisfactory maintenance levels are reached. In general, injections should not be given more often than every 3 days to avoid an increased risk of reaction (22). Conservative dose escalation uses 0.05-mL incremental increases up to 0.50 mL. Injection volumes larger than 0.50 mL are less comfortable, and thus usually not used. Instead, dose escalation is continued by mixing a new vial with antigens five times stronger (more concentrated). A 0.1-mL injection from this new vial is antigenically equivalent to the final 0.5 mL given from the original vial. However, because this new vial is stronger and contains fresher and thus potentially more potent antigens (21), if no vial test is given, it is recommended that the first dose from the new vial be halved by giving only 0.05 mL. Some clinicians both perform a vial test and reduce the first dose. Escalation then continues until a proper maintenance level (see later) is reached. The escalation dose increment can vary based on the clinical situation and judgment of the clinician. Conservative advancement by 0.05-mL increments in the beginning, and also when approaching maintenance, is suggested. More aggressive advancement by 0.1-mL increments can be entertained for average patients during the middle range of immunotherapy escalation. More rapid escalation allows the use of smaller-volume treatment vials, with savings of time, money, and effort and the potential for more rapid relief of symptoms. Accelerated schedules are appropriate for use by experienced clinicians, and for healthier, less sensitive patients (21).

Allergists who base therapy on prick testing usually prepare treatment vials using tenfold rather than fivefold dilutions. The initial dilution is either 1:10 or 1:5, so that dilutions from a 1:20 w/v concentrate of 1:200, 1:2,000, 1:20,000, and 1:200,000 (19,97), or 1:100, 1:1,000, 1:10,000, and 1:100,000 are produced (9). Creticos (49) and Van Metre and Adkinson (19) describe an escalation schedule for standardized short ragweed extract using once- or twice-weekly injections. The injection schedule is initiated at 0.1 mL of a $10^{-4}$ dilution, and progresses to dilutions of $10^{-3}$, $10^{-2}$, and $10^{-1}$. Doses are escalated by doubling the previous dose, with injection volumes ranging from 0.10 to 0.8 mL for each vial. However, when approaching maintenance, "the rate of increase commonly slows" (14). Ledford and Lockey (9) describe a very similar dose regimen that is administered on a weekly or twice-weekly schedule. It starts at 0.05 mL of a 1:10,000 w/v dilution, and progresses to dilutions of 1:1,000 w/v, and then 1:100 w/v. The doses are escalated in increments of 0.1 mL until reaching 0.5 mL. Escalation increments for the strongest vial (1:100) are reduced to 0.05 mL.

Both types of escalation schedules accomplish the same goals, and often in the same amount of time. Although it is true that in vitro– and SET-based techniques initiate therapy at higher doses in low-sensitivity patients, it also is true that progression through large dose ranges will be accomplished more quickly in techniques that use tenfold rather than fivefold dilution increments. Furthermore, as shown in Table 12.1, the starting doses for highly sensitive patients can be very similar regardless of which method is used, and reaching maintenance levels thus may take similar lengths of time (164). Therefore, clinicians should use whichever schedule is best for them, based on their experience and training.

### Rush Immunotherapy

One of the obvious disadvantages of the escalation methods described previously is that many weeks of injections are necessary before symptom-relieving and, ultimately, maintenance doses are reached. This is especially difficult for patients who for distance (9) or other reasons cannot come regularly to the office for injections. To address these issues, various forms of accelerated (rapid, rush, or cluster) immunotherapy have been used (9), even as early as 1926 (119, 165). The only real difference between this and other escalation methods is that the interval between accelerated injections is much shorter so as to reach maintenance quickly, in many cases in as little as 1 week. Because immunotherapy effectiveness is largely dose dependent, these schedules can be effective if essentially the same dose goals as with traditional techniques can be achieved (9). Various forms of accelerated immunotherapy schedules have been proposed, but, unfortunately, all involve a higher risk of anaphylaxis (117). Accelerated immunotherapy has been described for use in patients who were qualitatively tested, and normally is started at very low doses. Usually several injections are given on the first day and continued on more than 1 day a week (19,98,132,166). One method starts patients at 0.1 mL of a $1:10^7$ w/v dilution, and increases the dose four times a day until the MTD is reached, usually within 5 days (69). Another method begins with five injections on day 1, starting at 0.1 mL of $1:10^5$ w/v. Then, two injections are given on day 2, starting at 0.6 mL of $1:10^4$ w/v, then one injection on day 3 of 0.1 mL of 1:1,000 w/v, followed by maintenance injections of 0.2 mL of 1:1,000 w/v on day 7, and weekly thereafter. This method, however, was associated with a 20% incidence of systemic reactions (29). In private practice, rush schedules seldom are used, although they may be considered for use in cases of insect sting immunotherapy where there is a very high risk of another sting occurring within a short time.

## MAINTENANCE IMMUNOTHERAPY

Well before modern studies of immunotherapy efficacy (167–169), clinicians discovered that they were able to induce higher degrees of protection from allergen challenges when higher quantities of antigen were administered (11, 19). Further understanding of this relationship between cumulative dose and efficacy, as well as the development of improved techniques and confidence in treating injection reactions, has led to the evolution of more aggressive and effective maintenance dosing levels. The current goal of immunotherapy is to escalate antigen doses initially to a point of symptom relief, and ultimately to a point where long-lasting alteration of symptom thresholds and intensity occurs (21). In prior years, it was common to stop escalation once some symptom relief was observed. But a maintenance dose based only on symptom relief is now thought to be potentially inadequate because symptom relief can occur at antigen treatment levels that are below the range where changes in blocking antibodies can be demonstrated. Ideally, the maintenance dose level that achieves both immediate and prolonged symptom relief should be sought. To date, there is no known test method that can accurately predict either the optimal cumulative dose or the maintenance dose in any given patient (117). These treatment levels are now established through the individual clinical management of each patient, by closely monitoring clinical responses (8). Several different techniques that attempt to achieve adequate levels of maintenance dosing are presented in the following sections.

## Maintenance Dose Decisions Based on Clinical Responses

### Low-dose Treatment

The concept of low-dose immunotherapy (9,19) is discussed here to distinguish it from standard immunotherapy. There has been much criticism, confusion, and mislabeling of authors and techniques purported to be associated with low-dose immunotherapy. Low-dose immunotherapy has been in use since the 1920s, almost as long as immunotherapy has been available (119,143,146,147,169–176). Initially, low-dose immunotherapy was based on symptom relief, in an era when clinicians feared to use high antigen doses. Later, some physicians believed that a maintenance dose could be predetermined by quantitative skin testing, by advancing only to 0.5-mL doses of the endpoint dilution and no further (146,147,173). This low-dose immunotherapy method was incorrectly ascribed to the SET method developed by Rinkel, but was never taught by him. Rinkel's published works, in fact, emphasize the importance of continuing to escalate doses (177). This method had appeal because it achieved rapid, safe (144,172) relief without long escalation schedules (19). However, this technique was criticized because of its inability to improve allergy symptoms durably and to affect IgG and IgE antibody levels (19). Other forms of low-dose immunotherapy are currently in clinical use, including neutralization therapy (178) and enzyme-potentiated desensitization (179), but these do not elicit blocking antibody and are believed to act by directly affecting prostaglandin levels and T-cell regulatory mechanisms.

### Symptom-relieving Dose Treatment

The symptom-relieving maintenance dose is defined as the dose that is associated with patient-reported subjective symptom relief lasting for at least 1 week (21). Because this dose can theoretically maintain relief as long as regular injections are given, it often has been used as the maintenance dose, without further escalation. Questions about symptom relief should be an integral part of immunotherapy monitoring, to document the relationship between symptoms and antigenic stimulation. However, in most situations, symptom relief should not be used by itself to direct dose escalation decisions. There are two situations when symptom relief is the primary deciding factor. First, some

patients are so sensitive that a high maintenance dose cannot be achieved without unacceptable local or systemic reactions. Second, many patients exhibit a symptom-relieving dose range, and pushing to very high doses raises the dose above that range. In some of these patients, symptoms actually worsen at very high doses, which could indicate that an increased risk of anaphylaxis exists. Even under these circumstances, the clinician often can achieve maintenance levels that deliver at least 0.6 $\mu$g of antigen per dose (22), the minimum level that is known to cause the production of blocking antibodies in treatment of ragweed allergy (68) (Table 12.5). Using the fivefold dilution technique, this is accomplished by administering injections from a treatment vial to which #1 dilutions or concentrates have been added—that is, injections with a final antigen concentration of 1:2,500 w/v (dilution #3) or greater (Table 12.6). The lower limit of efficacy for immunotherapy doses is not known with any degree of accuracy (Tables 12.5 and 12.6), and it is possible that lower antigen doses may have some benefit in some patients. For example, patients often report significant relief at a treatment dose concentration of approximately 1:12,500 (dilution #4). Whenever benefits do occur at low doses, patients normally feel even better, and have longer relief, as treatment doses are further increased.

### Maximally Tolerated Dose Treatment

Most clinicians advocate the MTD as the maintenance dose (49). A series of reports has demonstrated a statistically significant improvement in symptom–medication scores and immunologic parameters in patients on ragweed immunotherapy escalated to the MTD (19,190). Unfortunately, similar excellent data are not available for any other antigen. The MTD technique attempts to determine clinically the highest tolerable escalation dose in each patient. This method requires close, regular monitoring of skin and symptom responses to progressively higher injection doses. One valuable clue that the MTD has not been reached is the complaint of a premature return of allergy symptoms before the next injection is due. King and Mabry define the MTD as "a point at which the local reaction produced signals that further advancement would be imprudent, while symptom relief is still being provided" (21). When multiple-vial immunotherapy is being administered, the MTD technique allows for individual adjustment of doses for each vial.

To determine the MTD, the dose is escalated first to the dose range where symptom relief is occurring. The clinician must remember that reactions may occur early during dose escalation, when IgE levels are still rising, and symptom relief has not yet developed. Doses must be cautiously pushed further, until IgE begins to drop and symptom relief is obtained. Further escalation in the range of doses that cause symptom relief eventually produces a dose that causes a local arm reaction, but not systemic symptoms. Then, doses are cautiously increased until an arm reaction between 25 and 50 mm in size occurs (191). A typical unacceptable

## TABLE 12.5. EFFECTIVE DOSES FOR ALLERGEN IMMUNOTHERAPY

### A. Ragweed, Antigen Amb a 1 in Whole-pollen Extract

| Maintenance Dose (μg) | Comments | References |
|---|---|---|
| 0.0001–0.006 | Not effective | (58) |
| 0.004–0.15 | Not effective | (148) |
| 0.6 | Not effective | (73,167,168) |
| >1 | Minimally effective | (19,68) |
| 2 | Effective, but not as effective as 24 μg | (167,168) |
| 6 | Effective, but not as effective as 12.4–24.8 μg | (180) |
| 11 | Effective | (58) |
| 10 | Suggested optimal dose range for asthma | (47) |
| 0.6–12.4 | Effective, but not as effective as 12.4–24.8 μg | (41,73,49) |
| 6–12 | Suggested optimal dose range for rhinitis | (49) |
| 4.7–25 | Effective | (167,168) |
| 12.4–24.8 | Effective, but more risk | (41,73,49) |

| Cumulative Dose (μg) | | |
|---|---|---|
| 3.1–3.7 | Not effective | (181) |
| 9.3 | Effective | (181) |
| 36 | More effective | (181) |

### B. Ragweed, Purified Amb a 1 (Antigen E)

| Cumulative Dose (μg) | Comments | References |
|---|---|---|
| 3.7–32 | Not effective | (181) |
| 252 | Effective | (181) |
| 400 | Effective | (181) |
| 743 | More effective | (181) |
| >1,000 | Effective, but more risk | (149,182) |

### C. Dust Mite, Antigen Der p 1 or Der f 1 in Mite Extract

| Maintenance Dose (μg) | Comments | References |
|---|---|---|
| 0.7 | Minimally effective for asthma | (183) |
| 6 | Effective | (167) |
| 7 | Optimal dose for asthma | (183,184) |
| 10 | Optimal dose for asthma | (184) |
| 11.9 | Effective | (44) |
| 6–12 | Effective, optimal dose range | (49) |
| 21 | Effective, but increased systemic reactions | (183) |

### D. Cat, Antigen Fel d 1 in Cat Extract

| Maintenance Dose (μg) | Comments | References |
|---|---|---|
| 6–12 | Effective | (49) |
| 13.2–13.8 | Effective for asthma | (185,186) |
| 15 | Effective | (167) |
| 8–16 | Effective for asthma | (186) |

### E. Pooid Grasses, Major Antigen in Whole-pollen Extract

| Maintenance Dose (μg) | Comments | References |
|---|---|---|
| 15 | Effective (orchard/rye) | (187) |
| 18.6 | Effective (timothy) | (34) |
| 18–36 | Effective (rye) | (167) |

**TABLE 12.6. EFFECTIVE DOSES FOR ALLERGEN IMMUNOTHERAPY: NONSTANDARDIZED POLLEN ANTIGENS**

| Maintenance Dose ($\mu$g of pollen) | Pollen Concentration (w/v), Volume (mL) | SET Equivalent 1:5 Dilution, Volume (mL) | Comments | References |
|---|---|---|---|---|
| 0.50 | $1:10^7$, 0.50 | #8, 0.40 | Not effective | (188) |
| <50 | 1:5,000, 0.25 | #4, 0.60 | Usually not effective | (21,51,98,189) |
| 100 | 1:5,000, 0.50 | #3, 0.25 | Effective | (128,159,188,189) |
| 1,000 | 1:500, 0.50 | #2, 0.50 | More effective, but more risk | (21,51,84) |
| 10,000 | 1:50, 0.50 | #1, 1.00 | Maximum dose | (128) |

SET, skin endpoint titration.

reaction is larger than 50 mm, is characterized by redness, warmth, itching, and induration, usually lasts for no more than 24 hours, and typically occurs with an injection from one vial, rather than all vials, during multiple-vial therapy (21,191). This reaction size should warn the clinician not to increase the dose on the next visit, but does not necessarily define the ultimate maximum maintenance dose. When a large arm reaction does occur, the clinician should decrease the next dose to one that previously caused less than a 25-mm reaction. A safe dose frequently is approximately one-half the unacceptable dose. Doses then should be cautiously reescalated to a point that does not cause more than a 25-mm reaction. Large arm reactions may be associated with a temporary provocation of allergic symptoms (21,22,191), and if this occurs, added caution is indicated during further attempts to reescalate the dose. Often on reescalation, doses can be raised further without the occurrence of either large arm reactions or symptoms. Because a patient's total environmental allergic load varies from day to day and month to month, the amount of injected immunotherapy antigens that are tolerated also varies. When environmental loads are high, such as during grass season or when a patient is eating a lot of a food to which he or she is allergic, the patient will not tolerate the same high immunotherapy dose as when the total load was less. Thus, periodic upward or downward adjustment of maintenance immunotherapy doses is required, using the steps outlined previously. Although all antigens cannot always be escalated to equally high doses, the clinician should continually search for the highest safe and comfortable dose levels.

## Optimal-dose Treatment

Because there is variation in practitioners' skills, there is variation in patient management. And, because the MTD technique takes the aggressive stance of using doses that are close to anaphylactic doses, it could lead to either uncomfortable reactions or, rarely, adverse outcomes, especially if patients are not being closely and thoughtfully monitored. Therefore, although we know that higher doses correlate with faster improvement in symptoms, a higher likelihood of symptom relief, and longer-lasting relief (186,192–194), it is possible that a slightly lower maintenance dose might produce most of these benefits, but at a lower risk. There also is clinical evidence suggesting that increasing doses beyond a certain high level does not necessarily produce any further improvement in symptoms (68). We also know that many clinicians have observed significant, long-lasting symptomatic improvement with immunotherapy doses below those that provoke local or systemic reactions (117). These observations have convinced many clinicians to adopt a more conservative, slightly less than MTD method for maintenance, which is called the *optimal-dose method*. In optimal-dose therapy, doses are escalated exactly as in MTD, but stop short of provoking large arm reactions. The goal in optimum-dose therapy is to relieve symptoms, not provoke symptoms, and deliver as high a dose as possible without causing arm reactions that exceed approximately 25 mm in size.

Physicians who use the optimum-dose method usually do not push immunotherapy doses above a treatment mix concentration of 1:500 w/v, a concentration obtained by adding 0.2 mL of concentrate to a 5-mL, ten-dose multiantigen treatment vial. This concentration determines the usual maximum dose range and allows up to 25 allergens to be placed into a single treatment vial. Physicians who prefer to escalate to MTD levels normally go one dilution stronger, to the optional maximum dose range. In addition to the greater risk of reaction, the other drawback to this higher dose range is that only five antigens can be mixed together, because 1 mL of each concentrate is added to a 5-mL treatment vial. When many allergens are being treated, multiple treatment vials therefore are required.

There are three main advantages to using the optimal-dose method. First, smaller arm reactions are much better tolerated by patients. Greater comfort helps patients stick with the desensitization schedule, rather than deciding to stop injections prematurely. Second, the doses are further away from the potential anaphylactic dose, which gives an added margin of safety. This is especially helpful if patients are not strictly adhering to a food allergy management program, and also when high levels of pollens or molds occur. Third, optimum doses normally do not exceed levels where treatment may be too high, thus precipitating increased symptoms. The potential drawback is the risk that a few patients may respond well only to very high treatment doses.

## Objective Measurement of Immunotherapy Doses

The potential variability in both outcomes and reaction rates in patient response–based immunotherapy has spurred surprisingly little research designed to quantitate and correlate immunotherapy treatment doses with outcomes. Effective immunotherapy antigen maintenance doses are known for only five clinically relevant antigens: *D. pteronyssinus*, *Dermatophagoides farinae*, cat, pooid grasses (e.g., timothy), and short ragweed (195), and minimally effective doses are known only for ragweed (68,73,181). A second significant limiting problem in rational immunotherapy dosing is the fact that, except for standardized extracts and most pollen extracts, the antigen concentrations in many other extracts are very low, raising the possibility that immunotherapy with these antigens may be of limited or no value (195). This was the thrust of Nelson's analysis of a survey of current immunotherapy maintenance doses used by practicing general allergists (195). Nelson was particularly concerned that possibly inadequate doses were being widely used for several important antigens, including Bermuda grass, cat, dog, and *Alternaria*. Dust mite immunotherapy was being used at minimally adequate levels, and there were no data reported for other nonpollen antigens (especially molds), which are not likely to be produced, or used, at concentrated levels. These observations reinforce the methodology outlined previously for choosing the MTD, and indicate that the MTD concept must be independently applied to every clinically important allergen. It is hoped that Nelson's admonishments, development of more standardized extracts (196, 197), and further research will take more of the guesswork out of immunotherapy dosing techniques (49,117). The goals are to improve teaching of immunotherapy techniques and achieve routine reproducibility and uniform success in immunotherapy practice.

Until adequate data are available for all antigens, clinicians have no choice but to rely on clinically determined symptom improvement dose ranges, optimal dose ranges, and cumulative dose ranges (49). These dose ranges would be associated with all of the symptom-relieving and immunomodulatory goals, but without the higher reaction rate associated with MTD techniques. In fact, Van Metre et al.

(49) discuss an optimal maintenance therapeutic dose range that is based on stepwise dose studies that identify a range, in micrograms, that has been shown reliably to induce measurable changes in the immune system that also correlate with symptom improvement (19). Thus far, the reported stepwise dose studies have identified similar effective antigen dose ranges for the few studied allergens. In theory, these studies should allow us to avoid the upper end of the dose range, just below the MTD, and thereby minimize systemic reactions without compromising efficacy.

Tables 12.5 and 12.6 summarize published stepwise studies addressing the issue of optimal dose ranges for effective immunotherapy. These studies have used measurements of the major allergenic protein moiety in each extract, or, in older work, the weight of whole pollens contained in the extracts, correlating these antigen doses with both clinical relief and laboratory evidence of immunomodulation. The effective maintenance dose range, based on measurement of the major antigen, for ragweed is approximately 6 to 24 μg; for dust mites, approximately 7 to 12 μg; for cat, approximately 11 to 17 μg; and for pooid grasses, approximately 15 to 19 μg (Table 12.5) (19,34,41,44,47,49,58,68, 73,148,149,167,168,180–187,195,198). For ragweed and dust mites, some effectiveness also was shown at major antigen levels as low as approximately 1 μg (19,68,183). For nonstandardized, whole-pollen extracts, the data (Table 12.6) show limited effectiveness in most patients at doses below approximately 50 to 100 μg, and there are no useful data regarding nonpollen antigens (21,51,84,117,128,139, 159,188,189,199).

### Identifying Minimally Effective Immunotherapy Doses

Based on these data, the lower end of the optimal dose range, which probably is near 100 μg of whole pollen, is 0.5 mL of a 1:5,000 w/v injection. This is equivalent to a 0.25-mL injection of 1:2,500 w/v (dilution #3), taken from a 5-mL treatment vial containing 0.2 mL of 1:100 w/v (dilution #1). Whenever possible, buildup immunotherapy doses should be escalated to a maintenance level that exceeds this minimal antigen dose. Because concentrates of nonpollen antigens often are available only at lower concentrations than are pollens, an attempt should be made to administer even higher doses of nonpollen antigens. How far beyond these minimal levels to advance continues to require experience-based clinical judgment. The experimentally derived maintenance dose levels presented previously should serve as rough guides only (21). They should be blended with individual patient clinical response assessments to arrive ultimately at the most effective maintenance dose for each patient. In general, minimum effective maintenance doses should be achieved when three criteria have been met. First, doses have been escalated until injections are being given from a 5-mL, ten-dose vial that contains at least 0.2 mL of a #1 dilution of each treatment antigen. Second, doses given from this vial are at or above a volume of 0.25 mL. Third, doses are not causing local reactions greater than 25 mm, and do not significantly provoke symptoms (4,117).

## Clinical Analysis of Ineffective Immunotherapy

If these criteria for delivering minimally effective doses have been met, and yet symptom relief is not being achieved, then the clinician should always reevaluate the patient to try to identify the reason for ineffective therapy (191). For most low- to moderate-sensitivity patients (endpoints on dilutions #1 to #3), symptom relief almost always occurs within 3 months of initiating therapy. For sensitive patients (endpoints on dilutions #4 to #6), advancement may be slow, and significant relief may take up to a year to develop. Certain patients never seem to benefit, no matter how much the treatment doses are raised. If this is the case after 12 (19) to 24 (69,101,200) months of treatment, and after careful review to try and identify other relevant allergic factors, then immunotherapy should be discontinued in search of other diagnoses and other possible solutions. Major sources of uncontrolled allergic load, such as a severely allergen-contaminated home or office, must be carefully searched for before abandoning allergy as the cause of symptoms. But, because immunotherapy is effective only for IgE-mediated allergy (19), could the patient's symptoms be related to something else? The clinical history and physical examination should corroborate the results of allergy testing, and should indicate the relevance of the particular allergens that test positive (49). Without this correlation, treatment may be given for irrelevant positive tests that are not contributing to clinical symptoms, so that immunotherapy will not be helpful, even if properly performed (19). This not only is wasteful, but may induce allergic reactions to previously unsensitized allergens (19,121). In addition, the clinician should always consider the possibility that autoimmune or other systemic diseases, such as hypothyroidism, may be producing symptoms that masquerade as allergy (201).

## Searching for the Optimum Maintenance Dose

The initial maintenance dose ascertained in any given patient may not turn out to be the final, ultimate maintenance dose. First, attempts to escalate further should be made once a patient enters the lower part of the symptom-relieving dose range. Second, how far advancement can continue is partly determined by the total allergic load at any point in time. Therefore, during escalation, the clinician should not be in a hurry to establish *the* maintenance dose. Many variable factors can influence a patient's allergic load over time, and what was initially thought to be the final maintenance dose, may, instead, represent a temporary plateau in escalation (21). This plateau sometimes may even be above the final optimal dose level. Thus, the escalation and maintenance phases of immunotherapy may overlap to some de-

gree because finding the optimum dose is always a dynamic clinical process. Clinicians should resist the temptation to define the maintenance dose with finality. Instead, thoughts are better focused on defining a maintenance dose range: a range that provides both symptom relief and immunomodulation, yet with minimal adverse reactions. In the SET-based study by Hurst et al., only 6.8% of patients were so brittle that they could never be advanced to maintenance doses above 1:12,500 w/v, and over 60% of all patients tolerated maximum-strength injections (1:500 w/v) from vials mixed with concentrates (162).

## IMMUNOTHERAPY AFTER MAINTENANCE

### Weekly Maintenance Phase of Immunotherapy

Once dose escalation has stabilized and a maintenance dose range has been reached, immunotherapy injections should be continued regularly at no longer than weekly intervals for at least 8 (21) to 12 months. Some physicians favor twice-weekly injections for a shorter period. During this time, the steady increase in cumulative antigen dose gives a progressive impetus to desirable immune system changes. At present, there are few objective data to guide decisions about how long to continue with weekly maintenance injections. For ragweed monotherapy, the data (Table 12.5) show that a cumulative pollen dose of approximately 9 to 36 times the minimally effective dose, or approximately 1.5 to 6 times the optimum maintenance dose, is required to initiate long-term favorable immune changes. In practice, physicians usually give weekly maintenance injections for as long as their prior training and experience has taught them is necessary, commonly for 1 year.

### Increasing the Interval between Injections

The withdrawal phase of immunotherapy begins with lengthening of the interval between injections. When feasible, these transition periods should begin after the patient's most significant allergen season has come to an end (21). As is the case with most other immunotherapy issues, there is no simple gold standard test that indicates the time to begin the withdrawal phase of immunotherapy. "Symptom improvement remains the standard response variable" (9); thus, symptom assessment should be the presiding influence over withdrawal decisions. When beginning to lengthen the interval between injections, continuing symptom relief is the primary measure of adequate immunomodulation. Both the clinician and patient should pay special attention during each attempt to increase the interval between injections. If symptom control decreases, the clinician should revert back to the old injection schedule (19), and try again at a later date (21). If attempts again fail, this may be because adequate maintenance doses were never reached during the previous weekly injections, and so adequate immunomodulation was never accomplished. Such doses may instead represent a plateau in escalation, and giving higher doses should be cautiously attempted before attempting again to increase intervals between injections.

When the injection interval has been successfully increased to 2 weeks, it usually is continued for 1 more year of therapy before further attempts to lengthen the interval. If the patient maintains good symptom relief through every allergy season of this second therapy year with a biweekly injection schedule, then increasing the interval even further, to 3 or 4 weeks (9,22,49), is reasonable. In the study by Hurst et al. during the second year of immunotherapy (162), approximately two thirds of patients were treated every 2 to 3 weeks, and by the third year, only 9% of patients still required weekly injections for symptom control, whereas an equal number were treated monthly. After the third year, two thirds of patients were controlled by treatment every 3 to 4 weeks (162). Many patients find a monthly injection interval to be convenient, particularly if they have any difficulty scheduling office visits. However, for some patients, stretching the interval beyond 2 weeks may lead to noncompliance (21). Marking the injection dates on the home calendar is one important way to enhance compliance. Some clinicians prefer to give a year of injections spaced at 3-week intervals before considering monthly treatment, whereas others rapidly advance to monthly injections after reaching maintenance treatment doses. Some physicians use maintenance intervals that exceed 1 month, but longer intervals raise the risk of an adverse reaction (106). According to Hurst et al., only a small minority of practices allowed patients to go as long as 5 or 6 weeks between maintenance injections, without requiring a dose reduction (162).

## Duration of Immunotherapy

How long to continue immunotherapy, and when to discontinue therapy, remain largely unstudied (9,49,202) and are unpredictable in any given patient (69). As always, patient symptoms should rule the decision making. If good practices have been followed, progressive symptomatic improvement should have occurred over the first 3 to 4 years of immunotherapy (19,49), and normally, improvement plateaus after this time. Practices surveyed by Hurst et al. reported that their patients were treated for 3 to 5 (mean, 3.8) years before an attempt was made to stop treatment (162). Complete withdrawal of immunotherapy can be considered in patients who have been symptom free for at least a year. However, many physicians believe that a 2- to 3-year period of reduced or symptom-free seasons (69,101, 200) is first necessary, and 3 to 5 years (49) of treatment may be desirable to effect lasting benefits (21,22). Another factor to consider is whether significant asthma is present.

Immunotherapy can be a significant steroid-sparing therapy; therefore, continuing monthly maintenance immunotherapy beyond 5 years may be advantageous in these patients. Also, some patients are encountered who have been treated previously with one or more courses of immunotherapy and have relapsed. These patients may prefer to remain on maintenance therapy rather than suffer another relapse. Similarly, patients with chronic sinusitis who have improved on immunotherapy may prefer not to change a successful therapy. In these types of situations there should be a careful discussion between clinician and patient about the pros and cons of continuing immunotherapy. King et al. recommend discontinuance if (a) injections have been administered for a minimum of 3 years (5 years for severe grass pollen allergy); (b) most of the injections have been in the maintenance range, with antigen concentrations of at least a #3 dilution or higher (0.2 mL of a #1 dilution or concentrate for each treated antigen, mixed into a 5-mL treatment vial); and (c) symptom relief has been enjoyed through all seasons of significance in the past year (21). However, the groundwork for the eventual successful discontinuance of immunotherapy must be laid much earlier, by proper diagnosis, aggressive escalation and maintenance dosing, achieving adequate symptom relief, and successful lengthening of injection intervals, without return of symptoms.

## Relapse After Immunotherapy

Unfortunately, an adequate and successful course of immunotherapy does not ensure a permanent cure after therapy is discontinued. In fact, discontinuance of immunotherapy causes IgG4 blocking antibodies to disappear rapidly (66). Both clinical experience and published studies have noted that efficacy can fade after immunotherapy is discontinued, requiring restarting of therapy (22,69,122). However, longterm relief after discontinuance is more likely when high antigen doses were administered for sustained periods. The discontinuance phase is another important transition time during which symptoms should be carefully monitored. Return of symptoms shortly after stopping immunotherapy is suggestive of inadequate immunomodulation. If this happens, the best time to intervene is earlier, rather than later, so that the immunologic changes that have been achieved can be preserved and enhanced, rather than starting all over. Thus, after withdrawal of therapy, the patient should be closely watched during the first 6 to 8 weeks (21). If symptoms recur during this time, immunotherapy should be reinstituted at one-half the previous maintenance dose, to be followed by gradual reescalation. If possible, the clinician should then strive to increase doses above those previously achieved, and resume weekly treatment. If longer than 2 months has gone by since discontinuance of immunotherapy, then an intradermal vial test (21) should be given before attempting to reinstitute subcutaneous injections. This same approach is used for patients who have gone for up to 1 year without allergy injections, by making a new vial based on their prior tests and checking sensitivity with a vial test. However, for periods over 1 year since stopping immunotherapy, reevaluation and retesting is the safest approach (21) because unpredictable changes in skin sensitivity, environment, and allergic load may have occurred.

## ALLERGY IMMUNOTHERAPY TROUBLESHOOTING

Since being introduced, immunotherapy has been practiced mainly as an art, and has been based on uncontrolled clinical observations (51,84,92,94,203,204). In the hands of those who are dedicated artists, outcomes usually are favorable. Dedication requires hard work, however, including undivided and focused attention on the patient, especially the problem patient. The following sections discuss some of the issues that require close attention at all times, but especially when the course and outcome of immunotherapy is less satisfactory than expected.

### Injections

The injection technique used should be methodical and consistent. The injection, if possible, should be given in the posterior area of the upper arm because this area can be easily observed and is more protected from local trauma (19, 21). The injection should be deep (22) and subcutaneous. If one injection is given per visit, then alternating arms is best (9). If more than one injection is given each visit, then administering in different arms and sites is best. Massaging the site after an injection should be avoided because it may lead to false-positive local reactions due to the trauma rather than to a real reaction (21). An ice pack can be applied to relieve local discomfort, and local pressure normally is sufficient to stop bleeding when a patient is taking a properly regulated anticoagulant.

### Injection Pain

Maintenance doses prepared primarily from concentrates may have glycerin concentrations that are significantly higher than 10%, and may therefore cause pain when injected. Glycerin-induced pain is primarily due to the osmotic effect, and is countered by drawing up at least an equal volume of sterile saline into the syringe with the treatment dose, lowering the glycerin concentration before administering the injection (21). Pain also may occur from large injection volume. In general, volumes under 0.5 mL are minimally uncomfortable, and pain increases as volumes approach or exceed 1 mL. Finally, pain will result from intradermal injection rather than subcutaneous injection. This can occur if the entire dose is not injected subcutane-

ously, but some antigen is still being injected as the needle is withdrawn from the arm.

### Predisposing Factors for Reactions

Some local reactions to immunotherapy injections are expected. These usually are characterized as small areas of redness and swelling that produce little discomfort (19). Reactions also may be associated with provocation of previous allergy symptoms. Injections during the early phase of immunotherapy, before the production of blocking antibody, may cause a worsening of preexistent symptoms (22); however, this should self-correct as dose escalation continues. The use of concomitant medications is another common reason for reactions and worsening allergy symptoms. Medication lists must be continually updated with specific searches for newly prescribed β-blockers or angiotensin-converting enzyme inhibitors, and the discontinuance of antihistamines or corticosteroids (22). Also, allergy injections given in the presence of respiratory infections are known to be associated with larger local reactions (21), and many clinicians therefore discourage the administration of injections when infections exist.

### Allergen Overload

In this circumstance, the patient is unexpectedly exposed to large quantities of aeroallergens, food allergens, chemicals, or a combination, causing an increase in circulating allergic mediators. Then, the addition of just a small added allergen challenge, such as an allergy immunotherapy injection, is enough to raise the mediators to symptom-producing levels. In such overloaded patients, a careful search for environmental, food, and chemical contacts usually is fruitful, and once the load is limited, new efforts to escalate the inhalant treatment dose can be made. Adverse reactions may arise after injections from a treatment vial containing any antigen, but especially when it contains antigens that cross-react with the external allergen exposure. When overload is suspected, patients should be carefully questioned about new or changing environmental or occupational exposures, including an inhalant in peak season or the seasonal consumption of a food allergen that is cross-reactive (see Chapter 3) (21,22,175,201). After food allergy exposures, the next most frequent causes of allergen overload are multiple pets in the home, heavy mold growth in the home or workplace, and continuing chemical exposure, especially to formaldehyde. A newly insulated attic, new carpets, new pet, broken dehumidifier, water leak, or new office building with sealed windows may be a factor. These factors are detected by careful history taking and selective retesting.

Allergen overload–induced symptoms, especially if temporary and controllable, do not always require immediate downward adjustment of immunotherapy doses (21). Dose adjustment may be necessary, however, because even patients who were previously under good control with long-term immunotherapy may need dose changes when exposed to high allergen levels (65,66,82,83,139,148,149,189,202, 205–209).

When one particular allergen or category of allergen is suspected or known to be in season, the best solution may be to isolate this allergen (or allergens) by splitting the treatment vial into two vials, one of which contains only the suspect allergen(s). Splitting the vial preserves the escalation levels already achieved with nonsuspect allergens, but allows easy changes in doses for the suspect allergens. During the first several months of immunotherapy, it is wise to anticipate a possible load problem and to put a highly sensitive allergen like ragweed or grass into a separate treatment vial. Dermatophyte allergens, such as *Candida albicans* (see Chapter 13), also often are easier to treat if they are placed in a separate treatment vial.

## Large Local Reactions

Skin reactions with induration and erythema of more than 25 mm should be monitored carefully (9), but there are no data to indicate that large local reactions are definite warning signs for the possible subsequent onset of systemic, anaphylactic reactions (89). Reactions of 3 to 4 cm, or larger, can be associated with systemic symptoms (19). Immediate treatment of large local reactions is by cold compresses, antihistamines (210–213), and, if severe, oral corticosteroids (9,19). The initial analysis of any significant reaction is to check that the dose given was correct, that there was no error in making the treatment vial, that the correct vial was used, and that the injection was given with good technique. Obviously, good records of vial manufacture and injections must be maintained to analyze what might have occurred. If all records are in order, and the vial is visibly normal, the clinician should consider giving a vial test before the next scheduled injection, or remake the vial. After making any corrections to a vial, a vial test should always be the initial dose. If the clinician does not suspect technical errors and chooses not to remix the vial or make a vial test, then the injection dose needs to be substantially cut back to either the previously tolerated dose, or further reduced to one tenth to one half of the reacting dose.

If local (not systemic) injection reactions cannot be reduced enough to allow adequate dose escalation, even when antihistamine pretreatment is used, and if immunotherapy is strongly indicated, then adding epinephrine or heparin to the treatment vial may rarely be of benefit. Amounts of these drugs that do not exceed the recommended single doses for the body mass of the patient should be added to the treatment vials, and small test doses, including vial testing, should be carried out (210). Pharmacologic prophylactic treatment of general or systemic reactions should never be relied on. A small number of patients may persist in having unacceptable local reactions no matter what attempts are made to minimize them. If the patient perceives significant relief, the clinician may, in this circumstance, have no choice but to settle for low-dose treatment. Otherwise, buildup immunotherapy may not be practical, and treatment with an alternate method such as neutralization or enzyme-potentiated immunotherapy may be considered (41).

## Allergen Potency

Allergenic extract potency must be maintained throughout the testing and treatment period. Large variations in potency can cause either reactions or poor efficacy. For maximum potency, aqueous extracts should be stored at a temperature of $4°C$ and should be discarded if allowed to either freeze or warm to greater than $40°C$ (9). Refrigerated concentrates and lyophilized antigens have extremely long potency half-lives, but after dilution or reconstitution, potency begins to decline. To ensure antigenic potency for at least 3 months, it is necessary to maintain a glycerin content of at least 10% in the treatment vial. This is ensured when all antigens used to manufacture a treatment vial are #1 dilution or concentrates. It also occurs if at least five concentrated antigens are added to a vial, which will also assure a concentration of at least 10% glycerin (0.2 mL $\times$ 5 = 1 mL @ 50% glycerin + 4 mL diluent = 5 mL @ 10% glycerin). Creating at least a 10% glycerin treatment vial concentration is a problem only when, early in immunotherapy, most of the vial components are high-dilution, weak antigens. Under these circumstances, 1 mL of 50% glycerin should be added to the treatment vial (21). It is not necessary to achieve glycerin concentrations that are exactly 10%. It is better to err on the high side rather than on the low side, which may result in low-potency extracts. It also is important to keep mixing instructions simple so that potential errors are prevented. In the practice survey of Hurst et al., all offices used phenol-containing normal saline diluent, and 30% added albumin to prevent surface adsorption of dilute antigens (162). Most practices used an average glycerin concentration of 12.5% w/v in treatment vials. Vials were refrigerated and outdated after 2 to 6 (mean 3.7) months from the date of mixing.

## Antigen Incompatibility

Many antigen extracts, including extracts of dust mites, pollens, and molds, are known to contain proteases (214–216). Mold proteases have been shown to cause antigen degradation in multiantigen vials (217,218). For this reason, some physicians advocate treating molds in a separate vial from other antigens. Because the stability of antigen mixes has not been determined for most storage conditions, it is prudent to use all feasible methods to ensure potency, including high glycerin content, refrigeration, and defined outdates for all treatment vials.

## Combining Antigens of Like Sensitivity

Antigens that differ quantitatively in their reactivity also normally differ in the time required to achieve successful maintenance levels, with more sensitive antigens requiring more time. However, antigens that are combined in the same treatment vial are subject to the same speed of escalation. Unless recognized, these facts can cause problems with immunotherapy. Antigens that test positive at low reactivity levels can be safely mixed into treatment vials at relatively high concentration, and usually can be raised quickly to maintenance doses. If these low-reactivity allergens are mixed with high-reactivity allergens, however, as the treatment dose is raised, injection reactions associated with the approach to maintenance by the low-sensitivity allergens will prevent adequate escalation of the high-reactivity allergens. Such mixing leads to ineffective immunotherapy for the high-sensitivity, low-concentration antigens (138,191, 219,220). This problem commonly occurs when all positive antigens are placed in a single treatment vial. The solution is to keep antigens of like reactivity together, based on quantitative testing. Therefore, "high reactors" (e.g., RAST level 3, 4, and 5 and SET endpoints 4, 5, and 6) should not be mixed in the same treatment vial as "low reactors" (e.g., RAST levels 0/1, 1, and 2 and SET endpoints 1, 2, and 3) (21). Ward suggests combining only those antigens that are within one dilution of each other (191).

## Allergen Mixes

The role of mixed allergens in allergy practice is controversial. There are five reasons why mixes can potentially cause immunotherapy problems. First, mixes of non–cross-reacting allergens may sensitize people to allergens to which they do not already react. Second, mixes cannot be used for treatment from in vitro testing results that are based on single antigens. Third, testing with large numbers of antigens in a mix is less sensitive than testing with single antigens, and therefore significant allergens may be overlooked. Fourth, some mixes, such as house dust, are crude preparations that contain undesirable contaminants. Use of single antigens for treating the major components of house dust gives equally good immunotherapy without the potential risks of injecting insecticides, or other nonallergenic substances, that may be present in the crude dust. Finally, during treatment with mixes, if both high- and low-sensitivity allergens are present, dose advancement may be limited by the low-sensitivity allergen, thus defeating the purpose of quantitation, and compromising results.

Mixes may be effectively used in a few very specific cases. One is the use of screening mixes to determine if full testing is required. Here, the key is to include only a few antigens in the screen, so loss of sensitivity is minimal. If the screen is positive, then all component antigens are tested for separately. A second example is to reduce the number of skin tests applied by including cross-reacting allergens in a diagnostic or treatment mix. For example, a mix composed of *D. farinae* and *D. pteronyssinus* or a mixture of several local oak species could be used, provided that the same ratio of allergens in the mix always is used for both diagnosis and for treatment.

## Glycerin Sensitivity

Completely removing glycerin from the treatment vial may be necessary in rare cases when patients are extremely glycerin sensitive. This should be done only when patients are warned about careful refrigerated storage and will adhere to a maximum vial life of 6 weeks. Before investing time and effort in preparing glycerin-free treatment sets, the clinician must be certain that the patient has true symptom production from glycerin. This can be suspected from SET testing with glycerin dilutions, where dilutions of #4 or greater show 7-mm or larger wheals. Significant glycerin sensitivity with symptom production is then proven by placebo-controlled subcutaneous challenges. Neutralization therapy can be used for glycerin sensitivity (see next section, Phenol Sensitivity). If neutralization is unsuccessful, glycerin-free lyophilized antigens can be purchased and reconstituted in sterile phenolated saline for use in these patients (210).

## Phenol Sensitivity

Very rarely, some patients may become phenol sensitive and mount either local or systemic reactions. When this is suspected, the degree of sensitivity is determined by SET using phenol diluted in pure saline. The condition is confirmed with placebo-controlled subcutaneous challenges. As initial treatment for phenol sensitivity, the clinician should attempt neutralization, in the same manner as neutralization for food allergens, with the neutralizing dose given by sublingual phenol drops just before administering the allergy injection (see Chapter 4). If there is inadequate relief with neutralization, and immunotherapy is strongly indicated, then lyophilized antigens can be reconstituted in saline for preservative-free treatment. If this method is elected, extreme care must be taken to prevent bacterial contamination of the solutions. Glycerin may be added to the treatment vial to enhance antigen stability, although glycerin is not an adequate bacteriostat. To minimize reentry into vials, use of only single-dose treatment vials is suggested (210). The practitioner should document carefully the antiseptic precautions that are taken if phenol is omitted from treatment sets.

## Allergy Retesting and Supplemental Testing

Routine retesting of patients on immunotherapy is neither necessary nor recommended (21,51). Some physicians customarily retest as part of the decision to end immunotherapy, believing that reduced skin sensitivity is a good indication that sufficient immunotherapy has been given. However, there are no good data to support the usefulness of this information, other than to confirm the observation that skin test sensitivity usually does gradually decline during immunotherapy. Instead, retesting should be reserved for situations where quantitation of the current allergic sensitivity of previously tested allergens is of paramount importance. This may be the case during an unrelenting or intractable phase of injection reactions, or if allergy symptoms increase without an obvious cause. Retesting also may be used to identify which of the antigens in a particular vial may be preventing advancement of the immunotherapy dose for that vial. It also is appropriate to retest any patient who has been off of allergy injections for more than a year and wishes to resume therapy (21,51). Retesting also may rarely be appropriate if factors known to affect skin test interpretation, such as medications, foods, pollutants, and stress (201), were not minimized at the time of initial skin testing, leading to possible test misinterpretation. Finally, retesting also may be appropriate in the occasional patient who has been on successful immunotherapy for years and suddenly has an unexplained worsening of symptoms. In many cases, retesting may be indicated for both previously positive and previously negative allergens because previously negative allergens may now be positive, and previously positive allergens may have shifted in sensitivity. For some allergens, skin sensitivity may change substantially with the season. Previously negative allergens are most likely to retest as positive if they were previously tested just before their season, and are now retested just after their season.

Because of the vast number of potential allergens available for testing, but limited time and resources, choices have to be made about what allergens are most important to test for in each patient (see Chapter 3). Supplemental allergy tests therefore are appropriate whenever it is suspected that significant allergens were not evaluated during initial testing. This issue most commonly arises during the first year or two of immunotherapy, when a patient who is otherwise improving complains of significantly worse symptoms during a particular season or in a particular location. It also may occur when a new, significant allergen is added to the office's normal test panel, and patients currently on immunotherapy may benefit from adding this new antigen to their treatment. Additional testing of the suspected new allergens is then ordered, and positive reactors are included in a new immunotherapy vial. If a good choice of supplemental antigens to test has been made, then, in subsequent years, further clinical improvement will occur.

## Adjunctive Pharmacotherapy

Use of antihistamines before injections is helpful, especially to decrease itching. There also is some evidence that antihis-

tamines reduce minor reactions without interfering with detection of potential serious reactions (162). Furthermore, antihistamines are known to affect lymphocytes, and a few studies have suggested that antihistamine treatment may enhance the effectiveness of immunotherapy. As a general precaution, asthmatic patients always should be on effective antiinflammatory therapy, and particularly during buildup immunotherapy. In complex patients with a serious allergic load, oral cromolyn may be used to reduce the food allergy load, antifungal drugs may be given to reduce the fungal load (in *Candida*-sensitive patients), and leukotriene inhibitors may be used to blunt delayed allergic reactions of any kind. In very ill patients, such as those with severe asthma, uncontrolled urticaria, or extensive eczema, oral corticosteroid therapy, with all of its potential side effects, may be the only method that can allow adequate testing and initiation of immunotherapy.

## In Vitro Monitoring of Immunotherapy

The routine use of either total IgE levels or allergen-specific IgE levels to monitor inhalant immunotherapy is not warranted because symptom levels during immunotherapy do not correlate closely with IgE levels (68). However, allergen-specific IgG levels are correlated with clinical improvement, and immunotherapy is not likely to be of benefit if not associated with increases in IgG (41). Thus, specific IgG testing may be of use to assess the effectiveness of the dose in a patient who is not responding to immunotherapy. Food-specific IgG levels also can be used to assess compliance with exclusion diets because specific IgG levels rapidly decline during food avoidance. Finally, in immunotherapy for *Hymenoptera* sting allergy, both specific IgE and specific IgG are critically important in determining the effectiveness of therapy, as well as in providing data to support a safe time for cessation of therapy.

## Monitoring and Communication

Because allergic patients have a chronic disorder that is being treated for years, physicians and nurses caring for these patients must appreciate the dynamic nature of the ongoing, never-ending history and physical examination that is required in such cases. Each clinician must inquire about the patient's health status at every encounter. Issues of concern include changes in home, work, and leisure environment, changes in medications (201), and the development of new allergies or new symptoms. Especially important is the response to therapy and the review of any reactions to injections or other treatments. Education also is important, both in training patients to recognize problems and in helping them learn to avoid allergens (21,162). Finally, good communication between the clinicians caring for the patient is as important as good communication with the patient. All of these elements can affect the success or failure of ongoing immunotherapy.

## IMMUNOTHERAPY SAFETY

The most important risk for patients treated with allergy immunotherapy is that of systemic anaphylactic reaction (162). The physician's obligation to all patients should be first to do no harm. Every effort in immunotherapy should be made with these two thoughts in mind. Unfortunately, history tells us that there have been anaphylactic deaths after allergy skin testing and therapeutic injections (89). However, based on published information, the numbers of serious reactions and deaths are very low. Most clinicians could probably agree on what constitutes a serious reaction, but reported reaction rates commonly also include less severe reactions, the incidence of which varies with inclusion criteria and capture techniques. With this caveat in mind, the reported incidence of immunotherapy reactions varies from less than 1% to greater than 36% (221). Retrospective data have identified a per injection adverse reaction rate of between 0.05% and 3.5% (100,222). Recent studies, however, would support the lower portion of this range, approximately 0.0007% to 0.4% for systemic reactions (106,223–225), and 0% to 0.002% for death rates (99,100, 162,223,224,226,227). These statistics also include those based on fivefold dilution quantitation techniques, and these are notable for very high safety (117,162,225,228).

These favorable statistics should not lull any physician into a false sense of security. Major systemic reactions from allergy immunotherapy, including death, are not unlike catastrophic complications from surgery, or those from recreational activities. The problem with all such disasters is that no one can predict when one will strike. Our only defense against these rare and unpredictable events is to learn the risk factors, minimize these factors, and be prepared at all times. The experienced and the inexperienced clinician alike must be familiar with the clinical risk factors, and be prepared for treating anaphylaxis. Diligent study, careful observation, and compulsive attention to safe practices should provide the safest possible environment for immunotherapy.

## Anaphylaxis Risk Factors

Many risk factors have been identified that influence immunotherapy safety (89,106,162,211,221,222,229–232). Those risks that are currently documented are shown in Table 12.7, and the more important of these are discussed here. Large local or mild systemic reactions that follow injections constitute early warning signs that immunotherapy doses may be close to the MTD and possible anaphylaxis can soon occur. Typical warning symptoms observed by Hurst et al., in order of frequency, were injection site wheal

**TABLE 12.7. RISK FACTORS FOR MAJOR SYSTEMIC REACTION FROM IMMUNOTHERAPY**

| Risk Factor | Authors |
|---|---|
| **Environment** | |
| High dose in pollen season | Van Arsdel and Sherman (222) |
| High dose in mold season | Tinkelman et al. (106) |
| High allergen exposure (load) | Gibofsky (230) |
| **Patient** | |
| Patient younger than age 5 y | Hejjaoui et al. (211) |
| Current increased symptoms | Gibofsky (230) |
| Prior systemic reaction | Van Arsdel and Sherman (222) |
| High sensitivity ("brittle") | Greineder (221) |
| Unstable asthma | Gibofsky (230) |
| β-Blocker treatment | Greineder (221) |
| **Technique** | |
| Error (wrong dose or vial) | Norman (232) |
| Inexperienced physician | Norman (232) |
| Buildup immunotherapy | Tinkelman (106) |
| Potent allergens | Lockey et al. (89) |
| Excessive allergen dose | Van Arsdel and Sherman (222) |
| Change to new allergy extract | Bosquet (231) |
| Initial injection from new treatment vial | Hurst et al. (162) |
| Treatment vial prepared by another office | Hurst et al. (162) |
| Injections closely spaced in time | Vervloet et al. (229) |
| Rush immunotherapy | Bosquet and Michel (231) |
| Injections less often than weekly | Tinkelman et al. (106) |

greater than 2 cm, arm swelling or local urticaria, sneezing or minor allergic symptoms, mild headache, flushing or burning feeling, or a lightheaded feeling (162). These minor reactions can be treated by observation or administration of an oral antihistamine, but they must be noticed so that extra care can be used in planning the next injection.

### Time After Injection

Although we cannot accurately predict if a major reaction will occur, we do know the range of time during which a reaction is likely to occur. Posttreatment anaphylactic reactions have presented from instantaneously with an injection, to 6 hours later (9,89,99,100,106,162,223,232–234). Most serious reactions occur within 15 to 20 minutes after exposure (106,162,235), so that, in the United States, this period normally is chosen for postinjection observation. For example, Hurst et al. found 87% of major reactions began within

20 minutes of injection (162), and Tinkelman et al. found six of seven severe reactions occurred within 20 minutes, and the seventh within 30 minutes of the injection (106). Yet, Greenberg et al. (233,234) reported that 38% of systemic reactions developed between 35 minutes and 6 hours postinjection, and during the first hour, some patients did acquire asthma that required epinephrine treatment. The British Committee on Safety of Medicines also identified late reactions when they reported on deaths and serious systemic reactions in the United Kingdom between 1957 and 1986 (223). Most fatalities occurred under the care of general practitioners who were not experienced in allergy management (232). Two fatalities occurred where symptoms first appeared between 30 and 90 minutes postinjection. The Committee concluded that these data warranted informed consent for allergy patients, treatment only where full resuscitation facilities were available, and a 2-hour observation period after injections. Therefore, although most serious systemic reactions do occur within 20 minutes, both physicians and patients should be prepared for possible late reactions, with a self-administered epinephrine kit available.

## Asthma

Patients who have uncontrolled asthma comprise one of the highest risk groups for anaphylaxis and anaphylaxis death (89,99). The clinician always should be cautious with these patients, as well as with highly sensitive patients (9,221), and those with a prior history of anaphylaxis (162). Part of the ongoing nursing assessment in allergy offices always should be concerned with the decision about when to give, when to change the dose of, and when to postpone allergy injections for patients with asthma.

## New Treatment Vial

Risk is increased with the first exposure to an antigen, such as during the initial injection from a new treatment vial (162). Any new vial has obvious potential for errors relating to improper mixing, higher potency, a newly added antigen, or a change in nonstandardized extract lot or manufacturer (89,162). Other errors can occur if vials are prepared outside of the physician's office (232) or are based on in vitro tests.

## High Allergen Load

Risk significantly increases with higher allergic load, such as during dose escalation (106), in-season pollen or mold therapy (89,106), spacing doses too closely together (162), excessive dose increase, (222), or mistaken overdose (232). Hurst et al., in a prospective safety study of over a million injections, found a larger than previously reported, 20-fold difference in risk between buildup and maintenance injections (162). In addition, a major increase in any allergy

symptoms should be a warning that a high allergen load may exist. For example, worsening asthma, urticaria, more frequent migraine headaches, and increased eczema all should raise suspicion.

## β-Blocker and Other Drug Treatment

Treatment with β-blockers both increases the risk for a reaction and complicates emergency treatment when a reaction occurs (see earlier). Consequently, these patients should be treated cautiously, like asthmatic patients. In the large study by Hurst et al., reactions while on β-blocker therapy were less than 10% as frequent as reactions in asthmatic patients, and less than half as frequent as reactions occurring from an injection from a new vial (162). Other potentially significant drugs are the angiotensin-converting enzyme inhibitors, which facilitate kinin-catalyzed reactions, and monoamine oxidase inhibitors, which sensitize to catecholamines (103). Occasionally, reactions even may occur because a patient discontinues a medication. For example, a patient may have taken an antihistamine before his or her initial skin testing, thus falsely reducing skin sensitivity, or a patient may recently have been tapered off of prednisone, with a consequent lessening of asthma control.

## Early Use of Epinephrine Is Important

There is evidence that physicians and nurses are not using epinephrine quickly enough when anaphylaxis does occur. Norman reported 24 recent immunotherapy deaths, in 40% of which epinephrine was never used (232). Hurst et al. found epinephrine was used only in 30% of systemic reactions, and also strongly supported early epinephrine use for suspected anaphylaxis (162). One of the reasons for failure to use epinephrine is thought to be fear of overdosing patients, causing tachycardia or arrhythmias. As a consequence, repeated administration of small (0.1- to 0.2-mL) doses of 1:1,000 epinephrine, rather than larger single doses, has been recommended by some authors (9). However, single doses of up to 1 mg (1 mL) are routinely used in adult cardiac resuscitation.

## Adequate Staffing and Training Is Important

In all offices surveyed by Hurst et al., injections were given only when two or more trained individuals were present. In addition, many offices now ensure that a physician, physician's assistant, or nurse practitioner is present during testing and injection hours. All studied practices had their physicians, and almost all practices had their nurses currently certified in basic cardiopulmonary resuscitation, and 40% of practices also had one or more people certified in advanced cardiac life support (162).

# IMMUNOTHERAPY INJECTIONS ADMINISTERED OUTSIDE OF THE SPECIALIST OFFICE

## Nonspecialist Health Care Facilities

Patients who are under the care of an allergy specialist often ask (or sometimes are required to ask by managed care) to receive their injections in health care facilities outside of the specialist's office. Although this practice adds patient convenience and enables more patients to receive immunotherapy, much of the art of immunotherapy, important to reliable and successful outcomes, can easily be lost. Nonspecialist facilities are rarely able to provide the expertise, experience, and knowledgeable observation that a trained allergy staff provides. In this situation, the proper management decisions necessary for successful escalation and achievement of maintenance, especially in the face of the variable allergen environment, can be difficult.

From a safety standpoint, immunotherapy in a nonspecialist health care office in the United States has only a slightly higher reaction risk than in a specialist's office (162). The most common error seen in nonspecialist offices is administering a tenfold overdose, by giving 0.5- or 1-mL injections, rather than 0.05 or 0.1 mL. An overdose of this magnitude in a patient who is not receiving very high doses usually results only in a large local reaction. Identification errors, fortunately, are much less common, because administering the wrong patient's allergen mix to a different patient could lead to a fatal reaction if there is a substantial difference in antigen content and concentration. Consequently, correct identification of patient, patient vial, and dose always must be stressed. It also is advisable to train patients to check their own vials and to become familiar with their own dose schedule.

The specialist should allow immunotherapy in other facilities only if there is good communication among all parties involved, including from office to office. When very complex patients are to be treated, direct physician-to-physician contact is suggested. In this setting, it is especially important that patients should be educated and reeducated about immunotherapy philosophy, goals, safety precautions, and emergency treatment because they must function as a check on their own treatment. Although the provision of this information in writing, for patients to read and study, does not eliminate the need for one-on-one instruction, such documentation should be provided at the beginning of treatment. It also is important that the nonspecialist provider be given documentation about the content of the treatment vials, the expected escalation schedule, and the management of local and systemic reactions (21,230). Patients also should be given a prescription for a self-administered epinephrine kit, and be instructed in its use.

## Home Immunotherapy

Patients also may ask to receive their injections at home. Again, home immunotherapy is convenient, and the inconvenience of office visits has been cited as a major reason for abandoning immunotherapy (236). This alternative then makes immunotherapy feasible to many patients for whom it otherwise would not be available. Home immunotherapy also is economical, another advantage for patients. Understandably, immunotherapy administered in the home environment has been controversial. The 1993 American Academy of Allergy, Asthma, and Immunology position statement on minimizing anaphylaxis (237) suggested that home therapy is likely to be less safe, and because resuscitation equipment is not available, they warned that anaphylaxis occurring at home is likely to be fatal. Their position statement therefore endorsed only office treatment, and only when facilities and personnel are prepared to treat anaphylaxis. However, that position statement has been challenged by clinicians who argue that it is possible to provide adequate precautions for home treatment (238,239).

Patients on home immunotherapy have now been studied in large numbers. The incidence of major systemic reactions actually has been found to be 26-fold lower than that associated with in-office treatment, and there were no deaths (162,224,228). Hurst et al., in 1999, completed a prospective, 1-year study of 25 otolaryngic allergy practices, observing approximately 600,000 home injections. This study showed a total reaction incidence of 0.028% with home injections, compared with 0.024% for office injections. This compares favorably with the 0.0007% to 0.4% modern rates reported for systemic reactions (106,223–225). In this study, only one major reaction occurred at home: a nonfatal exacerbation of asthma symptoms.

There are many factors responsible for the favorable safety record of home immunotherapy. The most important factor is probably the preferential selection of low-risk patients for home therapy. For instance, because of the higher reaction rate associated with escalation versus maintenance immunotherapy, patients on home immunotherapy (224, 228) are skewed rather heavily toward those on maintenance. For example, some practices always complete escalation in the office, and others begin escalation in the office, before allowing patients to go on home therapy. Higher-risk patients who have severe or poorly controlled asthma, are highly sensitive, are taking β-blockers, are on insect venom therapy, or are in the early buildup phase of immunotherapy are less likely to be allowed home injections.

The selection of appropriate patients for home treatment requires compulsive screening and special arrangements. The physician should have considerable experience in managing patients on immunotherapy in the office setting before embarking on home immunotherapy. Home immunotherapy success depends on effective communication, education, training, and equipping of the patient for safe and successful injections. Candidate selection criteria should begin with choosing capable patients. The physician must have trust in the patient's ability to respond to a reaction, willingness to report problems, and ability to maintain a written record of home injections (162). If the clinician and patient choose to escalate doses at home, there is the added responsibility for safe achievement of maintenance dose ranges that are proper and effective. When more than one patient in a household is on immunotherapy, color-coded or distinctively marked treatment vials are recommended. Patients on home immunotherapy should be prepared, each time that they administer their injection, with a functional, unoccupied telephone, and a responsible adult who could render aid. There also should be available epinephrine, an antihistamine, a tourniquet, and a bronchodilator (for asthmatic patients) (21). Because some patients find it more difficult and uncomfortable to self-administer injections in the posterior arm, they should be informed of alternative sites such as the anterior thigh (low enough so a tourniquet could be applied) (21). Finally, most practices require patients to begin home treatment with a vial test. Many physicians also require patients to return to the office for a vial test of each new treatment vial, or else the initial dose is reduced. A good alternative for patients who cannot return to the office several times a year is to provide single-dose treatment vials for home use.

## IMMUNOTHERAPY OUTCOMES

### Time to Symptom Relief

Despite the difficulty in measuring the severity of allergic disease, the natural variation in symptoms, and the possibility of spontaneous improvement, especially in younger children (9), there are published studies addressing the subject of immunotherapy outcomes. The onset of symptom relief after the initiation of immunotherapy is reported to range from 3 to 12 months (14,22,49). In one study of patients treated by immunotherapy for one to three inhalant allergens, over half had symptomatic improvement after 4 months, and a third had substantial decreases in spontaneous histamine release from leukocytes (240). In some cases, benefits of immunotherapy occur even earlier. For example, in a study of cat allergy, twice-weekly immunotherapy reduced skin test responses and symptoms in as little as 6 weeks (241).

### Range of Responses

Quality of life in patients with allergy, as assessed by objective questionnaires, improves significantly during 1 year of quantitative testing–based immunotherapy (242). According to a comparison study between dust mite immunotherapy and pharmacotherapy, symptom relief due to immuno-

therapy continues to improve every year for at least 5 years (243). In this study, pharmacotherapy was superior during the first year, equal with immunotherapy from the second to third year, and less effective than immunotherapy by the fifth year. Improvement due to immunotherapy treatment also can occur in specific allergic syndromes, such as Meniere's disease (244), or in chronic rhinosinusitis (48). In fact, Keenan suggests that only 5% to 10% of patients with inhalant allergy will not respond to immunotherapy (201). Significant long-term symptom relief is reported to be achievable in 80% to 90% of patients (22).

## Durability of Symptom Relief

Still incompletely determined is how durable are the results of immunotherapy. If permanent cure is defined as being able to discontinue therapy after 3 to 5 years without the recurrence of any allergy symptoms, then this occurs only rarely because relapses requiring restarting of therapy are observed frequently (69). However, King et al. (21) have suggested much higher long-term control rates of at least 80% when patients are treated with MTDs and a less strict definition of cure, allowing for intermittent use of pharmacotherapy after immunotherapy discontinuance, is applied (21). The remaining 20% of patients can be kept symptom free as long as immunotherapy is not stopped (21). Ebner et al. (245) similarly found that approximately 30% of patients on grass pollen immunotherapy relapsed within 3 years after completing therapy, but that the other 70% continued to show long-term symptomatic improvement. Most of the relapsed patients could be improved again by giving them a new, preseasonal booster series of immunotherapy injections (245). Ohashi et al. also identified some patients who, after 6 years of dust mite immunotherapy, had undetectable specific IgE, negative nasal provocations, and absence of rhinitis symptoms, and who remained well for at least 2 years without further immunotherapy (243).

Recently, two other groups studied patients who had received grass pollen immunotherapy, one group studied birch pollen immunotherapy, and another studied immunotherapy with cat and dog antigens. All studies found that, compared with untreated patients, substantial clinical improvement still could be observed 3 to 6 years after completing immunotherapy (246–249). In most patients, immune alterations in both immediate and delayed hypersensitivity persisted for long after the end of active immunotherapy (250), and results after 6 years were more durable for rhinitis (86%) than for asthma (68%) (248). After 5 years, 87% of asthmatic patients who had been treated with animal dander still were symptomatically improved, and their pulmonary histamine challenges remained improved, although challenges with animal dander had reverted to their original, pretreatment sensitivities (249). It appears that longer periods of symptomatic improvement follow longer courses of immunotherapy (249), but further research is required to verify this point.

## SUMMARY

The practice of effective clinical response–based immunotherapy can be traced to early allergists such as Curtis (251). At the beginning of the 20th century, Curtis achieved success in alleviating allergy symptoms using crude extracts and without producing severe complications. However, it became apparent that his technique could not be consistently duplicated and was associated elsewhere with unacceptable cases of anaphylaxis. Experiences like these spurred medical research to quantitate, and to correlate immunotherapy doses and techniques with outcomes. This chapter has stressed the advantages of using quantitative allergy testing methods for allergy treatment. The methodology for safe immunotherapy has been discussed, and potential pitfalls of the technique also have been outlined. Almost an entire century of research has now led to the development of methods that are easily understood and taught, and should have acceptable reproducibility, efficacy, and safety. As we enter a new century, improvements and new techniques in allergy care will continue to expand our capabilities and improve our understanding and use of allergy immunotherapy.

## ACKNOWLEDGMENTS

The authors thank Gwen Mayo, secretary, and Grace Sears, editor, from the University of Kentucky Chandler Medical Center, and Jeanie M. Vander Pyl, head librarian, June L. Bianchi, Phyllis J. Foley, and Sally C. Schumann, librarians, from the Cape Cod Hospital, all of whom contributed substantially to the quality of this manuscript.

## REFERENCES

1. Zeiss CR. Immunotherapy in allergic disease. In: Lockey RF, ed. *Allergy and clinical immunology.* Garden City, NY: Medical Examination Publishing, 1979:977–994.
2. Koessler KK. The specific treatment of hayfever by active immunization. *Ill Med J* 1914;25(August):120–127.
3. Noon L, Cantab BC. Prophylactic inoculation against hay fever. *Lancet* 1911;June 10:1572–1573.
4. Gordon BR. Allergy skin tests for inhalants and foods: comparison of methods in common use. *Otolaryngology Clinics North Am* 1998;31:35–54.
5. Besredka A, Steinhardt E. De l'anaphylaxie et de l'anaphylaxie vis-a-vis due serum de cheval. *Ann Inst Past* 1907;21:117–384.
6. Freeman J. Vaccination against hay fever. *Lancet* 1914;April 25: 1178–1180.
7. Cooke RA. The treatment of hay fever by active immunization. *Laryngoscope* 1915;25:108.
8. Cooke RA, Vander Veer A Jr. Human sensitization. *J Immunol* 1916;1:201–237.
9. Ledford DK, Lockey RF. Immunotherapy for allergic disease. In: Bierman CW, Pearlman DS, Shapiro GG, et al., eds. *Allergy, asthma, and immunology from infancy to adulthood,* 3rd ed. Philadelphia: WB Saunders, 1995:237–255.
10. Frankland AW, Augustin R. Prophylaxis of summer hayfever and asthma: a controlled trial comparing crude grass-pollen extracts with the isolated main protein component. *Lancet* 1954; 1:1055–1058.
11. Johnstone DE, Dutton A. The value of hyposensitization therapy for bronchial asthma in children: a 14 year study. *Pediatrics* 1968;42:793–802.
12. Hedlin G, Graff-Lonnevig V, Heilborn H, et al. Immunotherapy with cat- and dog-dander extracts: V. effects of 3 years of treatment. *J Allergy Clin Immunol* 1991;87:955–964.
13. Lowell FC, Frankland W. A double blind study of the effectiveness and specificity of injection therapy in ragweed hay fever. *N Engl J Med* 1965;273:675–679.
14. Fadal RG, Nalebuff DJ. A study of optimum dose immunotherapy in pharmacological treatment failures. *Arch Otolaryngol* 1980;106:38–43.
15. Hunt KJ, Valentine MD, Sobotka AK, et al. controlled trial of immunotherapy in insect sensitivity. *N Engl J Med* 1978;299: 157–161.
16. Malling HJ. Immunotherapy for mold allergy. *Clin Rev Allergy* 1992;10:237–251.
17. Kay AB. BSACI position paper on allergen immunotherapy. *Clin Exp Allergy* 1993;23[Suppl 3]:1–44.
18. Ohman JL Jr. Allergen immunotherapy: review of efficacy and current practice. *Med Clin North Am* 1992;76:977–991.
19. Van Metre TE Jr, Adkinson NF Jr. Immunotherapy for aeroallergen disease. In: Middleton JE, Reed CE, Ellis EF, et al., eds. *Allergy principles and practices,* 4th ed. St. Louis: Mosby, 1993: 1489–1509.
20. Anonymous. The veterinary services market. *J Am Vet Med Assoc* 1983;183:841–843.
21. King HC, Mabry RL, Mabry CS. Vial preparation and immunotherapy. *Allergy in ENT practice: a basic guide.* New York: Thieme Medical, 1998:201–262.
22. Gordon BR. Immunotherapy: rationale and mechanisms. *Otolaryngol Head Neck Surg* 1992;107:861–865.
23. Fell W, Mabry RL, Mabry CS. Quality of life analysis of immunotherapy for allergic rhinitis. *Ear Nose Throat J* 1997;76: 528–536.
24. Osterballe O. Immunotherapy in hay fever with two major allergens 19, 25 and partially purified extract of timothy grass pollen: a controlled double-blind study: in vivo variables, season 1. *Allergy* 1980;35:473–489.
25. Osterballe O, Lowenstein H, Prahl P, et al. Immunotherapy in hay fever with two major allergens 19, 25 and partially purified extract of timothy grass pollen: a controlled double-blind study: in vitro variables, season 1. *Allergy* 1981;36:183–199.
26. Munro-Ashman D, McEwen H, Feinberg JG. The patient self (P-S) test: demonstration of a rise in blocking antibodies after treatment with Allpyral. *Int Arch Allergy Appl Immunol* 1971; 40:448–453.
27. Ortolani C, Pastorello E, Moss RB, et al. Pollen immunotherapy: a single year double blind placebo-controlled study in patients with grass pollen induced asthma and rhinitis. *J Allergy Clin Immunol* 1984;73:283–290.
28. Reid MJ, Moss RB, Hsu YP, et al. Seasonal asthma in northern California: allergic causes and efficacy of immunotherapy. *J Allergy Clin Immunol* 1986;78:590–600.
29. Bousquet J, Hejjaoui A, Skassa-Brociek W, et al. Double blind, placebo-controlled immunotherapy with mixed grass-pollen allergoids: I. rush immunotherapy with allergoids and standard-

ized orchard grass-pollen extract. *J Allergy Clin Immunol* 1987; 80:591–598.

30. Bousquet J, Maasch H, Martinot B, et al. Double-blind, placebo-controlled immunotherapy with mixed grass-pollen allergoids: II. comparisons between parameters assessing the efficacy of immunotherapy. *J Allergy Clin Immunol* 1988;82:439–446.

31. Kuna P, Alam R, Kuzminska B, et al. The effect of preseasonal immunotherapy on the production of histamine-releasing factor (HRF) by mononuclear cells from patients with seasonal asthma: results of a double-blind, placebo-controlled, randomized study. *J Allergy Clin Immunol* 1989;83:816–824.

32. Varney VA, Hamid QA, Gaga M, et al. Influence of grass pollen immunotherapy on cellular infiltration and cytokine mRNA expression during allergen-induced late-phase cutaneous responses. *J Clin Invest* 1993;92:644–651.

33. Weyer A, Donat N, L'Heritier C, et al. Grass pollen hyposensitization versus placebo therapy: clinical effectiveness and methodological aspects of a pre-seasonal course of desensitization with a four-grass extract. *Allergy* 1981;36:309–317.

34. Varney VA, Gaga M, Frew AJ, et al. Usefulness of immunotherapy in patients with severe summer hay fever uncontrolled by antiallergic drugs. *BMJ* 1991;302:265–269.

35. Pence HL, Mitchell DQ, Greely RL, et al. Immunotherapy for mountain cedar pollenosis: a double-blind controlled study. *J Allergy Clin Immunol* 1976;58:39–50.

36. Parker WA, Whisman BA, Apaliski SJ, et al. The relationships between late cutaneous responses and specific antibody responses with outcome of immunotherapy for seasonal allergic rhinitis. *J Allergy Clin Immunol* 1989;84:667–677.

37. Viander M, Koivikko A. The seasonal symptoms of hyposensitized and untreated hay fever patients in relation to birch pollen counts: correlations with nasal sensitivity, prick tests and RAST. *Clin Allergy* 1978;8:387–396.

38. Rak S, Lowhagen O, Venge P. The effect of immunotherapy on bronchial hyperresponsiveness and eosinophilic cationic protein in pollen-allergic patients. *J Allergy Clin Immunol* 1988;82: 470–480.

39. Rak S, Hakanson L, Venge P. Immunotherapy abrogates the generation of eosinophil and neutrophil chemotactic activity during pollen season. *J Allergy Clin Immunol* 1990;86:706–713.

40. Bertelsen A, Andersen JB, Christensen J, et al. Immunotherapy with dog and cat extracts in children. *Allergy* 1989;44:330–335.

41. Creticos PS, Norman PS. Immunotherapy with allergens. *JAMA* 1987;258:2874–2880.

42. Dykewicz MS. Allergen immunotherapy for the patient with asthma. *Immunol Allergy Clin North Am* 1992;12:125–144.

43. Chapman MD, Platts-Mills TA, Gabriel M, et al. Antibody response following prolonged hyposensitization with *Dermatophagoides pteronyssinus* extract. *Int Arch Allergy Appl Immunol* 1980;61:431–440.

44. Ewan PW, Alexander MM, Snape C, et al. Effective hyposensitization in allergic rhinitis using a potent partially purified extract of house dust mite. *Clin Allergy* 1988;18:501–508.

45. McHugh SM, Lavelle B, Kemeny DM, et al. A placebo-controlled trial of immunotherapy with two extracts of *Dermatophagoides pteronyssinus* in allergic rhinitis, comparing clinical outcome with changes in antigen-specific IgE, IgG, and IgG subclasses. *J Allergy Clin Immunol* 1990;86:521–531.

46. Corrado OJ, Pastorello E, Ollier S, et al. A double-blind study of hyposensitization with an alginate conjugated extract of *D. pteronyssinus* (Conjuvac) in patients with perennial rhinitis: 1. clinical aspects. *Allergy* 1989;44:108–115.

47. Creticos PS, Reed CE, Norman PS, et al. Ragweed immunotherapy in adult asthma. *N Engl J Med* 1996;334:501–506.

48. Krouse JH, Krouse HJ. Efficacy of immunotherapy based on

skin end-point titration. *Otolaryngol Head Neck Surg* 2000;123: 183–187.

49. Creticos PS. Immunotherapy. In: Kaplan AP, et al., eds. *Allergy*, 2nd ed. Philadelphia: WB Saunders, 1997:726–739.

50. Tamir R, Castracane JM, Rocklin RE. Generation of suppressor cells in atopic patients during immunotherapy that modulate IgE synthesis. *J Allergy Clin Immunol* 1987;79:591–598.

51. Fadal RG. Experience with RAST-based immunotherapy. *Otolaryngol Clin North Am* 1992;25:43–60.

52. Rocklin RE, Sheffer AL, Greineder DK, et al. Generation of antigen-specific suppressor cells during allergy desensitization. *N Engl J Med* 1980;302:1213–1219.

53. Hsieh KH. Decreased production of cd8 (t8) antigen after immunotherapy. *J Clin Immunol* 1989;9:111–118.

54. Pastorello EA, Incorvaia C, Zanussi C. Specific immunotherapy: clinical efficacy and mechanisms of action. *Pharmacol Res* 1992;26[Suppl 2]:46–47.

55. Santrach PJ, Parker JL, Jones RT, et al. Diagnostic and therapeutic applications of a modified radioallergosorbent test and comparison with the conventional radioallergosorbent test. *J Allergy Clin Immunol* 1981;67:97–104.

56. Horst M, Hejjaoui A, Horst V, et al. Double-blind, placebo-controlled, rush immunotherapy with a standardized *Alternaria* extract. *J Allergy Clin Immunol* 1990;85:460–472.

57. Platts-Mills TAE, Von Maur RK, Ishizaka K, et al. IgA and IgG anti-ragweed antibodies in nasal secretions—quantitative measurements of antibodies in nasal secretions—quantitative measurements of antibodies and correlation with inhibition of histamine release. *J Clin Invest* 1976;57:1041–1050.

58. Van Metre TE, Adkinson NF Jr, Amodio FJ, et al. A comparison of immunotherapy schedules for injection treatment of ragweed pollen hay fever. *J Allergy Clin Immunol* 1982;69:181–193.

59. Lowenstein H, Graff-Lonnevig V, Hedlin G, et al. Immunotherapy with cat- and dog-dander extracts. *J Allergy Clin Immunol* 1986;77:497–505.

60. Muller UR, Morris T, Bischof M, et al. Combined active and passive immunotherapy in honeybee-sting allergy. *J Allergy Clin Immunol* 1986;78:115–122.

61. Lichtenstein LM, Holtzman NA, Burnett LS. A quantitative in vitro study of the chromatographic distribution of immunoglobulin characteristics of human blocking antibody. *J Immunol* 1968;101:317–324.

62. Nakagawa T. The Role of IgG subclass antibodies in response to house dust mite immunotherapy. *N Engl Reg Allergy Proc* 1987;8:423–428.

63. Creticos P, Reed CE, Norman PS, et al. The NIAID cooperative study of the role of immunotherapy in seasonal ragweed-induced adult asthma: 3rd year clinical endpoints: cost effectiveness. *J Allergy Clin Immunol* 1993;91:226(abst.).

64. Golden DB, Addison BI, Gadde J, et al. Prospective observations on stopping prolonged venom immunotherapy. *J Allergy Clin Immunol* 1989;84:162–167.

65. Sadan N, Rhyne MB, Mellits ED, et al. Immunotherapy of pollenosis in children: investigation of immunotherapy of pollenosis in children: investigation of immunologic basis of clinical improvement. *N Engl J Med* 1969;280:623–627.

66. Lichtenstein LM, Norman PS, Winkenwerder WL. A single year immunotherapy for ragweed hay fever: immunologic and clinical studies. *Ann Intern Med* 1971;75:663–671.

67. Peng Z, Naclerio RM, Norman PS, et al. Quantitative IgA and IgG subclass responses during and after long-term ragweed immunotherapy. *J Allergy Clin Immunol* 1992;89:519–529.

68. Creticos PS, VanMetre TE, Mardiney MR, et al. Dose response of IgE and IgG antibodies during ragweed immunotherapy. *J Allergy Clin Immunol* 1984;73:94–104.

69. Nalebuff DJ. In vitro-based allergen immunotherapy. In:

Krause HF, ed. *Otolaryngic allergy and immunology.* Philadelphia: WB Saunders, 1989:163–168.

70. Taylor CR. Immunoperoxidase techniques: practical and theoretical aspects. *Arch Pathol Lab Med* 1978;102:113–121.

71. Lichtenstein LM, Ishizaka K, Norman PS, et al. IgE antibody measurements in ragweed hay fever: relationship to clinical severity and the results of immunotherapy. *J Clin Invest* 1973;52:472–482.

72. Yunginger JW, Gleich GJ. Seasonal changes in serum and nasal IgE concentrations. *J Allergy Clin Immunol* 1973;51:174–186.

73. Creticos PS, Marsh DG, Proud D, et al. Responses to ragweed-pollen nasal challenge before and after immunotherapy. *J Allergy Clin Immunol* 1989;84:197–205.

74. Sparholt SH, Olsen OT, Schou C. The allergen specific B-cell response during immunotherapy. *Clin Exp Allergy* 1992;22:648–653.

75. Lichtenstein LM, Norman PS, Winkenwerder WL. Clinical and in vitro studies on the role of immunotherapy in ragweed hay fever. *Am J Med* 1968;44:514–524.

76. Lichtenstein LM, Norman PS, Winkenwerder WL. Antibody response following immunotherapy in ragweed hay fever: Allpyral vs. whole ragweed extract. *J Allergy* 1968;41:49–57.

77. Lichtenstein LM, Osler AG. Studies on the mechanism of hypersensitivity phenomena: IX. histamine release from human leukocytes by ragweed pollen antigen. *J Exp Med* 1964;120:507–530.

78. Brunet C, Bedard PM, Lavoie A, et al. Allergic rhinitis to ragweed pollen: I. reassessment of the effects of immunotherapy on cellular and hormonal responses. *J Allergy Clin Immunol* 1992;89:87–94.

79. Iliopoulos OD, Proud D, Adkinson NF Jr, et al. Effects of immunotherapy on the early late and rechallenge nasal reaction to provocation with allergen: changes in inflammatory mediators and cells. *J Allergy Clin Immunol* 1991;87:855–866.

80. Pienkowski MD, Norman PS, Lichtenstein LM. Suppression of late-phase skin reactions by immunotherapy with ragweed extract. *J Allergy Clin Immunol* 1985;76:729–734.

81. Mendoza GR, Minagawa K. Subthreshold and suboptimal desensitization of human basophils: I. kinetics of decay of releasability. *Int Arch Allergy Appl Immunol* 1982;61:101–107.

82. Van Metre TE, Adkinson NF Jr, Kagey-Sobotka A, et al. Immunotherapy decreases skin sensitivity to ragweed extract: demonstration by midpoint skin test titration. *J Allergy Clin Immunol* 1990;86:587–588.

83. Van Metre TE, Adkinson NF Jr, Kagey-Sobotka A, et al. How should we use skin testing to quantify IgE sensitivity? *J Allergy Clin Immunol* 1990;86:583–586.

84. Fadal RG, Nalebuff DJ, Ali M. The allergy problem. In: Spencer J, ed. *Allergy problems: current therapy.* Miami: Meded Publishers, 1981:13–59.

85. Price JF, Warner JO, Hey EN, et al. A controlled trial of hyposensitization with tyrosine adsorbed *Dermatophagoides pteronyssinus* antigen in childhood asthma: in vivo aspects. *Clin Allergy* 1984;14:209–219.

86. Naclerio RM, Kagey-Sobotka A, Lichtenstein LM, et al. Observations on nasal late phase reactions. *Immunol Invest* 1987–88;16:649–685.

87. Furin MJ, Norman PS, Creticos PS, et al. Immunotherapy decreases antigen-induced eosinophil migration into the nasal cavity. *J Allergy Clin Immunol* 1991;88:27–32.

88. Norman PS. Immunotherapy of IgE-mediated disease. *Hosp Pract* 1990;25:81–92.

89. Lockey RF, Benedict LM, Turkeltaub PC, et al. Fatalities from immunotherapy (IT) and skin testing (ST). *J Allergy Clin Immunol* 1987;79:660–677.

90. Gerrard JW. The biological importance of IgE. *Immunol Allergy Pract* 1984;6:381–385.

91. Fadal RG. Immunotherapy failure. *Otolaryngol Clin North Am* 1985;18:805–819.

92. Fadal RG. Immunotherapy failure. In: Fadal RG, Nalebuff DJ, eds. *RAST in clinical allergy.* Carlsbad, CA: Symposia Foundation, 1989:273–291.

93. Fadal RG, Nalebuff DJ, Ali M. An overview of immunotherapy. In: Fadal RG, Nalebuff DJ, eds. *RAST in clinical allergy.* Carlsbad, CA: Symposia Foundation, 1989:195–205.

94. Fadal RG, Nalebuff DJ, Ali M. RAST-based immunotherapy: a new and improved approach for effective allergen-specific treatment. In: Fadal RG, Nalebuff DJ, eds. *RAST in clinical allergy.* Carlsbad, CA: Symposia Specialists, 1989:247–253.

95. Johnstone DE. The case for hyposensitization: its rationale and justification. *Pediatr Clin North Am* 1975;22:239–249.

96. Bousquet J, Michel FB. Specific immunotherapy in asthma. *Allergy Proc* 1994;15:329–333.

97. Bush RK. Fungal extracts in clinical practice. *Allergy Proc* 1993;14:385–390.

98. Bush RK, Huftel MA, Busse WW. Patient selection. In: Lockey RF, Bukantz SC, eds. *Allergen immunotherapy.* New York: Marcel Dekker, 1991:25–50.

99. Reid MJ, Lockey RF, Turkeltaub PC, et al. Survey of fatalities from skin testing and immunotherapy 1985–1989. *J Allergy Clin Immunol* 1993;92:6–15.

100. Stewart GE, Lockey RF. Systemic reactions from allergen immunotherapy. *J Allergy Clin Immunol* 1992;90:567–578.

101. Bousquet J, Michel FB. Specific immunotherapy in asthma: is it effective? *J Allergy Clin Immunol* 1994;94:1–11.

102. Kaplan AP, Anderson JA, Valentine MD, et al. Beta-adrenergic blockers, immunotherapy, and skin testing. *J Allergy Clin Immunol* 1989;84:129–130.

103. Gordon BR. Prevention and management of office allergy emergencies. *Otolaryngol Clin North Am* 1992;25:119–134.

104. Toogood JH. Risk of anaphylaxis in patients receiving beta-blocker drugs. *J Allergy Clin Immunol* 1988;81:1–5.

105. Metzger WJ, Turner E, Patterson R. The safety of immunotherapy during pregnancy. *J Allergy Clin Immunol* 1978;61:268–272.

106. Tinkelman DG, Cole WQ, Tunno J. Immunotherapy: a one-year prospective study to evaluate risk factors of systemic reactions. *J Allergy Clin Immunol* 1995;95:8–14.

107. Schatz M, Hoffman CP, Zeiger RS, et al. The course and management of asthma and allergic diseases during pregnancy. In: Middleton E, Reed CE, Ellis EF, et al., eds. *Allergy: principles and practice,* 4th ed. St. Louis: Mosby, 1993:1301–1342.

108. Phanuphak P, Kohler PF. Onset of polyarteritis nodosa during allergic hyposensitization treatment. *Am J Med* 1980;68:479–485.

109. Yang WH, Dorval G, Osterland CK, et al. Circulating immune complexes during immunotherapy. *J Allergy Clin Immunol* 1979;63:300–307.

110. Katelaris CH, Walls RS. A study of possible ill effects from prolonged immunotherapy in treatment of allergic diseases. *Ann Allergy* 1984;53:257–261.

111. Wright DN, Nelson RP, Ledford DK, et al. Serum IgE and human immunodeficiency virus (HIV) infection. *J Allergy Clin Immunol* 1990;85:445–452.

112. Saxon A. AIDS: more common in allergy practice than once believed. *Respir News* 1989;9:2.

113. Mabry RL, Mabry CS. Allergic fungal sinusitis: the role of immunotherapy. *Otolaryngol Clin North Am* 2000;33:433–440.

114. Mabry RL, Marple BF, Mabry CS. Outcomes after discontinuing immunotherapy for allergic fungal sinusitis. *Otolaryngol Head Neck Surg* 2000;122:104–106.

115. Wide L, Bennich H, Johansson SGO. Diagnosis of allergy by an in vitro test for allergen antibodies. *Lancet* 1967;2:1105–1107.
116. Nalebuff DJ. In vitro testing methodologies: evolution and current status. *Otolaryngol Clin North Am* 1992;25:27–42.
117. Gordon BR. Allergy skin tests and immunotherapy: comparison of methods in common use. *Ear Nose Throat J* 1990;69:47–62.
118. AMA Council on Scientific Affairs, Panel on Allergy. In vivo diagnostic testing and immunotherapy for allergy. *JAMA* 1987; 258:1505–1508.
119. Phillips FW. Relief of hay fever by intradermal injections of pollen extract. *JAMA* 1926;86:182–184.
120. Mathews KP. Mediators of anaphylaxis, anaphylactoid reactions, and rhinitis. In: Settipane GA, ed. *Rhinitis,* 2nd ed. Providence, RI: OceanSide Publications, 1991:15–26.
121. Marsh DG, Lichtenstein LM, Norman PS. Induction of IgE-mediated immediate hypersensitivity to group I rye grass pollen allergens and allergoids in non-allergic man. *Immunology* 1972; 22:1013–1028.
122. Creticos PS. Immunotherapy with allergens. *JAMA* 1992;268: 2834–2839.
123. Lockey RF, Portnoy JM, Creticos PS. Forms use for skin testing and immunotherapy. In: Creticos PS, ed. *Immunotherapy: a practical guide to current procedures.* West Haven, CT: Miles, 1994:7–15, 49–50.
124. Fadal RG, Nalebuff DJ. Tools of the allergist: old and new. *Contin Educ Fam Physician* 1978;10:37–61.
125. Fadal RG, Nalebuff DJ, Ali M. Criticism of RAST reexamined. In: Fadal RG, Nalebuff DJ, eds. *RAST in clinical allergy.* Carlsbad, CA: Symposia Foundation, 1989:321–339.
126. Bierman CW, Pearlman DS, Berman BA. Injection therapy for allergic diseases. In: Bierman CW, Pearlman DS, ed. *Allergic diseases from infancy to adulthood.* Philadelphia: WB Saunders, 1988:279–293.
127. Frostad AB, Grimmer O, Sandvik L, et al. Clinical effects of hyposensitization using a purified preparation from timothy pollen as compared to crude aqueous extracts from timothy pollen and a four-grass pollen mixture respectively. *Clin Allergy* 1983;13:337–357.
128. Patterson R, Lieberman P, Irons JS, et al. Immunotherapy. In: Middleton E Jr, Reed CE, Ellis EF, eds. *Allergy: principles and practice,* 2nd ed. St. Louis: Mosby, 1983:1119–1142.
129. Nelson BL, Dupont LA, Reid MJ. Prospective survey of local and systemic reactions to immunotherapy with pollen extracts. *Ann Allergy* 1986;56:331–334.
130. Bernstein DI, Bernstein IL. Allergic rhinitis caused by house dust and other nonpollen allergens. In: Lichtenstein LM, Fauci AS, ed. *Current therapy in allergy, immunology, and rheumatology.* St. Louis: Mosby, 1985:8–16.
131. Grammer LC. Principles of immunologic management of allergic diseases due to extrinsic antigens. In: Patterson R, ed. *Allergic diseases diagnosis and management.* Philadelphia: JB Lippincott,1985:358–373.
132. Galant SP. Allergy shots for hay fever. *Postgrad Med* 1989;85: 203–209.
133. Barbee RA, Lebowitz MD, Thompson HC, et al. Immediate skin test reactivity in a general population sample. *Ann Intern Med* 1976;84:129–133.
134. Chipps BE, Talmo RC, Mellets DE, et al. Immediate (IgE-mediated) skin testing in the diagnosis of allergic disease. *Ann Allergy* 1978;41:211–215.
135. Fadal RG, Nalebuff DJ. RAST screening as a guide to immunotherapy: a study of 80 patients with allergic rhinitis and asthma. In: Johnson F, ed. *Allergy: including IgE in diagnosis and treatment.* Miami: Symposia Specialists, 1979:95–103.
136. Krouse HA, Klaustermeyer WB. Immediate hypersensitivity skin testing: a comparison of scratch, prick, and intradermal techniques. *Immunol Allergy Pract* 1980;2:13–20.
137. Reddy PM, Nagava H, Pascual HD, et al. Reappraisal of intracutaneous tests in the diagnosis of reaginic allergy. *J Allergy Clin Immunol* 1978;61:36–41.
138. Knicker WT. Clinical science and common sense in the diagnosis and immunotherapy of respiratory allergy. *Contin Educ Fam Physician* 1979;10:16–33.
139. Van Metre TE, Adkinson NF Jr, Lichtenstein LM, et al. A controlled study of the effectiveness of the Rinkel method of immunotherapy for ragweed pollen hay fever. *J Allergy Clin Immunol* 1980;65:288–297.
140. Lee LK, Knicker WT, Campos T. Aggressive coseasonal immunotherapy in mountain cedar pollen allergy. *Arch Otolaryngol* 1982;108:787–794.
141. Nalebuff DJ, Fadal RG. In vitro determination of initial immunotherapy dose: a new clinical application of the radioallergosorbent test. In: Johnson F, ed. *Allergy: including IgE in diagnosis and treatment.* Miami: Symposia Specialists, 1979:105–112.
142. Nalebuff DJ, Fadal RG, Ali M. Determination of initial immunotherapy dose for ragweed hypersensitivity with the modified RAST test. *Otolaryngol Head Neck Surg* 1981;89:271–274.
143. Hansel FK. *Allergy of the nose and paranasal sinuses.* St. Louis: Mosby, 1936:589–656, 739–774.
144. Furstenberg FF, Gay LN. The occurrence of constitutional reactions in the treatment of hay fever and asthma: analysis of the causative factors. *Bull Johns Hopkins Hosp* 1937;60:412–427.
145. Greene JE. Constitutional reactions in hay fever therapy. *Med Clin North Am* 1939;23:1255–1267.
146. Rinkel H. The management of clinical allergy: I. general considerations. *Arch Otolaryngol* 1962;76:491–508.
147. Willoughby JW. Serial dilution titration skin tests in inhalant allergy. *Otolaryngol Clin North Am* 1974;7:579–615.
148. Van Metre TE Jr, Adkinson NF Jr, Amodio FJ, et al. A comparative study of the effectiveness of the Rinkel method and the current standard method of immunotherapy for ragweed pollen hay fever. *J Allergy Clin Immunol* 1980;66:500–513.
149. Van Metre TE Jr, Adkinson NF Jr, Amodio FJ, et al. A comparison of immunotherapy schedules for injection treatment of ragweed pollen hay fever. *J Allergy Clin Immunol* 1982;69: 181–193.
150. Reisman RE. American Academy of Allergy position statement: controversial techniques. *J Allergy Clin Immunol* 1981;67: 333–338.
151. Smith MP. The use and interpretation of intradermal serial-dilution titration by general and specialized allergists. *Trans Am Soc Ophthalmol Otolaryngic Allergy* 1979;19:155–165.
152. Fadal RG, et al. Panel: RAST update. In: Spencer JT, ed. *Allergy: immunologic and management considerations.* Miami: Meded Publishers, 1982:59–68.
153. Yunginger JW, Gleich GJ. The impact of the discovery of IgE on the practice of allergy. *Pediatr Clin North Am* 1975;22:3–15.
154. Hoffman DR. Comparison of methods of performing the radio-allergosorbent test: Phadebas, Fadal-Nalebuff, and Hoffman protocols. *Ann Allergy* 1980;45:343–346.
155. Johansson SGO. The clinical significance of IgE. In: Franklin EC, et al. eds. *Clinical immunology update: reviews for physicians.* New York: Elsevier North Holland, 1981:123–145.
156. Nalebuff DJ. Predictive value of laboratory tests: diagnostic skin test and RAST models. In: Fadal RG, Nalebuff DJ, eds. *RAST in clinical allergy.* Miami: Symposia Specialists, 1989:165–179.
157. Nalebuff DJ, Fadal RG, Ali M. Development of the modified RAST. In: Fadal RG, Nalebuff DJ, eds. *RAST in clinical allergy.* Carlsbad, CA: Symposia Foundation, 1989:35–48.
158. Nalebuff DJ, Fadal RG. RAST, rhinitis, and Rinkel: epilogue. In: Johnson F, ed. *Allergy: including IgE in diagnosis and treatment.* Miami: Symposia Specialists, 1979:123–126.

159. Nalebuff DJ, Fadal RG. RAST-based immunotherapy. *Rhinology* 1984;22:11–19.

160. Nalebuff DJ, Fadal RG, Ali M. A logical approach to immunotherapy. In: Fadal RG, Nalebuff DJ, eds. *RAST in clinical allergy.* Carlsbad, CA: Symposia Foundation, 1989:207–221.

161. Ward WA. Immunotherapy dose based on skin endpoint titration. In: Mabry RL, ed. *Skin endpoint titration.* New York: Thieme Medical, 1992:39–42.

162. Hurst DS, Gordon BR, Fornadley JA, et al. Safety of home-based and office allergy immunotherapy: a multicenter prospective study *Otolaryngol Head Neck Surg* 1999;121:553–561.

163. Moyer DB, Nelson HS. Use of modified radioallergosorbent testing in determining initial immunotherapy doses. *Otolaryngol Head Neck Surg* 1985;93:335–338.

164. Freeman J. Rush inoculation. *Lancet* 1930;1:744–747.

165. Bousquet J, Braquemond P, Feinberg J, et al. Specific IgE response before and after rush immunotherapy with a standardized allergen or allergoid in grass pollen allergy. *Ann Allergy* 1986;56:456–459.

166. Stevens WJ, Verhelst JA, van den Bogaret W, et al. Clinical and biological evaluation of a semi-rush and ordinary immunotherapy schemes in type I allergic respiratory diseases. *Allergy* 1985;40:447–452.

167. Creticos PS. Effects of immunotherapy on the mediators of the allergic response. Address presented at the American Academy of Otolaryngic Allergy Advanced Course in Otolaryngic Allergy and Immunology, May 19, 1989, Baltimore, MD.

168. Creticos PS. Immunotherapy in asthma. *J Allergy Clin Immunol* 1989;83:554–562.

169. Lewis T, Grant RT. Vascular reactions of the skin to injury. *Heart* 1926;13:219–225.

170. Duke WW. *Allergy, asthma, hay fever, urticaria and allied manifestations of reaction.* St. Louis: CV Mosby, 1926.

171. Vaughan WT. Specific treatment of hay fever during the attack. *JAMA* 1923;80:245–246.

172. Anderson JM. Small dosage treatment for hay fever. *J Allergy* 1932;3:306–309.

173. Anderson JM. A new method of preparation of pollen extracts. *J Allergy* 1935;6:244–246.

174. Vaughan WT. An improved coseasonal therapy. *J Allergy* 1932;3:542–547.

175. Hansel FK. Coseasonal intracutaneous treatment of hay fever. *J Allergy* 1941;12:457–469.

176. Shambaugh GE. History of otolaryngologic regional allergy. *Otolaryngol Clin North Am* 1974;7:569–577.

177. Rinkel HJ. The management of clinical allergy part II: etiologic factors in skin titration. *Arch Otolaryngol* 1963;77:42–75.

178. Boris M, Schiff M, Weindorf S. Injection of low-dose antigen attenuates the response to subsequent bronchoprovocative challenge. *Otolaryngol Head Neck Surg* 1988;98:539–545.

179. Astarita C, Scala G, Sproviero S, et al. Effects of enzyme-potentiated desensitization in the treatment of pollinosis: a double-blind placebo-controlled trial. *J Investig Allergol Clin Immunol* 1996;6:248–255.

180. Creticos PS, Adkinson NF Jr, Kagey-Sobotka A, et al. Nasal challenge with ragweed pollen in hay fever patients. *J Clin Invest* 1985;76:2247–2253.

181. Creticos PS. Immunotherapy with allergens. *JAMA* 1992;268:2834–2839.

182. Turkeltaub PC, Campbell G, Mosimann JE. Comparative safety and efficacy of short ragweed extracts differing in potency and composition in the treatment of fall hay fever: use of allergenically bioequivalent doses by parallel line bioassay to evaluate comparative safety and efficacy. *Allergy* 1990;45:528–546.

183. Haugaard L, Dahl R, Jacobsen L. A controlled dose-response study of immunotherapy with standardized, partially purified extract of house dust mite: clinical efficacy and side effects. *J Allergy Clin Immunol* 1993;91:709–722.

184. Olsen OT, Larsen KR, Jacobsan L, et al. A 1-year, placebo-controlled, double-blind house-dust-mite immunotherapy study in asthmatic adults. *Allergy* 1997;52:853–859.

185. Alvarez-Cuesta E, Cuesta-Herranz J, Puyana-Ruiz J, et al. Monoclonal antibody-standardized cat extract immunotherapy: risk-benefit effects from a double-blind placebo study. *J Allergy Clin Immunol* 1994;93:556–566.

186. Van Metre TE Jr, Marsh DG, Adkinson NF Jr, et al. Immunotherapy for cat asthma. *J Allergy Clin Immunol* 1988;82:1055–1068.

187. Dolz I, Martinez-Cocera C, Bartolome JM, et al. A double-blind, placebo-controlled study of immunotherapy with grass-pollen extract Alutard SQ during a 3-year period with initial rush immunotherapy. *Allergy* 1996;51:489–500.

188. Johnstone DE. Study of the role of antigen dose in the treatment of pollenosis and pollen asthma. *Am J Dis Child* 1957;94:1–5.

189. Norman PS, Winkenwerder WL, Lichtenstein LM. Maintenance immunotherapy in ragweed hay fever: booster injections at six week intervals. *J Allergy* 1971;47:273–282.

190. Naclerio RM, Proud D, Moylan B, et al. A double-blind study of the discontinuation of ragweed immunotherapy. *J Allergy Clin Immunol* 1997;100:293–300.

191. Ward WA Jr. Skin endpoint immunotherapy. In: Krause HF, ed. *Otolaryngic allergy and immunology.* Philadelphia: WB Saunders, 1989:155–162.

192. Ohman JL, Findlay SR, Leiterman KM. Immunotherapy in cat-induced asthma: double-blind trial with evaluation of in vivo and in vitro responses. *J Allergy Clin Immunol* 1984;74:230–239.

193. Sundin B, Lilja G, Graff-Lonnevig V, et al. Immunotherapy with partially purified and standardized animal dander extracts: I. clinical results from a double-blind study on patients with animal dander asthma. *J Allergy Clin Immunol* 1986;77:478–487.

194. Taylor B, Sanders SS, Norman AP. A double-blind controlled trial of house mite fortified house dust vaccine in childhood asthma. *Clin Allergy* 1974;4:35–40.

195. Nelson HS. The use of standardized extracts in allergy immunotherapy. *J Allergy Clin Immunol* 2000;106:41–45.

196. Weber RW. Allergen immunotherapy and standardization and stability of allergen extracts. *J Allergy Clin Immunol* 1989;84:1093–1096.

197. Reed CE, Yunginger JW, Evans R. Quality assurance and standardization of allergy extracts in allergy practice. *J Allergy Clin Immunol* 1989;84:4–8.

198. Franklin W, Lowell FC. Comparison of two doses of ragweed extract in the treatment of pollenosis. *JAMA* 1967;201:915–917.

199. Bruce CA, Norman PS, Rosenthal RR, et al. The role of ragweed pollen in autumnal asthma. *J Allergy Clin Immunol* 1977;59:449–459.

200. Grammer LC, Shaughnessy MA, Patterson R. Administration of allergen extracts. In: Lockey RF, Bukantz SC, eds. *Allergen immunotherapy.* New York: Marcel Dekker, 1991:191–207.

201. Keenan JP. Management of problems and immunotherapy failures. In: Krause HF, ed. *Otolaryngic allergy and immunology.* Philadelphia: WB Saunders, 1989:209–214.

202. Norman PS, Winkenwerder WL, Lichtenstein L. Immunotherapy of hay fever with ragweed antigen E: comparisons with whole pollen extract and placebos. *J Allergy* 1968;42:93–108.

203. Norman PS. An overview of immunotherapy: implications for the future. *J Allergy Clin Immunol* 1980;65:87–96.

204. Norman PS. Specific therapy in allergy: pro (with reservations). *Med Clin North Am* 1974;58:111–125.

205. Norman PS, Winkenwerder WL, Lichenstein LM. Trials of alum-precipitated pollen extracts in the treatment of hay fever. *J Allergy Clin Immunol* 1972;50:31–44.

206. Norman PS, Lichtenstein LM, Marsh DG. Studies on allergoids from naturally occurring allergens: IV. efficacy and safety of long-term allergoid treatment of ragweed hay fever. *J Allergy Clin Immunol* 1981;68:460–470.

207. Norman PS, Lichtenstein LM, Kagey-Sobotka A, et al. Controlled evaluation of allergoid in the immunotherapy of ragweed hay fever. *J Allergy Clin Immunol* 1982;70:248–260.

208. Norman PS. A rational approach to desensitization. *J Allergy* 1969;44:129–145.

209. Norman PS, Lichtenstein LM. The clinical and immunologic specificity of immunotherapy. *J Allergy Clin Immunol* 1978;61: 370–377.

210. Gordon BR. Solving problems with escalation immunotherapy. AAOA Advanced Course Manual. Washington, DC: American Academy of Otolaryngic Allergy, 1996.

211. Hejjaoui A, Dhivert H, Michel FB, et al. Immunotherapy with a standardized *Dermatophagoides pteronyssinus* extract: IV. systemic reactions according to the immunotherapy schedule. *J Allergy Clin Immunol* 1990;85:473–479.

212. Portnoy J, Bagstad K, Kanarek H, et al. Premedication reduces the incidence of systemic reactions during inhalant rush immunotherapy with mixtures of allergenic extracts. *Ann Allergy* 1994; 73:409–418.

213. Nielsen L, Johnsen CR, Mosbech H, et al. Antihistamine premedication in specific cluster immunotherapy: a double-blind, placebo-controlled study. *J Allergy Clin Immunol* 1996;97: 1207–1213.

214. Bagarozzi DA, Travis J. Ragweed pollen proteolytic enzymes: possible roles in allergies and asthma. *Phytochemistry* 1998;47: 593–598.

215. John RJ, Rusznak C, Ramjee M, et al. Functional effects of the inhibition of the cysteine protease activity of the major house dust mite allergen Der p 1 by a novel peptide-based inhibitor. *Clin Exp Allergy* 2000;30:784–793.

216. Monod M, Jaton-Ogay K, Reichard U. *Aspergillus fumigatus*-secreted proteases as antigenic molecules and virulence factors. *Contrib Microbiol* 1999;2:182–192.

217. Rosenbaum MR, Esch RE, Schwartzman RM. Effects of mold proteases on the biological activity of allergenic pollen extracts. *Am J Vet Res* 1996;57:1447–1452.

218. Esch RE. Role of proteases on the stability of allergenic extracts. *Arb Paul Ehrlich Inst Bundesamt Sera Impfstoffe Frankf A M* 1992;85:171–177; discussion 177–179.

219. Sherman WB, Hebald S. A method of determining the probability of constitutional reactions during treatment of the ragweed hay fever patient. *Am J Med Sci* 1942;203:383–388.

220. Trevino RJ. IgG levels after treatment with antigen vials based on the scratch testing, intradermal testing, modified RAST testing. *Otolaryngol Head Neck Surg* 1986;95:307–311.

221. Greineder DK. Risk management in allergen immunotherapy. *J Allergy Clin Immunol* 1996;98:S330–S334.

222. VanArsdel PP Jr, Sherman WB. The risk of inducing constitutional reactions in allergic patients. *J Allergy* 1957;28:251–261.

223. Committee on Safety of Medicines. CSM update: desensitizing vaccines. *BMJ* 1986;293:948.

224. Davis WE, Cook PR, McKinsey JP, et al. Anaphylaxis in immunotherapy. *Otolaryngol Head Neck Surg* 1992;107:78–83.

225. Cook PR, Bryant JL, Davis WE, et al. Systemic reactions to immunotherapy: the American Academy of Otolaryngic Allergy Morbidity and Mortality Survey. *Otolaryngol Head Neck Surg* 1994;110:487–493.

226. Turkeltaub PC. Deaths associated with allergenic extracts. *FDA Med Bull* 1994;24(May):7.

227. Reid MJ, Lockey RF, Turkeltaub PC. Fatalities from immunotherapy. *J Allergy Clin Immunol* 1992;89:350(abstr).

228. Anon JB. Introduction to in vivo allergy testing. *Otolaryngol Head Neck Surg* 1993;109:593–600.

229. Vervloet D, Khairallah E, Arnaud A, et al. A prospective national study of the safety of immunotherapy. *Clin Allergy* 1980;10: 59–64.

230. Gibofsky A. Legal issues in allergy and clinical immunology. *J Allergy Clin Immunol* 1996;98:S334–S338.

231. Bosquet J, Michel FB. Safety considerations in assessing the role of immunotherapy in allergic disorders. *Drug Safety* 1994;10: 5–17.

232. Norman PS. Editorial: safety of allergen immunotherapy. *J Allergy Clin Immunol* 1989;84:438–439.

233. Greenberg MA, Kaufman CR, Gonzalez GE, et al. Late and immediate systemic allergic reactions to inhalant allergen immunotherapy. *J Allergy Clin Immunol* 1986;77:865–870.

234. Greenberg MA, Gonzalez GE, Trusewych ZP, et al. Late systemic allergic reactions to inhalant allergen immunotherapy. *J Allergy Clin Immunol* 1988;82:287–290.

235. U.S. Food and Drug Administration. Deaths associated with allergenic extracts. *FDA Med Bull* 1994;24(May):7.

236. Craig TJ, Moeckli, Donnelly A. Noncompliance with immunotherapy secondary to adverse effects. *Ann Allergy Asthma Immunol* 1995;75:290.

237. AAAAI Board of Directors. Guidelines to minimize the risk of systemic reactions caused by immunotherapy with allergenic extracts. *J Allergy Clin Immunol* 1994;93:811–812.

238. Falliers CJ. At-home administration of allergenic extracts. *J Allergy Clin Immunol* 1995;95:1061.

239. Wells JH. Home allergenic extract administration. *J Allergy Clin Immunol* 1995;95:1061–1063.

240. Wantke F, Gotz M, Jarisch R. Spontaneous histamine release in whole blood in patients before and after 4 months of specific immunotherapy. *Clin Exp Allergy* 1993;23:992–995.

241. Varney VA, Edwards J, Tabbah K, et al. Clinical efficacy of specific immunotherapy to cat dander: a double-blind placebo-controlled trial. *Clin Exp Allergy* 1997;27:860–867.

242. Derebery MJ, Berliner KI. Allergy and health-related quality of life. *Otolaryngol Head Neck Surg* 2000;123:393–399.

243. Ohashi Y, Nakai Y, Tanaka A, et al. A comparative study of the clinical efficacy of immunotherapy and conventional pharmacological treatment for patients with perennial allergic rhinitis. *Acta Otolaryngol* 1998;538[Suppl]:102–112.

244. Derebery MJ. Allergic management of Meniere's disease: an outcome study. *Otolaryngol Head Neck Surg* 2000;122: 174–182.

245. Ebner C, Kraft D, Ebner H. Booster immunotherapy (BIT). *Allergy* 1994;49:38–42.

246. Mosbech H, Osterballe O. Does the effect of immunotherapy last after termination of treatment? *Allergy* 1988;43:523–529.

247. Walker SM, Varney VA, Gaga M, et al. Grass pollen immunotherapy: efficacy and safety during a 4-year follow-up study. *Allergy* 1995;50:405–413.

248. Jacobsen L, Nuchel Petersen B, et al. Immunotherapy with partially purified and standardized tree pollen extracts: IV. results from long-term (6-year) follow-up. *Allergy* 1997;52: 914–920.

249. Hedlin G, Heilborn H, Lilja G, et al. Long-term follow-up of patients treated with a three-year course of cat or dog immunotherapy. *J Allergy Clin Immunol* 1995;96:879–885.

250. Durham SR, Walker SM, Varga EM, et al. Long-term clinical efficacy of grass-pollen immunotherapy. *N Engl J Med* 1999; 341:468–475.

251. Curtis HH. The immunizing cure of hay fever. *Med News* 1900; 77:16–18.

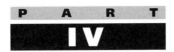
# OTOLOGIC ALLERGY

# 13

# ALLERGIC DISEASE AND THE EXTERNAL EAR

## STEVEN S. BALL
## HAROLD C. PILLSBURY III

Allergic diseases may affect the external ear. Such diseases are extremely common. In most cases, multiple skin-bearing areas of the body are affected. As a result, allergic diseases that affect the external ear are more commonly diagnosed and managed by generalists and specialists other than the otolaryngologist, such as dermatologists. However, the otolaryngologist often is consulted in cases limited to or severely affecting the external ear. The best described diseases of the external ear that have an allergic basis are atopic dermatitis and allergic contact dermatitis.

## ATOPIC DERMATITIS

The term *atopy* was coined in 1923 by Coca. Atopic diseases were later defined as noninfectious diseases, chiefly hay fever and asthma, that occurred in people who had a family history of the disease and increased serum immunoglobulin E (IgE) levels (1,2). Elevated serum IgE was presumed to be the primary immunologic abnormality of these people. Such elevated levels of IgE were later found in patients with atopic dermatitis; thus, atopic dermatitis was classified as an atopic disease (3).

Atopic dermatitis is a chronic, fluctuating disease of the skin, clinically characterized by intense pruritic lesions. It is extremely common, with a prevalence between 5% and 15% in children and 2% and 10% in adults (4,5). In 75% of cases, the onset is between 2 and 6 months of age. It may, however, start at any age. Initially, the lesions consist of intensely itchy, macular erythema and discrete or confluent papules. They may become exudative and crusted. Later, the erythema and papules tend to be replaced by lichenification. Although any skin surface may be affected, usually the disease begins on the face. At approximately 2 years of age,

the distribution of the rash frequently changes; the flexural surfaces of the neck, elbows, knees, wrists, and ankles become involved. Secondary infection with staphylococci or streptococci is common. When suprainfected, purulent exudate is not always present. Any acute vesicular eruption is suggestive of a secondary infection. Even in the absence of an infection, the skin of patients with atopic dermatitis frequently is colonized with staphylococci (6).

Atopic dermatitis commonly affects the external ear. A crusted, eczematous fissure involving the infraauricular crease is a reliable feature of atopic dermatitis in the infantile phase, when the face is most commonly involved. In addition, the tragal notch and, occasionally, the whole pinna may be affected (6).

The prognosis is variable. The severity of the disease in infancy does not correlate with the ultimate course of the disease. The prognosis is worse if both parents were at one time affected (7). In 30% to 50% of cases, asthma or allergic rhinitis develops in the patient (8,9). Finally, patients with atopic dermatitis are at greater risk from irritant contact dermatitis and less risk from allergic contact dermatitis (10).

The etiology of atopic dermatitis has been rigorously investigated and, to this date, is intensely debated. Early studies uncovered a family history in most cases. Indeed, a family history is obtained in 70% of patients with atopic dermatitis (11). Genetics is therefore presumed to play a major role in the etiology of this disease. Genetic analysis has not demonstrated simple mendelian inheritance patterns. And, although a link has been discovered between atopic respiratory diseases, such as asthma, and chromosome site 11q13, a link between atopic dermatitis and the same chromosome site has not been found. Atopic dermatitis likely is inherited polygenetically, and its expression influenced by environmental factors (12,13).

The mechanisms responsible for atopic dermatitis also have been extensively investigated. A vast number of immunologic abnormalities have been observed in these patients. However, the means by which these abnormalities interact and give rise to atopic dermatitis is as poorly understood today as it was when the disease was first recognized.

**S. S. Ball:** Division of Otolaryngology–Head and Neck Surgery, University of North Carolina, Chapel Hill, North Carolina.
**H. C. Pillsbury III:** Thomas J. Dark Distinguished Professor of Surgery, Division of Otolaryngology–Head and Neck Surgery, University of North Carolina, Chapel Hill, North Carolina.

Increased levels of total and specific IgE to antigens have long been associated with atopic dermatitis. Approximately 80% of patients with atopic dermatitis have elevated serum levels of IgE. The levels of IgE appear to correlate with the severity of the disease (14–16). Also, patients with higher levels are more likely to have increased anaphylactic sensitivity to food and inhaled allergens (17–19). Although IgE abnormalities clearly exist in patients with atopic dermatitis, IgE-mediated hypersensitivity is unlikely to be the fundamental defect responsible for the clinical findings for several reasons. First, people with atopic dermatitis may have no detectable IgE, and those without the disease may have abnormal levels. Likewise, patients with other atopic disorders may have levels of total and specific IgE similar to those in atopic dermatitis but not have skin disease. Furthermore, experimental evidence suggests that IgE-mediated allergic reactions induce transient wheal formation, not the dermatitis typical of atopic patients. Finally, allergen avoidance and desensitization rarely are helpful for the treatment of patients with atopic dermatitis. Thus, IgE abnormalities are unlikely to be the critical immunologic defect in atopic dermatitis (6).

Other immunologic abnormalities also have been identified in patients with atopic dermatitis. These patients demonstrate a lower incidence of delayed or cell-mediated immune reactions (20,21). For instance, atopic patients are harder to sensitize to dinitrochlorobenzene, a potent contact allergen in normal subjects (22,23). Such a reduction in delayed hypersensitivity response is correlated with the severity of the disease; the worse the disease, the greater the decreased responsiveness (22,23).

A number of lymphocyte abnormalities also have been noted. First, people with atopic dermatitis tend to have fewer T lymphocytes. This apparently is attributable to a lower number of CD8 cells. This reduction in CD8 cells also is responsible for an increased CD4/CD8 ratio (24–26). Other lymphocyte subpopulations, specifically natural killer cells, are also decreased in number (27,28). In addition to an absolute decrease in the number of lymphocytes, the lymphocytes may be less active; transformation tests have demonstrated decreased activity in vitro (29, 30). Furthermore, in atopic patients, CD4 cells respond to an antigen differently than in normal patients. In atopic patients, type 2 T helper (Th2) CD4 cells are preferentially stimulated; in contrast, in normal people, type 1 T helper (Th1) CD4 cells are activated to a greater degree. Activated Th2 cells synthesize interleukin-4 and interleukin-5, which stimulate B-cell proliferation and synthesis of IgE. Clearly, abnormalities in lymphocyte activation may contribute to the elevated levels of IgE found in most atopic patients (31–33). Although more and more immunologic abnormalities continue to be identified in patients with atopic dermatitis, their roles in the clinical manifestation of the disease are not well understood. The basic defects that give rise to atopic dermatitis likely have not been discovered. It is increasingly apparent that the etiology of this disease is extraordinarily complex.

The diagnosis of atopic dermatitis typically is based on a thorough history and physical examination. Measurement of serum IgE levels is not necessary. Twenty percent of patients with atopic dermatitis have normal levels, and approximately 15% of normal people have elevated levels (3). Furthermore, identification of antigen-specific IgE through in vitro testing to food or inhaled allergens is unlikely to assist in the management of the disease (34,35). Bacterial and viral cultures may be helpful during periods of exacerbation.

Other disorders may mimic atopic dermatitis of the external ear. In infancy, differentiating infantile seborrheic dermatitis from atopic dermatitis may be difficult. Early in the course of the diseases, both involve the face and, frequently, the external ear. However, seborrheic dermatitis typically appears earlier than atopic dermatitis, between 3 and 8 weeks of age, and the lesions are much less pruritic. With time, the distinction usually becomes clear. In seborrheic dermatitis, the axillae tend to be affected, unlike in atopic dermatitis, in which the proximal flexural surfaces usually are involved. Likewise, in infancy, scabies should be excluded, and, in severe cases, especially when associated with recurrent infections, immunodeficiency states should be considered. In adults, atopic dermatitis of the external ear may be confused with asteotic dermatitis, an eczematous condition associated with a decrease in skin lipids. Usually, asteotic dermatitis is seen in the elderly; atopic dermatitis rarely is seen in the elderly. Also, carcinoma of the external auditory canal, infectious otitis externa, seborrheic dermatitis, psoriasis, and contact dermatitis may mimic atopic dermatitis (6).

Topical steroids are the mainstay of treatment for atopic dermatitis. One strategy is to use a steroid strong enough to suppress the inflammation by twice-daily applications over a 1-week period. In most cases, we prescribe a medium-potency steroid such as 0.05% flurandrenolide (Cordran; Eli Lilly, Indianapolis, IN). Then, maintenance therapy should be instituted; either the frequency of application or the potency should be reduced. In children, the steroid potency should be less than in adults. In severe, recalcitrant cases, short-term oral steroids may be effective. Also, during exacerbations or overt infection, an antibiotic and steroid combination should be used. An oral antibiotic also may be beneficial (6).

Other topical medications are helpful in the management of atopic dermatitis. In general, ointments, as opposed to creams, are more effective in the treatment of chronic atopic lesions, especially lichenified lesions. However, if the lesions are exudative, creams or lotions may be more appropriate. The ointments should be applied immediately after washing to prevent drying and irritating the affected area. Because soaps may irritate the dermatitis, bathing with a dispersible bath oil, rather than soap, often is better. Moreover, a 1%

to 10% coal tar solution may be helpful as maintenance for chronic, lichenified lesions (6).

The value of allergen avoidance and desensitization for the treatment of atopic dermatitis is very limited. Based on history alone, diet may aggravate the dermatitis in approximately 10% of children, and much less in adults. However, it is controversial whether in vitro testing to specific foods and dietary manipulation is helpful in managing the disease; several studies have not shown a benefit to dietary changes, except in a few severe cases (36). A variety of inhaled irritants also have been implicated in exacerbations of atopic dermatitis. Of these, dust mites appear to be the most important (37–39). Although, in general, allergen avoidance and, even less so, desensitization are of limited benefit, in an occasional case, especially when mites are suspected, they are helpful (40,41). Oral antihistamines typically are not effective (42).

## ALLERGIC CONTACT DERMATITIS

Allergic diseases other than atopic dermatitis may affect the external ear. Allergic contact dermatitis is one example. The external ear is directly exposed to a variety of allergens on a frequent basis. Earrings, eyeglasses, and topical medications are a common source of these allergens. Typically, allergic contact dermatitis presents as a localized dermatitis at the site of contact with the allergen. The dermatitis is characterized by intensely pruritic, erythematous papules and vesicles. Frequently, the site is excoriated. Lichenification may develop later. In most cases, allergic contact dermatitis cannot be distinguished clinically from irritant contact dermatitis, the pathogenesis of which does not involve sensitization. Frequently, both types of contact dermatitis coexist (6).

The immunologic mechanisms responsible for allergic contact dermatitis are more clearly understood than for atopic dermatitis. Allergic contact dermatitis is due to a delayed or cell-mediated immune response. Critical to this response is the induction of sensitivity to the allergen. The allergen binds to major histocompatibility complex class II molecules on antigen-presenting cells in the skin. These cells travel to regional lymph nodes and stimulate the proliferation of antigen-specific Th1 CD4 lymphocytes, which disseminate throughout the body, including the skin. The person is thus sensitized to the allergen. When a sensitized person is reexposed to the allergen, the allergen binds to antigen-specific T lymphocytes in the skin. These lymphocytes trigger an inflammatory reaction. Clinically, this reaction manifests as dermatitis at the site of contact, usually 24 to 48 hours after reexposure. In addition, the allergen, after binding to antigen-presenting cells in the skin, may be carried to regional nodes and bind with antigen-specific T lymphocytes there. As a consequence, a systemic reaction may be generated (6).

Sensitization to an allergen depends on a number of factors: the susceptibility of the person to the allergen, the sensitizing properties of the allergen, the concentration of the allergen, and the frequency to which the person is exposed to the allergen (43). Why some people are more susceptible to sensitization is poorly understood. Susceptibility does not follow mendelian inheritance patterns; however, genetic factors are presumed to play a role (44). Different groups of people have different susceptibilities to sensitization. Atopic patients and blacks appear to have a lower risk for development of allergic contact dermatitis (10,45). In addition, it is difficult to predict whether a substance will induce sensitization, unless its chemical structure is similar to a known sensitizer. In general, the greater the amount of allergen to which a person is exposed and the more prolonged and frequent the contact, the greater the likelihood that sensitization will occur.

Local factors also affect the chance for development of sensitivity. Sensitization is more likely to occur if the allergen contacts damaged skin, which may enhance absorption of the allergen. Also, immune cells, previously recruited to irritated, traumatized skin, may prime the site for sensitization (6). Likewise, occlusive skin conditions promote sensitization (46). Both of these factors contribute to medication-induced contact dermatitis during the treatment of otitis externa.

Once acquired, contact sensitivity persists for variable lengths of time. Sensitivity may last for years or disappear rapidly. However, even sensitivity to weak allergens may persist if boosted by repeated exposure (47).

One of the most common allergens to cause contact dermatitis of the external ear is nickel. Ear piercing and wearing inexpensive metal earrings containing nickel are the sources of most cases of nickel contact dermatitis of the ear (48) (Fig. 13.1). Approximately 15% of those with pierced ears are estimated to have nickel sensitivity (49). Repeated exposure to jewelry that releases nickel at a rate of 0.5 $\mu g/cm^2/$ week involves a significant risk of nickel sensitization (50, 51). Nickel is the most common cause of allergic contact dermatitis in women, in large part because of ear piercing. However, even when controlled for ear piercing, nickel sensitization still is more common in women than in men (52).

Nickel dermatitis may simultaneously appear at sites of nickel contact other than the ear, such as under jean studs or bra fasteners. Less commonly, secondary eruptions on surfaces not directly associated with nickel contact, including the neck, eyelids, flexural surfaces of the arm, or anogenital areas, may develop. These reactions may occur simultaneously with, or shortly after, the dermatitis at the contact points (6).

Nickel sensitivity usually is diagnosed by a careful history. If uncertainty exists, patch testing with 5% nickel sulfate in petroleum may be performed. However, patch testing is not 100% sensitive and specific (53,54).

Because nickel is ubiquitous in the environment and repeated contact to some extent is unavoidable, sensitivity to

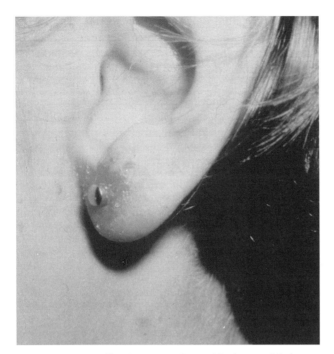

**FIG. 13.1.** Allergic contact dermatitis due to nickel.

nickel tends to persist. Sensitization to nickel should be considered a lifelong allergy. Despite persistence of the sensitivity, nickel-sensitized people usually have a good prognosis. If these people scrupulously avoid contact with nickel-containing objects, the contact dermatitis will likely clear and further outbreaks will usually be prevented (6). Most nickel-containing objects are readily apparent. If question exists, a dimethylglyoxime test can be used to detect levels of nickel capable of sensitizing a person (55).

Hand involvement, however, suggests a poor prognosis; the dermatitis may persist or relapse frequently, despite strict avoidance (6). In such cases, treatment with Antabuse (Wyeth-Ayerst, Philadelphia, PA), which chelates nickel, may be beneficial, although side effects to the medicine are common (56). Also, exposure of the oral mucosa to nickel through dental prosthetics may help desensitize these patients (57).

In addition to avoiding contact with the source of the allergy, the dermatitis should be treated acutely in a manner similar to atopic dermatitis. Irritants should be avoided. Emollients and topical steroids should be applied to moisturize and reduce inflammation. If suprainfection is suspected, topical or even oral antibiotics should be considered (6).

Metals other than nickel may cause allergic contact dermatitis of the external ear. Sensitization to cobalt, a frequent contaminant of nickel-containing objects, often occurs simultaneously with nickel sensitivity. Cobalt sensitivity may be responsible for cases in which nickel is suspected as causing the dermatitis but patch testing to nickel is negative

(58). Other metals used in earrings such as copper and chromium have been reported to trigger allergic contact dermatitis (59,60). Even gold, although less common, may cause a reaction. As a result, it is recommended that only surgical-grade stainless steel earrings be used for piercing, and gold earrings should be avoided for at least 6 weeks after piercing the ears (61).

In addition to the metals used in earrings, allergic contact dermatitis of the external ear may be caused by a number of other allergens. The external ear is exposed to allergens in spectacle frames, ear plugs, hearing aids, and earphones. Sensitizers that have been identified include epoxy and formaldehyde resins, acrylates, rubber, and plastic stabilizing compounds (62–65). These compounds are not only allergens, but irritants. In general, treatment requires topical medications, avoidance of the offending chemical, and management of aggravating factors such as acute otitis externa or canal debris (6). In cases involving hearing aids, a number of strategies are helpful to manage the dermatitis. A trend toward manufacturing silicon hearing aids containing no methacrylates has decreased the number of cases of allergic contact dermatitis due to hearing aids. However, silicon still may cause allergic contact dermatitis in a few people. Simply boiling the aid for 30 seconds to decrease its antigenicity may alleviate the problem. Another alternative is to mold the aid out of a material that is even less reactive than silicon, such as Lucite, although this material is more difficult to work with. Finally, in severe cases, coating the aid with a thin film of 14-karat gold usually resolves the problem.

Other sources of allergic contact dermatitis of the external ear exist. Topical medications frequently are used in the treatment of otitis externa and chronic otitis media. The damaged, inflamed, often occluded skin on which these medications are applied is especially susceptible to sensitization. Even weak sensitizers may cause allergic contact dermatitis when frequently applied under such circumstances (6). Sensitivity to neomycin, gentamicin, and bacitracin has been well documented (6) (Fig. 13.2). More recently, sensitivities to imidazoles (66,67) and topical steroids (68,69) have been noted. The diagnosis of medication-induced allergic contact dermatitis can be difficult, particularly when the skin on which the medication is applied is already inflamed, as in the case of otitis externa. Medication-induced allergic contact dermatitis, however, should be suspected in refractory cases of otitis externa for which a topical medication has been used frequently. Furthermore, dermatitis at sites that may have been contacted by the medication but should not be involved by the underlying condition for which the medication is being used are diagnostic clues. Examples of such sites include the concha in chronic otitis media or areas on the neck where the medication may have dripped. In difficult cases, patch testing may be beneficial. The treatment is similar to that for other cases of allergic contact dermatitis (6). In addition, patients must be warned about the potential for cross-sensitivity. Cross-reactivity has

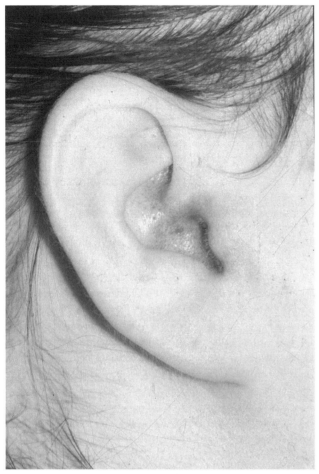

**FIG. 13.2.** Allergic contact dermatitis due to neomycin in Corti-cosporin drops (GlaxoWellcome, Research Triangle Park, NC).

Another example of an allergic disease of the external ear is the dermatophytid (id) reaction. The id reaction is an allergic skin eruption that occurs in specifically sensitized people who have a fungal infection at a site remote from that of the id reaction. The id reaction commonly affects the external ear for unknown reasons. The id reaction may present as pruritic vesicles on the external ear, or the reaction may more closely resemble the erythematous, scaling, maculopapular lesions typically associated with chronic dermatitis. Common sites of the fungal infection include the nails, skin, and vagina. The most common fungus involved is *Trichophyton.* Other types include *Candida* and *Epidermophyton* (71). According to classic descriptions of the id reaction, a positive skin test demonstrating a type I IgE-mediated reaction to fungal antigens is present, and eradication of the fungal infection results in spontaneous resolution of the id reaction (72). Although identification and treatment of the fungal infection remains the mainstay of therapy, in some instances, a clear fungal infection may not be obvious. In these patients, a yeast-free diet and desensitization with fungal extracts may be beneficial (73).

## CONCLUSION

A number of allergic diseases affect the external ear. They may affect multiple areas of the body and therefore may be managed by many physicians, including internists, pediatricians, dermatologists, and otolaryngologists. These diseases typically are diagnosed by a thorough history and physical examination. In general, they are treated with topical steroids and emollients, and, in the case of allergic contact dermatitis, the offending allergen must be avoided.

been noted to occur between the aminoglycosides, for instance (70).

## OTHER ALLERGIC DISEASES OF THE EXTERNAL EAR

Allergic diseases other than atopic dermatitis and allergic contact dermatitis may affect the external ear, and these diseases should be included in the differential diagnosis of chronic otitis externa refractory to standard therapy. For instance, a few cases of chronic otitis externa may be caused by food allergies. As previously noted, diet may exacerbate atopic dermatitis in a small percentage of patients. Also, foods have been associated with vasodilation of the auricle. Typically, this is self-limited. In addition, foods, which have been linked to all types of Gell and Coombs reactions, may potentially cause type III immune complex reactions that affect the external ear. These reactions may be diagnosed by oral challenge food tests or intradermal progressive dilutional food tests.

## REFERENCES

1. Coca AF, Cooke RA. On the classification of phenomena of hypersensitiveness. *J Immunol* 1923;8:163–182.
2. Coca AF, Grove EF. Studies in hypersensitiveness: XII. a study of the atopic reagins. *J Immunol* 1925;10:445–464.
3. Juhlin L, Johanson SGO, Bennich H, et al. Immunoglobulin E in dermatoses. *Arch Dermatol* 1969;100:12–16.
4. Diepgen TL, Fartasch M. Recent epidemiological and genetic studies in atopic dermatitis. *Acta Derm Venereol Suppl (Stockh)* 1992;176:13–18.
5. Johnson ML, Johnson KG, Engel A. Prevalence, morbidity, and cost of dermatologic diseases. *J Am Acad Dermatol* 1984;11:930–936.
6. Champion RH, Breathnach SM. *Rook/Wilson/Ebling textbook of dermatology.* Oxford: Blackwell Science, 1998.
7. Rystedt I. Prognostic factors in atopic dermatitis. *Acta Derm Venereol Suppl (Stockh)* 1985;114:87–92.
8. Quielle Roussel C, Raynaud F, Saurat HJ. A prospective computerised study of 500 cases of atopic eczema in childhood: I. initial analysis of 250 parameters. *Acta Derm Venereol Suppl (Stockh)* 1985;114:87–92.
9. Pasternak B. The prediction of asthma in infantile eczema: a statistical approach. *J Pediatr* 1965;66:164–165.

10. Cronin E, Bandmann J-J, Calnan CD, et al. Contact dermatitis in the atoptic. *Acta Derm Venereol* 1970;50:183–187.
11. Schultz-Larsen F. The epidemiology of atopic dermatitis. In: Burr ML, ed. *Epidemiology and clinical allergy.* Monographs in allergy 31. Basel: Karger, 1993:9–28.
12. Cookson WOCM, Sharp PA, Faux JA, et al. Lindage between immunoglobulin E responses, underlying asthma, rhinitis and chromosome 11q. *Lancet* 1989;1:1292–1295.
13. Coleman R, Trembath RC, Harper JI. Chromosome iiq13 atopy underlying atopic eczema. *Lancet* 1993;341:1121–1122.
14. Ohman S, Johansson SGO. Immunoglobulins in atopic dermatitis, with special reference to IgE. *Acta Derm Venereol* 1974;53:193–202.
15. Ohman S., Johansson SGO. Allergen-specific IgE in atopic dermatitis. *Acta Derm Venereol* 1974;54:283–290.
16. Jones HE, Inouye JC, McGerity JL, et al. Atopic disease and serum immunoglobulin-E. *Br J Dermatol* 1975;92:17–25.
17. Sampson HA, McCaskill CM. Food hypersensitivity and atopic dermatitis: evaluation of 113 patients. *J Pediatr* 1985;107:669–675.
18. Guillet G, Guillet M-H. Natural history of sensitizations in atopic dermatitis: a 3-year follow-up in 250 children—food allergy and high risk of respiratory symptoms. *Arch Dermatol* 1992;128:187–192.
19. Adinoff AD, Teller P, Clar RAF. Atopic dermatitis and aeroallergen contact sensitivity. *J Allergy Clin Immunol* 1988;81:736–742.
20. Raika G. *Essential aspects of atopic dermatitis.* Berlin: Springer-Verlag, 1989.
21. De Groot AC. The frequency of contact allergy in atopic patients with dermatitis. *Contact Dermatitis* 1990;22:273–277.
22. Lobitz WC, Honeyman JF, Winkler NW. Suppressed cell-mediated immunity in two adults with atopic dermatits. *Br J Dermatol* 1972;86:317–328.
23. Rogge JL, Hanifin JM. Immunodeficiencies in severe atopic dermatitis: depressed chemotaxis and lymphocyte transformation. *Arch Dermatol* 1976;112:1391–1399.
24. Braathen LR. T cell subsets in patients with mild and severe atopic dermatitis. *Acta Derm Venereol Suppl (Stockh)* 1985;114:133–136.
25. Faure MR, Nicolas JF, Thivolet J. Studies on T cell subsets in atopic dermatitis: human T cell subpopulation defined by specific monoclonal antibodies. *Clin Immunopathol* 1982;22:139–146.
26. Willemze R, De Graff-Reitsma CG, Crossen J. Characterization of T cell subpopulations in sking and peripheral blood of patients with cutaneous T cell lymphomas and benign inflammatory dermatitis. *J Invest Dermatol* 1983;80:60–66.
27. Jensen JR. Reduction of active natural killer cells in patients with atopic dermatitis estimated at single cell level. *Acta Derm Venereol Suppl (Stockh)* 1985;114:105–108.
28. Reinhold V, Wehrman W, Bauer R. Defizit natuerlicher Killerzellen (NK-zellen) im peripheral Blut bei atopishcer Dermatitis. *Hautarzt* 1986;37:438–443.
29. Leung DYM, Wood N, Dubey D, et al. Cellular basis of defective cell-mediated lympholysis in atopic dermatitis. *J Immunol* 1983;72:1482–1486.
30. Chan S, Henderson WR, Li S-H, et al. Prostaglandin E2 control of T cell cytokine production is functionally related to the reduced lymphocyte proliferation in atopic dermatitis. *J Allergy Clin Immunol* 1996;97:85–94.
31. Péne JF, Rousset F, Briére F, et al. IgE production by normal human B cells induced by alloactive T cell clones is mediated by IL-4 and suppressed by IFN-γ. *J Immunol* 1988;141:1218–1224.
32. Wierenga EA, Snoek M, de Groot C, et al. Evidence for compartmentalization of functional subsets of CD2 + T lymphocytes in atopic patients. *J Immunol* 1990;144:4651–4656.
33. Parronchi P, Macchia D, Picini MP, et al. Allergen- and bacterial antigen-specific T cell clones established from atopic donors show a different profile of cytokine production. *Proc Natl Acad Sci USA* 1991;88:4538–4542.
34. David TJ. Conventional allergy tests. *Arch Dis Child* 1991;66:281–282.
35. Pryzbilla B, Ring J. Food allergy and atopic eczema. *Semin Dermatol* 1990;9:220–225.
36. Mabin DC, Sykes AE, David TJ. Controlled trial of a few foods diet in severe atopic dermatitis. *Arch Dis Child* 1995;73:202–207.
37. August PJ. House dust mite causes atopic eczema: a preliminary study. *Br J Dermatol* 1984;111[Suppl 26]:10–11.
38. Arshad SH, Matthews S, Grant C, et al. Effect of allergen avoidance on development of allergic disorders in infancy. *Lancet* 1992;339:1493–1497.
39. Platts-Mills TAE, Mitchell EB, Rowntree S, et al. The role of house dust mite allergens in atopic dermatitis. *Clin Exp Dermatol* 1983;8:233–247.
40. Champion RH, Lachmann PJ. Specific desensitization in dermatology. In: Champion RH, ed. *Recent advances in dermatology.* Edinburgh: Churchill Livingstone, 1986:233–250.
41. Kay AB. Allergen injection immunotherapy (hyposensitization) on trial. *Clin Exp Allergy* 1989;119:591–596.
42. Healsmith M, Berth-Jones J, Graham-Brown RAC. Histamine, antihistamines, and atopic dermatitis. *J Dermatol Treat* 1991;1:325–330.
43. Friedmann PS, Moss C, Shuster S, et al. Quantitative relationships between sensitivity, dose of DNCB and reactivity in normal subjects. *Clin Exp Immunol* 1983;53:709–715.
44. Menné T, Holm V. Genetic susceptibility in human allergic sensitization. *Semin Dermatol* 1986;5:301–306.
45. Anderson KE, Maibach HI. Black and white human skin differences. *J Am Acad Dermatol* 1979;1:276–282.
46. Holmes RC, Johns AN, Wilkinson JD, et al. Medicament contact dermatitis in patients with chronic inflammatory ear disease. *J R Soc Med* 1982;75:27–30.
47. Valsecchi R, Ross A, Bigardi A, et al. The loss of contact sensitization in man. *Contact Dermatitis* 1991;24:183–186.
48. McDonagh AJF, Wright AL, Cork MJ, et al. Nickel sensitivity: the influence of ear piercing and atopy. *Br J Dermatol* 1992;126:16–18.
49. Nielsen NH, Menné T. Nickel sensitization and ear piercing in an unselected Danish population. *Contact Dermatitis* 1993;29:16–21.
50. Emmett EA, Risby TH, Jiang L, et al. Allergic contact dermatitis to nickel: the influence of ear piercing and atopy. *Br J Dermatol* 1992;126:16–18.
51. Menné T, Christophersen J, Green A. Epidemiology of nickel dermatitis. In: Maibach HI, Menné T, eds. *Nickel and the skin: immunology and toxicology.* Boca Raton, FL: CRC Press, 1989:109–115.
52. Nielsen NH, Menné T. Allergic contact sensitization in an unselected Danish population: the Glostrup Allergy Study, Denmark. *Acta Derm Venereol* 1992;72:456–460.
53. Fullerton A, Anderson JR, Hoelgaard A, et al. Permeation of nickel salts through human skin in vitro. *Contact Dermatitis* 1986;15:173–177.
54. Uehara M, Takahashi C, Ohiji S. Pustular patch test reactions in atopic dermatitis. *Arch Dermatol* 1975;111:1154–1157.
55. Menné T, Andersen KE, Kaaber K, et al. Evaluation of the dimethyl-glyoxime test for detection of nickel. *Berufsdermatosen* 1987;35:128–130.
56. Kaaber K, Menné T, Tjell JC, et al. Antabuse treatment of nickel dermatitis. Chelation—a new principle in the treatment of nickel dermatitis. *Contact Dermatitis* 1979;5:221–228.
57. Van Hoogstraten IMW, Andersen KE, Von Blomberg BME, et

al. Preliminary results of a multicentre study on the incidence of nickel allergy in relationship to previous oral and cutaneous contacts. In: Frosch P, Dooms-Goossens A, LaChapelle J-M, et al., eds. *Current topics in contact dermatitis.* Berlin: Springer-Verlag, 1989:178–183.

58. Marcussen PV. Cobalt dermatitis: clinical picture. *Acta Derm Venereol* 1963;43:231–234.
59. Karlberg AT, Boman A, Wahlberg JE. Copper—a rare sensitizer. *Contact Dermatitis* 1983;9:134–139.
60. Burrows D. The dichromate problem. *Int J Dermatol* 1984;23:215–220.
61. Fisher AA. Allergic contact dermatitis due to gold earring. *Cutis* 1990;39:473–475.
62. Fregert S, Dahlquist I, Persson K. Sensitizing capacity of substances related to epoxy resin oligomer MW340 (DCIBA). *Contact Dermatitis* 1984;10:47–48.
63. Hamply EM, Wilkinson DS. Contact dermatitis to butyl acrylate in spectacle frames. *Contact Dermatitis* 1978;4:115.
64. Logan WP, Perry HO. Contact dermatitis due to formaldehyde sensitivity. *Arch Dermatol* 1973;106:717–721.
65. Jordan WP, Dahl MV. Contact dermatitis from cellulose ester plastics. *Arch Dermatol* 1972;105:880–885.
66. Raulin C, Frosch PJ. Contact allergy to imidazole antimycotics. *Contact Dermatitis* 1998;18:76–80.
67. Jelen G, Tennstedt D. Contact dermatitis from topical imidazole antifungals: 15 new cases. *Contact Dermatitis* 1989;21:381–382.
68. Wilkinson SM. Hypersensitivity to topical corticosteroids. *Clin Exp Dermatol I* 1994;19:1–11.
69. Jagodzinski LJ, Taylor JS, Oriba H. Allergic contact dermatitis from topical corticosteroid preparations. *Am J Contact Dermatitis* 1995;6:67–74.
70. Forstrom L, Pirilä V. Cross-sensitivity within the neomycin group of antibiotics. *Contact Dermatitis* 1978;4:312.
71. Becker GD. Treatment of chronic otitis externa with *Trichophyton, Oidiomycetes, Epidermophyton* antigen. *Otolaryngol Head Neck Surg* 1980;88:293–294.
72. Rook A. Mycology: dermatophytide reactions. In: Ebeling FJG, Wilkinson DS, eds. *Textbook of dermatology.* Oxford: Davis, 1968:840–842.
73. Derebery MJ, Berliner KI. Foot and ear disease: the dermatophytid reaction in otology. *Laryngoscope* 1996;106:181–186.

# ALLERGIC DISEASE AND THE MIDDLE EAR

## JOEL M. BERNSTEIN

The role of immunoglobulin E (IgE)-mediated hypersensitivity in the development of otitis media (OM) is still controversial. Although hypersensitivity to inhalant allergens, foods, and other foreign substances in humans has been recognized for almost a century, there is considerable disagreement as to how this immunologic mechanism produces inflammation and fluid in the middle ear cleft. The middle ear cleft can be defined as the eustachian tube, middle ear, and mastoid. For purposes of this chapter, the term *allergy* is defined specifically as type I hypersensitivity—that is, the release of inflammatory mediators from mast cells or basophils secondary to specific antigen–IgE binding on the surface of these basophiloid cells and the subsequent recruitment of other inflammatory cells, collectively referred to as *allergic inflammation* (1). Although an in-depth discussion of the release of inflammatory mediators and the interaction of cytokines with both the cell surface integrins and counterreceptors on the surface of vascular endothelial cells is not provided, the reader must keep in mind that allergic inflammation consists of many diverse, sophisticated molecular biologic interactions. These molecular biologic mechanisms are just beginning to be unraveled and obviously involve both cellular surface and intracellular biochemical mechanisms, including sodium and calcium channels and secondary messengers in the cells (2).

Immunoregulation of the allergic reaction in the upper as well as lower respiratory tract is now believed to be a direct reflection of the type of T cell that dominates specific immunologic "memory": a predominantly type 2 T helper (Th2) cell–like response potentially leading to allergic reactivity, versus apparent "unresponsiveness" if the memory pool is dominated by type 1 T helper (Th1) cells (3). Under this scheme, it is envisaged that the allergy-specific immune response in atopic patients is dominated by CD4$^+$ T cells of the Th2-like phenotype, which secrete interleukin (IL)-4/IL-5, potentially driving immune responses characterized by IgE and eosinophilia (4,5). In contrast, normal subjects have predominantly antigen-specific Th1-like cells that respond to allergen by interferon-$\gamma$ secretion, which results in little other than low-grade IgG production. Accordingly, the key question in relation to the etiology of allergic respiratory diseases is, what determines whether individual allergen-specific T-cell responses are diverted toward Th1 or Th2? It is not the purpose of this chapter to discuss the immunoregulation of the allergic reaction in the respiratory tract, but to emphasize that understanding the allergic response requires evaluation of the regulatory mechanisms that are functioning in the relatively early stages of immune responses in children. In addition, in the future, this information potentially may be exploited for the development of novel immunoprophylactic strategies to prevent primary allergic sensitization in humans at a stage when allergen-specific immune responses are in theory most susceptible to regulation (i.e., during early childhood) (6).

This chapter reviews clinical and experimental evidence relating the role of IgE-mediated hypersensitivity to the development of OM and OM with effusion (OME). Other immunologic mechanisms as a cause of middle ear effusion, however, such as immune complex disease with foods, may exist and are briefly discussed in this chapter.

Most otologists would agree that the pathogenesis of OM and OME is multifactorial, with infection and eustachian tube blockage representing perhaps the best-documented primary causes (7). The factors leading to inflammation of the middle ear cleft include viral infection, allergic reactivity of the host, the overuse and inappropriate use of antibiotics for viral-like infections of the upper respiratory tract, (8) and genetic predisposition to infectious diseases secondary to poor development of various IgG subclasses and IgA in particular (9). These factors are schematically outlined in Fig. 14.1. Although this chapter deals exclusively with the role of allergy, the other predisposing factors as well as other immunologic mechanisms also must be considered to play some role in the development of inflammation of the middle ear.

Historically, the role of allergy in the development of OM had been suggested in many publications in the otolar-

**J. M. Bernstein:** Professor of Clinical Otolaryngology and Pediatrics, Department of Otolaryngology, State University of New York at Buffalo, Buffalo, New York.

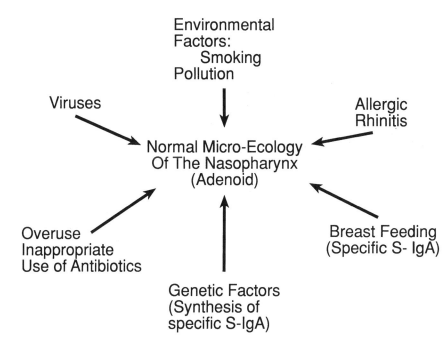

**FIG. 14.1.** Schematic diagram of the multiple variables that contribute to alteration of the normal microecology of the nasopharynx or adenoid. Viral infections and allergic rhinitis play a major role, although environmental factors such as cigarette smoking, pollution in the environment, and day care center attendance also are important. The indiscriminate and inappropriate use of antibiotics may change the normal flora, and genetic factors and breast-feeding which lead to specific secretory IgA in the nasopharynx also are important variables.

yngic literature in the 1940s and 1950s (10). These reports have been criticized because the allergic diagnoses used in these studies were based on different criteria and most reports lacked a formal and accepted definition of allergy. Furthermore, most studies reporting a good response to antiallergy therapies were not blinded or placebo controlled and failed to appreciate the consequences of the natural history of OME, which now is recognized to include a variable time course of complete resolution without therapy. At the most recent International Symposium on Otitis Media with Effusion, held in Ft. Lauderdale, Florida, in June of 1999, not one epidemiologic report from investigators throughout the world included allergy as a risk factor. It may be that clinical studies on the role of allergy in OM that have been published by well-meaning clinicians have not been acceptable to epidemiologists because they have not been carefully controlled with placebo or subjected to acceptable statistical methods.

The following questions are addressed in this chapter:

1. Is OM with effusion an allergic disease?
2. What percentage of children with OME are allergic?
3. What anatomic parts of the upper respiratory tract are involved in the allergic process and OME (e.g., nose, nasopharynx, eustachian tube, middle ear mucosa)?
4. What is the most likely pathophysiologic mechanism by which allergy affects the middle ear cleft?

## PHYSIOLOGIC DEFINITION OF THE MIDDLE EAR

Most clinicians would define the middle ear cleft on an anatomic basis, with the lateral wall as the tympanic mem-

brane and the medial wall as the basal turn of the cochlea formed by the promontory of the middle ear. The eustachian tube is located anteroinferiorly. Posteriorly, the middle ear communicates with the aditus ad antrum, and superiorly, the middle ear is associated with the attic or epitympanum. However, the physiologic definition of the middle ear is more important in terms of the role of immunologic reactivity. The middle ear is a sterile, modified gas pocket (11). It is essentially immunoincompetent in that in the normal healthy state, it possesses very few lymphocytes or other immunocompetent cells. Therefore, the middle ear can be defined as a modified physiologic sterile gas pocket maintained by bidirectional gas exchange across the middle ear mucosa, bidirectional gas exchange through the eustachian tube, and, finally, bidirectional gas exchange between the mastoid cavity and the middle ear. Although most competent clinicians consider that the middle ear is filled with atmospheric air, this concept is incorrect because the middle ear gases are similar to those of mixed venous blood, and therefore the middle ear cleft possesses significantly lower oxygen tension than atmospheric gases and a markedly higher carbon dioxide partial pressure (Fig. 14.2). Most of the gas laws can be applied to oxygen, carbon dioxide, and nitrogen, which are the major gases present in the middle ear space. Only 1 to 2 $\mu$L of gas is exchanged with each swallow (12). Thus, during a 24-hour period, if one considers somewhere between 100 and 200 swallows per day to be approximately normal, only approximately 1 to 2 mL of gas enters the middle ear with the opening of the eustachian tube. Furthermore, if the middle ear cleft and mastoid in the normal person are taken to be somewhere between 4 to 8 mL, the amount of gas entering the middle ear with each

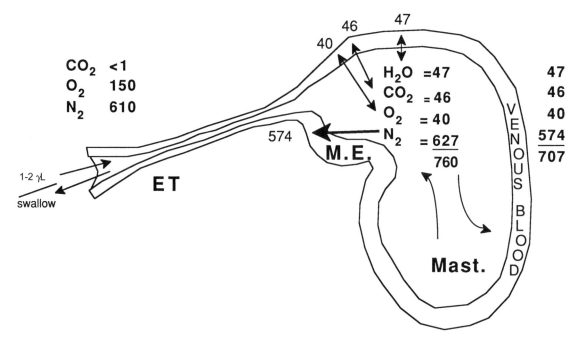

**FIG. 14.2.** Schematic diagram of the pathways of gas exchange in the middle ear cleft. The partial pressure of gases in the middle ear most resembles that of mixed venous blood. The oxygen content is much lower than that of atmospheric air, and the carbon dioxide content is much higher. There always is a slightly greater amount of nitrogen in the middle ear space. There is a constant slow movement of nitrogen from the middle ear space into the tissue surrounding the middle ear. The function of the eustachian tube is intermittently to regulate the partial pressure of gases in the middle ear to keep them at approximately atmospheric pressure. This requires primarily the introduction of nitrogen into the middle ear. Eustachian tube blockage secondary to allergic inflammation could result in underpressure of the middle ear. The mastoid also is important as a buffer. In general, the larger the mastoid cavity, the less likely it is for a child to have otitis media.

swallow is extremely small. Oxygen and carbon dioxide are quickly equilibrated between the middle ear tissue and the middle ear space, whereas nitrogen diffuses across the middle ear space much more slowly. The nitrogen content of the middle ear is higher than that of the tissue space, and therefore the ultimate movement of gas from the middle ear into the tissue involves the slow but steady migration of nitrogen molecules out of the middle ear into the surrounding tissue (7). The opening of the eustachian tube therefore plays a critical role in replenishing the middle ear space with nitrogen so that the middle ear maintains atmospheric pressure and the tympanic membrane does not collapse.

These concepts of gas exchange in the middle ear are critical to an understanding of the role of allergy in OM, because if the allergic response produces changes in eustachian tubal function as a result of edema and mucous blockage of the tube, then the eustachian tube cannot equilibrate the appropriate gas exchange to compensate for the continuous but slow removal of nitrogen from the middle ear space (7).

The problem becomes more complicated during inflammation when there is an increase in blood flow in the middle

ear mucosa. Because nitrogen also is a perfusion-related gas, inflammation results in a faster movement of nitrogen out of the middle ear space (13). The ability of the eustachian tube to equilibrate middle ear underpressure therefore is compromised in an inflamed middle ear and an underpressure develops more quickly, resulting in a fluid transudation. Thus, one of the important roles of the allergic response in OM may be the development of eustachian tubal edema with resultant blockage, thus preventing normal physiologic gas exchange between the nasopharynx and the middle ear space. The resulting underpressure and the eventual formation of a serous transudation from the middle ear mucosa into the middle ear space may be the major result of allergic rhinitis or allergic nasopharyngitis.

## POSSIBLE TARGET SITES FOR IMMUNOGLOBULIN E–MEDIATED HYPERSENSITIVITY AND OTITIS MEDIA

Figure 14.3 is a schematic diagram demonstrating four possible areas of the upper respiratory tract that may be the target sites for an allergic reaction. These include (a) the

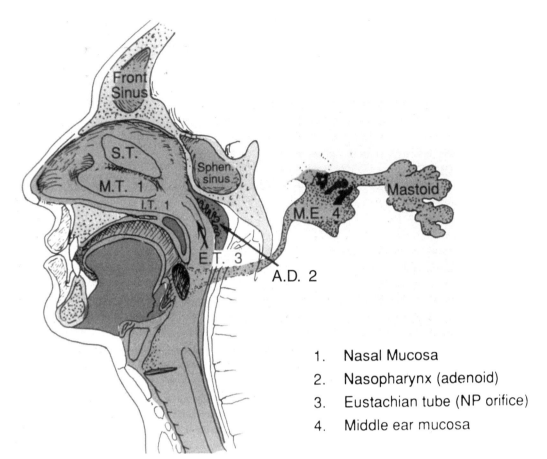

1. Nasal Mucosa
2. Nasopharynx (adenoid)
3. Eustachian tube (NP orifice)
4. Middle ear mucosa

**FIG. 14.3.** Diagram of possible targets for IgE-mediated hypersensitivity and otitis media. The four possible targets include (a) the nasal mucosa, (b) the nasopharyngeal or adenoidal mucosa, (c) the eustachian tube mucosa, and (d) the middle ear mucosa. The clinical and experimental data suggest that the nasal, nasopharyngeal, and eustachian tube mucosa are the most likely targets for allergic disease. The middle ear mucosa is the least likely site, except for the rare possibility of circulating immune complexes deposited by the bloodstream.

nasal mucosa; (b) the nasopharynx or adenoidal tissue; (c) the eustachian tube, both the nasopharyngeal orifice as well as the more distal opening into the middle ear; and (d) the middle ear mucosa itself.

## The Middle Ear Mucosa

Although a number of clinical and animal experimental investigations have suggested that the middle ear mucosa may act as a target organ for allergy, this scenario can be questioned on the basis of biomechanical constraints. Specifically, local allergic reactions require that antigen be delivered more or less continuously to the middle ear space. Low levels of antigen delivery or limited exposure times have been shown in animals to result in local, transient inflammation without the accumulation of significant effusion (14, 15). Because the eustachian tube offers the only potential pathway for antigen access to the middle ear and the tube usually is closed, with opening occurring during noninspira-

tory events such as swallowing or yawning, it is unlikely that inhalant antigens are deposited during inspiration, and it would not be expected that aerosolized antigens could reach the middle ear mucosa. Thus, there is no established vehicle for introducing antigens in any quantity or with any regularity to the middle ear space. Further, as discussed previously, nasal allergic reactions provoking tubal blockage would more completely isolate the middle ear space from the environment. Consequently, without a proven pathway for antigen delivery, the mechanism of the middle ear mucosa as a target tissue lacks sufficient foundation to be considered as playing a major role in relating allergy to OME. The studies of Hurst and Venge (16), which demonstrate eosinophilic cationic protein to be elevated in middle ear fluid, are interesting, but do not necessarily prove IgE-mediated hypersensitivity to be present in the middle ear space. The presence of eosinophils and eosinophilic mediators might suggest only that chronic inflammation is present. A similar scenario is true in nasal polyposis, where eosinophils

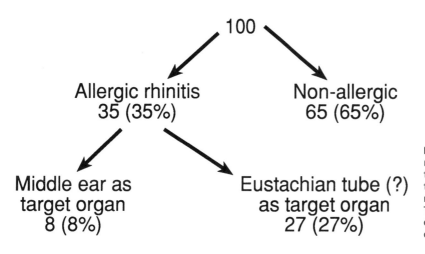

**FIG. 14.4.** Of 100 patients with persistent otitis media (requiring at least two tympanostomy tubes) followed prospectively, approximately one third or 35% had allergic rhinitis. This figure is significantly greater than in the normal population. Therefore, it is likely that nasal allergy is a significant factor in the development of otitis media or otitis media with effusion.

and inflammatory mediators from eosinophils are abundant, yet most patients with massive nasal polyposis are not allergic (17). For example, the highest numbers of eosinophils are found in the aspirin-intolerant patient. This disease is not considered to be IgE mediated, but rather a metabolic disease in which leukotriene synthesis appears to be abnormal.

In several prospective studies from our laboratory, 100 children with recurrent OME requiring at least two tympanostomies with tubes (children with more serious and more likely otitis-prone disease) were studied (18). A summary of these findings is shown in Fig. 14.4. Of 100 children with recurrent OME, approximately one third or 35% had allergic rhinitis, as established by history, physical examination, skin prick testing, radioallergosorbent testing (RAST), and family history. Of these children with allergic rhinitis, only in a very small number could the middle ear mucosa be considered a target organ. Thus, in the overall spectrum of OME, we believe the middle ear mucosa is a target organ in less than 10% of children. It is possible that circulating immune complexes with food antigen could trigger the development of middle ear effusion if they reached the middle ear mucosa from the bloodstream. This hypothesis has yet to be established.

### The Nasal Mucosa

The nasal mucosa is the most likely target organ for allergic disease in the middle ear because allergic rhinitis produces significantly increased mucus and inflammatory mediators that can be transmitted to the nasopharynx by mucociliary transport. In a study by Mogi and Suzuki (19), allergic rhinitis was found in 42% of children with OME. Furthermore, OME was found in 36% of children with allergic rhinitis, whereas in the control group, 17% had allergic rhinitis and 6% had OME. This study strongly suggests that there is a relationship between allergic rhinitis and OME. These findings indicate that the frequency of allergy in patients with OME is significantly higher than that reported in similarly aged, normal children of the general population.

Inflammatory mediators such as histamine and other products of mast cell degranulation could cause eustachian tube edema and mucus obstruction. Therefore, the nasal mucosa is a most likely target organ in the development of OME. It is even more likely that the eustachian tube mucosa itself is a major anatomic site for the development of allergic reactivity. Many studies have been conducted by both conventional and otolaryngic allergists demonstrating that nasal inhalation of allergens in the allergic patient significantly increases eustachian tube obstruction (20–24). Nevertheless, most of these elegantly performed studies, as well as some studies with extremely high doses of antigen in nasal provocation tests, have failed to produce OM or OME. Even in the natural ragweed season, our laboratory has conducted studies demonstrating a significant increase in eustachian tube obstruction (25), but few, if any of these children acquired inflammation of the middle ear or middle ear effusions during the ragweed season.

Temporal bones studied by Sadé and Luntz clearly demonstrate the middle ear mucosa to be the primary region of inflammation compared with the eustachian tube in patients with OM (26). Epidemiologic and anatomic studies therefore do not support blockage of the eustachian tube alone as a cause of OM, although prolonged blockage of this tube, as mentioned previously, may lead to underventilation of the middle ear and serous effusion. Therefore, most studies on the role of allergy and OM support the concept that the eustachian tube can be blocked as a result of allergic inflammation. The development of middle ear inflammation and middle ear effusion or OM, however, requires other factors, the most common being viral–bacterial interaction at the level of the nasopharynx, ascent of these infectious agents through the eustachian tube (most likely in the mucus blanket into the middle ear space), and the development of an infection of the middle ear space (27). As mentioned earlier, long-term eustachian tube blockage eventually leads to middle ear effusion because of abnormal gas exchange rather than because of the allergen itself reaching the middle ear mucosa as a target organ. Although it is not the purpose of this chapter to discuss the physiology of mastoid gas exchange, it should be mentioned that the smaller the mastoid, the more likely a child will have recurrent OM. One of the possible reasons for this relationship is the lack of the mastoid acting as a gas buffer to provide gas exchange into the attic and middle ear (28).

The data suggest that allergy as an immunologic mechanism is present in at least 35% to 40% of children, and that a major role for this immunologic mechanism is mechanically to block the eustachian tube. One hypothesis, then, might suggest that viral–bacterial interaction at the level of the nasopharynx is responsible for the production of acute OM, and that in most but certainly not all cases, acute OM resolves with therapeutic modalities such as antibiotics and by normal immunologic mechanisms resulting in a sterile middle ear effusion that is painless and referred to clinically as OME. Because acute challenge exposures or more chronic seasonal exposures rarely result in OM or OME, it is alternatively suggested that the tubal obstruction associated with nasal allergy is not associated with the pathogenesis of OME, but rather contributes to the persistence of the effusion. Honjo et al. (29) and Mogi et al. (30) have shown that active tubal opening promotes the clearance of fluids from the middle ear space. Thus, failure to dilate the tube promotes the persistence of middle ear effusion. This result is consistent with the epidemiologic data presented by Pukander and Karma (31). They studied 753 infants with acute OM and reported a significantly longer persistence of the effusion in those with a history of allergy compared with the nonallergic control subjects. This hypothesis is attractive, and, if supported by the results of future experiments, could well explain the observed relationship between allergy and OME.

## The Eustachian Tube

A blocked eustachian tube not only causes a significant underpressure of the middle ear due to the slow absorption of nitrogen, but impairs the inability of the inflamed middle ear to evacuate fluid. Hence, there are at least two ways in which the eustachian tube can be involved in allergy.

One mechanism is direct allergic inflammation as a result of antigen–IgE complexes on the surface of the eustachian tube mucosa with resultant edema, increased capillary permeability, increased inflammation, and influx of both acute and chronic inflammatory cells with their inflammatory mediators, producing the net result of eustachian tube edema and obstruction. Once this obstruction occurs and the middle ear is infected with bacteria or virus with the develop-

ment of middle ear effusion, the effusion cannot be relieved because of allergic inflammation of the eustachian tube.

## The Nasopharynx

Like the eustachian tube and the nasal mucosa, the mucosa of the nasopharynx, and especially the adenoid, can become involved in allergic inflammation. One mechanism for this is simply allergic inflammation, which could cause inflammation and blockage of the nasopharyngeal orifice of the eustachian tube. In those children with a genetic predisposition to IgE-mediated hypersensitivity, it is likely that the lymphocytes in the nasopharyngeal tonsil (adenoid) are programmed to produce IL-4 and IL-5. These cytokines are particularly important in the development of tissue eosinophilia or, more specifically, allergic inflammation. This inflammation would involve the nasopharyngeal area and, specifically, the nasopharyngeal orifice of the eustachian tube.

In summary, the four areas could be considered as follows. The middle ear mucosa is an unlikely site for allergic inflammation because it would be very difficult for antigen to reach the area once the eustachian tube is blocked. Furthermore, the middle ear in the normal state is an immunoincompetent tissue in which there are very few lymphocytes.

The nasal, nasopharyngeal, and eustachian tubal mucosae may all be involved in allergic inflammation as a result of specific airborne antigen reaching them. The development of allergic inflammation in any of these mucosae leads to eustachian tube blockage, edema, and inflammation. Eustachian tube inflammation results in the inability to equilibrate pressure in the middle ear, as well as the inability to clear the fluid that results from middle ear inflammation caused by bacteria or viral–bacterial interaction at the level of the middle ear mucosa.

## Viral Infection and Allergy and Their Relation to Otitis Media

The two most common respiratory viruses associated with OM are respiratory syncytial virus (RSV) and rhinovirus. These viruses may be associated with the release of histamine in the nasopharyngeal secretions as a result of their eliciting an anti-virus IgE–mediated reaction on the surface of both mast cells and epithelial cells. This interaction results in the release of mediators of allergic inflammation that in turn can elicit inflammation of the eustachian tube mucosa, and increased mucus secretion. This anti-viral IgE–mediated reaction is identical to an allergen IgE-mediated reaction in the nose or nasopharynx. Thus, it is possible that viruses associated with OM produce IgE-mediated reactivity that mimics the allergic reactivity caused by other allergens, as described previously. Virus-specific IgE also has been observed in patients infected with parainfluenza, herpes sim-

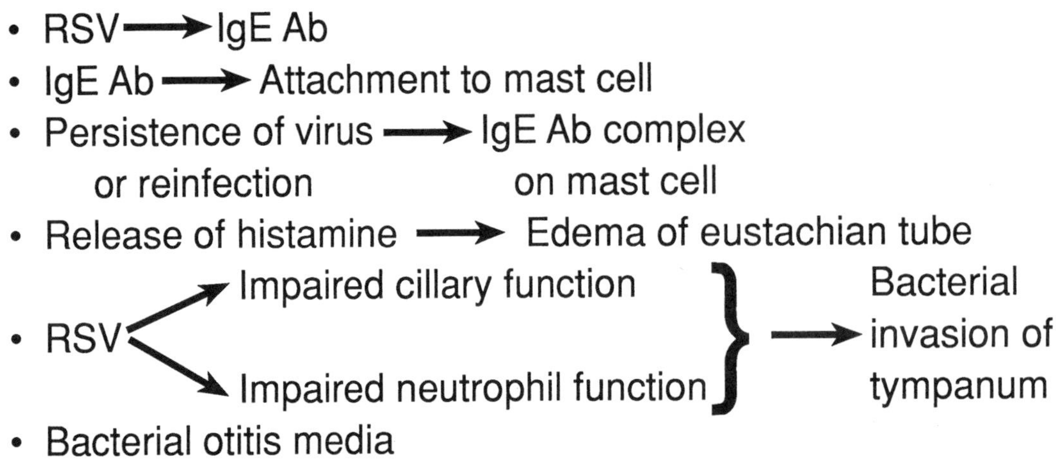

- RSV⟶IgE Ab
- IgE Ab ⟶ Attachment to mast cell
- Persistence of virus ⟶ IgE Ab complex
  or reinfection          on mast cell
- Release of histamine ⟶ Edema of eustachian tube

```
           Impaired cillary function     Bacterial
• RSV                               }  ⟶ invasion of
           Impaired neutrophil function   tympanum
```

- Bacterial otitis media

**FIG. 14.5.** Potential mechanisms of viral-induced bacterial otitis media. Respiratory syncytial virus may react with IgE on mast cells in the nasopharynx. IgE antibody complexes on the mast cell release inflammatory mediators, resulting in eustachian tube blockage. Impaired ciliary function or neutrophil function also may result from viral infection. Finally, bacterial invasion of the middle ear space leads to bacterial otitis media.

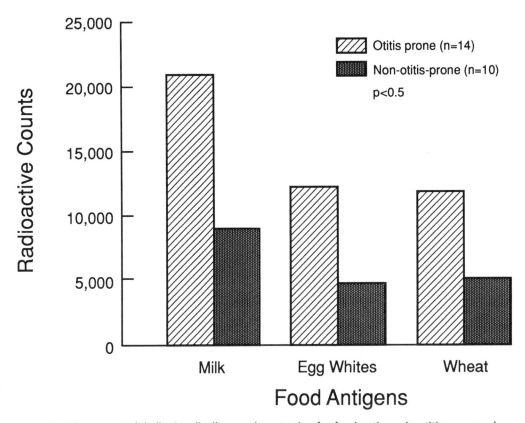

**FIG. 14.6.** Immunoglobulin G radioallergosorbent testing for food antigens in otitis-prone and non–otitis-prone children. There is an elevation of IgG to various foods in the middle ear fluid of otitis-prone children. Although there is a significant difference between the otitis-prone and non–otitis-prone children, the numbers are small and it remains to be proved that the elevation of IgG in the middle ear and serum in otitis-prone children is biologically significant as a cause of otitis media.

plex, and rubella viruses (32). Finally, leukotriene C4 (LTC4) also may be elevated as a result of viral-specific IgE reactivity in the respiratory tract of RSV-infected infants manifesting wheezing (33). These findings suggest that respiratory viral infections may be involved in the activation of mast cells during acute-phase reactions and of other effector cells during late-phase reactions in a manner similar to type I allergic reactions. Because the presence and level of LTC4 in the nasopharynx are directly related to the degree of eustachian tube obstruction in patients with allergic rhinitis (34), viral infection may contribute to the pathogenesis of OME in a manner similar to that of respiratory tract allergy. A schematic representation of the potential mechanism of virus-induced bacterial OM is outlined in Fig. 14.5.

## Possible Role of Food Allergy in Otitis Media with Effusion

There have been no studies demonstrating the presence of food immune complexes in the middle ear in both otitis-prone and non–otitis-prone children. In 1988, our laboratory studied the middle ear effusions and sera of otitis-prone and non–otitis-prone children and measured IgG–food immune complexes using milk, egg white, and wheat. We found a significantly increased amount of IgG by RAST in the otitis-prone child compared with the non–otitis-prone child (35). Whether these findings are biologically significant remains to be determined, but the data suggest that food antigen immune complexes can activate complement in the middle ear and cause inflammation. Although this is a different type of immunologic response than type I hypersensitivity, it is nevertheless a possible cause of recurrent middle ear effusion in young children. However, further studies need to be performed in this interesting area of IgG–food immune complexes to determine whether these complexes are of any clinical or biologic significance. Figure 14.6 summarizes our data.

## SUMMARY

This chapter has reviewed the possible pathophysiologic mechanisms of IgE-mediated allergy in the development of OM and OME. It is emphasized early in the chapter that the risk factors for OM are multiple and include viral infection, allergic rhinitis, eustachian tube blockage, cigarette smoking, genetic immunologic deficiencies, and day care center attendance. It is extremely disappointing that the most current epidemiologic studies, reported in 1999, do not include allergy as a risk factor, yet it is obvious to those of us who treat children with recurrent OM that allergy plays a role in as much as 40% to 50% of children. Although allergy itself may not be responsible for the development of OM or OME, it certainly contributes to it. The most likely pathophysiologic mechanisms are eustachian tube blockage

causing abnormalities of gas exchange in the middle ear cleft, or prevention of the clearance of middle ear mucus related to viral–bacterial interaction in the middle ear cleft.

Viral infection, particularly with RSV, has a predilection to produce IgE-mediated hypersensitivity and cause an allergic reaction at the level of the nasopharynx and eustachian tube. Finally, it is cautiously suggested that food antigen immune complexes could lead to middle ear inflammation in a small number of children allergic to milk, egg white, or wheat, or possibly other foods. Additional basic data are needed to develop adequately these more complex interactive models. Regardless of the theoretic mechanism, the relationship between allergy and OM will remain controversial until well controlled clinical studies are conducted documenting that, in select populations, antiallergy therapy is efficacious in preventing or limiting the duration of OME. Lacking these data, the results of the various experiments will remain an interesting set of physiologic observations without focused relevance to the pathogenesis of OME in children.

## REFERENCES

1. Ishizaka T, Ishizaka K. Biology of immunoglobulin-E: molecular basis of reaginic hypersensitivity. *Prog Allergy* 1975;19:60–72.
2. Lichtenstein LM, DeBernardo R. The immediate allergic response: in vitro action of cyclic AMP active and other drugs on the two stages of histamine release. *J Immunol* 1971;107:1131–1138.
3. Holt PG. Immunoregulation of the allergic reaction in the respiratory tract. *Eur Respir J* 1996;9:85–89.
4. Mosmann TR, Coffman RL. Th1 and Th2 cells: different patterns of lymphokine secretion lead to different functional properties. *Annu Rev Immunol* 1989;7:145–173.
5. Holt PG. Immunoprophylaxis of atopy: life at the end of the tunnel? *Immunol Today* 1994;15:484–489.
6. Hattevig G, Kjellman B, Bjorksten B. Appearance of IgE antibodies to ingested and inhaled allergens during the first 12 years of life in atopic and non-atopic children. *Pediatr Allergy Immunol* 1993;4:182–186.
7. Bernstein JM, Doyle WJ. Role of IgE-mediated hypersensitivity in otitis media with effusion: pathophysiologic considerations. *Ann Otol Rhinol Laryngol Suppl* 1994;163:15–19.
8. Bernstein JM, Reddy MS, Scannapieco FA, et al. The microbial ecology and immunology of the adenoid: implication for otitis media. *Ann NY Acad Sci* 1997;830:19–31.
9. Harabuchi Y, Faden H, Yamanaka N, et al. Nasopharyngeal colonization with non-typable *Haemophilus influenzae* and recurrent otitis media. *J Infect Dis* 1994;170:862–866.
10. Senturia BH. Symposium on prophylaxis and treatment of middle ear effusions. *Laryngoscope* 1972;82:1622–1624.
11. Doyle WJ, Seroky JT. Middle ear gas exchange in rhesus monkeys. *Ann Otol Rhinol Laryngol* 1994;103:636–645.
12. Mover-Lev H, Priner-Barenholtz R, Sadé J. Quantitative analysis of gas losses and gains in the middle ear. *Respir Physiol* 1998;114:143–151.
13. Alper CM, Doyle WJ, Seroky JT. Higher rates of pressure decrease in inflamed compared with non-inflamed middle ears. *Otolaryngol Head Neck Surg* 1999;121:98–102.
14. Miglets A. The experimental production of allergic middle ear effusions. *Laryngoscope* 1973;83:1355–1384.

15. Doyle WJ, Takahara T, Fireman P. The role of allergy in the pathogenesis of otitis media with effusion. *Arch Otolaryngol* 1985; 111:502–506.

16. Hurst DS, Venge P. Levels of eosinophil cationic protein and myeloperoxidase from chronic middle ear effusion in patients with allergy and/or acute infection. *Otolaryngol Head Neck Surg* 1996;114:531–544.

17. Hamilos DL, Leung DY, Wood R, et al. Eosinophil infiltration in non-allergic chronic hyperplastic sinusitis with nasal polyposis is associated with endothelial VCAM-1 upregulation and expression of TNF-alpha. *Am J Respir Cell Mol Biol* 1996;15:443–450.

18. Bernstein JM, Lee J, Conboy K, et al. Further observations on the role of IgE-mediated hypersensitivity in recurrent otitis media with effusion. *Otolaryngol Head Neck Surg* 1985;93:611–615.

19. Mogi G, Suzuki M. The role of IgE-mediated immunity in otitis media: fact or fiction? *Ann NY Acad Sci* 1997;830:61–69.

20. Friedman RA, Doyle WJ, Casselbrant ML, et al. Immunologic mediated eustachian tube obstruction: a double blind crossover study. *J Allergy Clin Immunol* 1983;71:442–447.

21. Ackerman M, Friedman RA, Doyle WJ, et al. Antigen-induced eustachian tube obstruction: an intranasal provocative challenge test. *J Allergy Clin Immunol* 1984;73:604–609.

22. Skoner DP, Doyle WJ, Chamovitz AH, et al. Eustachian tube function after provocative challenge with house dust mite. *Arch Otolaryngol* 1986;112:840–842.

23. Georgitis JW, Gold SM, Bernstein JM. Eustachian tube function associated with histamine-induced and ragweed-induced rhinitis. *Ann Allergy* 1988;61:234–238.

24. Toyama Y, Chiyonori I, Honda K, et al. Effective nasal allergy on eustachian tube function. In: Lim DJ, Bluestone CD, Klein JO, et al., eds. *Proceedings of the 4th International Symposium on Recent Advances in Otitis Media.* Toronto, Canada: BC Decker, 1988;69–71.

25. Osur SL, Volovitz, V, Dickson S, et al. Eustachian tube dysfunction in children with ragweed hay-fever during nature pollen exposure. *Allergy Proc* 1989;10:1333–1339.

26. Sadé J, Luntz M. Eustachian tube lumen: a comparison between normal and inflamed specimens. *Ann Otol Rhinol Laryngol* 1988; 98:630–634.

27. Miyamoto N, Bakaletz LO. Kinetics of the ascension of NTHi from the nasopharynx to the middle ear coincident with adenovirus-induced compromise in the chinchilla. *Microb Pathog* 1997; 23:119–126.

28. Elam M, Harrell M, Luntz M, et al. Middle ear pressure variations during 50% N$_2$O anesthesia as a function of mastoid pneumatization. *Am J Otol* 1998;19:709–711.

29. Honjo I, Hayashi M, Ito S, et al. Pumping and clearance function of the eustachian tube. *Am J Otolaryngol* 1985;6:241–244.

30. Mogi G, Chaen T, Tomonaga K. Influence of nasal allergic reactions on the clearance of middle ear effusion. *Arch Otolaryngol* 1990;116:331–334.

31. Pukander JS, Karma PH. Persistence of middle ear effusion and its risk factors after an acute attack of otitis media with effusion. In: Lim DJ, Bluestone CD, Klein JO, et al., eds. *Proceedings of the 4th International Symposium on Recent Advances in Otitis Media.* Toronto, Canada: BC Decker, 1988:8–11.

32. Ida S, Hooks JJ, Siraganian PP, et al. Enhancement of IgE-mediated histamine release from human basophils by viruses: role of interferon. *J Exp Med* 1977;145:892–906.

33. Volovitz B, Welliver RC, DeCastro G, et al. The release of leukotrienes in the respiratory tract during infection with respiratory syncytial virus: role in obstructive airway disease. *Pediatr Res* 1988;24:504–507.

34. Volovitz B, Osur SL, Bernstein JM, et al. Leukotriene C4 release in upper respiratory mucosa during natural exposure to ragweed in ragweed-sensitive children. *J Allergy Clin Immunol* 1988;82: 414–418.

35. Bernstein JM. Recent advances in immunological reactivity in otitis media with effusion. *J Allergy Clin Immunol* 1988;81: 1004–1009.

# 15

# ALLERGIC DISEASE AND THE INNER EAR

## M. JENNIFER DEREBERY
## KAREN I. BERLINER

Although we know that the labyrinth is not an immunoprivileged organ, and that an allergic basis for some cases of inner ear disease was proposed as early as 1893 (1), we are disadvantaged by the inability to sample for biopsy the suspected target organ of affected people to assess evidence of actual immune-mediated damage. Evidence to date is largely based on animal studies or on case histories of patients, as well as on improved outcomes after treatment for specific allergens.

It is likely that there is more to an "allergic" reaction involving the labyrinth than a classic type I hypersensitivity reaction. Autoimmune responses involving the inner ear range from the patient with Meniere's disease who has a clear seasonal component to his or her symptoms, to the patient with a true organ-specific response characteristic of autoimmune inner ear disease.

The temporal relationship between ingestion of a suspect food and the development of vertigo or hearing loss in an affected person, as well as the well documented evidence of increased circulating immune complexes in the serum of patients with Meniere's disease, all hint strongly at a type III immune complex–mediated hypersensitivity (2,3).

Failure to consider the possible spectrum of autoimmune manifestations of patients with labyrinthine symptoms attributed to allergy may result in permanent hearing loss and disabling vertigo. The clinician is advised to consider the possibility that the labyrinth itself, most probably the endolymphatic sac, is a target organ of an allergic reaction, which may respond well to allergic desensitization for inhalant allergens or dietary elimination of food allergens.

However, we do not believe that "all" autoimmune inner ear disease is allergic, but rather there is truly an organ-specific autoimmune disease involving the labyrinth, which is best treated by immunosuppressive or immunomodulating medications.

This chapter deals with common symptoms and syndromes that may be caused or influenced by an underlying allergic etiology. We use the term *allergy* here in relationship to food ingestion somewhat broadly, recognizing that immune symptoms produced by food ingestion may involve other Gell and Coombs reactions besides a classic type I reaction.

## IMMUNOLOGY

Why was the inner ear said in the past to be immunologically privileged? Many elements of the immune response of the labyrinth are similar to that of the brain, which enjoys a blood–brain barrier, contributing to the unique extracellular environment that allows neurons and other brain elements to function.

The labyrinth also exhibits a blood–labyrinthine barrier, analogous to the blood–brain barrier, which helps to maintain the ionic characteristics that are unique to the cochlear environment. In a manner similar to the brain, there is no lymphatic drainage from the inner ear. Although immunoglobulins are present in the perilymph, the amount is only 1/1,000 of that in the serum (4).

However, in many ways, the inner ear is more immunoresponsive than the brain. The inner ear demonstrates both cellular and humoral immunity, with the seat of immunoactivity in the inner ear appearing to reside in the endolymphatic sac and duct. Immunoglobulin G (IgG), IgM, and IgA, as well as secretory component, are all found in the endolymphatic sac, and numerous plasma cells and macrophages are found in the perisaccular connective tissue (5).

Far from being isolated from allergic reactions, the labyrinth has been found to have active components of allergic reactivity as well. Mast cells have been identified in the perisaccular connective tissue. After sensitization, IgE-mediated degranulation of the mast cells has resulted in eosinophilic infiltration of the perisaccular connective tissue and the clinical production of endolymphatic hydrops (6).

The endolymphatic sac has been shown to be capable

**M. J. Derebery:** House Ear Clinic and House Ear Institute, Los Angeles, California.

**K. I. Berliner:** Clinical Studies Department, House Ear Institute, Los Angeles, California.

**TABLE 15.1. INNER EAR SYMPTOMS THAT MAY HAVE AN ALLERGIC COMPONENT**

| |
|---|
| Meniere's disease |
| Vestibular hydrops |
| Cochlear hydrops |
| Dizziness |
| Tinnitus |

both of processing antigen, as well as producing its own local antibody response (7,8). Antigen and inflammatory responses are both noted to be decreased after the surgical destruction of the endolymphatic sac or the obliteration of the endolymphatic duct (8). The endolymphatic sac has a highly vascular subepithelial space containing numerous fenestrated blood vessels (9). Arterial branches of the posterior meningeal artery supply the endolymphatic sac and duct (10). Although the labyrinth is similar to the rest of the central nervous system in being protected by this blood–labyrinthine barrier, the posterior meningeal artery is fenestrated, offering a peripheral portal of circulation. In other parts of the body, fenestrated vessels supplying organs involved in absorption (e.g., kidney, choroid) are especially susceptible to damage by immune complex deposition.

From this abbreviated background of otoimmunology, we now review some specific symptom complexes in the labyrinth that may be caused or influenced by an underlying allergic reaction (Table 15.1).

## MENIERE'S DISEASE

The first published report of Meniere's disease secondary to allergy was in 1923 (11). Both inhalant and food allergies have been linked with symptoms of Meniere's disease and cochlear hydrops (12). Changes in electronystagmography and electrocochleography recordings have been noted in patients injected with food extracts during provocative food testing. (13,14). Gibbs et al. reported the production of electrocochleographic changes in patients with known inhalant allergies and Meniere's disease after nasal provocation of inhalant antigens (15).

Many of the clinical characteristics of Meniere's disease suggest an underlying autoimmune etiology. Its notorious propensity to wax and wane, becoming active again after long periods of remission, suggests an inflammatory component. It is bilateral in a significant number of cases. A delayed Meniere's-like picture may develop in a normal ear after trauma to the contralateral ear. It often is responsive—at least initially—to steroid treatment. An increased level of circulating immune complexes has been found in 96% of patients with Meniere's disease (3).

Despite the aforementioned evidence of immune activ-

ity, only 30% of patients with Meniere's disease show evidence of a true autoantibody response to specific anti-cochlear antibody by Western blot assay (16). Results of tests of abnormal cell-mediated immunity, such as the lymphocyte transfer test and the lymphocyte migration inhibition assay, either have been inconsistent or have been found to be normal even in patients with known causes of autoimmune dysfunction of the inner ear, such as Cogan's syndrome (16).

The suggestion is strong that Meniere's disease can be caused or influenced by autoimmune factors, yet the most accurate tests available to diagnose an autoimmune abnormality give normal results. However, there may be other immune-mediated causes for the development of symptoms. With an incidence of 20%, allergy is the most common "autoimmune" disease clinically. We found in a survey of 734 patients with Meniere's disease that the incidence of concurrent allergic disease is 41%, twice the incidence in the general population (17).

An elevated level of circulating immune complexes has been reported in patients with allergic rhinitis and asthma, as well as those with Meniere's disease (3,18). The tendency for allergic reactions to be intermittent, as Meniere's disease symptoms are, led to the original misdiagnosis of allergy as an "effluvium" emanating from freshly mown hay. The whole concept of a sudden influx of fluid into the endolymphatic sac, producing a rupture of Reissner's membrane, and the resulting production of Meniere's disease symptoms would be very consistent with the vasodilatation, fluid transudation, and inflammatory reaction that are the hallmarks of an allergic reaction.

If we accept that 40% of patients with Meniere's disease also are allergic, how do we distinguish which patients should undergo diagnostic testing and treatment for allergy? Table 15.2 lists the type of symptoms that should alert the clinician to the possibility that an underlying problem with allergies may cause or contribute to Meniere's disease symptoms in a given patient.

There have been several studies from our institution to assess the profile and treatment outcome in patients with

**TABLE 15.2. INDICATIONS FOR ALLERGY TESTING**

| |
|---|
| Childhood history of allergy |
| Family history of allergy |
| Patient suspects food reaction |
| Symptoms seasonal |
| Symptoms weather related |
| Nasal congestion |
| Rhinitis |
| Pharyngitis |
| Other allergic symptoms |
| Failure to respond to conventional treatments |

Meniere's disease and allergy treated with specific immunotherapy and dietary elimination.

In a first study, 93 patients with Meniere's disease, diagnosed according to American Academy of Otolaryngology–Head and Neck Surgery (AAOHNS) standards, were tested for allergies (19). Criteria for patients in the testing group included a history of Meniere's disease symptoms related to seasons, weather changes, or a suspect food; a known history of allergy; a significant childhood history of allergy; bilaterality of symptoms; or refractoriness to usual methods of treatment.

After control skin testing with histamine, saline, and glycerin, patients underwent serial endpoint titration (SET) skin testing for inhalant allergens. Radioallergosorbent test (RAST) screening also was performed in selected cases. Patients were asked to keep a food diary for 1 to 2 weeks before undergoing food testing with the subcutaneous provocative food test (PFT). In addition, IgG, IgE, and RAST tests were performed for selected foods.

Nearly a third (32.6%) of the patients thought that a reaction to a food provoked their Meniere's symptoms. Many patients also believed that their symptoms were related to weather (23.7%) or seasonal changes (47.3%). Most patients had significant symptoms of a systemic disorder suggesting allergies; 87% had a history of nasal congestion. Nine percent of patients had a history of a known autoimmune disease.

Eighty-two percent of patients had a normal total serum IgE (100 ng/mL). Levels of antigen-specific IgE as measured by SET also tended to be low, with most of the endpoint dilutions to weed, grass, and tree pollens, as well as dust and mold, occurring in dilution #2 (1 to 500 w/v). The most common foods identified by PFT included wheat, milk, corn, egg, yeast, and soy.

After immunotherapy, 56 of the 90 patients with follow-up (62%) reported a decrease in both frequency and severity of vertigo attacks. Fifty percent also reported an improvement in tinnitus and 59% in other (extralabyrinthine) symptoms, the most common of which was nasal congestion. Complete or substantial control of vertigo, using the AAOHNS definition, occurred in 86% of those patients for whom sufficient information was available to calculate the number of spells per month. None was worse.

In a more recent study, we evaluated the effect of specific allergy immunotherapy and food elimination of suspected food allergens on the course of patients with Meniere's disease. (20) Patients with Meniere's disease for whom allergy treatment had been recommended were identified and were mailed a questionnaire regarding their symptoms. Of those returned complete enough for inclusion, 113 had received allergy treatment; 24 did not have treatment and served as a control group. The 113 patients treated for symptoms of allergy using desensitization and diet showed a significant improvement from pretreatment to posttreatment, not only in allergy symptoms, but in Meniere's disease symptoms

(Table 15.3). The patient ratings of frequency, severity, and interference with everyday activities of their Meniere's symptoms also appeared better after allergy treatment than ratings from the control group of untreated patients. Vertigo control results, using the AAOHNS classification, were 47.9% class A or B. Hearing was stable or improved in 61.4%. Results indicate that patients with Meniere's disease can show improvement in their symptoms of tinnitus and vertigo when receiving specific allergy therapy, and suggest that the inner ear also may be the target, directly or indirectly, of an allergic reaction.

The symptoms of Meniere's disease—vertigo, hearing loss, and tinnitus—are thought to be produced by a sudden influx of fluid into the endolymphatic sac, producing a rupture of Reissner's membrane in the cochlea. The resulting potassium intoxication of the auditory and vestibular nerves causes the local neurologic changes. This increase in fluid could be caused by a sudden cessation of endolymph resorption in the endolymphatic sac, or could be secondary to the rapid production of endolymph in either the stria vascularis or the endolymphatic sac. The site is more likely the endolymphatic sac; the sac is capable of secretion as well as absorption, and the response of the sac to inner ear disturbance actually appears to be an increase in its secretory activity (21).

It also may be necessary to have an anatomic variant to contract Meniere's disease. It has been noted that the endolymphatic sac is smaller in patients with Meniere's disease than in normal control subjects (22). We could theorize that perhaps a smaller sac in the presence of a patient with allergy would predispose that person to being less able to handle the sudden secretion of endolymph that could be stimulated by an underlying problem with allergy.

There may be different possible mechanisms by which an allergic reaction results in the production of Meniere's disease symptoms. These have been discussed in detail elsewhere, but are briefly summarized here (20).

First, the endolymphatic sac itself could be a target organ of the allergic reaction. The sac's peripheral and fenestrated blood vessels could allow the entry of an antigen, which would then stimulate mast cell degranulation in the perisaccular connective tissue. The resulting inflammatory mediator release could affect the sac's filtering capability, resulting in a toxic accumulation of metabolic products and interfering with hair cell function. In addition, the fenestrated blood vessels to the sac could be pharmacologically vulnerable to the effects of the vasoactive mediators, such as histamine, that are released in an allergic reaction elsewhere in the body. The unique blood supply of the interosseus sac would serve as a portal for these mediators to exert a direct pharmacologic effect. The potent vasodilating effects of histamine or other mediators could affect the resorptive capacity of the sac.

A second proposed mechanism involves the production of a circulating immune complex, such as a food antigen,

**TABLE 15.3. PAIRED COMPARISON OF MENIERE'S DISEASE SYMPTOMS PRETREATMENT AND POSTTREATMENT FOR THE ALLERGY TREATED GROUP**

| Variables | $N^a$ | Pretreatment Median | Pretreatment Mean | Pretreatment SD | Posttreatment Median | Posttreatment Mean | Posttreatment SD | p Value |
|---|---|---|---|---|---|---|---|---|
| **Frequency of symptoms**[b] | | | | | | | | |
| Vertigo | 72 | 2.5 | 4.6 | 6.9 | 0.5 | 1.6 | 4.5 | <0.005 |
| Tinnitus | 84 | 5.0 | 4.1 | 1.2 | 5.0 | 3.8 | 1.3 | <0.005 |
| Unsteadiness | 84 | 3.0 | 3.0 | 1.0 | 2.0 | 2.4 | 1.0 | <0.001 |
| Running nose | 83 | 3.0 | 3.4 | 1.1 | 3.0 | 2.7 | 0.9 | <0.001 |
| Sore throat | 82 | 2.0 | 2.3 | 1.1 | 2.0 | 1.8 | 0.8 | <0.001 |
| Ear infection | 79 | 1.0 | 1.9 | 1.1 | 1.0 | 1.6 | 0.9 | <0.001 |
| Eczema | 84 | 1.0 | 1.9 | 1.2 | 1.0 | 1.8 | 1.0 | <0.03 |
| Asthma | 80 | 1.0 | 1.5 | 1.0 | 1.0 | 1.4 | 1.0 | |
| **Severity of symptoms**[c] | | | | | | | | |
| Vertigo | 45 | 4.0 | 4.2 | 0.9 | 2.0 | 2.7 | 1.6 | <0.001 |
| Tinnitus | 72 | 3.0 | 2.9 | 1.1 | 2.0 | 2.1 | 1.2 | <0.001 |
| Unsteadiness | 61 | 3.0 | 3.0 | 1.1 | 2.0 | 2.0 | 1.2 | <0.001 |
| **Interference with everyday activites**[d] | | | | | | | | |
| Vertigo | 49 | 4.0 | 3.8 | 0.9 | 3.0 | 2.8 | 1.3 | <0.001 |
| Tinnitus | 78 | 2.0 | 2.4 | 1.1 | 2.0 | 2.0 | 1.0 | <0.001 |
| Unsteadiness | 65 | 3.0 | 3.3 | 1.0 | 2.0 | 2.3 | 1.1 | <0.001 |
| Hearing loss | 86 | 3.0 | 3.5 | 1.2 | 3.0 | 2.8 | 1.3 | <0.001 |
| **Disability**[e] | | | | | | | | |
| Unsteadiness | 61 | 2.0 | 2.6 | 1.0 | 2.0 | 1.8 | 0.9 | <0.001 |

SD, standard deviation.
[a]Patients with missing data were excluded pairwise; therefore, the N for each variable can differ.
[b]Frequency: 1 = never, 2 = almost never, 3 = sometimes, 4 = almost always, 5 = always; frequency of vertigo (days/mo) ranges from 0 = never to 30 = always.
[c]Severity: 1 = not at all severe, 2 = somewhat severe, 3 = moderately severe, 4 = quite severe, 5 = extremely severe.
[d]Interference: 1 = never, 2 = almost never, 3 = sometimes, 4 = almost always, 5 = always.
[e]Disability: 1 = no disability, 2 = mild disability, 3 = moderate disability, 4 = severe disability.
From Derebery MJ. Allergic management of Ménière's disease: an outcome study. *Otolaryngol Head Neck Surg* 2000;122:174–182, with permission.

which is then deposited through the fenestrated blood vessels of the endolymphatic sac, producing inflammation. As previously noted, an increased incidence of circulating immune complexes in the serum has already been described in both Meniere's disease and allergic rhinitis. The inflammatory response resulting from the deposition of immune complexes along vascular basement membranes is the hallmark of an immune complex disease. Although the binding of the complexes to the cell membranes facilitates their phagocytosis, it also results in the release of tissue-damaging enzymes. This is believed to be the mechanism of unexplained sensorineural hearing loss in patients with a prototype immune complex–mediated disease, Wegener's granulomatosis. When the temporal bones of patients with Wegener's granulomatosis and unexplained sensorineural hearing loss have been studied, the cochlea is found to be normal; the pathologic process is found in the endolymphatic sac (23).

Alternatively, circulating immune complexes may be deposited in the stria, causing the normally intact blood–labyrinthine barrier to leak as a result of increased vascular permeability. In addition to disrupting normal ionic and fluid balance in the extracapillary spaces, this could facilitate the entry of autoantibodies into the inner ear. Harris and Ryan found a 30% incidence of a positive 68-kd autoantibody in the serum of patients with Meniere's disease (16). This antibody is presumed to be heat-shock protein 70, a constitutive protein that serves to chaperone other endogenous proteins during times of stress or damage to tissue. They also found that some human subjects with a known autoimmune disease have elevated levels of this circulating autoantibody, without evidence of hearing loss, suggesting that the antibody had not yet entered the inner ear. Harris and Sharp theorize that another factor must be present to facilitate its expression (24). This may well be the role played by a food antigen.

A third mechanism is of a viral antigen/allergic interaction. A predisposing viral infection in childhood, such as mumps or herpes, is carried to the inner ear, where it sets up a chronic low-grade inflammation. Although this is not enough to result in hearing loss, it does produce a mild impairment of sac absorption. "Something" in the system then stimulates excess fluid production. Shambaugh theorized that allergies or metabolic abnormalities, such as thyroid or hormonal dysfunction, were likely culprits, causing the sac to decompensate with the resulting production of endolymphatic hydrops (25).

Viral infections have been assumed by several investigators to play a direct or indirect role in the etiology of Meniere's disease. They are capable of exacerbating allergic symptoms by several mechanisms. Both live and ultraviolet light-inactivated viruses also have been shown to enhance histamine release, an effect believed to be mediated by interferon. Viruses also can damage epithelial surfaces, thereby enhancing antigen entry and increasing the responsiveness of target organs to histamine.

It appears that the most effective treatment for allergic endolymphatic hydrops is the prevention of mast cell degranulation. Several mediators are released when the mast cell degranulates, including histamine, serotonin, bradykinin, and slow-reacting substance of anaphylaxis. Clinically, the antihistamine treatments (e.g., meclizine, diphenhydramine) commonly used as an adjunct to lessen the clinical severity of vertigo in affected patients do not change the underlying pathologic process of a hydropic distention of the endolymphatic space. Pharmacologically, these antihistamines do not block the effects of the other inflammatory mediators that are released with mast cell degranulation.

Effective immunotherapy, with its induced immunologic changes, including the production of an antigen-specific IgG-blocking antibody, can prevent mast cell degranulation. The use of an appropriate elimination diet for documented food allergies obviously can prevent an immune-mediated reaction from occurring at all.

This is not to say that there may not be a true organ-specific autoimmune response against inner ear antigens. However, most autoimmune diseases are not by themselves "pure" entities, but rather a mixture of different hypersensitivity reactions with the type named being the most predominant. The clinical and histologic evidence is that a classic type I hypersensitivity reaction, a food antigen type III circulating immune complex reaction, or both together may play a role in the production of endolymphatic hydrops.

By the same presumed mechanism described previously, allergies also can play a role in the production of cochlear and vestibular hydrops (13).

## DIZZINESS

Allergic patients also may complain of vague dizziness rather than true vertigo, or a sensation of floating (26). Typically, these are young adults with a normal neurotologic examination and audiogram. Their symptoms usually are perennial, but their complaint of dizziness almost always is accompanied by other symptoms suggestive of allergy, especially nasal congestion or chronic rhinitis.

Other metabolic conditions, such as thyroid dysfunction or hypoglycemia, may give rise to similar complaints and need to be ruled out by appropriate laboratory tests. These patients often have been treated with various medications with no relief of their symptoms. That, along with the almost universal association of other allergic symptoms, should suggest a possible underlying atopic cause for symptoms, which will markedly improve after the institution of specific allergic treatment.

## TINNITUS

Allergic patients also may complain of tinnitus. Two studies evaluating tinnitus in patients with other allergic symptoms severe enough to warrant skin testing found that nearly 40% of all such patients reported the presence of significant tinnitus (27). In one study, a tinnitus questionnaire was completed by a sample of allergic patients with tinnitus. Results indicated that tinnitus was rated as usually being of moderate or loud intensity, but did not interfere greatly with daily life. In the second study, patients with Meniere's disease described their tinnitus before and after treatment for allergy (20). Ratings regarding the frequency of occurrence of tinnitus, the severity, and the interference with daily activities after treatment for allergy were significantly better than ratings describing tinnitus before treatment. Tinnitus appeared less severe in the treated patients than in a group of patients who did not receive treatment.

An indirect cause of tinnitus in the allergic patient may be an exaggeration of symptoms produced by the side effects of the decongestant drugs that often are used as an adjunct in treatment. Many of these medications have vasoconstricting properties similar to caffeine, which has long been recognized for its ability to exacerbate tinnitus.

## SUMMARY

Far from being an immunoprivileged organ, the inner ear demonstrates evidence of active immunosurveillance and immunoreactivity. Histopathologic studies support the concept, first published over 100 years ago, that allergic reactions may play a role in the production of labyrinthine symptoms. As many recent outcome studies have shown, those patients with allergy and Meniere's disease often have an excellent clinical response when the underlying allergic problem is recognized and appropriately treated.

## REFERENCES

1. Quincke H. Über meningitis serosa. *Samml Klin Vortr Innere Med* 1893;67:655.

2. Brookes GB. Circulating immune complexes in Ménière's disease. *Arch Otolaryngol Head Neck Surg* 1986;112:536–540.

3. Derebery MJ, Rao VS, Siglock TJ, et al. Ménière's disease: an immune complex-mediated illness? *Laryngoscope* 1991;101:225–229.

4. Harris JP. Immunology of the inner ear: response of the inner ear to antigen challenge. *Otolaryngol Head Neck Surg* 1983;91:18–23.

5. Altermatt HJ, Gebbers JO, Müller C, et al. Human endolymphatic sac: evidence for a role in inner ear immune defense. *ORL J Otorhinolaryngol Relat Spec* 1990;52:143–148.

6. Uno K, Miyamura K, Kanzaki Y, et al. Type I allergy in the inner ear of the guinea pig. *Ann Otol Rhinol Laryngol* 1992;101[Suppl 157]:78–81.

7. Harris JP. Immunology of the inner ear: evidence of local antibody production. *Ann Otol Rhinol Laryngol* 1984;93:157–162.

8. Tomiyama S, Harris JP. The role of the endolymphatic sac in inner ear immunity. *Acta Otolaryngol* 1987;103:182–188.

9. Wackym PA, Friberg U, Linthicum FH Jr, et al. Human endolymphatic sac: morphologic evidence of immunologic function. *Ann Otol Rhinol Laryngol* 1987;96:276–281.

10. Gadre AK, Fayad JN, O'Leary MJ, et al. Arterial supply of the human endolymphatic duct and sac. *Otolaryngol Head Neck Surg* 1993;108:141–148.

11. Duke WW. Ménière's syndrome caused by allergy. *JAMA* 1923;81:2179–2181.

12. Powers WH. Allergic factors in Ménière's disease. *Trans Am Acad Ophthalmol Otolaryngol* 1973;77:22–29.

13. Powers WH, House WF. The dizzy patient-allergic aspect. *Laryngoscope* 1969;79:1330–1338.

14. Viscomi GJ, Bojrab DI. Use of electrocochleography to monitor antigenic challenge in Ménière's disease. *Otolaryngol Head Neck Surg* 1992;107:733–737.

15. Gibbs SR, Mabry RL, Rolnad PS, et al. Electrocochleographic changes after intranasal allergen challenge: a possible diagnostic tool in patients with Ménière's disease. *Otolaryngol Head Neck Surg* 1999;121:283–284.

16. Harris JP, Ryan AF. Fundamental immune mechanisms of the brain and inner ear. *Otolaryngol Head Neck Surg* 1995;112:639–653.

17. Derebery MJ, Berliner KI. Prevalence of allergy in Ménière's disease. *Otolaryngol Head Neck Surg* 2000;123:69–75.

18. Yang WH, Dorval F, Osterland CK, et al. Circulating immune complexes during immunotherapy. *J Allergy Clin Immunol* 1979;63:300–307.

19. Derebery MJ, Valenzuela S. Ménière's syndrome and allergy. *Otolaryngol Clin North Am* 1992;25:213–224.

20. Derebery MJ. Allergic management of Ménière's disease: an outcome study. *Otolaryngol Head Neck Surg* 2000;122:174–182.

21. Rask-Andersen H, Bredberg G, Stahle J. Structure and function of the endolymphatic duct. In: Vosteen KH, Schuknecht H, Pfaltz CR, et al., eds. *Ménière's disease: pathogenesis, diagnosis, and treatment.* New York: Thieme-Stratton, 1981:99–109.

22. Hebbar GK, Rask-Andersen H, Linthicum FH Jr. Three dimensional analysis of the endolymphatic ducts and sacs in ears with and without Ménière's disease. *Ann Otol Rhinol Laryngol* 1991;100(3):2215–2225.

23. Leone CA, Feghali JG, Linthicum FH Jr. Endolymphatic sac: possible role in autoimmune sensorineural hearing loss. *Ann Otol Rhinol Laryngol* 1984;93:208–209.

24. Harris JP, Sharp PA. Inner ear autoantibodies in patients with rapidly progressive sensorineural hearing loss. *Laryngoscope* 1990;100:516–524.

25. Shambaugh GE Jr, Wiet RJ. The endolymphatic sac and Ménière's disease. *Otolaryngol Clin North Am* 1980;13:585–588.

26. Powers WH. Allergic phenomena in the inner ear. *Otolaryngol Clin North Am* 1971;4:557–564.

27. Derebery MJ, Berliner KI. Allergic aspects of tinnitus. In: Reich FE, Vernon HA, eds. *Proceedings of the Fifth International Tinnitus Seminar.* Portland, OR: 1995:447–484.

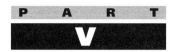

PART

V

# RESPIRATORY ALLERGY

# 16

# SEASONAL AND PERENNIAL RHINITIS

## JOHN H. KROUSE

Rhinitis is a common clinical problem that affects a large number of people around the world. By definition, rhinitis involves an inflammatory condition affecting the nasal mucosa that may be caused by a variety of different pathologic processes. It may present in affected people with a variety of different symptom patterns, ranging from mildly bothersome and inconsequential to severe and disabling. Because there is no broadly accepted uniform definition, the presence of rhinitis usually is diagnosed on the basis of the patient's history, supplemented by an examination of the nasal membranes and neighboring structures (1). Additional testing can be of use in further delineating the nature of the rhinitis.

Rhinitis may be related to allergic causes, or may be unrelated to atopic disease. The various types of infectious and noninfectious nonallergic rhinitis may share clinical symptom patterns with allergic rhinitis, but the pathophysiologic process involved in these syndromes is different from that seen in allergic patients. In addition, the treatment of these conditions also differs in several important ways. This chapter reviews the epidemiology, anatomy, pathophysiology, and diagnosis of both allergic and nonallergic rhinitis, and reviews various approaches to treatment of these common conditions.

## EPIDEMIOLOGY

Rhinitis is the most common clinical problem noted in patients with allergies (2). It is consistently ranked among the top six chronic diseases in the United States (3). When taken in combination with its comorbid diseases, such as otitis media, asthma, and rhinosinusitis, this cluster of disease entities comprises the most common, frequently noted chronic conditions in the United States (3). In addition, a number of additional factors contribute to the morbidity

of the disease, including sleep dysfunction, infection, and adverse effects of medications (4). The effect of chronic rhinitis on the patient's quality of life can be profound (5).

## Prevalence

Although a number of studies have investigated the prevalence of allergic rhinitis, the true prevalence of nonallergic rhinitis is unknown (6). It has been suggested that of patients with symptoms of rhinitis, approximately half have nonallergic disease (7,8). There is frequent overlap of allergic and nonallergic symptoms, however, and studies have not been done to differentiate the prevalence of the two disorders using either in vitro or skin assessments of immunoglobulin E (IgE).

The prevalence of allergic rhinitis has been well studied, and estimates of its prevalence vary based on the age, location, and methodology of the study design. Allergic rhinitis affects people of all ages, from infancy through adulthood, although it often is first diagnosed in childhood. The mean age of diagnosis has been estimated at between 9 and 11 years of age (9). Although the disease usually begins in early childhood, its peak symptoms usually occur between the ages of 10 and 40 years (10).

In 1974, a large study was conducted in which the entire 10,000-person population of a small town in Michigan was examined for the presence of allergic rhinitis. The cumulative prevalence of allergic rhinitis in this population was approximately 10% for both men and women (11). In a study examining twins in Sweden, prevalence rates of allergic rhinitis were noted at 15% in men and 14% in women (12). Rates have been estimated at 20% in a more recent series of studies (9).

In an ongoing prospective study, 747 healthy children have been followed from birth in a large Health Maintenance Organization in Tucson, Arizona (13). These children have been examined prospectively from birth to evaluate the cumulative prevalence of a number of childhood illnesses over time. In this study, 42% of these 747 children were diagnosed by their physicians with allergic rhinitis by

J. H. Krouse: Department of Otolaryngology, Wayne State University, Detroit, Michigan.

the time they were 6 years of age. The Tucson experience suggests that the true prevalence of allergic rhinitis actually may be greater than the 20% often quoted in the literature.

By several indicators, the prevalence of allergic rhinitis steadily increased throughout the 20th century. Although allergic rhinitis was reportedly rare in the 19th century (14), it has become progressively more commonplace. It has been debated whether the increased number of patients with allergic rhinitis reflects a true increase in the prevalence of the disease, or only an increase in the awareness and diagnosis of the condition.

Several studies have suggested the association of environmental factors with the increasing prevalence of allergic rhinitis. In one such study, schoolchildren from Aberdeen, Scotland were examined in 1964 and compared with a group examined 25 years later in 1989 using the same instruments. The authors found that not only did the prevalence of allergic rhinitis increase from 3% to 12% over the 25-year period, but that similar increases were noted in other atopic diseases such as eczema and asthma (15). The researchers attributed this increased prevalence to chemical agents found in air pollution. The same authors argued that noxious agents such as ozone, nitrogenous compounds, and sulfur dioxide can affect cellular mechanisms, making them more sensitive to aeroallergens (16).

## Etiology

As with many conditions, allergic rhinitis involves an interaction between environmental factors and a genetic predisposition toward development of the disease (17,18). Allergic rhinitis is not distinct among the atopic diseases in this interaction, however, and conditions such as asthma and dermatitis share similar characteristics.

There is a well described genetic component known to be present in the expression of allergic rhinitis. Multiple genetic factors appear to be involved. Although a genetic predisposition to development of atopic reactions and hypersensitization to antigens has been described, specific antigenic sensitivities or the type of allergic disease do not appear to be inherited in a simple manner (19). The relationship between parental allergy and the development of allergic disease in children has been described from population studies. It has been estimated that allergic disease occurs in approximately 13% of children if neither parent is atopic, in 30% of children if one parent is atopic, and in 50% of children if both parents are atopic (10).

As noted earlier, environmental factors appear to be important in the pathogenesis of allergic diseases. Noxious chemicals present in air pollution affect cellular physiology, leading to an increase in proinflammatory mediators and an increased expression of allergic rhinitis (16). In addition, among children with a genetic predisposition toward atopy, the exposure to viral infections can be a direct precipitant of allergic rhinitis (20). Other factors that have been postu-

lated to be involved in the expression of allergic rhinitis include decreased ventilation in homes, schools, and offices, dietary factors, and more sedentary lifestyles (21).

## NASAL ANATOMY AND PHYSIOLOGY

### Nasal Anatomy

The external nose consists of a supporting framework in the shape of a pyramid. The paired nasal bones form the superior portion of this pyramid, meeting in the midline. More inferiorly, the paired upper and lower lateral cartilages continue this pyramid, and provide contour to the lower nose. The upper lateral cartilages are firmly attached to the inferior border of the nasal bones. In the midline of the nose is the nasal septum, again consisting of the bony perpendicular plate of the ethmoid, the vomer, and the cartilaginous septum. These structures provide the skeleton for nasal projection and its position on the face.

Attached to the lateral nasal walls are bony prominences covered with mucosa known as the *turbinates* (Fig. 16.1). These structures protrude into the nasal airway, altering the flow of inspired air as it passes from the anterior nose to the posterior choanae. The turbinates create a turbulent flow of air, and allow this inspired air to pass over a large surface area as it is drawn posteriorly into the pharynx, providing warmth and humidification.

The external nose is covered with skin and subcutaneous tissue that is contiguous with the skin of the face. The anterior portion of the inner nose, referred to as the *nasal vestibule,* is lined with a thin, lightly keratinized, stratified squamous epithelium. This vestibular area is covered with numerous fine hairs known as *vibrissae,* which intercept large particles as they are inspired. The vestibule then communicates with the nasal valve region, where the mucosa changes to a ciliated pseudostratified columnar epithelium. This epithelium then continues throughout the nose and sinuses, and is similar histologically to the mucosa that lines the lower airway. The nasal valve is a slitlike region that is formed by the upper lateral cartilage, the nasal septum, and the anterior portion of the inferior turbinate. This region provides the greatest resistance to flow in the entire airway (10). The posterior portion of the nose is contiguous with the nasopharynx, and opens from the nasal cavities through a bony arch known as the *posterior choana.*

There is an extensive blood supply to the nose, fed from both the internal and external carotid circulations. The ethmoidal arteries, branches of the ophthalmic artery, enter the nose superiorly and course through the orbit to enter the nose. The inferior blood supply to the nose is through branches of the external carotid circulation, including the internal maxillary artery and the facial artery. The venous drainage of the nose is through the pterygoid and ophthalmic plexuses.

The turbinates are lined with cavernous tissue that reacts

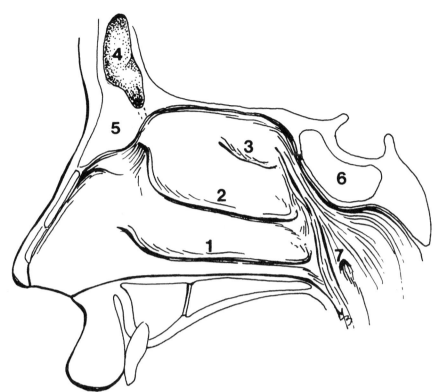

**FIG. 16.1.** View of the lateral wall of the nose. 1, Inferior turbinate; 2, middle turbinate; 3, superior turbinate; 4, frontal sinus; 5, agger nasi cell; 6, sphenoid sinus; 7, torus tubarius. (From Figueroa RE, Kuhn FA. Imaging evaluation for functional endoscopic sinus surgery. In: Taveras J, Ferucci R, eds. *Radiology: diagnosis, imaging, intervention.* Philadelphia: JB Lippincott, 1995:232–244, with permission.)

physiologically to various types of stimulation. This erectile tissue can become engorged, leading to nasal obstruction. Negus (22) described how the superficial vessels and deep cavernous tissues can act independently in response to air temperature, humidity, and irritation by foreign substances. These responses can cause either nasal swelling or decongestion.

The nasal mucosa is innervated by both sensory and autonomic fibers. It is the autonomic innervation of the nasal membranes that is important in the physiology of the nose. Sympathetic (adrenergic) fibers are found diffusely in the nose, and their function is mediated by norepinephrine. Parasympathetic (cholinergic) fibers also are found diffusely in the nose, and their function is mediated by acetylcholine. In general, the effects of these two systems on nasal physiology are antagonistic, and their balance is responsible for both the control of nasal congestion and the periodicity of the nasal cycle (23).

## Nasal Physiology

The functions of the nose are numerous, but all are related to its central role in the inspiration of air. The nose is involved in both olfaction and respiration. This chapter focuses only on the latter. The respiratory functions of the nose involve its role as an airway, a mechanism for warming and humidification of inspired air, and a filter for particulate matter and microorganisms.

The nasal airway functions as a much more effective breathing apparatus than does the mouth. Airflow through the nose has been described as more efficient in gas exchange, and as requiring the expenditure of less energy than mouth breathing (24). Resistance to air flow occurs within the nasal cavities, and is influenced by both dynamic and adynamic factors. Cyclical changes occur in the cavernous tissues of the turbinates owing to rhythmic changes in blood flow. The resultant nasal cycle can alter air flow in one nostril by up to 80%, yet total airflow usually is maintained in a compensatory fashion by mucosal changes in the contralateral nostril.

In addition to the cyclical changes that occur in the nasal mucosa, the nasal tissues are very responsive to both internal and external stimulation. Vasomotor reactions due to parasympathetic stimulation lead to an increase in nasal congestion, and can be stimulated by hormones such as estrogen, emotional influences, and various chemical and pharmacologic agents. Sympathetic stimulation results in vasoconstriction and mucosal shrinkage and is mediated by either endogenous or exogenous adrenergic agents. Irritation by noxious agents such as chemical fumes also can cause changes in the physiology of the nasal mucosa.

In addition to the airway functions of the nose, the nasal apparatus is involved in the humidification and temperature regulation of inspired air. As ambient air is inspired through the nose, it contacts the moist mucosa that lines the septum and nasal turbinates. The turbulent flow created by these structures allows inspired air to come into contact with a large surface area of mucosa, facilitating transfer of water to the air stream. Further, cold air is warmed toward body temperature concurrently with its humidification. In very hot, arid conditions, the nose is unable adequately to moisturize the inspired air, leading to irritation and inflammation of the upper and lower airways. In addition, aggressive surgical therapy of the turbinates creates a similar condition, leading to increased dryness and causing chronic changes in the larynx and lower respiratory tree (25). Because of these adverse effects of aggressive turbinate surgery, care must be taken in the preservation of normal physiologic function during turbinate procedures.

Finally, the nose serves a filtering function in protecting the lower airway and systemic circulation from particulate matter and inspired microorganisms. Because of the turbulent air flow through the nose, and with the assistance of the nasal vibrissae, most particles larger than 1 μm are retained in the nose. These particles are either cleared externally or swept into the pharynx by the mucus blanket and swallowed. This mucus blanket is swept through the nose with the assistance of the ciliated epithelium in a process known as *mucociliary clearance.* This active mechanism also is involved in clearance of mucus and particulate matter from the sinus chambers.

This nasal mucus is secreted by goblet cells in the mucosa under parasympathetic cholinergic control. Nasal fluids also are secreted by serous and seromucous glands, and diluted by a tissue transudate expressed through the capillaries of the mucosa (26).

In addition to the filtering properties of the nose, there is an active immune mechanism involved in the protection of the body from microorganisms. The major factor involved in this mechanism is secretory immunoglobulin A (IgA). Other immunoglobulins such as IgG and cytokines such as the antiviral substance interferon also appear to be involved in the protective function of the nasal membranes.

## PATHOPHYSIOLOGY OF RHINITIS

### Allergic Rhinitis

The primary mechanism involved in the development of allergic rhinitis is the deposition of foreign inhalant antigens onto the nasal mucosa. These antigens come into contact with antigen-presenting cells—macrophages and dendritic cells—which process the foreign antigens. These antigens are then presented to T helper lymphocytes, which respond to these foreign proteins and in turn secrete chemical mediators known as *cytokines.* The classes of cytokines include interleukins, interferons, and tumor necrosis factors (27, 28). These chemical mediators act as messengers, communicating with B lymphocytes and signaling them to synthesize *IgE,* the primary immunoglobulin involved in the allergic response. Interleukin (IL)-4 and IL-13 appear to be particularly important in this initial phase of allergic sensitization. Allergen-specific IgE synthesized by B cells then binds to receptors located on basophils and mast cells, which are found in the nasal mucosa as well as in the systemic circulation.

Once attached to mast cells and basophils, IgE molecules remain quiescent, awaiting subsequent exposure to antigens. On subsequent exposure to previously encountered allergens, the antigen particle attaches to two adjacent IgE molecules, cross-linking these molecules and triggering a prompt release of histamine and other proinflammatory mediators (29). This degranulation process leads to the immediate hypersensitivity response characteristic of allergy.

On release of histamine, both immediate and delayed effects of allergic stimulation take place. Histamine mediates a rapid response through a variety of local cellular and tissue effects. The blood vessels in the nose become engorged with red blood cells owing to local dilatation. The nasal membranes rapidly swell as a result of leakage of plasma from capillaries and venules. Mucus glands are stimulated to secrete mucin, and neural responses mediated by substance P and other neurotransmitters contribute to the development of local inflammation. The consequence of these physiologic effects is the cluster of symptoms characteristic of allergic rhinitis, including sneezing, itching, rhinorrhea, and nasal obstruction (30).

In addition to the immediate effects of antigen stimulation and histamine release, there is a second, late-phase reaction that occurs between 2 and 4 hours after antigen exposure. This late-phase reaction consists of a cellular infiltration by eosinophils and neutrophils. Additional mediators are both released and produced, in part because of the effects of IL-4 and IL-5, and include arachidonic acid metabolites such as prostaglandin $D_2$ and the leukotrienes $LTC_4$, $LTD_4$, and $LTE_4$. These late-phase processes continue to stimulate allergic inflammation in the nose beyond the initial acute phase of histamine release.

A common phenomenon among patients with allergic rhinitis is known as *priming.* Priming occurs in hypersensitive people as the result of exposure to nonspecific irritant stimuli such as irritant particles, noxious fumes, and strong odors. This phenomenon appears to be related to epithelial injury caused by exposure to antigen and the inflammatory processes that are triggered by that exposure.

### Nonallergic Rhinitis

There is no uniform simple mechanism involved in the pathogenesis of the rhinitis that occurs independent of allergic hypersensitization. Various physiologic processes lead to the syndrome described as *nonallergic rhinitis,* producing a symptom complex similar to that seen with allergic rhinitis.

Both intrinsic and extrinsic factors are involved in the pathophysiologic process of nonallergic rhinitis.

Exposure to a variety of external stimuli can lead to irritation of the nose with resultant rhinitis. Irritants in the form of particulate matter, odors, fumes, and noxious agents can be inhaled directly into the nose and cause a local inflammatory reaction of the mucosa. In addition, foods, chemicals, and pharmaceutical agents can be ingested orally and exert their effects on the nose. Infectious agents also can produce rhinitis, but are not discussed here.

Intrinsic factors that lead to rhinitis include hormonal effects, vasoactive mediators, and autonomic nervous system influences. In addition, endocrine disturbances such as hypothyroidism and hyperthyroidism and normal hyperendocrine states such as pregnancy are common triggers of rhinitis. An interaction between extrinsic and intrinsic factors also is important in nonallergic rhinitis, such as that seen with antihypertensive agents that block sympathetic function and increase nasal congestion and rhinorrhea.

## Rhinitis Medicamentosa

A very common type of nonallergic rhinitis is *rhinitis medicamentosa*. This condition is a drug-induced rhinitis that is characterized primarily by the prolonged use of topical vasoconstricting agents. Drugs such as oxymetazoline and phenylephrine are available as over-the-counter preparations, and are used as topical nasal sprays to reduce nasal congestion and secretion. They are α-adrenergic stimulators, and work directly on the nasal mucosa to cause constriction of the nasal vasculature, resulting in decreased nasal resistance and secretion. The prolonged use of these agents results in tachyphylaxis, in which more frequent application of the drugs is necessary to maintain control of symptoms. In addition, periods between use are characterized by rebound vasodilatation, which creates profound nasal congestion and rhinorrhea. This cycle of dependency can begin with as little as 5 days of consecutive use. For this reason, prolonged use of vasoconstrictive nasal sprays is to be avoided. Other drugs reported to cause rhinitis medicamentosa are listed in Table 16.1.

## Rhinitis of Pregnancy

Pregnancy is characterized by a steady increase in the systemic concentration of estrogen in the mother. Estrogens have been shown to increase the amount of hyaluronic acid in the tissues of the nose, causing increased tissue edema and congestion (31). In addition, during pregnancy there is an increase in mucus glands in the nasal mucosa with increased cavernous tissues in the nose and decreased cilia. As a result, there is increased congestion in the nose, increased mucus production, and decreased mucus clearance (31). The rhinitis seen in pregnancy is characterized by nasal

### TABLE 16.1. DRUGS ASSOCIATED WITH RHINITIS MEDICAMENTOSA

**Systemic**
  Antihypertensive agents
    Methyldopa
    Guanethidine
    Reserpine
    Hydralazine
    Prazosin
  β-Blockers
    Propranolol
    Nadalol
  Antidepressants and tranquilizers
    Thioridazine
    Chlordiazepoxide
    Amitryptyline
    Perphenazine
    Alprazolam
  Oral contraceptives and estrogens
  Aspirin and nonsteroidal antiinflammatory agents
  Ergot alkaloids
  Antithyroid drugs
  Iodides
  Alcohol
  Tobacco
  Hashish
  Marijuana
**Topical**
  Vasoconstrictors
    Oxymetazoline
    Xylometazoline
    Phenylephrine
    Ephedrine
    Cocaine

From Gluckman JL, Stegmoyer R. Nonallergic rhinitis. In: Paparella MM, Shumrick DA, Gluckman JL, et al., eds. *Otolaryngology*. Philadelphia: WB Saunders, 1991:1889–1898, with permission.

congestion without sneezing or itching. It is primarily seen in the second and third trimesters of pregnancy.

## Vasomotor Rhinitis

A very common, yet very frustrating type of rhinitis is vasomotor rhinitis. This condition involves a diagnosis of exclusion, once other allergic and nonallergic causes for rhinitis have been eliminated. It is very common in elderly patients, and appears to increase in prevalence with aging.

In vasomotor rhinitis, the patient is bothered by nasal congestion accompanied by postnasal discharge and paroxysmal rhinorrhea. There is no pruritus or sneezing associated with vasomotor rhinitis, and there usually is no associated pain. Frequently the symptoms in these patients can be triggered by exposure to exogenous stimulants such as odors, aromas of foods, or temperature changes. These triggers are thought to stimulate parasympathetic expression in susceptible patients, leading to a hyperresponsive mucosa. Vasomotor rhinitis therefore is believed to reflect an autonomic dysregulation of nasal function (32).

## CLINICAL PRESENTATION
### Allergic Rhinitis

Allergic rhinitis can be subdivided into two classes: seasonal and perennial. Allergic rhinitis is characterized by a classic set of symptoms that include sneezing, nasal and conjunctival pruritus, congestion, clear rhinorrhea, epiphora, and palatal itching (33). In addition, many patients complain of frontal and periorbital headaches, loss of taste or smell, and pressure in the ears.

### Seasonal Allergic Rhinitis

In seasonal allergic rhinitis, a direct association can be noted between exposure to the antigenic pollens and the onset of symptoms. Symptoms begin shortly after exposure to seasonal antigens in direct response to increased antigen-specific IgE stimulated by IL-4 release from type 2 T helper lymphocytes (34,35). In response to IL-4–mediated sensitization, IL-5 is synthesized, leading to the expression of allergic symptoms (35). These symptoms usually are expressed most significantly at the peak of pollen season, and both clinical symptoms and physical signs are most prominent at this time.

It is quite common for allergic rhinitis to be accompanied by systemic symptoms in addition to those experienced in the head and neck. Patients often complain of fatigue, malaise, and weakness, and these symptoms can be manifested by decreased alertness, impaired psychomotor performance, and lack of concentration (36). The effects of allergic rhinitis and related disease on quality of life are discussed in Chapter 26.

It is important for the physician treating patients with seasonal allergic rhinitis to be aware of the seasonal fluctuations that characterize various pollens in the local geographic region. In general, there are three seasons that are important in the clinical presentations of patients with seasonal allergic rhinitis: spring, summer, and fall. Tree pollination occurs in the late winter and spring months, with a peak time of March in the southern United States to May in more northern temperate climates. The summer months are characterized by grass pollens, reaching a peak in June and July. Weed pollens are primarily noted in the fall, beginning around the time of Labor Day in the northern temperate climates and decreasing sharply with the first frost. The winter months are free of these seasonal allergens because of the lack of pollination and the ground cover of snow and frost. Fungal antigens are perennial antigens in much of the warmer United States, but have a seasonal peak in the summer months as well (10).

### Perennial Allergic Rhinitis

Allergens that cause perennial allergic rhinitis are present in the environment throughout the year, with little or no seasonal fluctuation. Without the clear seasonal component of the patient's exposure history, it often is more difficult to diagnose perennial allergy than it is to characterize a seasonal disorder. Perennial allergens include molds, as noted previously, as well as animal danders, dust mites, cockroach, and other animal proteins. There is no difference in the pathophysiologic process of seasonal and perennial allergic rhinitis in either immunologic mechanisms or mediators (10).

Patients with perennial allergic rhinitis may have a different clinical presentation from the patient with seasonal allergy. The sneezing that is characteristic of seasonal exposure often is absent in the patient with perennial allergic rhinitis. Nasal obstruction and nasal congestion alone are frequently the primary manifestations of hypersensitivity to perennial antigens. As a result, the diagnosis of allergic rhinitis in these patients often is confused with related presentations such as vasomotor rhinitis or chronic rhinosinusitis. Careful history and confirmatory studies are necessary to diagnose the condition accurately.

A patient with hypersensitivity to an ingested food sometimes can present with allergic nasal manifestations as well. These food reactions can be quite complex and difficult to characterize, and often are mediated by processes other than IgE-related hypersensitivity (37). Substances such as milk, beer, brewer's yeast, baker's yeast, and other antigenic foods have been commonly implicated in the development of rhinitic symptoms. A thorough discussion of food sensitivities and their treatments is found elsewhere in this text.

## Nonallergic Rhinitis

When the patient presents with symptoms of rhinitis and no clear allergic cause can be elicited by history and judicious use of testing, the diagnosis of nonallergic rhinitis is reached by exclusion. There is no universally accepted definition of nonallergic rhinitis, although the patient often presents with several characteristic symptoms. In general, patients with nonallergic rhinitis complain of increased clear rhinorrhea, sometimes copious and paroxysmal, accompanied by nasal obstruction. Sneezing is unusual among patients with nonallergic rhinitis, as is the ocular, nasal, and palatal itching seen in allergic rhinitis. In addition, there is an increasing incidence of nonallergic rhinitis with advancing age (38).

### Vasomotor Rhinitis

Vasomotor rhinitis is characterized by a clinical presentation of symptoms associated with changes in temperature, use of alcohol, eating, or exposure to odors. The symptoms are variable, and primarily consist of increased secretion of mucus and nasal obstruction. In some of these patients, there has been a vagal mechanism described after ingestion of foods (39). In addition, chemical sensitivities and various pharmaceutical agents can exacerbate this condition.

## Nonallergic Rhinitis with Eosinophilia

Nonallergic rhinitis with eosinophilia (NARES) has been described as affecting approximately 15% of patients with nonallergic rhinitis (40). In this condition, first described in 1981 (41), patients present with symptoms of chronic perennial allergic rhinitis with frequent exacerbations of more severe symptoms. They have marked eosinophilia on nasal smears, but are not allergic to any inhalant allergens on either skin testing or serum measures of IgE. In fact, there is no significant difference in specific or total IgE between patients with NARES and nonallergic subjects (42). Although some authorities continue to assume that this disease process is allergic, others do not. The etiology of NARES remains unknown.

### Rhinitis Medicamentosa

The patient with rhinitis medicamentosa presents to the physician with worsening nasal obstruction over a period of months to years. Accompanying this advancing obstruction is the more frequent use of topical vasoconstrictive nasal sprays. Patients begin using these nasal sprays to relieve the obstructive symptoms accompanying an allergic diathesis or an upper respiratory infection. The rapid decongestant effect of these medications provides reinforcement to the patient, who continues to use the medication on a more regular basis. Unfortunately, the regular use of topical vasoconstrictors is accompanied by tachyphylaxis, and the patient begins to use the medications more frequently.

Prolonged use of these agents results in a syndrome known as *rebound rhinitis,* where the patient experiences severe nasal obstruction as the effects of the topical agents wear off. In fact, this obstruction usually is more severe than the congestion for which the patient began using the medications initially. The patient complains of a dry, irritated nose, which fluctuates with periods of severe congestion when the drugs are not used. Nasal examination demonstrates a beefy red mucosa with punctate hemorrhage and dry mucosa. The patient finds it extremely difficult to cease using the medication because of dependency on the chemical to provide nasal decongestion.

## DIAGNOSTIC TESTS IN THE WORKUP OF RHINITIS

### History

As with all medical illnesses, the history of the patient's illness is the primary mechanism through which the physi-

cian can reach a working diagnosis. Patients with rhinitis usually present with the chief complaint of nasal obstruction, sneezing, postnasal drainage, rhinorrhea, nasal irritation, headache, or ear pressure. It is important for the physician to pay careful attention to the precise cluster of symptoms described by the patient, and to note any seasonality to the complaints or any antecedent triggers that stimulate symptoms. This history also should include a description of when the condition began, and whether there were any allergic symptoms in childhood. These childhood symptoms may not only be nasal in character, but might include those of related allergic illnesses such as otitis media or asthma. In addition to the individual history, it is important to note the patient's family history as well. Because there is a higher prevalence of allergy among children of allergic parents, a description of allergic diseases in the parents is vital. A thorough discussion of the allergic history is found in Chapter 5.

### Physical Examination

It is important for the patient with rhinitis to have a thorough otolaryngologic evaluation, as well as some examination of the lower airway. The face should be examined for signs of puffiness, edema, or periorbital discoloration. Allergic patients commonly have puffiness of the lower lids with fine creases known as *Dennie's lines* parallel to the lid border. The conjunctivae are examined for injection, hyperemia, or edema. If epiphora is present, its character is noted.

The external nose is examined for any obvious structural deformity. The caudal septum is examined for any deviation or deformity, and the presence of any gross external rhinorrhea is noted. Examination of the internal nose is then undertaken. The position of the cartilaginous septum is noted with anterior rhinoscopy, as are the size of the turbinates and the condition of the overlying mucosa. The presence and character of rhinorrhea is noted, as well as whether there are any masses or polyps present. In patients with rhinitis, it is useful to examine the nose both with and without topical vasoconstriction.

It also is important to examine the oral cavity and oropharynx for any postnasal discharge or drainage, and for any hypertrophy of the lymphoid tissue. Prominent lymphoid tissue in the pharyngeal bands of the posterior pharyngeal wall, also known as *cobblestoning,* is characteristic of allergic disease. If the patient complains of hoarseness, indirect or fiberoptic examination of the larynx and lower pharynx is indicated.

Finally, because many patients with upper airway disease also have pulmonary illnesses, auscultation of the chest is important in patients with rhinitis. Concurrent asthma can occur in 15% to 20% of patients with rhinitis, and allergic rhinitis has been considered a predisposing factor to the development of asthma (43). It therefore is important to examine the lungs for any rhonchi or wheezes that may suggest lower respiratory disease.

## Nasal Endoscopy

Nasal endoscopic examination has become a valuable part of the diagnostic workup of patients with rhinitis, and can be of benefit in differentiating infectious and noninfectious pathologic processes of the nose and sinuses. In addition, the posterior aspect of the nasal cavity is not demonstrated well on anterior rhinoscopy. The use of both rigid and flexible fiberoptic endoscopes allows a more thorough examination of the nasal cavity than does anterior rhinoscopy alone. Because patients with rhinitis often have concurrent rhinosinusitis, it is important to use endoscopic examinations to assist in the diagnosis of these conditions.

## Nasal Cytology

An examination of the nasal mucus can be of assistance in the diagnosis of allergic versus nonallergic rhinitis. Nasal swabs or scrapings can be collected from the inside of the nose and examined microscopically. The main utility of this procedure has been to differentiate infectious from noninfectious rhinitis. The nasal cytogram in patients with infection is characterized predominantly by increased number of neutrophils, whereas allergic rhinitis presents with an increased number of eosinophils. The nasal cytogram is of variable utility and frequently yields inaccurate findings (44).

## Allergy Testing

In the patient with suspected allergic disease, the use of specific antigen testing can be confirmatory and can assist with treatment planning. Both in vivo or skin tests and in vitro or serum tests are in clinical use for the diagnosis of inhalant allergy. Allergy testing is discussed in detail elsewhere in this textbook.

## Tests of Nasal Patency

Measurement of airway patency and airway resistance can be of benefit in objectively assessing the flow of air through the nose. Several procedures have been described to measure nasal airflow and nasal resistance. Rhinomanometry, or measurement of airway resistance in the nose, is one such commonly used procedure. A more recent method for assessing nasal patency is acoustic rhinometry, a procedure in which a sound is directed into the nasal chamber and its reflection from various nasal structures is assessed. This procedure is easily conducted with relatively inexpensive equipment, and appears to be a more sensitive and specific measure than rhinomanometry for the diagnosis of nasal disease (45). Despite the ability of acoustic rhinometry to assess

structural lesions, its findings do not correlate well with self-recorded symptom scores (45).

## TREATMENT OF ALLERGIC AND NONALLERGIC RHINITIS

### Environmental Controls

The use of environmental controls is an important adjunct in the therapy of both allergic and irritative rhinitis. Avoidance of antigens to which the patient is known to be allergic can decrease the total allergic load and reduce symptoms accordingly (46). It may be easier to avoid indoor perennial antigens than seasonal airborne pollens, but patients can clearly arrange their outdoor activities to decrease exposure during peak pollen times. A more thorough discussion on the use of environmental controls is found in Chapter 10.

### Saline Irrigations

Saline rinses to cleanse the nasal mucosa have been used as effective adjuncts for the treatment of rhinitis for many years. Studies have examined the use of both hypertonic saline rinses (47) and physiologically normal saline (48) in the therapy of rhinitis, and have found improvement in symptoms in both allergic and nonallergic disease. Saline rinses not only cleanse the nose and allow topical medications to have increased efficacy at the mucosal level, they improve ciliary function and mucociliary clearance (49,50). Saline rinses can be a very effective ancillary treatment for both rhinitis and rhinosinusitis.

### Exercise

The use of vigorous physical exercise has been shown to cause a significant decrease in nasal congestion through stimulation of adrenergic receptors in the nasal mucosa. In fact, exercise is the most commonly used adjuvant therapy in patients with rhinosinusitis (51,52).

### Pharmacologic Therapies

#### Antihistamines

The mainstay of treatment for allergic rhinitis over the past 50 years has been the use of oral antihistamines. Antihistamines can be administered systemically through either oral or parenteral routes, or can be used topically in ocular preparations or nasal sprays. Antihistamines were initially used for the treatment of allergic rhinitis in the 1940s and have been widely used ever since that time.

First-generation antihistamines include such agents as diphenhydramine, chlorpheniramine, and clemastine. The primary limitation to the use of these agents is their strong central nervous system depressant activity due to their significant lipophilicity and their free crossing of the blood–brain barrier. These effects are expressed not only in self-reported sedation and drowsiness, but in performance, cognitive, and psychomotor impairment (53). In addition, these agents have significant anticholinergic effects, causing dryness of the mucosa in both the upper and lower airways, as well as increased tenacity of mucus.

Because of these performance effects, newer agents have been developed in an attempt to maintain antihistaminic efficacy but without the deleterious effects on alertness and psychomotor function. The first two of these agents to be widely used were terfenadine and astemizole, introduced to the market in the mid-1980s. Although these drugs were effective in reducing the symptoms of allergic rhinitis, they were found to have serious cardiac side effects, resulting in malignant arrhythmias and death. These cardiac effects were due to the manner in which the agents were metabolized through the hepatic cytochrome p450 enzymes (54,55). As a result of these fatal complications, neither terfenadine nor astemizole is currently available in the United States.

There are three second-generation antihistamines available for the treatment of allergic rhinitis in the United States: loratadine, fexofenadine, and cetirizine. Although loratadine and fexofenadine are classified as nonsedating antihistamines, cetirizine does maintain some sedative effects, although to a lesser degree than that seen with first-generation antihistamines. There have not been any cardiac events noted with any of these agents.

Histamine release is of importance only in the pathophysiologic process of allergic rhinitis, not in nonallergic disease. For that reason, antihistamines have little or no utility in the treatment of nonallergic or vasomotor rhinitis. An exception may be in the treatment of NARES, where loratadine has been shown to have some efficacy in symptom reduction (40). In addition, antihistamines have little or no decongestant effect. A more thorough discussion of antihistamines and other pharmacologic agents is contained in Chapter 11.

## Decongestants

α-Adrenergic agents are used both orally and topically to treat the nasal obstruction and congestion common in both allergic and nonallergic rhinitis. A number of studies have shown the efficacy of these agents in reducing the symptomatic congestion noted in these patients (56,57). The primary adverse effect of topical decongestants is rhinitis medicamentosa, which was discussed earlier. Oral decongestants such as pseudoephedrine and phenylpropanolamine have a number of significant, dose-related adverse effects, including tremulousness, irritability, palpitations, tachycardia, hypertension, insomnia, anxiety, and urinary obstruction. Although these agents have good efficacy, they should be used in the lowest dose capable of relieving symptoms, and for the shortest possible time.

## Mast Cell Stabilizers

As noted previously, sensitized mast cells degranulate, releasing histamine and other inflammatory mediators. Cromolyn sodium and nedocromil sodium are two agents that can be applied intranasally to stabilize mast cell membranes and inhibit degranulation. These agents must be given before exposure to offending antigens because they have little effect once mast cells have acutely degranulated. In addition, these agents have relatively short half-lives, and therefore must be given frequently. These drugs, however, are quite safe and well tolerated, and cromolyn sodium is available over the counter for nasal use in the United States. Again, mast cell stabilizers are effective only for rhinitis due to allergy.

## Corticosteroids

Steroid preparations are available for use in both topical intranasal and systemic forms. Although systemic corticosteroids are effective in the reduction of symptoms of allergic rhinitis, they are limited in their utility by the wide range of potentially serous side effects that accompany their use. For this reason, oral and parenteral steroids should be used only judiciously, for the shortest time possible to gain symptomatic relief, and with the full informed consent of the patient.

Topical intranasal corticosteroids are widely used for the treatment of both allergic and nonallergic rhinitis, and provide prompt, effective, and safe relief of symptoms. These agents work in the nasal mucosa to decrease neutrophil and eosinophil chemotaxis, reduce inflammation, suppress mast cell–mediated reactions, and reduce intracellular edema (58). They also inhibit the expression of both IL-4 and IL-5. Rare reports of increased intraocular pressure, cataract formation, and septal perforations have been noted, especially with older agents.

The newer nasal steroids, such as fluticasone and mometasone, are characterized by long half-lives and very low systemic bioavailability. This decreased systemic absorption is very important in that suppression of the hypothalamic–pituitary axis is possible with systemic absorption. In addition, growth retardation has been reported with the use of budesonide (59) in orally inhaled form for asthma and with beclomethasone (60) for both allergic rhinitis and asthma. No such growth retardation has been noted with mometasone nasal spray (61). Additional research is necessary further to characterize these findings and to assess their long-term effects on growth, especially among susceptible patients.

## Anticholinergic Medications

The administration of anticholinergic agents such as atropine to the nasal mucosa blocks parasympathetic input, resulting in decreased rhinorrhea. The primary agent available for use is ipratropium bromide, available in both a 0.03% concentration for noninfectious rhinitis and a 0.06% concentration for viral rhinitis. These medications do appear safe, but are of limited efficacy in the treatment of rhinitis. Their primary use is in acute viral rhinosinusitis and in nonallergic rhinitis.

### Leukotriene Inhibitors

Agents that interfere with leukotriene metabolism have been demonstrated to be effective in reducing the inflammation associated with asthma. They therefore have become more widely used for the treatment of lower respiratory disease, either alone or in combination with other agents. Some studies have also begun to demonstrate the effectiveness of leukotriene inhibitors as adjuvant agents in the treatment of allergic rhinitis. In one such study, the concomitant use of montelukast and loratadine demonstrated better symptom reduction among patients than did either agent alone (62). Leukotriene modifiers also have been demonstrated to have efficacy in the reduction of symptoms in patients with chronic rhinosinusitis (63) and nasal polyposis (64).

## Immunotherapy

Immunotherapy involves the subcutaneous, oral, or sublingual administration of small but increasing amounts of antigens to which the patient has tested positive to effect the gradual desensitization of the patient to those antigens. There have been numerous studies that have demonstrated the efficacy of immunotherapy. Several studies have specifically examined the effectiveness of skin endpoint titration (SET), and shown that immunotherapy based on SET can be safe and effective (65,66). Immunotherapy is discussed in detail in Chapter 12.

## Surgery

The surgical treatment of rhinitis is designed to correct any structural abnormalities that may be contributing to patient symptoms. The primary focus of surgical attention in rhinitis is the inferior turbinates. Once any significant septal deformity is corrected and after any obstructing lesions or polyps are removed, the reduction of the inferior turbinate is undertaken through one of a number of approaches. These procedures include superficial and intraturbinate cautery, cryosurgery, laser surgery, radiofrequency ablation, submucous resection, partial turbinectomy, and total inferior turbinectomy. The type and extent of surgery have been of major controversy for many years, and continue to be debated (67,68). In general, the trend has been toward more conservative resections of the inferior turbinate, with the preservation of adequate turbinate tissue to retain normal physiologic function.

Superficial cautery of the inferior turbinates primarily causes an injury to the mucosa without submucosal tissue reduction. As a result, there is minimal long-term change in the bulk of the inferior turbinates. Submucosal cautery is more effective in that it improves the nasal airway by reducing submucosal tissue. Similar effects are seen with cryosurgery of the turbinates. The effects of cryosurgery and cautery, however, appear to be short-lived (69,70). with recurrence of symptoms common within 1 year or less.

Laser surgery, with $CO_2$, potassium titanyl phosphate (KTP)-532, yttrium–aluminum garnet (YAG), and Ho-YAG lasers, has been used in the surgical treatment of rhinitis for several decades. One advantage that has been shown with laser turbinectomy has been the maintenance of treatment effects for prolonged periods (71). In part, these findings are due to the ability of the lasers to create not only mucosal reduction, but reduction in submucosal soft tissue and bone. Laser turbinectomy can result in necrosis of the underlying bone, and can be accompanied by prolonged healing and the need for frequent debridement of sequestrum.

A more recent approach to the surgical treatment of rhinitis has been the use of radiofrequency ablation of the inferior turbinate. In this approach, a submucosal radiofrequency probe is placed in the inferior turbinate and a predetermined amount of energy is delivered to the tissue. This energy causes a specific, predictable injury to the submucosal soft tissues, resulting in scar retraction and reduction of bulk. This procedure is safe and easily accomplished, and has shown significant improvement in nasal symptoms that persists for greater than 1 year (72,73). Longer follow-up of these patients is needed to assess maintenance of treatment effects.

Finally, "cold steel" approaches to the inferior turbinate continue to be used with good efficacy. One such approach that has been used widely is the submucous resection of the inferior turbinate, first described many years ago (74). In this procedure, an incision is made in the turbinate edge, and a portion of the bony structure of the inferior turbinate is removed. Attention is paid primarily to the anterior portion of the inferior turbinate, which is the major site of obstruction in most patients because of its contribution to the nasal valve. A recent adaptation of this technique has been described in which the microdebrider is used to remove submucosal bone and soft tissue with good success and minimal morbidity (75).

Both subtotal and total resections of the inferior turbinate also have been described for the treatment of rhinitis (76,77). These procedures are described by their proponents as being safe and effective in the reduction of nasal airway obstruction and nasal rhinorrhea. Although these procedures are technically easy to perform, they can be accompanied by significant postoperative hemorrhage and crusting, and require the use of nasal packing for several days. The major concern with this technique has been the development of a very dry, atrophic nose. Significant complications have been noted with this technique, and its use has been condemned by several authors (78,79).

## CONCLUSION

Rhinitis is a significant problem for many patients, and presents with symptoms of nasal obstruction, rhinorrhea, sneezing, and pruritus. It is associated with a variety of illnesses, including rhinosinusitis, asthma, and otitis media. It is critical to examine the nature of each patient's symptoms to determine the underlying mechanisms involved in that rhinitis, and to develop a plan of treatment that will maximize relief with minimal adverse effects.

## REFERENCES

1. Weeke ER. Epidemiology of hay fever and perennial allergic rhinitis. *Monogr Allergy* 1987;21:1–20.
2. Evans R. Epidemiology and natural history of asthma, allergic rhinitis, and atopic dermatitis. In: Middleton E Jr, Reed C, Ellis E, et al., eds. *Allergy: principles and practice,* 4th ed. St. Louis: Mosby; 1993:1109–1136.
3. National Center for Health Statistics. *Prevalence of selected chronic conditions.* Hyattsville, MD: Public Health Service, 1994.
4. Young T, Finn L, Kim H. Nasal obstruction as a risk factor for sleep-disordered breathing. *J Allergy Clin Immunol* 1997;99: 757–762.
5. Juniper EF. Measuring health-related quality of life in rhinitis. *J Allergy Clin Immunol* 1997;99:S742–S749.
6. Druce HM. Rhinitis and inhalant allergens. In: Middleton E Jr, Reed C, Ellis E, et al., eds. *Allergy: principles and practice,* 4th ed. St. Louis: Mosby, 1993:1005–1016.
7. Jacobs RL. Nonallergic chronic rhinitis syndromes. *Immunol Clin North Am* 1987;7:93–100.
8. Jones AS. Non-allergic perennial rhinitis. *Biomed Pharmacother* 1988;42:499–505.
9. Settipane GA. Allergic rhinitis: update. *Otolaryngol Head Neck Surg* 1986;94:470–474.
10. Naclerio R, Solomon W. Rhinitis and inhalant allergens. *JAMA* 1997;278:1842–1848.
11. Broder I, Higgins MW, Mathews KP, et al. Epidemiology of asthma and allergic rhinitis in a total community. *J Allergy Clin Immunol* 1974;54:100–105.
12. Edifors-Lubs ML. Allergy in 7,000 twin pairs. *Acta Allergol* 1971; 26:249–255.
13. Wright AL, Holberg CJ, Martinez FD, et al. Epidemiology of physician-diagnosed allergic rhinitis in childhood. *Pediatrics* 1994;94:895–901.
14. Emanuel EB: Hayfever, a post-industrial revolution epidemic: a history of its growth during the 19th century. *Clin Allergy* 1988; 18:295–304.
15. Rusznak C, Devalia JL, Davies RJ. The impact of pollution on allergic disease. *Allergy* 1994;49:21–27.
16. Davies RJ, Rusznak C, Devalia JL. Why is allergy increasing?—environmental factors. *Clin Exp Allergy* 1998;28[Suppl 6]:8–14.
17. Ownby D. Environmental factors versus genetic determinants of childhood inhalant allergies. *J Allergy Clin Immunol* 1990;86: 279–284.
18. Aberg N. Familial occurrence of atopic disease: genetic versus environmental factors. *Clin Exp Allergy* 1993;23:829–834.
19. Huang SK, Marsh DG. Genetics of allergy. *Ann Allergy Asthma Immunol* 1993;70:347–359.
20. Weeke ER, Pedersen PA, Backman A, et al. Epidemiology. In: Mygind N, Weeke B, eds. *Allergic and vasomotor rhinitis.* Copenhagen: Munksgaard, 1985:15.
21. Schoenwetter WF. Allergic rhinitis: epidemiology and natural history. *Allergy Asthma Proc* 2000;21:1–6.
22. Negus V. *The comparative anatomy and physiology of the nose and paranasal sinuses.* London: Livingston, 1958.
23. Kimmelman CP, Ali GHA. Vasomotor rhinitis. *Otolaryngol Clin North Am* 1986;19:65–74.
24. Ogura JH, Unno T, Nelson JR. Baseline values in pulmonary mechanics for physiologic surgery of the nose: preliminary report. *Ann Otol* 1968;77:367–397.
25. Homes EM. Clinical classification of ethmoiditis. *JAMA* 1914; 63:2097–2100.
26. Connell JT. Nasal disease: mechanisms and classification. *Ann Allergy* 1983;50:227–232.
27. Abbas AK, Lichtman AH, Pober JS. *Cellular and molecular immunology.* Philadelphia: WB Saunders, 1991.
28. Pearlman DS. Pathophysiology of the inflammatory response. *J Allergy Clin Immunol* 1999;104:S132–S137.
29. Gomez E, Corrado OH, Baldwin DL, et al. Direct in vivo evidence for mast cell degranulation during allergen-induced reactions in man. *J Allergy Clin Immunol* 1986;78:637–645.
30. Naclerio RM. Allergic rhinitis. *N Engl J Med* 1991;325:860–869.
31. Topposada H, Topposada M, El-Ghazzami I, et al. The human respiratory nasal mucosa in females using contraceptive pills. *J Laryngol Otol* 1984;98:43–50.
32. Bickmore JT. Vasomotor rhinitis: an update. *Laryngoscope* 1981; 91:1600–1605.
33. Naclerio RM. Pathophysiology of perennial allergic rhinitis. *Allergy* 1997;52:7–13.
34. Moverare R, Elfman L, Bjornsson E, et al. Changes in cytokine production in vitro during the early phase of birch-pollen immunotherapy. *Scand J Immunol* 2000;52:200–206.
35. Nakai Y, Ohashi Y, Kakinoki Y, et al. Allergen-induced mRNA expression of IL-5, but not of IL-4 and IFN-gamma, in peripheral blood mononuclear cells is a key feature of clinical manifestation of seasonal allergic rhinitis. *Arch Otolaryngol Head Neck Surg* 2000;126:992–996.
36. Blaiss MS. Cognitive, social, and economic costs of allergic rhinitis. *Allergy Asthma Proc* 2000;21:7–13.
37. Dixon HS. Treatment of delayed food allergy based on specific immunoglobulin G RAST testing. *Otolaryngol Head Neck Surg* 2000;123:48–54.
38. Sanico A, Togias A. Noninfectious, nonallergic rhinitis (NINAR): considerations on possible mechanisms. *Am J Rhinol* 1998;12:65–72.
39. Mullarkey MF. The classification of nasal disease: an opinion. *J Allergy Clin Immunol* 1981;67:251–254.
40. Purello-D'Ambrosio F, Isola S, Ricciardi L, et al. A controlled study on the effectiveness of loratadine in combination with flunisolide in the treatment of nonallergic rhinitis with eosinophilia (NARES). *Clin Exp Allergy* 1999;29:1143–1147.
41. Jacobs RL, Freedman PM, Boswell RN. Nonallergic rhinitis with eosinophilia (NARES syndrome): clinical and immunologic presentation. *J Allergy Clin Immunol* 1981;67:253–262.
42. Schiavino D, Nucera E, Milani A, et al. Nasal lavage cytometry in the diagnosis of nonallergic rhinitis with eosinophilia syndrome (NARES). *Allergy Asthma Proc* 1997;18:363–366.
43. Corren J. The relationship between allergic rhinitis and bronchial asthma. *Curr Opin Pulm Med* 1999;5:35–37.
44. Mullarkey MF, Hill JS, Webb DR. Allergic and nonallergic rhini-

tis: their characterization with attention to the meaning of nasal eosinophilia. *J Allergy Clin Immunol* 1980;65:22–26.

45. Passali D, Mezzedimi C, Passali GC, et al. The role of rhinomanometry, acoustic rhinometry, and mucociliary transport time in the assessment of nasal patency. *Ear Nose Throat J* 2000;79:397–400.

46. Derebery MJ. Otolaryngic allergy. *Otolaryngol Clin North Am* 1993;26:593–611.

47. Tomooka LT, Murphy C, Davidson TM. Clinical study and literature review of nasal irrigation. *Laryngoscope* 2000;110:1189–1193.

48. Nuutinen J, Holopainen E, Haahtela T, et al. Balanced physiological saline in the treatment of chronic rhinitis. *Rhinology* 1986;24:265–269.

49. Talbot AR, Herr TM, Parsons DS. Mucociliary clearance and buffered hypertonic saline solution. *Laryngoscope* 1997;107:500–503.

50. Homer JJ, England RJ, Wilde AD, et al. The effect of pH of douching solutions on mucociliary clearance. *Clin Otolaryngol* 1999;24:312–315.

51. Krouse JH, Krouse HJ. Patient use of traditional and complementary therapies in treating rhinosinusitis before consulting an otolaryngologist. *Laryngoscope* 1999;109:1223–1227.

52. Krouse HJ, Krouse JH. Complementary therapeutic practices in patients with chronic sinusitis. *Clin Excell Nurse Pract* 1999;3:346–352.

53. Kay GG. The effects of antihistamines on cognition and performance. *J Allergy Clin Immunol* 2000;105:S622–S627.

54. Renwick AG. The metabolism of antihistamines and drug interactions: the role of cytochrome P450 enzymes. *Clin Exp Allergy* 1999;29:116–124.

55. Ament PW, Paterson A. Drug interactions with the nonsedating antihistamines. *Am Fam Physician* 1997;56:223–231.

56. Ferguson BJ. Cost-effective pharmacotherapy for allergic rhinitis. *Otolaryngol Clin North Am* 1998;31:91–110.

57. Hendeles L. Selecting a decongestant. *Pharmacotherapy* 1993;13:129S–134S.

58. Pipkorn U, Proud D, Lichtenstein LM, et al. Inhibition of mediator release in allergic rhinitis by pretreatment with topical glucocorticosteroids. *N Engl J Med* 1987;316:1506–1512.

59. Skoner DP, Szefler SJ, Welch M, et al. Longitudinal growth in infants and young children treated with budesonide inhalation suspension for persistent asthma. *J Allergy Clin Immunol* 2000;105:259–268.

60. Skoner DP, Rachelefsky GS, Meltzer EO, et al. Detection of growth suppression in children during treatment with intranasal beclomethasone dipropionate. *Pediatrics* 2000;105:E23.

61. Schenkel EJ, Skoner DP, Bronsky EA. Absence of growth retardation in children with perennial allergic rhinitis after one year of treatment with mometasone furoate aqueous nasal spray. *Pediatrics* 2000;105:E22.

62. Meltzer EO, Malmstrom K, Lu S, et al. Concomitant montelukast and loratadine as treatment for seasonal allergic rhinitis: a randomized, placebo-controlled clinical trial. *J Allergy Clin Immunol* 2000;105:917–922.

63. Ulualp SO, Sterman BM, Toohill RJ. Antileukotriene therapy for the relief of sinus symptoms in aspirin triad disease. *Ear Nose Throat J* 1999;78:604–613.

64. Parnes SM, Chuma AV. Acute effects of antileukotrienes on sinonasal polyposis and sinusitis. *Ear Nose Throat J* 2000;79:18–20, 24–25.

65. Krouse JH, Krouse HJ. Efficacy of immunotherapy based on skin end-point titration. *Otolaryngol Head Neck Surg* 2000;123:183–187.

66. Trevino RJ. Comparison of results of immunotherapy based on skin end-point titration, prick testing, and scratch testing. *Otolaryngol Head Neck Surg* 1994;111:550–552.

67. Mabry RL. Surgery of the inferior turbinates: how much and when? *Otolaryngol Head Neck Surg* 1984;92:571–576.

68. Jackson LE, Koch RJ. Controversies in the management of inferior turbinate hypertrophy: a comprehensive review. *Plast Reconstr Surg* 1999;103:300–312.

69. Rakover Y, Rosen G. A comparison of partial inferior turbinectomy and cryosurgery for hypertrophic inferior turbinates. *J Laryngol Otol* 1996;110:732–735.

70. McCombe AW, Cook J, Jones AS. A comparison of laser cautery and sub-mucosal diathermy for rhinitis. *Clin Otolaryngol* 1992;17:297–299.

71. Cook JA, McCombe AW, Jones AS. Laser treatment of rhinitis—1 year follow-up. *Clin Otolaryngol* 1993;18:209–211.

72. Utley DS, Goode RL, Hakim I. Radiofrequency energy tissue ablation for the treatment of nasal obstruction secondary to turbinate hypertrophy. *Laryngoscope* 1999;109:683–686.

73. Smith TL, Correa AJ, Kuo T, et al. Radiofrequency tissue ablation of the inferior turbinates using a thermocouple feedback electrode. *Laryngoscope* 1999;109:1760–1765.

74. Saunders WH. Surgery of the inferior nasal turbinates. *Ann Otol Rhinol Laryngol* 1982;91:445–447.

75. Friedman M, Tanyeri H, Lim J, et al. A safe, alternative technique for inferior turbinate reduction. *Laryngoscope* 1999;109:1834–1837.

76. Ophir D, Shapira A, Marshak G. Total inferior turbinectomy for nasal airway obstruction. *Arch Otolaryngol* 1985;111:93–98.

77. Martinez SA, Nissen AJ, Stock CR, et al. Nasal turbinate resection for relief of nasal obstruction. *Laryngoscope* 1983;93:871–876.

78. Moore GF, Freeman TJ, Ogren FP, et al. Extended follow-up of total inferior turbinate resection for relief of chronic nasal obstruction. *Laryngoscope* 1985;95:1095–1098.

79. Berenholz L, Kessler A, Sarfati S, et al. Chronic sinusitis: a sequela of inferior turbinectomy. *Am J Rhinol* 1998;12:257–261.

# 17

# RHINOSINUSITIS AND ALLERGY

## JOHN H. KROUSE

Acute and chronic rhinosinusitis are among the most common illnesses in the world. It is estimated that 30% of Americans experience the symptoms of rhinosinusitis, at a direct medical cost of over $2 billion annually (1). In fact, it is generally believed that the incidence and prevalence of rhinosinusitis in adults are increasing (2). The symptoms of acute and chronic rhinosinusitis are varied, and contribute significantly to patient morbidity through decreased productivity and impaired quality of life (3). The association between allergic inflammation of the nose and sinuses and the symptoms of chronic rhinosinusitis has been postulated for many years, although the influence of allergic disease in the pathogenesis of rhinosinusitis remains a subject of intense debate. This chapter reviews the research that relates allergic rhinitis and rhinosinusitis, and discusses a framework for further examination of this important topic.

## DEFINITION OF RHINOSINUSITIS

One of the difficulties in all research related to the pathogenesis and treatment of sinus disease is the vast differences that exist in the classification and definition of what constitutes a case of "sinusitis." To this end, the American Academy of Otolaryngology-Head and Neck Surgery (AAOHNS) in 1996 convened a Task Force on Rhinosinusitis to discuss this disease and offer a uniform definition that could improve communication and guide research. The Task Force presented its consensus statement in August of that year, offering working definitions for acute rhinosinusitis, subacute rhinosinusitis, recurrent acute rhinosinusitis, chronic rhinosinusitis, and acute exacerbation of chronic rhinosinusitis. These recommendations were subsequently approved by both the American Rhinologic Society (ARS) and the American Academy of Otolaryngic Allergy (AAOA), and reflect the positions of the three major otolaryngologic associations with interests in sinus disease (2).

Sinusitis, in a broad sense, can be viewed as an inflamma-

tory response of the mucous membranes of the nose and sinuses, the fluids in these areas, or the underlying bony framework. The symptoms of the disease are quite broad as well, involving such diverse presentations as nasal congestion, nasal discharge, facial pressure and pain, cough, fever, halitosis, eustachian tube dysfunction, anosmia or hyposmia, and headache. Because the mucosa of the nose and sinuses is one epithelium in continuity, inflammatory effects of one area frequently are expressed in contiguous areas as well (4). In fact, sinusitis often is preceded by rhinitis, and rarely occurs without involvement of the nose (5).

Because of this common association between inflammatory and infectious diseases of the nose and sinuses, the Task Force on Rhinosinusitis concluded that the correct term used to classify this spectrum of diseases should be *rhinosinusitis* rather than *sinusitis*. This terminology has been generally accepted by the AAOHNS, the ARS, and the AAOA, and is used currently in research and clinical practice by the otolaryngology community at large. In addition, a conjoint conference held with the AAOHNS and the American Academy of Allergy, Asthma and Immunology (AAAAI) also has suggested that "rhinosinusitis may be a more appropriate term than either rhinitis or sinusitis alone" (p. S830) (4). For these reasons, the term *rhinosinusitis* is used in the remainder of this chapter.

Chronic rhinosinusitis has been reported through much of the 1990s as the most common chronic illness in the United States (1). It is estimated from this survey that 15% of the American population is bothered by symptoms of rhinosinusitis for at least 3 months yearly. In fact, as many as half of all patients seen by primary care physicians present with some form of viral, bacterial, or allergic rhinosinusitis (6). There is a higher incidence of reported cases of rhinosinusitis in the Midwest and South compared with the Northeast and Western United States (4).

## CLASSIFICATION OF RHINOSINUSITIS

According to the Task Force on Rhinosinusitis, rhinosinusitis is clinically defined as "a condition manifested by an inflammatory response involving the following: the mucous

**J. H. Krouse:** Department of Otolaryngology, Wayne State University, Detroit, Michigan.

## TABLE 17.1. FACTORS ASSOCIATED WITH A DIAGNOSIS OF RHINOSINUSITIS

**Major factors**
  Facial pain/pressure[a]
  Facial congestion/fullness
  Nasal obstruction/blockage
  Nasal discharge/purulence/discolored postnasal drainage
  Hyposmia/anosmia
  Purulence in nasal cavity on examination
  Fever (acute rhinosinusitis only)[b]
**Minor factors**
  Headache
  Fever (all nonacute)
  Halitosis
  Fatigue
  Dental pain
  Cough
  Ear pain/pressure/fullness

[a]Facial pain/pressure alone does not constitute a suggestive history for rhinosinusitis in the absence of another major nasal symptom or sign.
[b]Fever in acute sinusitis alone does not constitute a strongly suggestive history for acute rhinosinusitis in the absence of another major nasal symptom or sign.

membranes (possibly including the neuroepithelium) of the nasal cavity and paranasal sinuses, fluids within these cavities, and/or underlying bone" (p. S4) (1). The Task Force described a group of major and minor symptoms that are necessary to confirm a clinical diagnosis of rhinosinusitis (Table 17.1). Major factors include facial pain or pressure, facial congestion or fullness, nasal obstruction, nasal discharge, hyposmia/anosmia, purulence in the nasal cavity on examination, and fever. Minor factors include headache, nonacute fever, halitosis, fatigue, dental pain, cough, and ear pain, pressure, or fullness. A similar system relying on major and minor clinical criteria was suggested by a group from the American College of Allergy and Immunology (7).

Based on a review of various presenting symptoms and signs of patients with rhinosinusitis, the Task Force concluded that there were five distinct classifications for rhinosinusitis in adults. The Task Force presented a series of characteristics for each of these five classifications in which the duration of the illness, the patterns of its symptoms and signs, and the physical examination are used to establish a diagnosis of a specific type of rhinosinusitis. Radiologic findings are *not* required to establish a clinical diagnosis of rhinosinusitis. These five classifications are presented in Table 17.2, and are discussed in the following sections.

## Acute Rhinosinusitis

Acute rhinosinusitis in adults is a very common condition that has a sudden onset of symptoms, and lasts from 1 day to 4 weeks (1,8,9). A strong history is necessary to entertain the diagnosis of acute rhinosinusitis. This history includes

two or more major factors or one major factor and two minor factors (Table 17.1). One of the major concerns regarding the diagnosis of acute rhinosinusitis is the distinction between the acute viral upper respiratory infection (common cold) and bacterial rhinosinusitis. Because a large number of patients experience common colds yearly, and because there are many similarities in the symptoms of these two disorders, it is important to consider criteria that distinguish viral processes from bacterial so that therapy can be properly prescribed. Studies have shown that when symptoms worsen after 5 days and then persist longer than 10 days, this presentation is more consistent with a bacterial rather than a viral rhinosinusitis (10).

Certain symptoms and physical signs also are suggestive of a diagnosis of acute bacterial rhinosinusitis. Facial erythema or edema and maxillary tooth pain are strongly associated with acute rhinosinusitis, although they are relatively uncommon presenting findings (11). In addition, the finding of purulence in the nose on physical examination also is strongly indicative of acute rhinosinusitis (1).

## Subacute Rhinosinusitis

The AAOHNS Task Force has defined an interim category of disease that it has labeled as *subacute rhinosinusitis*. This process does not represent a discrete pathologic entity, but rather reflects a "continuum of the natural progression of acute rhinosinusitis that has not resolved" (p. S6). It is defined as a continued presentation of acute disease beyond the 4-week period and lasting up to 12 weeks. The symptoms are less severe in magnitude but similar in character to those seen with acute rhinosinusitis. Fever is not considered a major factor in the diagnosis, similar to the classification of chronic rhinosinusitis. Subacute rhinosinusitis is treated with medical therapy, and usually resolves completely with treatment (1).

## Recurrent Acute Rhinosinusitis

Recurrent acute rhinosinusitis reflects a pattern of frequent, repetitive periods of acute rhinosinusitis, occurring four or more times yearly. Between episodes the patient is symptom free. Some authors have suggested that this period of quiescence must be at least 8 weeks or more (12). The diagnostic criteria are similar to those for acute rhinosinusitis, although there are recurrent episodes. It is not clear at this time whether recurrent acute rhinosinusitis represents a distinct disease entity or the random occurrence of repeated episodes of acute rhinosinusitis.

## Chronic Rhinosinusitis

Chronic rhinosinusitis has been defined as a prolonged inflammatory condition of the nose and sinuses. Various authors have suggested that to be considered chronic it must persist for greater than 8 (13) to 12 weeks (14). The

**TABLE 17.2. CLASSIFICATION OF ADULT RHINOSINUSITIS**[a]

| Classification | Duration | History | Include in Differential | Special Notes |
|---|---|---|---|---|
| Acute | ≤4 wk | ≥2 major factors, 1 major factor and 2 minor factors, or nasal purulence on examination | 1 major factor or ≥2 minor | Fever or facial pain does not constitute a suggestive history in the absence of other nasal signs or symptoms. Consider acute bacterial rhinosinusitis if symptoms worsen after 5 days, if symptoms persist for >10 days, or in presence of symptoms out of proportion to those typically associated with viral infection. |
| Subacute | 4–12 wk | Same as chronic | Same as chronic | Complete resolution after effective medical therapy. |
| Recurrent acute | ≥4 episodes per year, with each episode lasting ≥7–10 days, and absence of intervening signs and symptoms of chronic rhinosinusitis | Same as acute | | |
| Chronic | ≥12 wk | ≥2 major factors, 1 major factor and 2 minor factors, or nasal purulence on examination | 1 major factor or ≥2 minor factors | Facial pain does not constitute a suggestive history in the absence of of other nasal signs or symptoms. |
| Acute exacerbations of chronic | Sudden worsening of chronic rhinosinusitis, with return to baseline after treatment | | | |

[a]Rhinosinusitis may be clinically defined as the condition manifested by an inflammatory response involving the mucous membranes (possibly including neuroepithelium) of nasal cavity and paranasal sinuses, fluids in these cavities, or underlying bone. Fluids in these cavities are dynamic and are related to dynamic pathologic changes in bone and soft tissues of nasal cavity and paranasal sinuses. Symptoms associated with rhinosinusitis include nasal obstruction, nasal congestion, nasal discharge, nasal purulence, postnasal drip, facial pressure and pain, alteration in sense of smell, cough, fever, halitosis, fatigue, dental pain, pharyngitis, otologic symptoms (e.g., ear fullness and clicking), and headache (1).

AAOHNS Task Force states that chronic rhinosinusitis must last greater than 12 weeks (1). To confirm a diagnosis of chronic rhinosinusitis, the patient must have a clinical presentation with either two or more major factors or one major factor and two minor factors as noted in Table 17.1. Facial pain does not constitute a diagnosis of chronic rhinosinusitis in the absence of nasal symptoms and signs. Changes in the appearance of computed tomography (CT) scans can be of assistance in making the diagnosis (14), but the Task Force criteria do not require CT abnormalities in the diagnosis of chronic rhinosinusitis.

## Acute Exacerbation of Chronic Rhinosinusitis

The final category of rhinosinusitis involves acute exacerbations of chronic disease. There is a baseline of chronic symptoms of rhinosinusitis, with acute flares lasting less than 4 weeks.

## PATHOPHYSIOLOGY OF THE PARANASAL SINUSES

The paranasal sinuses are paired air-containing spaces in the bony framework of the skull. They develop sequentially from birth through adolescence, and reach their full size by adulthood. The bony framework of the sinuses is lined with a ciliated pseudostratified columnar epithelium that is contiguous with the mucosa of the nasal cavity and nasopharynx. Goblet cells in the sinus mucosa secrete mucus that bathes the membranes and is swept by an active mechanism toward the sinus ostia and posteriorly into the pharynx. This normal physiologic mechanism is known as *mucociliary*

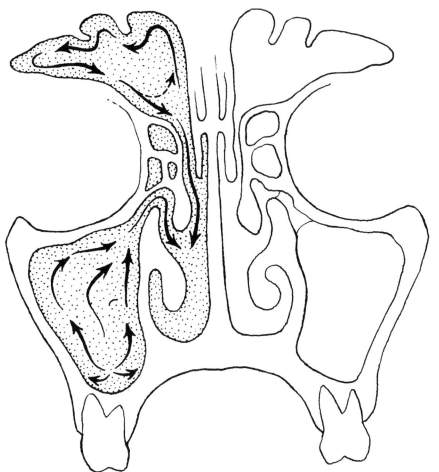

**FIG. 17.1.** Coronal diagram showing direction of flow of mucous blanket in frontal and ethmoid sinuses. (Reprinted from Rice DH, Schaefer SD. *Endoscopic paranasal sinus surgery.* New York: Raven Press, 1993:52, with permission.)

*clearance.* The process of mucociliary clearance is a vital component in the healthy functioning of the sinuses. The orientation of this active transport is genetically directed toward the natural ostium of each sinus (15) (Fig. 17.1).

The anatomy of the sinuses defines two specific patterns of flow: anteriorly and posteriorly. The anterior sinuses, including the maxillary sinuses, the anterior ethmoid cells, and the frontal sinuses, drain into an area know as the *infundibulum.* This region, lateral to the middle turbinate, with the inclusion of the uncinate process, an extension of the ethmoid bone, is referred to as the *ostiomeatal complex* (OMC). The OMC is thought to be the major anatomic region involved in the pathogenesis of acute and chronic sinus disease (16). The more posterior sinuses, including the posterior ethmoid cells and the sphenoid sinus, drain posteriorly into the sphenoethmoidal recess and back into the nasopharynx.

Although acute rhinosinusitis usually is thought to be secondary to a viral upper respiratory infection, the pathophysiologic process of chronic rhinosinusitis is less well understood. The generally accepted position regarding chronic rhinosinusitis is that it reflects a long-standing bac-

terial infection that is unresolved. Obstruction of the OMC is thought to be of central importance in its pathogenesis (9,16,17), and both medical and surgical treatments have been directed to relieving this obstruction. The evidence to support this presumed pathologic process is circumstantial, and the cause of rhinosinusitis remains an object of controversy.

In its generally accepted pathophysiologic model, chronic rhinosinusitis represents a chronic bacterial infection that is in large part due to obstruction of the OMC. The reduction in the cross-sectional area of the ostia creates an increased resistance to both air exchange and drainage, resulting in a disruption in the normal physiology of the sinus chambers (18). This impairment in air exchange results in a relative decrease of the oxygen tension in the sinuses and a relative increase in the carbon dioxide content, leading to decreased mucociliary function and increased recruitment of inflammatory cells (19,20).

Acute and chronic rhinosinusitis traditionally have been considered bacterial diseases. Although acute episodes of rhinosinusitis favor common organisms such as *Streptococcus pneumoniae, Haemophilus influenzae,* and *Moraxella catar-*

*rhalis,* chronic rhinosinusitis is represented by a far wider range of bacteria, including both gram-positive and gram-negative aerobes and anaerobes. Culture patterns vary widely, especially in chronic disease. Recent research has suggested that fungal organisms may play a much more central role in the pathogenesis of chronic rhinosinusitis. In fact, fungal organisms were demonstrated to be present in nearly all cases of chronic rhinosinusitis, with a resultant non–type I-mediated inflammatory response to the organisms (21). Clearly, the view of chronic rhinosinusitis as purely a chronic bacterial infection seems inadequate.

The role of allergy in both acute and chronic rhinosinusitis has been controversial as well. The next portion of this chapter examines research related to this important clinical question.

## ROLE OF ALLERGY IN RHINOSINUSITIS

### Clinical Studies

A link between allergic disease and rhinosinusitis was described as early as 1971 by Sanders, who believed that allergic rhinitis was an important component of the pathogenesis of rhinosinusitis (22). Others over the years have reviewed the literature and reached similar conclusions (23). Similar links also were noted among children with allergy and rhinosinusitis (24).

One major study to investigate the association between allergic disease and rhinosinusitis was conducted by Pelikan and Pelikan-Filipek (25). In this investigation, the authors performed nasal antigen challenges on 37 patients with confirmed chronic rhinosinusitis. The authors noted that 29 of the 37 patients mounted positive responses with increased nasal and sinus symptoms such as pressure and otalgia, and 32 demonstrated changes on sinus radiographs. The authors concluded that exposure to antigen in allergic patients "leads to an edematic [*sic*] obstruction of the nasal ostia, decreased paranasal sinus ciliary action, and increased mucus production" (p. 488). They thought that nasal allergy "may regularly play a role in changes of the mucosal membrane in maxillary sinuses" (p. 490).

In another study, 79 patients with chronic rhinosinusitis were tested for allergy (26). Of this group, 31 patients had perennial allergic rhinitis and 48 patients did not, for a prevalence of allergy of 39%. The authors found that among patients with chronic rhinosinusitis and allergy, there was a significant increase in the number of eosinophils and activated eosinophils, suggesting a pivotal role for type I allergic disease among these patients. In addition, there was a significantly higher level of interleukin (IL)-5 among the allergic patients, again suggesting their allergic etiology. The authors concluded that allergic changes in the nose and sinuses were an important component in the pathogenesis of rhinosinusitis among these patients, both through local inflammatory mechanisms and through edematous obstruction of the sinus ostia.

Slavin and colleagues examined the role of allergy in rhinosinusitis in several investigations. In their methodology, single-photon emission CT (SPECT) scanning was used to assess metabolic activity in the sinuses related to antigen exposure. In one study, increased metabolic activity and hyperemia of the sinuses was noted in season among a group of ragweed-allergic patients, but after ragweed season this activity returned to normal (27). In a related study, a patient who was skin-test positive for ragweed antigen had a nasal challenge with ragweed into one nostril. The patient noted symptoms of rhinitis with increased inflammation on physical examination. SPECT imaging revealed increased activity in the maxillary sinus on the ipsilateral side, but not in the contralateral antrum. No such inflammation was seen in a nonallergic patient with nasal challenge (28).

In another investigation, 224 young healthy adults who had been diagnosed with acute maxillary sinusitis by physical examination and confirmed with sinus radiography and 103 young, healthy adults without maxillary sinusitis were tested with standard skin prick techniques using 12 seasonal and perennial antigens (29). Skin testing yielded positive allergic responses in 102 of 224 patients with rhinosinusitis (45%) and 34 of 103 control subjects (33%). Patients with chronic rhinosinusitis had a higher incidence of allergy on skin testing than patients without chronic rhinosinusitis. The authors concluded that "acute sinusitis seems to be more common in allergic than in non-allergic individuals" (p. 122).

A major, well constructed study was conducted by Newman and associates on 104 patients undergoing surgery for chronic rhinosinusitis (14). In this study, patients were diagnosed with chronic rhinosinusitis based on a combination of history, CT appearance, and physical examination. Patients completed symptom questionnaires and had thorough medical histories taken. CT scans were completed on all patients, and were staged for severity of disease. Specific immunoglobulin E (IgE) antibodies to eight inhalant allergens were assessed by in vitro methodology, and bacterial and fungal cultures were taken at the time of surgery. In addition, peripheral and tissue eosinophilia was assessed. The findings of this study demonstrated that there was a strong association between the extent of disease as assessed by CT scan and the presence of both eosinophilia and IgE antibodies to inhalant allergens. The authors concluded that "allergic individuals . . . are at increased risk for extensive sinus disease . . . than nonallergic patients" (p. 366). Similar findings also were reported by Krouse (30).

Berrettini and colleagues examined the prevalence of abnormal CT appearance of the sinuses in both allergic and nonallergic patients in another study (31). CT scans were scored independently for severity of disease using the Lund-Mackay system (13). Of the 40 allergic patients studied, 27 (67.5%) had sinus stages ranging from 1 to 17. Among the

30 nonallergic patients, only 10 (33.3%) had a CT stage greater than 0. The mean CT stage among patients with allergic disease was 5.5, and among patients without allergic disease, 2.5. These findings were significantly different, demonstrating the presence of worse sinus abnormalities among allergic than nonallergic patients. The authors concluded that "allergic patients exhibit more extensive sinusitis than the general population" (p. 247).

Two other studies have noted similar findings. Lavigne and associates examined the response to surgery among 15 atopic patients undergoing ethmoidectomy and maxillary antrostomy for chronic rhinosinusitis (32). The authors examined both clinical indicators of outcome and immunologic mediators at 0, 6, and 24 months after surgery. Two important findings were noted in the study. Only 7 of the 15 patients with allergic rhinitis who underwent sinus surgical intervention improved after surgery, whereas 8 patients were either unchanged or worse after surgical treatment. In addition, among patients that were worse after surgery, there was a significantly higher level of IL-5 in the ethmoid sinuses at the time of surgery. The authors concluded that patients with elevated levels of IL-5 in their ethmoid sinuses, a marker of symptomatic activity in allergic rhinitis, are likely to have a poorer outcome after sinus surgery.

In a second study, Stewart and associates examined 57 patients undergoing surgical treatment for chronic rhinosinusitis (33). The authors used clinical measures of disease-specific symptom severity and examined various factors as they affected the outcome of surgery. Among these factors, using a multivariate analysis, only two elements of the patient's history correlated with outcome. First, patients with worse CT staging before surgery had the most change in their symptoms after surgery, demonstrating greater improvement and lower postoperative symptomatology. Second, those patients with significant allergic rhinitis had less change after surgery than predicted by the severity of the CT scan. The authors concluded that allergic rhinitis was an independent predictor of success in patients undergoing surgery for chronic rhinosinusitis, and that these patients could expect less improvement after surgery than patients without allergic rhinitis.

Finally, Kennedy studied prognostic factors among patients treated with endoscopic sinus surgery for chronic rhinosinusitis (34). He examined 120 patients over an 8-month postoperative period on both objective measures such as appearance of the surgical site, and on subjective measures such as symptomatic improvement. Although he noted no significant difference between allergic and nonallergic patients in the objective outcome of endoscopic sinus surgery, he did not comment on postoperative subjective symptoms or quality-of-life factors. An important finding in Kennedy's report is the high prevalence of allergy in his surgical patients. Among his group of 120 patients undergoing surgery for chronic rhinosinusitis, 57% were positive for inhalant allergy on either skin or in vitro tests. Kennedy

concludes that "it would appear that allergy may well be a predisposing cause of chronic sinusitis" (p. 12).

## Immunologic Studies

Studies have examined the immunologic mechanisms in allergic disease and their relationship to rhinosinusitis. In one such study, 42 patients with chronic rhinosinusitis were selected for skin testing with inhalant allergens, measurement of serum IgE, and assessment of IgE in sinus mucosa (35). The authors noted that there were significantly higher numbers of eosinophils in the sinus mucosa of allergic patients than there were in the mucosa of nonallergic patients. There was no increase in specific IgE in the sinus tissues themselves. The authors concluded that "allergy may be a predisposing factor to sinusitis and that the pathologic change of the sinus mucosa is mainly secondary, due to sinus ostial obstruction" (p. 252).

Armenaka and colleagues performed an additional study, examining the association of specific IgG to dust mite with the presence of sinus disease (36). The authors reviewed the literature, and noted that rhinosinusitis may be related not to IgE-mediated immune disease, but rather to another immune mechanism. They examined 63 adults with symptomatic chronic rhinosinusitis, obtaining CT scans of the sinuses and measuring dust mite–specific IgG in the serum of these patients. They divided these patients into three groups on the basis of their CT scans: patients without CT changes (rhinitis alone), patients with mild CT changes, and patients with severe CT changes. They compared these three groups of patients with asymptomatic control subjects. The authors noted that serum levels of IgG specific for dust mite antigen were significantly higher in patients with rhinosinusitis than in normal control subjects. This difference was most notable in the patients with severe disease. There was no significant difference in skin testing for dust mites among the patients. The authors believed that their findings suggested an immune-mediated mechanism involved with IgG sensitivity to aeroallergens such as dust mite, and concluded that "there is a statistically significant association between elevated mite IgG and both chronic rhinitis and chronic sinusitis, that is unrelated to mite allergy" (p. 675).

Two studies have demonstrated an elevated level of IL-8 among patients with chronic rhinosinusitis. Takeuchi and colleagues examined levels of IL-8 in nasal and sinus tissues among patients with both chronic rhinosinusitis and allergic rhinitis (37). They noted that IL-8 had been demonstrated to be involved in allergic rhinitis in that it encourages chemotaxis of inflammatory cells important in the pathogenesis of the disease (38,39). Among their patients, they noted that IL-8 also was recovered from the maxillary antral mucosa of patients with chronic rhinosinusitis. They concluded that IL-8 was involved in the chronic inflammatory changes seen in the mucosa of patients with chronic rhinosinusitis, and suggested that IL-8 activation may be related in part to allergic rhinitis.

In a related study, Rhyoo and associates assessed the sinus mucosa among 22 patients undergoing surgery for chronic rhinosinusitis and 9 control subjects for the presence and amount of IL-8 (40). They also obtained CT scans and symptom scores on patients undergoing surgery. The authors found that IL-8 was present in the sinus mucosa of 12 of the 22 patients with chronic rhinosinusitis, but in none of the 9 control subjects. In addition, they noted that there was a significant association between disease severity and levels of IL-8. The authors concluded that IL-8 appeared to be a marker for the severity of symptoms in patients with chronic rhinosinusitis.

Wright and associates examined the role of IL-4 and IL-5 in patients with chronic rhinosinusitis in another study (41). Both IL-4 and IL-5 have been shown in many studies to be important mediators of the allergic response, being secreted by type 2 T helper (Th2) cells in response to antigenic stimulation (42). Although IL-4 had been demonstrated to be of major significance in allergic sensitization, IL-5 was more correlated with symptoms in patients with allergic rhinitis (43). In Wright and colleagues' study, sinus mucosa from patients with chronic rhinosinusitis with and without allergic sensitivity was compared with sinus mucosa harvested from control subjects (41). Results demonstrated that IL-4 was found only among allergic patients with chronic rhinosinusitis, whereas IL-5 was found in both allergic and nonallergic patients. From this study, it would appear that similar Th2-mediated mechanisms may be involved in the expression of symptoms in both chronic rhinosinusitis and allergic rhinitis.

## CONCEPTUAL FRAMEWORK

The aforementioned studies strongly suggest the contributory role of allergic disease among patients with chronic rhinosinusitis. It is clear that chronic rhinosinusitis is not a bacterial disease alone, and that treatments designed to address infection only will fail in many cases. In addition, surgical intervention alone will also be inadequate in many cases because it does not address the underlying inflammatory disease. These findings were described in a study by Krouse and Krouse, who demonstrated that in as many as 26% of patients treated for chronic rhinosinusitis who fail treatment, undiagnosed allergic disease is a major factor in their pathophysiologic process (44). This section discusses a conceptual model of the pathophysiologic process and treatment of patients with chronic rhinosinusitis.

The pathophysiologic process of chronic rhinosinusitis can best be described as an interaction between two broad factors: *adynamic* or fixed or anatomic factors, and *dynamic*

**TABLE 17.3. DYNAMIC AND ADYNAMIC FACTORS IN CHRONIC RHINOSINUSITIS**

**Dynamic factors**
  Allergy
    Inhalant
    Food
  Infection
    Bacterial
    Fungal
    Viral
  Mucosal irritation
  Environmental effects of mucosal condition
    Heat
    Humidity
    Deposition of particulate matter
**Adynamic factors**
  Anatomic abnormalities
    Deviated nasal septum
    Ostiomeatal stenosis
  Postoperative scarring
    Synechiae
    Restenosis
    Lateralization of the middle turbinate
  Ciliary dyskinesias
  Foreign body
  Nasal polyps
  Obstructing neoplasms
  Accessory ostia with recirculation

or variable or physiologic factors (Table 17.3). These factors work synergistically to create underlying conditions in the sinus mucosa that predispose the patient to chronic inflammatory disease. Although in some patients adynamic factors appear to predominate, in others dynamic forces appear to be more central. To understand the pathologic process among individual patients in a clinical setting, this interaction must be considered and treatment directed toward alleviating the relevant dysfunction.

Adynamic or fixed anatomic factors are important in contributing to the pathophysiologic process of chronic rhinosinusitis in that they lead to fixed obstruction of the narrow communicating passages between the sinuses and the nose. As the diameter of the ostia decreases, the resistance to flow of both air into the sinuses and mucous secretion out of the sinuses increases by the fourth power of the radius of the opening. Small changes in ostial diameter therefore can lead to significant resistance to flow through these openings. In addition, as the diameter of the sinus ostia decreases, any swelling of the mucosa lining the bony ostia becomes a more critical factor in pathogenesis. Because patency of the OMC, the infundibulum, and the sphenoid ostium is critical to sinus health, small changes in the passages can be clinically significant. Although the exact dimensions of the ostia necessary to provide normal function are not known, it appears that the creation of large openings is not necessary, and may actually be counterproductive to normal function (45).

Other anatomic abnormalities are known to contribute to the pathophysiologic process of chronic rhinosinusitis. A deviated nasal septum can be displaced into the middle turbinate and middle meatus, narrowing the middle meatus significantly and leading to anatomic obstruction and chronic rhinosinusitis. Abnormal pneumatization can occur during development, leading to obstructive aerated cells such as Haller's cells and agger nasi cells that obstruct the maxillary and frontal ventilation and drainage, respectively. Repeated infection with ostial obstruction can lead to the development of secondary ostia for drainage into the nose, usually through the posterior fontanelle of the lateral nasal wall. These secondary ostia can lead to a phenomenon known as *recirculation,* in which mucous secretion from the maxillary antrum exits the natural ostium only to reenter the secondary ostium, leading to chronic infection.

In addition, postoperative changes frequently lead to fixed obstructions in the nose and sinus ostia. Common complications of sinus surgery include lateralization of the middle turbinate, in which the floppy turbinate shifts in position to obstruct the middle meatus, leading to secondary ethmoid, maxillary, or frontal sinusitis. This complication is seen when the superior attachment of the middle turbinate is destabilized, resulting in the turbinate being drawn into the meatus. An additional complication of surgery is restenosis of the sinus ostia due to hypertrophic scarring. Circumferential removal of tissue and excessive trauma to the mucosa during surgery are predisposing factors to restenosis. In addition, synechiae can form between areas of surgical resection, resulting in narrowness and stenosis of sinus outflow tracts. It is critical in surgical treatment to perform the minimum surgery necessary to improve the patient's anatomic disease and retain normal, healthy mucosa.

Finally, masses in the nose and sinuses, including nasal polyps, can be viewed as adynamic factors. Although polyps clearly have an inflammatory etiology, it is their physical bulk that is critical in the pathogenesis of chronic rhinosinusitis. Obstructing masses such as polyps, inverted papillomas, and other neoplasms can become large enough to obstruct the ostia of the sinuses, and secondary infection and inflammation can occur behind these obstructions.

These adynamic or fixed factors in the pathogenesis of chronic rhinosinusitis are treated primarily with surgical interventions. Little, if any therapeutic effect can be obtained through the use of nonsurgical treatments in these conditions, in that these anatomic factors, with the exception of polyps, are not responsive to topical or systemic medications. It is important, therefore, for the physician to assess the presence of significant anatomic disease and judiciously to recommend surgical treatment when indicated.

In addition to adynamic factors, chronic rhinosinusitis also has as a major component physiologic or dynamic factors that contribute to its pathophysiologic process. As

noted, allergy is one of the primary dynamic factors in the development of chronic sinus disease. As a result of the mucosal edema generated by the allergic response, the narrow sinus ostia become increasingly occluded and predisposed to increasing chronic infection. In addition, IL-5 generated in response to allergic stimulation promotes inflammation and increases symptoms among allergic patients. Increased eosinophilic influx also is stimulated by IL-4 and IL-5, increasing local mucosal inflammation and predisposing to mucosal infection with bacterial and fungal organisms. Allergic stimulation is considered a dynamic factor in that it affects nasal and sinus physiology, and can fluctuate as a function of allergy exposure.

Infection is another dynamic factor in the pathogenesis of chronic rhinosinusitis. Viral, bacterial, and fungal processes commonly affect the sinuses, and can either occur acutely or persist chronically. Acute bacterial rhinosinusitis often follows a viral upper respiratory infection, and responds well to antibiotic therapy with rapid and complete resolution. Chronic rhinosinusitis is a much more complex illness, and does not respond predictably to any discrete treatment. Not only is the infectious component of the disease a pathologic outcome of chronic inflammation, it provides continued stimulation to the chronic disease state. Mucosal inflammation persists in response to the infectious process, causing persistent edema and OMC obstruction. This obstruction in turn prevents clearance of the bacterial component of the process, leading to a vicious cycle of disease. Successful treatment of the bacterial infection through a combination of antimicrobial therapy and surgical drainage and ventilation assists in the resolution of the rhinosinusitis, but in many cases does not bring about complete symptomatic relief. Attention to any adynamic or anatomic abnormalities and other physiologic factors such as allergy is essential in maximizing treatment outcome.

Finally, any environmental factors that contribute to mucosal inflammation in the nose and sinuses must be addressed in the comprehensive treatment of chronic rhinosinusitis. Many agents play a role in sinus health and illness, and attention to these factors can assist in the treatment of chronic rhinosinusitis. Factors as diverse as tobacco smoke, air pollution, and chemical exposures can contribute to mucosal inflammation and interfere with the clearance of chronic rhinosinusitis. These issues need to be considered in the treatment of patients with this disease.

Chronic rhinosinusitis, then, can be conceptualized as an inflammatory disorder with both anatomic and physiologic components that leads to a symptom pattern of chronic disease. There is a complex interaction between these two groups of dynamic and fixed factors that influences the chronicity and resolution of the disease process. Each patient with chronic rhinosinusitis may have a different balance between these two interacting processes, with either anatomic or physiologic components predominating. When considering treatment options for patients, health care providers need to evaluate thoroughly all relevant contributing factors before recommending one specific course of action.

## TREATMENT OF CHRONIC RHINOSINUSITIS

Treatment of chronic rhinosinusitis depends on an adequate diagnosis of the contributing factors to the disease in each patient. Acute rhinosinusitis is easily treated and its management is not discussed in this chapter. The treatment of chronic rhinosinusitis is much more controversial and complex, and receives attention in this portion of the chapter.

The primary treatment of chronic rhinosinusitis has been well described in several major reviews. As Benninger and colleagues discuss (46), rhinosinusitis is multifactorial, and initial medical therapy needs to address these various components of the disease process. Aggressive medical therapy remains the mainstay of treatment for chronic rhinosinusitis. Certainly antibiotic therapy is indicated in the primary treatment of most cases. Broad-spectrum antibiotics such as amoxicillin-clavulanate and quinolones usually are recommended as primary antimicrobial agents, and should be used in the treatment of chronic rhinosinusitis for 4 to 6 weeks.

In addition to addressing the bacterial component of the disease, adjuvant therapies are indicated in the treatment of chronic rhinosinusitis. The use of saline rinses and irrigations can be important in clearing viscous secretions from the nose, moisturizing the nasal mucosa, and improving mucociliary clearance (47). Oral decongestants can be of benefit in alleviating some of the bothersome nasal congestion experienced by these patients. The use of mucolytics and antihistamines remains controversial. Topical nasal steroids, however, have been shown to have good utility in chronic rhinosinusitis, both in the reduction of mucosal edema and in the inhibition of immunomodulatory agents such as IL-4 and IL-5 (48).

McNally and colleagues examined 200 cases of chronic rhinosinusitis treated with aggressive medical therapy (49) Diagnosis of chronic sinusitis was made using criteria similar to those suggested by the AAOHNS Task Force. Treatment consisted of 4 weeks of oral antibiotics, nasal corticosteroids, nasal lavage, and topical decongestants. All symptoms improved with medical therapy, but 12 patients (6%) did not achieve adequate resolution and required endoscopic surgery for treatment of their disease. The authors concluded that medical therapy is appropriate and effective in most patients with chronic rhinosinusitis.

In another review of the treatment of sinusitis, Calhoun also recommended aggressive medical therapy as the primary management of chronic rhinosinusitis (50). She also noted the importance of adjuvant therapy in the treatment of this disease, with more aggressive therapy in patients with allergic rhinitis. Calhoun recommended that antibiotic treatment be accompanied by nasal lavage, decongestants,

mucolytics, and corticosteroids, with consideration given to the use of antihistamines among allergic patients. She also recommended the limited, judicious use of surgery, stating that "sinus surgery to facilitate drainage and permit appropriate ventilation should be reserved for patients no longer responsive to pharmacotherapy and those with anatomic deformities" (p. 850).

Slavin discussed the treatment of chronic rhinosinusitis, and noted that allergic rhinitis was a common predisposing factor to this disease (51). He noted the relationship between mucosal edema and ostial obstruction, as well as the impairment in ciliary function seen in allergic disease and rhinosinusitis. Slavin recommended antibiotic therapy along with adjuvant therapy, including increased fluid intake to decrease mucous tenacity, decongestants, and mucolytics. He also recommended the use of topical corticosteroids to reduce both edema and leukocyte infiltration of the mucosa. The author concluded that surgical therapy is indicated when "sinusitis is persistent or recurs despite appropriate medical therapy" (p. 954).

The use of immunotherapy as an adjuvant modality in the treatment of allergic patients with chronic rhinosinusitis also shows efficacy. Nishioka and colleagues demonstrated that allergic patients who underwent immunotherapy had better long-term outcomes after sinus surgery than did patients whose allergies were not treated (52). Krouse and Krouse, as discussed earlier, noted that the failure to treat allergic disease in patients with chronic rhinosinusitis is associated with poorer outcomes among those patients as well (44). Similar findings were noted by Stewart and associates (33). The strong association between allergic rhinitis and chronic rhinosinusitis suggests that among allergic patients with chronic rhinosinusitis, immunotherapy should be considered as an important component of the comprehensive treatment in this disease. Mabry also states that the failure to treat allergy in these patients may jeopardize the results of endoscopic sinus surgery (53). Because of this significant association and its implications, all patients who are being considered for endoscopic sinus surgery should have a thorough allergy evaluation before undergoing surgery.

Surgical therapy in the treatment of chronic rhinosinusitis has a definite role in the management of severe and refractory disease, and in disease in which severe anatomic factors prevent resolution of the disease with medical management alone. Absolute indications for surgery have been presented by the AAOHNS Task Force, and are displayed in Table 17.4 (54). According to these guidelines, surgery is absolutely indicated in the presence of orbital or intracranial complications of rhinosinusitis, mucocele formation, neoplasm, allergic or invasive fungal sinusitis, and cerebrospinal fluid rhinorrhea. In cases without these severe complications, the primary indication for surgery is failure of aggressive, appropriate medical therapy.

Current surgical strategies rely on functional endoscopic surgical approaches to the sinuses, as discussed by Kennedy

## TABLE 17.4. ABSOLUTE INDICATORS FOR SURGERY IN RHINOSINUSITIS

Bilateral extensive and massive obstructive nasal polyposis with complications
Complications of adult rhinosinusitis
   Subperiosteal or orbital abscess
   Pott's puffy tumor
   Brain abscess
   Meningitis
Chronic adult rhinosinusitis with mucocele or mucopyocele formation
Invasive or allergic fungal adult rhinosinusitis
Diagnosis of tumor of nasal cavity and paranasal sinuses
Cerebrospinal fluid rhinorrhea

From Anand VK, Osguthorpe JD, Rice D. Surgical management of adult rhinosinusitis. *Otolaryngol Head Neck Surg* 1997;117:550–552, with permission.

(55) and Stammberger (16,56). In these techniques, the goal is to reestablish normal patency of occluded areas critical to the function of the affected sinuses. The methods rely on preservation of normal mucosa to enhance healing, decrease crusting and scarring, and encourage restoration of normal mucociliary function. Surgical treatment and specific techniques of surgery are discussed extensively elsewhere, and are not included here.

## CONCLUSION

Chronic rhinosinusitis is a common disorder affecting a large number of adults and children in the United States and throughout the world. Extensive evidence exists to support the central role of allergy in the pathophysiologic process of this chronic disease. Allergy acts as a predisposing factor in the pathogenesis of chronic rhinosinusitis, and contributes to the ongoing cycle of inflammation that is characteristic of this multifaceted disease.

Chronic rhinosinusitis can be viewed as a complex interaction between two broad factors: dynamic or physiologic factors, and adynamic or anatomic factors. The relative contributions of each of these factors differ from patient to patient, and their balance determines the role for various modalities in the treatment of the chronic process. Dynamic factors require attention to the various physiologic agents and processes involved in the development of chronic rhinosinusitis, whereas adynamic factors primarily are related to the structure and patency of the bony and cartilaginous framework of the nose and sinuses. The treatment of dynamic factors involves pharmacotherapy, environmental management, and immunotherapy, whereas anatomic abnormalities may require surgical treatment.

It is critical for physicians to understand this conceptual framework for chronic rhinosinusitis, and to implement di-

agnostic and treatment protocols with appreciation for the various contributing factors to the illness. Surgery is indicated primarily in the case of severe anatomic deformity with obstruction, complications of sinusitis, and failure of aggressive and adequate medical management. Before considering surgery, and with an appreciation of the common presence of allergic disease in patients with chronic rhinosinusitis, all patients for whom surgical intervention is planned require allergy evaluation and appropriate allergy management if indicated.

## REFERENCES

1. National Center for Health Statistics. *Vital and health statistics: current estimates from National Health Interview Survey No. 190.* Washington, DC: U.S. Department of Health and Human Services, 1994.
2. Lanza DC, Kennedy DW. Adult rhinosinusitis defined. *Otolaryngol Head Neck Surg* 1997;117:S1–S7.
3. Gliklich RE, Metson R. The health impact of chronic sinusitis in patients seeking otolaryngologic care. *Otolaryngol Head Neck Surg* 1995;113:104–109.
4. Kaliner MA, Osguthorpe JD, Fireman P, et al. Sinusitis: bench to bedside—current findings, future directions. *J Allergy Clin Immunol* 1997;99:S829–S847.
5. Lund VJ, Kennedy DW. Quantification for staging sinusitis: the staging and therapy group. *Ann Otol Rhinol Laryngol Suppl* 1995; 167:17–21.
6. Reilly JS. The sinusitis cycle. *Otolaryngol Head Neck Surg* 1990; 103:856–862.
7. Shapiro GG, Rachelfsky GS. Introduction and definition of sinusitis. *J Allergy Clin Immunol* 1992;90:417–418.
8. Stankiewicz J, Osguthorpe JD. Medical treatment of sinusitis. *Otolaryngol Head Neck Surg* 1994;110:361–362.
9. Ferguson BJ. Acute and chronic sinusitis. *Postgrad Med* 1995; 97:45–57.
10. Evans FO, Sydnor JB, Moore WEC, et al. Sinusitis of the maxillary antrum. *N Engl J Med* 1975;293:735–739.
11. Williams JW, Simel DL. Does this patient have sinusitis? Diagnosing acute sinusitis by history and physical examination. *JAMA* 1993;270:1242–1246.
12. International Rhinosinusitis Advisory Board. Infectious rhinosinusitis in adults: classification, etiology, and management. *Ear Nose Throat J* 1997;76:1–22.
13. Lund VJ, Kennedy DW. Staging and therapy group: quantification for staging sinusitis. *Ann Otol Rhinol Laryngol Suppl* 1995; 104:17–21.
14. Newman LJ, Platts-Mills TAE, Phillips D, et al. Chronic sinusitis: relationship of computed tomographic findings to allergy, asthma, and eosinophilia. *JAMA* 1994;271:363–367.
15. Stammberger H. *Functional endoscopic sinus surgery.* Philadelphia: Decker, 1991.
16. Stammberger H. Endoscopic endonasal surgery—concepts in treatment of recurring rhinosinusitis. Part I: anatomic and pathophysiologic considerations. *Otolaryngol Head Neck Surg* 1986;94: 143–147.
17. Gwaltney JM Jr, Scheld WM, Sande MA, et al. The microbial etiology and antimicrobial therapy of adults with acute community-acquired sinusitis: a fifteen-year experience at the University of Virginia and review of other selected studies. *J Allergy Clin Immunol* 1992;90:457–462.
18. Aust R, Stierna P, Drettner B. Basic experimental studies of ostial

patency and local metabolic environment of the maxillary sinus. *Acta Otolaryngol Suppl (Stockh)* 1994;515:7–11.

19. Norlander T, Westrin KM, Stierna P. The inflammatory response of the sinus and nasal mucosa during sinusitis: implications for research and therapy. *Arch Otolaryngol Suppl (Stockh)* 1994;515:38–44.

20. Westrin KM, Stierna P, Soderlund K. Microorganisms and leukocytes in purulent sinusitis: a symbiotic relationship in metabolism. *Acta Otolaryngol Suppl (Stockh)* 1994;515:18–21.

21. Ponikau JU, Sherris DA, Kern EB, et al. The diagnosis and incidence of allergic fungal sinusitis. *Mayo Clin Proc* 1999;74:877–884.

22. Sanders SH. Allergic rhinitis and sinusitis. *Otolaryngol Clin North Am* 1971;4:565–578.

23. Spector SL. The role of allergy in sinusitis in adults. *J Allergy Clin Immunol* 1992;90:518–520.

24. Furukawa CT. The role of allergy in sinusitis in children. *J Allergy Clin Immunol* 1992;90:515–517.

25. Pelikan Z, Pelikan-Filipek M. Role of nasal allergy in chronic maxillary sinusitis: diagnostic value of nasal challenge with allergen. *J Allergy Clin Immunol* 1990;86:484–491.

26. Suzuki M, Watanabe T, Suko T, et al. Comparison of sinusitis with and without allergic rhinitis: characteristics of paranasal sinus effusion and mucosa. *Am J Otolaryngol* 1999;20:143–150.

27. Slavin RG, Zilliox AP, Samuels LD. Is there such an entity as allergic sinusitis? *J Allergy Clin Immunol* 1988;81:284.

28. Borts MR, Slavin RG, Samuels LD, et al. Spectral positron emission computerized tomography (SPECT). *J Allergy Clin Immunol* 1989;83:302.

29. Savolainen S. Allergy in patients with acute maxillary sinusitis. *Allergy* 1989;44:116–122.

30. Krouse JH. CT stage, allergy testing, and quality of life in sinusitis. *Otolaryngol Head Neck Surg* 2000;123:389–392.

31. Berrettini S, Carabelli A, Sellari-Franceschini S, et al. Perennial allergic rhinitis and chronic sinusitis: correlation with rhinologic risk factors. *Allergy* 1999;54:242–248.

32. Lavigne F, Nguyen CT, Cameron L, et al. Prognosis and prediction of response to surgery in allergic patients with chronic sinusitis. *J Allergy Clin Immunol* 2000;105:746–751.

33. Stewart MG, Donovan DT, Parke RB Jr, et al. Does the severity of sinus computed tomography findings predict outcome in chronic sinusitis? *Otolaryngol Head Neck Surg* 2000;123:81–84.

34. Kennedy DW. Prognostic factors, outcomes and staging in ethmoid sinus surgery. *Laryngoscope* 1992;102[Suppl 57]:1–18.

35. Liu CM, Shun CT, Song HC, et al. Investigation into allergic response in patients with chronic sinusitis. *J Formos Med Assoc* 1992;91:252–257.

36. Armenaka MC, Grizzanti JN, Oriel N, et al. Increased immune reactivity to house dust mites in adults with chronic rhinosinusitis. *Clin Exp Allergy* 1993;23:669–677.

37. Takeuchi K, Yuta A, Sakakura Y. Interleukin-8 gene expression in chronic sinusitis. *Am J Otolaryngol* 1995;16:95–102.

38. Leonard EJ, Skeel A, Yoshimura T, et al. Leukocyte specificity and binding of human neutrophil and attractant/activating protein. *J Immunol* 1990;144:1323–1330.

39. Lee HS, Majima Y, Sakakura Y, et al. Quantitative cytology of nasal secretions under various conditions. *Laryngoscope* 1993;103:533–537.

40. Rhyoo C, Sanders SP, Leopold DA, et al. Sinus mucosal IL-8 gene expression in chronic rhinosinusitis. *J Allergy Clin Immunol* 1999;103:395–400.

41. Wright ED, Frenkiel S, Al-Ghamdi K, et al. Interleukin-4, interleukin-5, and granulocyte-macrophage colony-stimulating factor receptor expression in chronic sinusitis and response to topical steroids. *Otolaryngol Head Neck Surg* 1998;118:490–495.

42. Moverare R, Rak S, Elfman L. Allergen-specific increase in interleukin (IL)-4 and IL-5 secretion from peripheral blood mononuclear cells during birch-pollen immunotherapy. *Allergy* 1998;53:275–281.

43. Nakai Y, Ohashi Y, Kakinoki Y, et al. Allergen-induced mRNA expression of IL-5, but not of IL-4 and IFN-gamma, in peripheral blood mononuclear cells is a key feature of clinical manifestation of seasonal allergic rhinitis. *Arch Otolaryngol Head Neck Surg* 2000;126:992–996.

44. Krouse JH, Krouse HJ. Patient use of traditional and complementary therapies in treating rhinosinusitis before consulting an otolaryngologist. *Laryngoscope* 1999;109:1223–1227.

45. Setliff RC III. The small-hole technique in endoscopic sinus surgery. *Otolaryngol Clin North Am* 1997;30:341–354.

46. Benninger MS, Anon J, Mabry RL. The medical management of rhinosinusitis. *Otolaryngol Head Neck Surg* 1997;117:S41–S49.

47. Nuutinen J, Holopainen E, Haaketela T, et al. Balanced physiologic saline in the treatment of chronic sinusitis. *Rhinology* 1986;24:265–269.

48. Meltzer EP, Orgel HA, Backhaus JW, et al. Intranasal flunisolide spray as an adjunct to oral antibiotic therapy for sinusitis. *J Allergy Clin Immunol* 1993;92:812–823.

49. McNally PA, White MV, Kaliner MA. Sinusitis in an allergist's office: analysis of 200 consecutive cases. *Allergy Asthma Proc* 1997;18:169–175.

50. Calhoun K. Diagnosis and management of sinusitis in the allergic patient. *Otolaryngol Head Neck Surg* 1992;107:850–854.

51. Slavin RG. Sinusitis in adults and its relation to allergic rhinitis, asthma, and nasal polyps. *J Allergy Clin Immunol* 1988;82:950–956.

52. Nishioka GJ, Cook PR, McKinsey JP. Immunotherapy in patients undergoing functional endoscopic sinus surgery. *Otolaryngol Head Neck Surg* 1994;110:406–412.

53. Mabry RL. Allergic and infective rhinosinusitis: differential diagnosis and interrelationship. *Otolaryngol Head Neck Surg* 1994;111:335–339.

54. Anand VK, Osguthorpe JD, Rice D. Surgical management of adult rhinosinusitis. *Otolaryngol Head Neck Surg* 1997;117:S50–S52.

55. Kennedy DW, Zinreich SJ, Rosenbaum A, et al. Functional endoscopic sinus surgery: theory and diagnosis. *Arch Otolaryngol* 1985;111:576–582.

56. Stammberger H. Endoscopic endonasal surgery—concepts in the treatment of recurring rhinosinusitis. Part II: surgical technique. *Otolaryngol Head Neck Surg* 1986;94:147–156.

# 18

# ALLERGIC FUNGAL SINUSITIS

## BRADLEY F. MARPLE
## RICHARD L. MABRY

In less than two decades, allergic fungal sinusitis (AFS) has evolved from a curiosity to an increasingly recognized condition. The combination of polyposis, crust formation, and sinus cultures yielding *Aspergillus* was first noted in 1976 by Safirstein (1), who observed the clinical similarity that this constellation of findings shared with allergic bronchopulmonary aspergillosis. This description was followed by reports of "allergic aspergillosis of the paranasal sinuses" (2), and "allergic *Aspergillus* sinusitis" (3–5). The term *allergic fungal sinusitis* was introduced by Robson and colleagues (6) in 1989 after reports that this condition could be caused by a number of different fungi, most of them classified as darkly pigmented, or dematiaceous.

## ASSOCIATED FUNGI: THE ROLE OF DEMATIACEOUS FUNGI

A word of explanation should be given regarding the difference between "fungi" and "molds." The term *fungus* is more inclusive, and embraces yeasts, smuts, rusts, and mushrooms. Fungi other than mushrooms usually are collectively called *molds*. The molds of allergenic significance are contained in the group called *fungi imperfecta,* and it is to this group that most allergists refer when they use the term *mold*. The organisms typically cultured in AFS, such as *Bipolaris* and *Aspergillus,* are usually called *fungi*. Although we most often speak of *fungi* when dealing with a causative organism, and *molds* when dealing with antigens for immunotherapy, the terms may be used interchangeably.

Because of the limited resources for fungal cultures available in most laboratories and the intrinsic difficulty posed by performing fungal cultures, initial attempts at culturing fungi from patients with AFS resulted in low growth rates. It was the morphologic appearance of the fungal hyphae identified in eosinophilic mucin of AFS, coupled with the recognized clinical and immunologic similarities shared between AFS and allergic bronchopulmonary aspergillosis (ABPA), that understandably led to the early implication of *Aspergillus* species as the primary causative fungal pathogen. This notion was further supported by early serologic testing, published by Katzenstein et al., demonstrating elevated specific immunoglobulin E (IgE) to *Aspergillus flavus* in two patients with AFS (5). As more culture-specific fungal information regarding AFS was published, it became apparent that many fungal species could be associated with the disease (7).

Most human fungal disease is caused by three groups of fungi; Zygomycetes, *Aspergillus,* and the dematiaceous family. Zygomycetes, and to some extent *Aspergillus,* are primarily associated with invasive fungal disease in immunocompromised hosts, whereas most allergic fungal disease is associated with *Aspergillus* and the dematiaceous fungi. Dematiaceous fungi, long recognized for the role they play in inhalant allergy, consist of the genera *Bipolaris, Curvularia, Exserohilum, Alternaria, Drechslera, Helminthosporium,* and *Fusarium*. In a 1996 review of the English literature performed by Manning, 263 cases of AFS were identified, of which 168 cases yielded positive fungal cultures. Of these 168 positive cultures, 87% were from the dematiaceous genera, whereas only 13% yielded *Aspergillus* (8). Similar observations led Robson et al. to introduce the broader term, *AFS* (6).

## CONTROVERSY: INFECTIOUS OR ALLERGIC?

The presence of fungi in the paranasal sinuses has raised questions concerning the potential for tissue invasion. Early attempts to treat AFS were influenced by the belief that fungi in the paranasal sinuses represented a potentially fatal variant of invasive fungal sinusitis. As a result, extensive surgical debridement followed by therapy with systemic and topical antifungal agents was routine. Gungor et al. (9) reported an occurrence of invasive fungal sinusitis after renal transplantation in a patient who had previously been treated for a fungus ball, suggesting a potential risk of progressive fungal invasion arising from noninvasive disease in an im-

**B. F. Marple and R. L. Mabry:** Department of Otolaryngology, University of Texas Southwestern Medical Center, Dallas, Texas.

munocompromised host. Aside from a few anecdotal reports, evidence supportive of AFS acting as a preliminary step in the development of invasive disease has been lacking. Clarification of this controversy, however, is critical to choices about treatment for AFS, as Corey et al. have noted (10). If AFS truly represents an allergic disease, then the use of systemic antifungal medications, such as amphotericin B or itraconazole, would provide little benefit and could result in potentially significant toxic side effects. On the other hand, corticosteroids could be counterproductive if AFS acts as a precursor to invasive fungal disease.

This controversy was objectively addressed by Manning and Holman (11) in two separate studies. In the first study, eight patients with culture-positive *Bipolaris* AFS were prospectively compared with ten control subjects who did not have AFS. Both groups were evaluated with (a) radioallergosorbent (RAST) and enzyme-linked immunosorbent assay (ELISA) inhibition to *Bipolaris*-specific IgE and IgG antibodies; and (b) skin testing with *Bipolaris* antigen. All eight patients had positive skin test reactions to *Bipolaris* antigen as well as positive RAST and ELISA inhibition to *Bipolaris*-specific IgE and IgG. Eight of the ten control subjects had negative results on both skin and serologic testing, implicating the importance of allergy to fungal antigens (both in vivo and in vitro) in the pathogenesis of AFS.

In a complementary study (11), sinus mucosal specimens from 14 patients with AFS were compared with those from 10 control subjects who did not have AFS. Immunohistochemical analysis for eosinophilic mediators (major basic protein and eosinophilic-derived neurotoxin) and a neutrophil-derived mediator (neutrophil elastase) was done to assess the underlying nature of inflammation. Eosinophilic-derived mediators were much more common ($p < 0.00001$) than neutrophil-derived mediators in the AFS group, whereas significant differences were not seen in the control group. The predominance of eosinophilic-derived mediators further supports the association between noninfectious (i.e., allergic) inflammation and AFS.

The concept of eosinophilic activation associated with

AFS was further emphasized by Feger et al. (12), who studied eosinophilic cationic protein levels in the serum and mucin of patients with AFS. No differences in serum eosinophilic cationic protein were detected between patients with AFS and control subjects, but eosinophilic cationic protein levels were significantly higher in the mucin of patients with AFS ($p < 0.01$).

Studies such as those by Manning and Holman (11) and Fager et al. (12) offer strong immunologic and histologic data to support the argument that AFS represents an immunologically mediated disorder rather than a point on the spectrum of infectious fungal disease.

## PATHOPHYSIOLOGY

It is postulated that the pathophysiologic process of AFS is similar to that of allergic bronchopulmonary fungal disease (a term replacing *bronchopulmonary aspergillosis*). Manning and colleagues (13) have suggested that several interrelated factors and events lead to the development and perpetuation of AFS (Fig. 18.1). First, an atopic host is exposed to fungi, theoretically through normal nasal respiration, which provides the initial antigenic stimulus. An initial inflammatory response ensues as the result of both a Gel and Coombs type I (IgE mediated) and type III (immune complex mediated) reaction, causing subsequent tissue edema. The resulting obstruction of sinus ostia, which may be accentuated by anatomic factors such as septal deviation or turbinate hypertrophy, results in stasis in the sinuses. This creates an ideal environment for further proliferation of the fungus, thus increasing the antigenic exposure to which the host is allergic. At some point, the cycle becomes self-perpetuating, resulting in the eventual product of this process, allergic mucin—the material that fills the involved sinuses of patients with AFS. The accumulation of this debris obstructs the involved sinuses and propagates the process.

It is the production of this allergic mucin and its eventual clinical, histologic, and radiographic characteristics that are

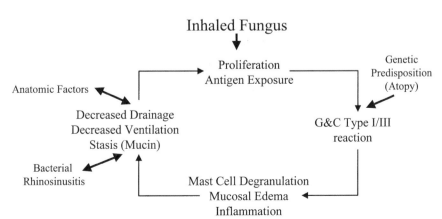

**FIG. 18.1.** Pathogenic cycle of allergic fungal sinusitis, as proposed by Manning et al. (11), with permission.

unique to AFS, and serve as a hallmark of the disease. Grossly, allergic fungal mucin is thick, tenacious, and highly viscous in consistency; its color may vary from light tan to brown or dark green (14,15). Its characteristic gross appearance has resulted in the use of such descriptive terms as *peanut butter* and *axle grease* when referring to allergic fungal mucin.

## EPIDEMIOLOGY

Allergic fungal sinusitis usually is recognized as a disease distinct from other fungal forms of sinusitis. Most common among adolescents and young adults (mean age at diagnosis, 21.9 years) (11), it is invariably associated with nasal polyposis and the presence of allergic fungal mucin. It is estimated that approximately 5% to 10% of patients with chronic rhinosinusitis actually carry a diagnosis of AFS (15–18). Atopy is characteristic of the disease: roughly two thirds of patients report a history of allergic rhinitis, and 90% show elevated specific IgE to one or more fungal antigens. Approximately 50% of the patients in a series by Manning et al. had asthma. No linkage to aspirin sensitivity has been established (11).

The incidence of AFS appears to be affected by geographic factors. Review of the world's literature reveals most sites reporting cases of AFS to be located in temperate regions of relatively high humidity (9,18). Ferguson et al. (19) performed a questionnaire-based study to assess the regional incidence of AFS. This information was compared with respective local mold counts. Insufficient mold spore data during the reporting period of this study resulted in no discernible correlation between the regional incidence of AFS and available mold counts. The incidence of AFS, however, varied remarkably based on the location of reporting sites. AFS in the United States was most commonly encountered in the Mississippi basin, the Southeast, and the Southwest. The reason for this geographic difference remains unexplained.

## CLINICAL PRESENTATION

### History and Physical

Occasionally, the presentation of AFS may be dramatic, giving rise to acute visual loss (20), gross facial dysmorphia (13,21), or complete nasal obstruction. Patients may alternatively present with extensive nasal polyposis, chronic sinusitis (unilateral at first but often becoming bilateral), or recalcitrant disease, often recurring despite several surgeries. More often, the presentation of AFS is subtle. Patients typically complain of gradual nasal airway obstruction and production of semisolid nasal crusts that, on inquiry, match the gross description of allergic fungal mucin. The develop-

ment of nasal airway obstruction may have been so gradual that the patient is unaware of its presence. Likewise, if facial dysmorphia is present, its progression often is so slow that its identification escapes the patient and family members. Pain is uncommon among patients with AFS and suggests the concomitant presence of a bacterial rhinosinusitis (14, 22).

Patients with AFS are atopic but usually have been unresponsive to antihistamines, intranasal corticosteroids, and prior immunotherapy. The use of systemic corticosteroids may produce some relief of symptoms, but relapse is typical after completion of therapy. In contrast to patients with invasive fungal sinusitis, patients with AFS are axiomatically immunocompetent (22).

The range of physical findings on examination typically is broad, ranging from nasal airway obstruction resulting from intranasal inflammation and polyposis to gross facial disfigurement (Fig. 18.2) and orbital or ocular abnormalities. The slow accumulation of allergic fungal mucin imparts unique and rather predictable characteristics to the disease. Allergic fungal mucin is sequestered in involved paranasal sinus cavities. As its quantity increases, the involved parana-

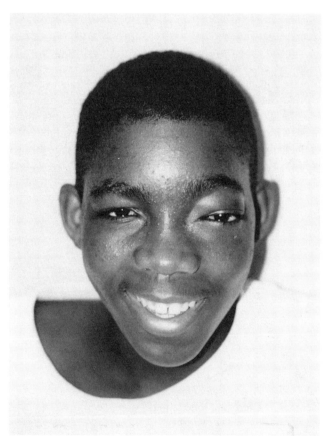

**FIG. 18.2.** Left malar prominence resulting from the expansile growth of left-sided ethmoid and maxillary allergic fungal sinusitis.

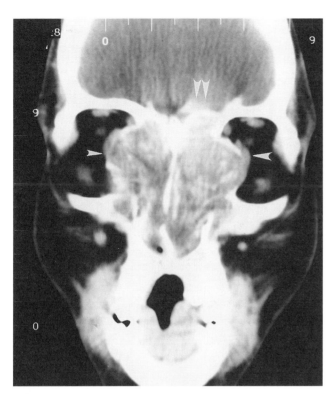

**FIG. 18.3.** Coronal computed tomography (CT) scan demonstrating expansion of allergic fungal sinusitis into the orbits *(single arrows)* and anterior cranial fossa *(double arrows)*. Despite the massive encroachment noted on this CT scan, no fungal invasion of tissue was present.

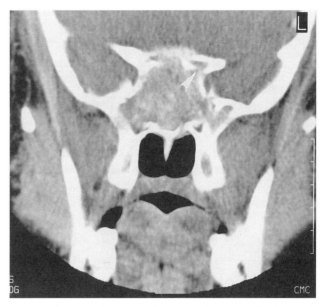

**FIG. 18.4.** Coronal computed tomography scans of sphenoethmoid allergic fungal sinusitis. Note encroachment into the optic canal *(arrow)* responsible for visual loss.

sal sinus begins to resemble and behave in a way consistent with a mucocele (sometimes referred to as a *fungal mucocele*) (20). With time, bony remodeling and decalcification may occur, causing the disease to mimic "invasion" into adjacent anatomic spaces (Fig. 18.3). The location of bone destruction seems to be determined simply by the location of the disease, and this destruction often gives rise to exophthalmos, facial dysmorphia, or intracranial extension without tissue invasion (23).

At times, the extension of AFS into adjacent anatomic spaces can produce a dramatic clinical presentation. Highlighting the ocular manifestations of AFS, Carter et al. (24) reported six affected patients who presented with objective unilateral proptosis. This led them to report proptosis as the most common ophthalmologic manifestation of AFS. In a study by Marple et al. (20), 82 patients with AFS were reviewed for specific ophthalmologic complications. Orbital involvement without visual loss was found in 14.6% of the patients and most commonly resulted in proptosis (encountered in 6.1% of patients) and telecanthus (7.3%). Visual loss from AFS, encountered in 3.7% of the patients in this series, was reversible with immediate surgical treatment of the underlying disease (Fig. 18.4).

## Radiologic Findings

The accumulation of allergic fungal mucin eventually leads to the increasingly well recognized radiographic findings characteristic of AFS. A study of sinus computed tomography (CT) scans from 45 patients with AFS objectively supports several previous clinical observations (25). AFS, although bilateral in 51% of the cases reviewed, caused asymmetric involvement of the paranasal sinuses in 78% of the cases. Bone erosion and extension of disease into adjacent anatomic areas was encountered in 20% of the patients and was more likely to occur in the presence of bilateral, advanced disease. No difference was detected in the incidence of intracranial and orbital extension. Expansion, remodeling, or thinning of involved sinus walls was common (and was thought to be due to the expansile nature of the accumulating mucin). Areas of high attenuation were found in the expanded paranasal sinuses in all patients (Fig. 18.5). The authors point out that the CT specificity of diagnosing AFS could not be inferred from these findings because of the retrospective design of the study. Similar radiographic findings can be caused by rare osteoid/chondroid matrix–producing sinonasal sarcomas or meningiomas.

To characterize further the patterns of bone erosion associated with AFS, Nussenbaum et al. (23) reviewed CT scans of 142 patients treated for AFS at a single institution. As seen in prior studies, bone erosion was encountered in approximately 20% of the patients studied. A statistically significant association was identified between expansion of paranasal sinuses involved with disease and the presence of bone erosion. The ethmoid sinus was the most commonly

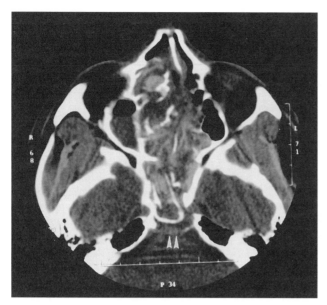

**FIG. 18.5.** Axial computed tomography scan demonstrating several characteristics of allergic fungal sinusitis, including asymmetric involvement, expansion and remodeling of bony walls, areas of varied signal intensity in involved sinuses, and bone erosion *(double arrows).*

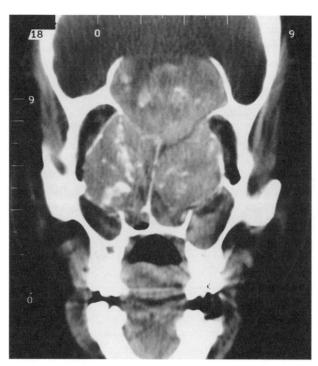

**FIG. 18.6.** Coronal computed tomography scans demonstrating areas of signal heterogeneity in sinuses filled with allergic fungal mucin.

involved sinus, whereas the adjacent lamina papyracea was the most common bone to exhibit demineralization. Extension of AFS beyond the confines of the paranasal sinuses most commonly occurred into the orbit, followed by the anterior, middle, and posterior cranial fossae, respectively. Despite the sometimes remarkable extension into adjacent anatomic spaces, no cases of histologic invasion were identified.

Heterogeneous areas of signal intensity in paranasal sinuses filled with allergic fungal mucin are frequently identified on CT scans (Fig. 18.6). Although these findings are not specific for AFS, they remain relatively characteristic of the disease, and may provide preoperative information supportive of a diagnosis of AFS. This characteristic, which is best identified using soft tissue algorithms on CT, has been the focus of some interest. An initial theory proposed that hemosiderin in inspissated mucin was responsible for the areas of increased signal intensity. This was disputed by Zinreich et al. (26), who were unable to identify increased hemosiderin in typical allergic fungal mucin (25). Current evidence points to the presence of accumulations of heavy metals (e.g., iron and manganese) and calcium salt precipitation in inspissated allergic fungal mucin (25) as the most likely cause of these radiographic findings.

Magnetic resonance imaging (MRI) also can provide information useful in preoperative identification of allergic fungal mucin. Som and Curtin (27) have pointed out that protein concentrations exceeding 28% cause a decreased signal on both T1 and T2- weighted MRIs because of pro-

tein cross-linking and slower macromolecular motion. This effect is more pronounced on T2-weighted images as a result of prolonged magnetic field relaxation times. The high protein and low water concentration of allergic fungal mucin, coupled with the high water content in surrounding edematous paranasal sinus mucosa, give rise to rather specific MR characteristics (Fig. 18.7). Manning et al. (28), in a series of 10 cases of AFS, demonstrated that hypointense central T1 signal, central T2 signal void, and the presence of increased peripheral T1/T2 enhancement was highly specific for AFS compared with other forms of fungal sinusitis (invasive fungal sinusitis and fungal ball) and mucocele. The combined CT and MRI findings provided a radiographic appearance that was highly specific for AFS (28).

## Laboratory Findings

### Immunologic Testing

Total IgE values usually are elevated in AFS, often to more than 1,000 U/mL. The total IgE level has traditionally been used to follow the clinical activity of allergic bronchopulmonary fungal disease. Based on similar IgE behavior associated with recurrence of AFS, total IgE levels have been proposed as a useful indicator of AFS clinical activity (12,29–31).

Patients with AFS usually demonstrate positive skin test and in vitro (RAST) responses for both to fungal and nonfungal antigens (Table 18.1). The sensitivity of RAST was

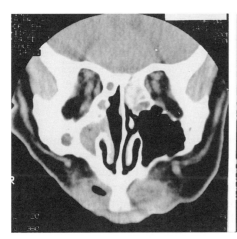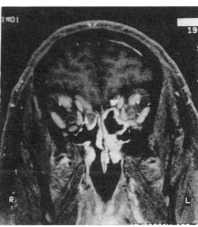

**FIG. 18.7.** Comparison of computed tomography scan and T1-weighted magnetic resonance image (MRI) of the same patient with allergic fungal sinusitis. Note that MRI *(right)* results in a decrease of signal intensity in involved paranasal sinuses filled with allergic fungal mucin. (Reprinted with permission from Manning et al. [11].)

first demonstrated by Manning et al. (32), who compared 16 patients with histologically confirmed AFS with a control group with chronic rhinosinusitis. Levels of fungal-specific IgE were uniformly elevated in all patients with AFS and corresponded with the results of fungal cultures; in contrast, levels of fungal-specific IgE were not elevated in the control group. Moreover, patients with AFS appear to demonstrate a broad sensitivity to a number of fungal and nonfungal antigens. Mabry et al. (33) reported their experience indicating that patients wit AFS are allergic to multiple fungal antigens, as well as many typical nonfungal antigens.

Preliminary information suggests that methods of quantitative skin testing (in vivo) may provide even greater sensitivity ratings than RAST (33) in patients with AFS. RAST traditionally has been considered less sensitive than skin testing for the investigation of atopy involving fungi. This has been attributed to technical problems, such as difficulty in binding the mold antigen to the carrier substrate. To study the validity of this concept, Mabry et al. (33) prospectively evaluated 10 patients with AFS for sensitivity to 11 pertinent fungi by both RAST and dilutional intradermal testing. A predictable correlation between RAST and skin test scores was observed in many, but not all, cases. Most often, this disparity was in the form of greater sensitivity indicated by skin testing than by RAST, sometimes differing by as many as three classes. The lack of concordance was not confined to testing for fungi cultured from the sinuses, nor was it more or less pronounced in the case of dematiaceous fungi. The most likely causes for the disparity were thought to involve subtle differences in antigens used in skin test material compared with RAST standards. In addition, skin testing allowed for observation of delayed and late-phase reactions, a measure not possible by specific IgE testing with RAST. This study appears to emphasize the importance of both skin testing and specific IgE testing by RAST in the initial evaluation of patients with suspected AFS.

Gell and Coombs type I hypersensitivity in patients with AFS can be been demonstrated by both elevation of serum total and fungal-specific IgE, (31,32), as well as by positive skin test results for both fungal and nonfungal antigens. This reaction does not, however, appear to be fungal specific. Sensitivity to numerous fungi has been indicated by both in vitro (RAST) and in vivo methods (skin testing), although usually only a single fungus is isolated by culture of corresponding allergic fungal mucin. This has been thought previously to represent either a common fungal epitope or a genetic predisposition toward fungal allergy in AFS. Chrzanowski et al. (34) identified the presence of an 18-kd protein in allergic mucin obtained from patients with AFS, which may represent such a "pan-antigen."

### Histologic Examination of Allergic Fungal Mucin

Allergic fungal mucin normally is first encountered at the time of surgery; therefore, recognition of its presence is the

**TABLE 18.1. FUNGAL ANTIGENS IN CURRENT TESTING AND TREATMENT PROTOCOL AT THE UNIVERSITY OF TEXAS SOUTHWESTERN MEDICAL CENTER AT DALLAS**[a]

| |
|---|
| Helminthosporium |
| Alternaria |
| Stemphyllium |
| Curvularia |
| Aspergillus |
| Epicoccum |
| Fusarium |
| Mucor |
| Pullularia |
| Cladosporium |
| Penicillium |

[a]In approximate relative order of local (Dallas, TX) importance. From Mabry RL, Marple FB, Folker RJ, et al. Immunotherapy for allergic fungal sinusitis: three years' experience. *Otolaryngol Head Neck Surg* 1998;119:648–651, with permission.

initial step in establishing an accurate diagnosis of AFS. It is the mucin, rather than paranasal sinus mucosa, that demonstrates the histologic appearance consistent with AFS (35–38). Examination of mucosa and polyps obtained from involved paranasal sinuses reveals findings consistent with the inflammation of a chronic inflammatory process, and should be done to establish that no fungal invasion is present (36).

Once mucin is collected, both culture and pathologic examination is undertaken.

Initially described by Millar et al. (2), Lamb et al. (3), and Katzenstein et al. (5), histologic examination of allergic mucin reveals a constellation of characteristic findings. Branching noninvasive fungal hyphae are identified in sheets of eosinophils and elongated eosinophilic bodies (Charcot-Leyden crystals), which represent the product of eosinophilic degradation. Use of various histologic staining techniques helps to identify the variety of components in allergic fungal mucin. Hematoxylin and eosin (H&E) staining accentuates the mucin and cellular components of allergic fungal mucin. Using this stain, background mucin often takes on a chondroid appearance, whereas eosinophils and Charcot-Leyden crystals are heavily stained and become easily detected. Fungi fail to stain using this technique and may therefore be difficult to identify. The presence of fungi may be implicated on H&E stain by their resulting negative image against an otherwise stained background. Fungal hyphae and elements, however, often are rare, scattered, and fragmented in allergic mucin, rendering identification difficult unless specific histologic stains are used. Fungal elements are recognized for a unique ability to absorb silver. This property is the basis for various silver stains, such as

Grocott's or Gomori's Metamine silver stain, which turns fungi black or dark brown (Fig. 18.8). The use of a fungal stain complements the findings of initial H&E staining, and is extremely important in the identification of fungi.

### Culture of Fungi

Fungal cultures of allergic fungal mucin, typically obtained at the time of surgery, may provide some supportive evidence helpful in the diagnosis and subsequent treatment of AFS. However, the diagnosis of AFS is not established, nor is it eliminated, based on the results of this culture. This is due to the variable yield of fungal cultures (64% to 100%) (8) and the recognized saprophytic nature of fungi. When positive, fungal cultures from allergic fungal mucin of patients with AFS often, but not always, isolate a single species. In a 1996 review of the English literature performed by Manning (8), 263 cases of AFS were identified, of which 168 yielded positive cultures. Of these 168 positive cultures, 87% were dematiaceous genera, including *Bipolaris* (including *Drechslera*) (45%), *Curvularia* (26%), *Alternaria* (7%), and *Exserohilum* (5%), whereas only 13% yielded *Aspergillus*.

### DIAGNOSTIC CRITERIA

Consensus is lacking about diagnostic criteria for AFS. Allphin and colleagues (16) described certain features they thought differentiated AFS from other forms of fungal sinusitis: radiographic presence of multiple, opacified parana-

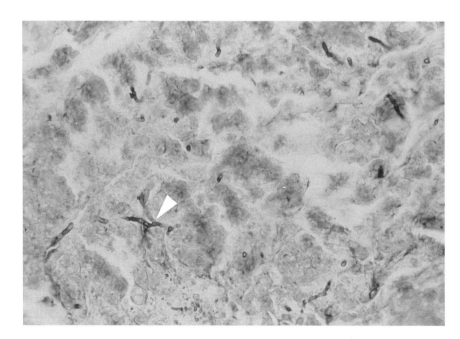

**FIG. 18.8.** Gomori's Metamine silver stain of allergic mucin reveals a darkly stained fungal hypha *(arrow)* in a cellular background (black and white).

## TABLE 18.2. BENT AND KUHN CRITERIA FOR ALLERGIC FUNGAL SINUSITIS

I. Type I hypersensitivity (history, skin test, or serology)
II. Nasal polyposis
III. Characteristic radiographic findings
IV. Eosinophilic mucus demonstrating fungus without tissue invasion

From Bent J, Kuhn F. Diagnosis of allergic fungal sinusitis. *Otolaryngol Head Neck Surg* 1994;111:580–588, with permission.

sal sinuses; characteristic histologic findings of allergic mucin; and laboratory evidence of allergy.

Laury and Schaefer (39) proposed multiple diagnostic criteria: eosinophilia, immediate skin reactivity or serum IgG antibodies to fungal antigen, elevated total IgE level, nasal mucosal edema or polyposis, histopathologic findings of allergic mucin containing noninvasive fungal hyphae, and characteristic CT or MRI findings. Cody et al. (7), in reporting the Mayo Clinic experience, simplified the diagnostic criteria to include only characteristic allergic mucin and either noninvasive fungal hyphae in the collected mucin or positive fungal cultures.

Based on the analysis of 15 cases of AFS, Bent and Kuhn (17) demonstrated 5 common characteristics: Gell and Coombs type I (IgE mediated) hypersensitivity, nasal polyposis, characteristic radiographic findings, eosinophilic mucin without fungal invasion into sinus tissue, and positive fungal stain of sinus contents removed at the time of surgery (Table 18.2). A similar set of five criteria was proposed by de Shazo (40): radiographic evidence of sinusitis, the presence of allergic mucin (identified grossly or histopathologically), positive fungal stain or culture from the patient's sinus at the time of surgery, the absence of contributory factors (e.g., diabetes mellitus or immunodeficiencies), and the absence of fungal invasion.

It is notable that a positive fungal culture does not confirm the diagnosis of AFS, nor does a negative culture rule it out. For example, fungi may proliferate as saprophytic growth in diseased sinuses. Furthermore, mycology laboratories vary in capability, and specimen handling significantly influences the rate of positive fungal cultures in a clinical setting (22). Allergic mucin remains the most reliable indicator of AFS.

### Differential Diagnosis

Given that nasal polyposis is not unique to AFS, and that fungi may be present in the nose and paranasal sinuses in multiple diseases, AFS must be differentiated from other mycotic diseases of the sinuses:

### Invasive Fungal Sinusitis

This condition typically is encountered in patients who are immunocompromised or have diabetes mellitus and is char-

acterized by angioinvasive fungal penetration of tissue. Hypesthesia, local pain, and intranasal necrosis (in an immunocompromised person) strongly suggest invasive fungal sinusitis and help to differentiate this disease from AFS.

### Saprophytic Fungal Growth

This growth may be found in one or more paranasal sinus cavities of patients with chronic suppurative rhinosinusitis (41). Similar growth may occur in nasal debris of patients who have undergone aggressive sinonasal surgery or those with rhinitis sicca. Although fungal cultures may be positive, the absence of gross and histiologic findings of allergic mucin and the lack of clinical manifestations of invasive fungal sinusitis suggest saprophytic fungal growth.

### Mycetoma, Aspergilloma, or Fungus Ball of the Sinuses

This clinical entity differs from AFS in presentation. Rather than involving multiple sinuses, a fungus ball typically involves a single sinus, most often the maxillary antrum or sphenoid. Patients with this condition are not necessarily allergic and usually do not exhibit nasal polyps. On histologic examination, the material removed from the sinuses demonstrates only fungal hyphae without eosinophils. Surgery in such cases usually is curative (42).

### Eosinophilic Mucin Sinusitis

Pansinusitis, polyposis, and mucin that is clinically indistinguishable from that of AFS are characteristic. However, examination of mucin reveals no fungal hyphae (43). Allergy is not as constant a feature as in AFS, but asthma is more frequently seen. It has been suggested by Ferguson (personal communication, 1998) that this condition may represent a variant of Samter's triad.

## TREATMENT

Based on a postulated schema of the pathophysiologic process of AFS, a variety of treatment plans addressing its multiple contributing factors have emerged. Medical control of the disease has made use of various combinations of antifungal medications, corticosteroids, and immunotherapy with varying degrees of disease control. Attempts to control this disease by only partially addressing the underlying causes have likely contributed to a high rate of recidivism. Successful treatment of AFS requires that the treatment plan account for each factor responsible for the propagation of the disease. The "AFS cycle," as described earlier in this chapter (Fig. 18.9), suggests that atopy, continuous antigenic exposure, and inflammation all have key roles in the perpetuation

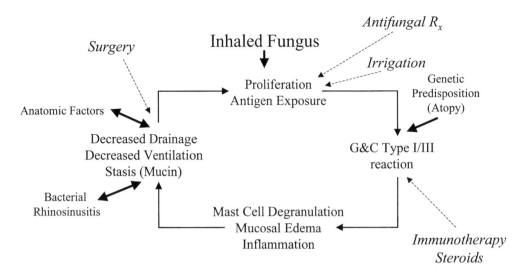

**FIG. 18.9.** Rationale for various therapeutic interventions.

of the disease. In theory, individually accounting for each of these factors will provide for the best chance of long-term disease control (14). This comprehensive approach to management depends on complete removal of all fungal mucin (usually requiring surgery) and long-term prevention of recurrence though either immunomodulation (immunotherapy or corticosteroids) or fungistatic antimicrobials (Fig. 18.10).

### Traditional Surgical Therapy

The single invariable component of combination therapy remains surgical removal of the inciting fungal allergic mucin and marsupialization of the involved sinuses. For this reason, surgery has played an important role in the management of AFS since its earliest reports. An aggressive surgical posture was adopted initially owing to a perceived risk of fungal invasion. In 1979, reporting their experience of four patients with "paranasal aspergillosis," McGuirt et al. (44) stated, "without question, the treatment of paranasal sinus aspergillosis is surgical–the key to successful surgical treatment is the removal of diseased mucosa and aeration and drainage of the involved sinus."

This frequently was accomplished through the use of open antrostomies with radical removal of mucosa, intranasal sphenoethmoidectomies, and Lynch frontoethmoidec-

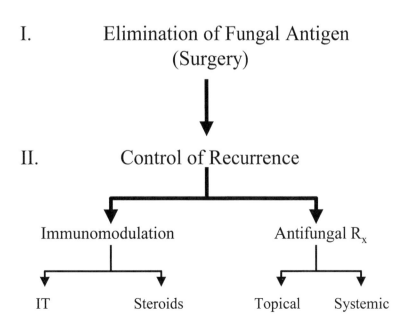

**FIG 18.10.** Treatment principles. Long-term control of allergic fungal sinusitis requires both elimination of fungal antigen and control of its recurrence.

tomies. Despite such aggressive therapy, recidivism remained high and most patients required multiple surgical procedures (45).

The clinical appearance of the disease often confused the underlying diagnosis, further influencing surgeons to adopt a more radical stance. Radiographic evidence of "invasion" into adjacent spaces, such as the orbit or intracranial cavity, frequently was interpreted as evidence of malignancy or invasive fungal disease. It logically followed that surgical approaches appropriate for these serious conditions, such as lateral rhinotomy, facial degloving approaches, and craniofacial resection, would be performed. Sarti et al. (46), in 1988, reported a case of "paranasal aspergillosis" with extension into the anterior cranial fossa and sella turcica. Although no histologic invasion of mucosa was demonstrated, the presence of fungal hyphae coupled with dramatic radiographic bony erosion yielded a diagnosis of "invasive aspergillosis." The patient unfortunately died as a result of a pulmonary embolus after a craniofacial resection.

Increased acceptance of specific immunologic hypersensitivity as the cause for AFS has led to changes in its management. These changes have involved both the medical and surgical arms of therapy. Whereas systemic use of antifungal medications has largely been replaced by immunomodulation, radical surgery for AFS has given way to more conservative, tissue-sparing approaches. Mabry et al. (47) refer to this surgery as "conservative, but complete," relying almost completely on endoscopic techniques.

## Surgical Implication of the Physical Characteristics of Allergic Fungal Sinusitis

The slow accumulation of allergic fungal mucin over an extended period in involved paranasal sinuses imparts unique and rather predictable characteristics to the disease. As the quantity of mucin increases, the involved paranasal sinus begins to resemble a mucocele, (sometimes referred to as a *fungal mucocele*). With time, bony remodeling and decalcification may occur, causing the disease to mimic "invasion" into adjacent anatomic spaces (46,48–51). The location of bone demineralization and extension appears to be determined by the location of the expansile disease, and is thought to occur as a result of a combination of pressure and local inflammatory mediators. As mentioned earlier in this chapter, the process often gives rise to exophthalmos, facial dysmorphia, and intracranial extension (51).

It is the physical characteristics of AFS that influence its surgical treatment. By the very nature of the disease, AFS creates a series of local inflammatory responses, each capable of producing polyposis and allergic mucin. The clinical and radiographic involvement can be extensive at times, causing large-scale bone dissolution and encroachment into adjacent anatomic spaces. These typical features of AFS, once used

to justify radical surgical approaches, actually can aid in the pursuit of a more conservative surgical approach (52).

Nasal polyposis is inherent to AFS (53) and can range from subtle to extensive, causing distortion of local anatomy and loss of useful surgical landmarks. Bleeding often occurs in response to surgical manipulation of the polyps, increasing the potential for disorientation. The operating surgeon must recognize that these factors, in combination with the high likelihood of bony dehiscence, increase the risk of iatrogenic injury.

Aside from these problems, polyps can provide an important intraoperative role by serving as a marker of disease. AFS causes a relatively consistent configuration of disease. The involved paranasal sinus, acting as a reservoir for allergic fungal mucin, is the epicenter of the disease process. Allergic fungal mucin completely occupies the sinus cavity, whereas the lining mucosa, demonstrating only mild to moderate inflammation, remains an intact barrier to the fungus (14, 36). More significant inflammation located at the sinus ostia gives rise to polyps that extend into the infundibulum, middle meatus, sphenoethmoid recess, and nasal cavity. Recognition of this allows the surgeon to "follow the polyps to the disease" (52).

The resulting nasal polyposis can facilitate the surgical treatment of AFS in another fashion. The expansile behavior of AFS increases access to involved paranasal sinuses. As revealed radiographically, the combination of slowly growing nasal polyps and accumulating allergic fungal mucin expands the involved paranasal sinuses as well as the surgical route to the involved sinuses. Enlargement of the nasal cavity, middle meatus, and frontal recess provides the surgeon with access adequate to deal with the disease in even the most difficult areas, such as the frontal sinus (14).

After surgical access to the involved sinus is achieved, a dilated cavity filled with allergic fungal mucin is encountered. As described earlier in this chapter, this material is thick, tenacious, and viscous, and may vary in color from light tan to black. Because of its noninvasive behavior, it may be removed in a blunt fashion, leaving the involved sinus completely lined with intact mucosa (Fig. 18.11). Preservation of mucosa provides protection of adjacent anatomic structures, even in the face of large areas of bony dehiscence.

## Surgical Technique

To minimize recurrence of disease, treatment of AFS is directed at removal of the inciting antigenic material by complete surgical removal of allergic mucin and debris, while also ameliorating the underlying inflammatory process through the use of limited systemic and topical steroid preparations. Other forms of adjunctive medical therapy are discussed later in this chapter. One accepted preoperative medical regimen is to initiate systemic corticosteroid therapy (prednisone, 0.5 to 1.0 mg/kg/day) approximately 1

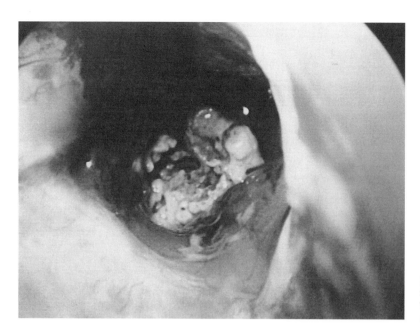

**FIG. 18.11.** Allergic fungal mucin in the sphenoid sinus. Note that surrounding mucosa is intact and without significant signs of inflammation. The mucin lies adjacent to the mucosa, without invasion.

week before surgery to decrease intranasal inflammation and nasal polyp volume. In addition, preoperative antibiotics are instituted because of the frequency of concomitant post-obstructive bacterial sinusitis (14).

At surgery, three goals should be achieved. First, surgery should result in complete extirpation of all allergic mucin and fungal debris, thus greatly reducing or eliminating the antigenic inciting factor in the atopic patient. At times this may be challenging. Access to the frontal sinus and other potentially involved spaces, such as extramural ethmoid cells, or a pneumatized pterygoid of the sphenoid, may be limited. However, as noted previously, the expansile behavior of the disease tends to widen natural tracts into these normally limited areas, facilitating surgical manipulation.

The next goal of surgery is to produce permanent drainage and ventilation of the affected sinuses, while preserving the integrity of the underlying mucosa. This has been greatly aided by the advent of tissue-sparing instrumentation (54). Even in the setting of significant dissolution of the fovea ethmoidalis, lamina papyracea, clivus, and sphenoid planum, wide marsupialization of diseased areas can be achieved without causing trauma to the underlying mucosa. Careful preservation of mucosa ensures that underlying periosteum, dura, or periorbita remains free of penetrating injury. Sinonasal polyposis may initially preclude orientation, but removal in a controlled fashion using powered microdissection provides the operating surgeon with eventual access to areas of fungal presence. After adequate ventilation and drainage are achieved, the preserved underlying mucosa is able to revert to its normal state.

Adequate ventilation and drainage also provide for the final goal of surgery: postoperative access to the previously diseased areas. Even under ideal conditions, small residua of fungus may remain in situ, inciting recurrence if not controlled after surgery. Surgery should be performed with facilitation of postsurgical care in mind. This goal can be reliably attained in most cases while preserving the integrity of important intranasal structures, such as the middle and inferior turbinates.

These surgical goals can be accomplished through a number of approaches and techniques, the choice of which ultimately is influenced by the experience and training of the surgeon. Endoscopic powered instrumentation has demonstrated its effectiveness through the ability, using this technique, to remove soft tissue and thin bone while maintaining superb visibility. Great care should be exercised when using powered instrumentation, however, because the well recognized bone dissolution associated with AFS increases the potential risk of inadvertent orbital or intracranial penetration. In the event of extensive remodeling or bone erosion, image-guided systems (e.g., Landmarx, Medtronic Xomed, Jacksonville, FL) may be of benefit (52).

Postoperative care begins immediately after surgery in the form of nasal saline irrigation. Weekly clinic visits initially are required to allow regular inspection of the operative site and debridement of crusts and retained fungal debris. Systemic corticosteroids, which were initiated before surgery, are continued during the postoperative period and slowly tapered during the process of healing. The length of corticosteroid treatment is based on the discretion of the managing physician as well as the form of postoperative adjunctive medical management used to control the disease. The period of postoperative corticosteroid coverage may be used to initiate other forms of medical management.

## Complications of Surgery

In most cases, surgery is performed without incident, but the pathologic behavior of AFS theoretically increases surgical risk. Nasal polyposis, expansile accumulations of allergic mucin, as well as poor intraoperative hemostasis may increase spatial disorientation. In addition, areas of bony dehiscence may confuse or distort anatomic boundaries while offering little protection to the orbit and intracranial cavities. On the other hand, a less-than-complete surgical procedure (in an attempt to decrease iatrogenic injury) is likely to lead to incomplete retrieval of allergic fungal mucin and rapid recurrence of AFS.

Based on the currently accepted pathophysiologic process of AFS, little risk of fungal invasion into adjacent tissues should exist in the immunocompetent host. It appears that rare exceptions may occur. Tsimakas et al. (55) report a single case of an *Aspergillus* frontal lobe abscess occurring after surgical treatment of AFS that had expanded into the anterior cranial fossa. This case may represent seeding of the intracranial cavity as a result of inadvertent dural penetration, and emphasizes the importance of mucosal preservation.

In addition to fungal or bacterial seeding, penetration of the dura or periorbita results in injury of structures in the orbit or intracranial cavities. Such transgressions can cause diplopia, blindness, hemorrhage, stroke, intracranial hemorrhage, or cerebrospinal fluid rhinorrhea. The patient shown in Fig. 18.12 illustrates this point. She was referred to our clinic after surgical treatment of AFS. Violation of the left periorbita had resulted in trauma and fibrosis of the ipsilateral medial rectus muscle, causing subsequent perma-

nent diplopia. Violation of the anterior cranial fossa dura resulted in development of an encephalocele. Avoidance of such an injury requires careful attention to anatomic orientation and strict preservation of mucosa and underlying tissues (55).

Erosion by AFS of the osseous boundaries separating the intracranial fossa from the sinonasal cavities may increase the risk of subsequent encephalocele formation. It is commonly accepted in the otologic community that dural exposure in the absence of dural injury along the tegmen mastoideum rarely results in the development of an encephalocele (56). Unfortunately, no analogous information in the rhinologic literature exists. It is logical to assume, however, that eventual encephalocele formation may occur as a result of a combination of factors, including dural injury, location of bony dehiscence, or size of the bony dehiscence. In rare cases, accumulations of allergic fungal mucin may appear actually to support intracranial structures. Figure 18.13 shows a patient who presented with extensive erosion of the planum sphenoidale and ethmoid roof. Her disease was addressed endoscopically, during which strict mucosal preservation was observed. Postoperative CT scan revealed the encephalocele shown in Fig. 18.14. Monitoring for development of encephaloceles is important because their occurrence may require subsequent repair of bony dehiscence.

## Medical Therapy

### Corticosteroids

The origin of corticosteroid therapy for the long-term management of AFS arose directly from the success of this strat-

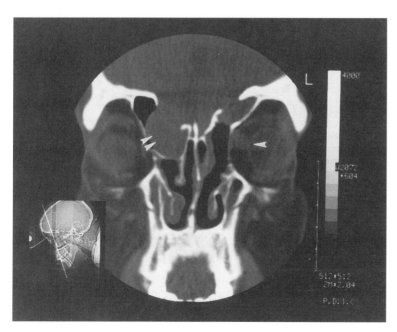

**FIG. 18.12.** Coronal computed tomography scan of patient after endoscopic surgery for allergic fungal sinusitis. Violation of mucosa and dura of the anterior cranial fossa resulted in encephalocele formation *(double arrows)*, whereas violation of the contralateral periorbita produced trauma and fibrosis of the medial rectus muscle *(single arrow)*.

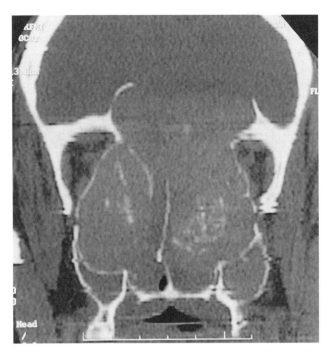

**FIG. 18.13.** Coronal computed tomography scan of extensive ethmoid root and planum sphenoidale erosion resulting from allergic fungal sinusitis.

egy in the treatment of ABPA. The potent antiinflammatory and immunomodulatory effects of corticosteroids appear to be well suited to controlling recurrence of disease. This concept was emphasized by Bent et al. (57), who noted eventual universal recurrence of AFS in their patients who were not treated with systemic corticosteroids. Schubert and

Goetz (30) further studied the role of systemic corticosteroids in the postoperative management of AFS, demonstrating a significant increase in the time to revision sinus surgery in those patients with AFS who received prolonged courses of postoperative corticosteroids. Postoperative corticosteroid therapy in this study ranged from 2 to 12 months, with improved outcomes recorded among those patients who were placed on longer courses of therapy. At present, however, the optimal dosing regimen and length of therapy remain unclear.

Topical corticosteroids are accepted as a standard therapy in the postoperative treatment of AFS, but they possess a limited benefit before surgery because nasal access is restricted. After surgery, however, they may be effective in controlling local inflammation.

**Complications of Corticosteroids**

The well recognized benefits of systemic corticosteroids are counterbalanced by numerous potential adverse effects, including growth retardation, diabetes mellitus, hypertension, psychotropic effects, gastrointestinal side effects, cataracts, glaucoma, osteoporosis, and aseptic necrosis of the femoral head. Schubert and Goetz (30) noted no adverse effects among their series of 67 patients with AFS treated for up to 1 year with systemic corticosteroids, but long-term follow-up for this form of therapy is lacking. The side effect profile of systemic corticosteroids warrants careful consideration when they are used in a long-term fashion to control AFS.

Topical corticosteroids usually present fewer side effects than systemic corticosteroids, based on their limited bioavailability. Long-term use, especially at high dosages or in combination with inhaled corticosteroids, presents a risk of

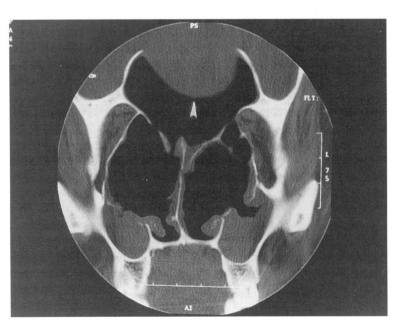

**FIG. 18.14.** Coronal computed tomography scan obtained after surgical removal of allergic fungal mucin. Note herniation of encephalocele *(arrow)*.

hypothalamic–pituitary–adrenal axis suppression, cataract formation, growth retardation, nasal bleeding, and nasal septal perforation in rare cases. As with any form of chronic therapy, topical corticosteroid sprays should be monitored.

## Immunotherapy

The similarity between AFS and ABPA led to an empiric (and theoretic) concern that immunotherapy using specific fungal antigens in patients with either of these diseases might incite further allergic reactions by adding to the patients' fungal antigenic stimulus (58). This concern specifically addressed the possible exacerbation of immune complex development and deposition. However, in the case of AFS, surgery is able to remove the inciting fungal load from the paranasal sinuses; therefore, it was postulated that immunotherapy may be beneficial, rather than harmful, as a component of treatment for AFS (58,59).

To investigate the safety of fungal immunotherapy as an adjunct to AFS treatment, a prospective study was performed to examine the response of patients with AFS, after adequate surgery, to immunotherapy with all antigens (fungal and nonfungal) to which the patients were sensitive (58). In the first year of this study, clinical status was not shown to worsen, the patients did not require systemic corticosteroids, most patients were able to discontinue topical corticosteroid therapy, and AFS recurrence was markedly diminished among those patients compliant with the regimen. Follow-up revealed similar findings at 2 and 3 years (47, 59). A complementary study retrospectively compared 11 patients treated in this manner with 11 age- and diseased-matched control subjects who received the same surgical and medical treatment but no immunotherapy. A statistically significant difference was noted between the two groups. The cohort receiving immunotherapy as part of their treatment performed better in quality-of-life scores as well as objective endoscopic measures of mucosal edema (60).

In a series of eight patients in whom immunotherapy was given for 3 to 5 years and then discontinued, no recurrences were seen up to 17 months after discontinuation (61). Additional study is necessary, but initial work suggests that a role may exist for immunotherapy in the overall treatment strategy for AFS.

## Technique of Immunotherapy in Allergic Fungal Sinusitis

In initial studies, only immunotherapy for positive fungal antigens was administered for the first 6 months to be certain that any effects (either positive or negative) on the disease process were due to the administration of fungal antigens. Later, both fungal and nonfungal antigens to which the patient was found to be allergic were included in the treatment mix. However, it remains advisable to administer these in two separate vials for the first several months of treatment to assess more easily the source of any untoward

**TABLE 18.3. PROTOCOL FOR IMMUNOTHERAPY IN ALLERGIC FUNGAL SINUSITIS**

1. After successful surgical exenteration of sinuses and confirmation of diagnosis, perform allergy evaluation and testing (RAST or quantitative skin test) for typical panel of nonfungal antigens appropriate for the area. Test (RAST or quantitative skin test) for all relevant molds (fungi) available. Discuss treatment protocol with patient and obtain informed consent.
2. Instruct patient in avoidance measures for molds. Adjust pharmacotherapy as necessary.
3. Prepare vial of all positive nonfungal antigens, and second vial of all positive fungal antigens. Perform vial test with each.
4. Administer immunotherapy weekly, with dosage advancement as tolerated, placing one injection from each vial in a different arm. This allows for accurate recognition of cause of any local reactions noted.
5. Observe patient regularly, adjust dosage as necessary if local reactions or adverse changes in nasal signs/symptoms occur. Patient should be examined regularly by endoscopy to watch for reaccumulation of allergic mucin or reformation of polyps, and cleaning, medical management, and so forth carried out.
6. As dosage advancement permits (usually by second vial), may combine antigens into one vial and continue for a 3- to 5-year regimen as per standard practice.

RAST, radioallergosorbent test.

local reaction and more efficiently advance treatment dosage. After maintenance levels are achieved, the fungal and nonfungal antigens may be combined into one vial (Table 18.3).

A common misconception is that only immunotherapy for those fungi identified by culture from allergic fungal mucin should be included in the testing/treatment regimen for a patient. Because of variability in mycology laboratories and circumstances, a positive culture is not obtained in all cases. Conversely, the presence of fungi on culture of sinus contents does not make the diagnosis of AFS. One successful approach has been to test for a wide variety of molds (the choice being dictated by experience gained in testing and treating allergic patients in the region), and to include all positive reactors in the treatment set (47).

Advancement and adjustment of dosage is carried out in the usual fashion (62). Although late local reactions (induration >30 mm in diameter occurring 24 to 48 hours after an injection) are said to be more common when administering immunotherapy for molds than for other antigens, this has not been the reported experience in treating patients with AFS (33). Systemic reactions to immunotherapy likewise have not been observed in the University of Texas Southwestern experience.

Based on experience, it currently is recommended that immunotherapy be administered to patients with AFS for the same duration as recommended for patients with allergy in general: 3 to 5 years (61).

**Complications of Immunotherapy**

At the time of this publication, no treatment-related complications have been identified when immunotherapy follows appropriate surgical extirpation of all allergic mucin. This, however, should not promote a sense of false security concerning this form of therapy because immunotherapy continues to represent a new and incompletely understood treatment modality. In general terms, immunotherapy potentially may lead to worsening of local or systemic disease, specifically if the patient continues to be exposed to a significant antigenic load.

Ferguson (63) reported seven patients who received immunotherapy for the treatment of AFS. The five patients who received immunotherapy before surgical removal of all allergic mucin either symptomatically worsened or failed to improve in response to therapy. In contrast to these findings, the two patients who underwent surgery before initiation of immunotherapy responded well to this treatment modality. This small study supports the concept that immunotherapy administered in the presence of an ongoing antigenic load (in this case fungus) raises the risk of untoward complications of therapy (e.g., immune complex deposition, delayed or late-phase reactions, local reactions).

Another permutation of this concern occurs when AFS presents concomitantly with ABPA (64). Unlike the situation in AFS, the fungi in the lower respiratory tract of patients with ABPA cannot be surgically removed, thus resulting in a retained antigenic load. Moreover, although the clinical manifestations of AFS sometimes are dramatic, they are rarely life threatening. The threat of ABPA is potentially much greater. Given the lack of information regarding the effects of immunotherapy on ABPA, great care should be taken when immunotherapy is given in this situation (65).

*Antifungals*

Systemic antifungal therapy for AFS initially was proposed to control the theoretic potential for progression to invasive forms of fungal sinusitis. As the unacceptably high rate of recidivism after surgery alone was recognized, antifungal therapy often was used in an attempt to provide some degree of control over recurrence of AFS. The early use of amphotericin B yielded to the use of less toxic agents, such as ketoconazole, itraconazole, and fluconazole, but the poor in vivo activity of these agents against dematiaceous fungi was soon discovered (11). Objective data on the effects of this form of therapy for AFS have been limited. Denning et al. (66) studied the effect of systemic itraconazole in patients with ABPA and showed a decrease in both total IgE (used as a marker of disease severity) and systemic corticosteroid requirements. Anecdotal reports of systemic itraconazole to prevent AFS recurrence offer mixed results. Ferguson (67) points out that the expense, limited available data, and potential drug related morbidity of systemic antifungal ther-

apy may limit the usefulness of this form of treatment for noninvasive fungal disease.

Topical application of antifungal agents may hold some benefit in the control of postoperative recurrence, and studies of this form of treatment are underway. Bent and Kuhn (68) studied the in vitro susceptibility of fungi commonly encountered in patients with AFS and determined that minimal inhibitory concentrations can be exceeded with certain antifungal agents when applied topically. Similarly, Ponikau et al. (69) suggest the use of topical antifungal agents. Supportive data are pending.

**Complications of Antifungal Therapy**

Antifungal medications are recognized for some potentially serious side effects that warrant consideration when these drugs are used as a form of treatment for AFS. The well known complications associated with amphotericin B include acute renal failure, anemia, agranulocytosis, acute liver failure, cardiopulmonary hypertension, and hemorrhagic gastroenteritis. Itraconazole and fluconazole offer a slightly safer form of antifungal therapy, but still may give rise to drug-induced cardiac dysrhythmias, hepatic dysfunction, urticaria, and anaphylaxis (70).

**Recurrence of Disease**

The potential for AFS recidivism is well respected and ranges from 10% (71) to nearly 100%. Published rates of AFS recurrence, however, can be misleading and are highly dependent on length of follow-up. To emphasize the importance of long-term surveillance, Bent and Kuhn (57) pointed out that in their experience, the often dramatic initial response to surgical therapy was eventually replaced by recurrence of AFS in the absence of ongoing therapy. Similarly, Kupferburg et al. (72) followed the appearance of sinonasal mucosa in 24 patients treated with combined medical and surgical therapy for AFS. Nineteen of the 24 eventually had recurrence of disease after discontinuation of systemic corticosteroids, but the authors observed that endoscopic evidence of disease usually preceded return of subjective symptoms.

Allergic fungal sinusitis recidivism appears to be influenced by long-term postoperative therapy. Schubert and Goetz (30) reported the long-term clinical outcome of 67 patients after initial surgical therapy for AFS. Patients treated with at least 2 months of oral corticosteroids were compared with those who received no corticosteroids. At 1 year after initial surgery, patients treated with oral corticosteroids were significantly less likely to have experienced recurrent AFS (35%) than those who had not (55%). AFS recidivism, however, remains high despite appropriate postoperative medical therapy. As addressed earlier in this chapter, fungal- and non–fungal-specific immunotherapy holds some potential as a form of postoperative treatment in patients with AFS, but clinical failures can arise during immunotherapy.

Marple et al. (71), in a review of 42 patients who had received immunotherapy after surgery, reported 4 recurrences of disease, which were attributed to either noncompliance with immunotherapy or inadequate operative extirpation of allergic fungal mucin.

## CONCLUSION

Allergic fungal sinusitis is a relatively newly characterized disease entity that commands a great deal of interest. Large amounts of information are being generated addressing the underlying etiology of the disease, its clinical presentation, and forms of treatment. Although controversy still exists, recent evidence supports the theory that AFS represents an immunologic, rather than infectious, disease process. An improved understanding of this underlying disease process has led to evolution in the treatment of AFS. Medical therapy has begun to shift from an emphasis on systemic antifungal therapy to various forms of topical treatment and immunomodulation. Likewise, surgical treatment of AFS, still a crucial component of the overall treatment plan of the patient, has shifted from a radical to a more conservative but complete approach. Although important, surgery alone does not lead to a long-term disease-free state. A comprehensive management plan incorporating both medical and surgical care remains the most likely way to provide long-term disease control for AFS.

## REFERENCES

1. Safirstein B. Allergic bronchopulmonary aspergillosis with obstruction of the upper respiratory tract. *Chest* 1976;70:788–790.
2. Millar J, Johnston A, Lamb D. Allergic bronchopulmonary aspergillosis of the maxillary sinuses. *Thorax* 1981;36:710(abstr).
3. Lamb D, Millar J, Johnston A. Allergic aspergillosis of the paranasal sinuses. *J Pathol* 1982;137:56.
4. Sher T, Schwartz H. Allergic aspergillus sinusitis with concurrent allergic bronchopulmonary aspergillus: report of a case. *J Allergy Clin Immunol* 1988;81:844–846.
5. Katzenstin A, Greenberger P, Sale S. Allergic aspergillus sinusitis: a newly recognized form of sinusitis. *J Allergy Clin Immunol* 1983;72:89–93.
6. Robson J, Hogan P, Benn R, et al. Allergic fungal sinusitis presenting as a paranasal sinus tumor. *Aust N Z J Med* 1989;19:351–353.
7. Cody D, Neel H, Gerreiro J, et al. Allergic fungal sinusitis: the Mayo Clinic experience. *Laryngoscope* 1994;104:1074–1079.
8. Manning SC. *Allergic fungal sinusitis*. Thesis submitted for fellowship in the American Academy of Laryngology, Rhinology, and Otology.
9. Gungor A, Adusmilli V, Corey JP. Fungal sinusitis: progression of disease in immunosuppression: a case report. *Ear Nose Throat J* 1998;77:207–215.
10. Corey J, Delsupehe K, Ferguson B. Allergic fungal sinusitis: allergic, infectious, or both? *Otolaryngol Head Neck Surg* 1995;113:110–119.
11. Manning SC, Holman M. Further evidence for allergic fungal sinusitis. *Laryngoscope* 1998;108:1485–1496.
12. Feger T, Rupp N, Kuhn F, et al. Local and systemic eosinophil activation. *Ann Allergy Asthma Immunol* 1997;79:221–225.
13. Manning S, Vuitch F, Weinberg A, et al. Allergic aspergillosis: a newly recognized form of sinusitis in the pediatric population. *Laryngoscope* 1989;99:P681–P685.
14. Marple BF, Mabry RL. Comprehensive management of allergic fungal sinusitis. *Am J Rhinol* 1998;12:263–268.
15. Corey JP. Allergic fungal sinusitis. *Otolaryngol Clin North Am* 1992;25:225–230.
16. Allphin L, Strauss M, Abdul-Karim F. Allergic fungal sinusitis: problems in diagnosis and treatment. *Laryngoscope* 1991;10:815–820.
17. Bent J, Kuhn F. Diagnosis of allergic fungal sinusitis. *Otolaryngol Head Neck Surg* 1994;111:580–588.
18. Deshpande RB, Shaukla A, Kirtane MV. Allergic fungal sinusitis: incidence and clinical and pathological features of seven cases. *J Assoc Physicians India* 1995;43:98–100.
19. Ferguson BJ, Barnes L, Bernstein JM. Geographic variation in allergic fungal sinusitis. *Otolaryngol Clin North Am* 2000;33:441–449.
20. Marple BF, Gibbs SR, Newcomer MT, et al. Allergic fungal sinusitis—induced visual loss. *Am J Rhinol* 1999;13:1915.
21. Manning S, Schaefer S, Close L, et al. Culture-positive allergic fungal sinusitis. *Arch Otolaryngol Head Neck Surg* 1991;117:174–178.
22. Marple BF. Allergic fungal sinusitis. *Curr Opin Otolaryngol* 1999;7:383–387.
23. Nussenbaum B, Marple BF, Schwade ND. Characteristics of bony erosion in allergic fungal sinusitis. *Otolaryngol Head Neck Surg* 2001;124:150–154.
24. Carter KD, Graham SM, Carpenter KM. Ophthalmologic manifestations of allergic fungal sinusitis. *Am J Ophthalmol* 1999;127:189–195.
25. Makherjig SK, Figueroa R, Ginsberg LE, et al. Allergic fungal sinusitis: CT findings. *Radiology* 1998;207:417–422.
26. Zinreich SJ, Kennedy DW, Fullerton GD. Fungal sinusitis: diagnosis with CT and MR imaging. *Radiology* 1988;169:439–444.
27. Som PM, Curtin HD. Chronic inflammatory sinonasal disease including fungal infections: the role of imaging. *Radiol Clin North Am* 1993;31:33–44.
28. Manning SC, Merkel M, Kreisel K, et al. Computed tomographic and magnetic resonance diagnosis of allergic fungal sinusitis. *Laryngoscope* 1997;107:170–176.
29. Schubert MS, Goetz DW. Evaluation and treatment of allergic fungal sinusitis: I. demographics and diagnosis. *J Allergy Clin Immunol* 1998;102:387–394.
30. Schubert MS, Goetz DW. Evaluation and treatment of allergic fungal sinusitis: II. treatment and follow-up. *J Allergy Clin Immunol* 1998;102:395–402.
31. Manning S, Mabry R, Schaefer S, et al. Evidence of IgE-mediated hypersensitivity in allergic fungal sinusitis. *Laryngoscope* 1993;103:717–721.
32. Mabry R, Manning S. Radioallergosorbent microscreen and total immunoglobulin E in allergic fungal sinusitis. *Otolaryngol Head Neck Surg* 1995;113:721–723.
33. Mabry RL, Marple BF, Mabry CS. Mold testing by RAST and skin test methods in patients with allergic fungal sinusitis. *Otolaryngol Head Neck Surg* 1999;121:252–254.
34. Chrzanowski RR, Rupp NT, Kuhn FA, et al. Allergenic fungi in allergic fungal sinusitis. *Ann Allergy Asthma Immunol* 1997;79:431–435.
35. Schanadig VJ, Rassekh CH, Gourley WK. Allergic fungal sinusitis: a report of two cases with diagnosis by intraoperative aspiration cytology. *Acta Cytol* 1999;43:268–272.

36. Torres C, Rule out JY, el-Naggar AK, et al. Allergic fungal sinusitis: a clinicopathologic study of 16 cases. *Hum Pathol* 1996;27: 793–799.

37. Gourley DS, Whisman BA, Jorgensen NL, et al. Allergic *Bipolaris* sinusitis: clinical and immunopathologic characteristics. *J Allergy Clin Immunol* 1990;85:583–591.

38. Katzenstein A, Sale S, Greenberger P. Pathologic findings in allergic aspergillus sinusitis. *Am J Surg Pathol* 1983;7:439–443.

39. Loury MC, Schaefer SD. Allergic aspergillus sinusitis. *Arch Otolaryngol Head Neck Surg* 1993;119:1042–1043.

40. deShazo R, Scwain R. Diagnostic criteria for allergic fungal sinusitis. *J Allergy Clin Immunol* 1995;96:24–35.

41. Berrettini S, Carabelli A, Papini M, et al. Sellari Franceschini allergic fungal sinusitis: is this rare disease an allergy or infection? *Acta Otorhinolaryngol Ital* 1996;16:447–454.

42. deShazo RD, O'Brien M, Chapin K, et al. Criteria for the diagnosis of sinus mycetoma. *J Allergy Clin Immunol* 1997;99: 4755–4785.

43. Ramadan HH, Quraishi HA. Allergic mucin sinusitis without fungus. *Am J Rhinol* 1997;11:145–147.

44. McGuirt WF, Harrill JA. Paranasal sinus aspergillosis. *Laryngoscope* 1979;89:1563–1568.

45. Kupferberg SB, Bent JP, Kuhn FA. The prognosis of allergic fungal sinusitis. *Otolaryngol Head Neck Surg* 1997;117:35–41.

46. Sarti EJ, Blaugrund SM, Lin PT, et al. Paranasal sinus disease with intracranial extension: aspergillosis versus malignancy. *Laryngoscope* 1988;98:632–635.

47. Mabry RL, Marple BF, Folker RJ, et al. Immunotherapy for allergic fungal sinusitis: three years' experience. *Otolaryngol Head Neck Surg* 1998;119:648–651.

48. Pratt MF, Burnett JR. Fulminant *Drechslera* sinusitis in an immunocompetent host. *Laryngoscope* 1988;97:1343–1347.

49. Lydiatt WM, Sobba-Higley A, Huerter JV, et al. Allergic fungal sinusitis with intracranial extension and frontal lobe symptoms: a case report. *Ear Nose Throat J* 1994;73:402–404.

50. Young CN, Swart JG, Ackermann D, et al. Nasal obstruction and bone erosion caused by *Drechslera hawaiiensis*. *J Laryngol Otol* 1978;92:137–143.

51. Klapper SR, Lee AG, Patrinely JR, et al. Orbital involvement in allergic fungal sinusitis. *Ophthalmology* 1997;104:2094–2100.

52. Marple BF. Allergic fungal rhinosinusitis: surgical management. *Otolaryngol Clin North Am* 2000;33:409–419.

53. Schweitz LA, Gourley DS. Allergic fungal sinusitis. *Allergy Proc* 1992;13:3–6.

54. Mirante JP, Krouse JH, Munier MA. The role of powered instrumentation in the surgical treatment of allergic fungal sinusitis. *Ear Nose Throat J* 1998;77:678–682.

55. Tsimakas S, Hollingsworth HM, Nash G. Aspergillus brain abscess complicating allergic aspergillus sinusitis. *J Allergy Clin Immunol* 1994;94:264–267.

56. Jackson CG, Pappas DG, Manolidis S, et al. Is brain herniation into the middle ear and mastoid: concepts in diagnosis and surgical management. *Am J Otol* 1997;18:198–206.

57. Bent JP III, Kuhn FA. Allergic fungal sinusitis/polyposis. *Allergy Asthma Proc* 1996;17:259–268.

58. Mabry RL, Manning SC, Mabry CS. Immunotherapy in the treatment of allergic fungal sinusitis. *Otolaryngol Head Neck Surg* 1997;116:31–35.

59. Mabry RL, Mabry CS. Immunotherapy for allergic fungal sinusitis: the second year. *Otolaryngol Head Neck Surg* 1997;117: 367–371.

60. Folker RJ, Marple BF, Mabry RL, et al. Treatment of allergic fungal sinusitis: a comparison trial of postoperative immunotherapy with specific fungal antigens. *Laryngoscope* 1998;108: 1623–1627.

61. Mabry RL, Marple BF, Mabry CS. Outcomes after discontinuing immunotherapy for allergic fungal sinusitis. 2000;122:104–105.

62. King HC, Mabry RL, Mabry CS. *Allergy in ENT practice.* New York: Thieme Medical, 1998:227–242.

63. Ferguson BJ. Immunotherapy and antifungal therapy in allergic fungal sinusitis. Presented at the 1993 Annual Meeting of the American Academy of Otolaryngic Allergy, Minneapolis, MN, September 29, 1993.

64. Travis WK, Kwon-Chung KJ, Kleiner DE, et al. Unusual aspects of allergic bronchopulmonary fungal disease: report of two cases due to *Curvularia* organisms associated with allergic fungal sinusitis. *Hum Pathol* 1991;22:1240–1248.

65. Greenberger P, Atkinson NF Jr, Yuninger JW, et al. Allergic bronchopulmonary aspergillosis. In: Middleton E, Reed C, Ellis E, et al., eds. *Allergy principles and practice.* St. Louis: Mosby, 1993:1395–1414.

66. Denning DW, Van Wye JE, Lewiston NJ. Adjunctive treatment of allergic bronchopulmonary aspergillosis with itraconazole. *Chest* 1991;100:813–819.

67. Ferguson BJ. What role do systemic corticosteroids, immunotherapy, and antifungal drugs play in the therapy of allergic fungal rhinosinusitis? *Arch Otolaryngol Head Neck Surg* 1998;124: 1174–1177.

68. Bent JP III, Kuhn FA. Antifungal activity against allergic fungal sinusitis organisms. *Laryngoscope* 1996;106:1331–1334.

69. Ponikau JU, Sherris DA, Kern EB, et al. The diagnosis and incidence of allergic fungal sinusitis. *Mayo Clin Proc* 1999;74: 877–884.

70. *Physicians' Desk Reference,* 53rd ed. Des Moines: Medical Economics, 1999.

71. Marple BF, Mabry RL. Allergic fungal sinusitis: learning from our failures. *Am J Rhinol* 2000;14:223–226.

72. Kupferberg SB, Bent JP, Kuhn FA. Prognosis for allergic fungal sinusitis. *Otolaryngol Head Neck Surg* 1997;117:35–41.

# THE PHARYNX AND LARYNX

## STEPHEN J. CHADWICK

Though the pharynx is a multi-structured organ, it is not an isolated one. Its functions are related to and dependent on other organs . . . While some of the pathologic processes of the pharynx are well understood, others continue to be the object of investigation. The clinician is frequently challenged in his effort to differentiate those processes which are restricted to certain structures and those which mirror or reflect disease in the other organs of the body (1).

In 1953, Hollender made these remarks as part of the preface to his edited work, *The Pharynx.* The tenor of these statements echoes into the present. The laryngopharynx often is at the center of many common presenting otolaryngic complaints. Hoarseness, voice change, globus, dysphagia, postnasal drainage, and ear/throat pain are only a few of the disorders that are seen daily in the general otolaryngology practice. The laryngopharynx is located upstream from the lower respiratory and the upper gastrointestinal tracts (i.e., in the extrathoracic and supraesophageal aerodigestive tract), while sitting downstream from the sinonasal tract. The laryngopharynx and these contiguous organ systems may be simultaneously or separately affected by allergic inflammation or related processes.

Questions to be considered for this discussion then are (a) how does allergy affect the larynx, pharynx, laryngopharynx, and their (its) function; (b) what are and how can the plethora of interrelated complaints be appraised in a complete and yet concisely efficient manner; and (c) what is currently known, what is not known, what are some of the working models, and what are some of the directions for further investigation? The answers to these questions require an examination of a broad spectrum of topics, including applied regional anatomy and physiology, the current understanding of the biology of inflammation (especially allergic inflammation), and how these contiguous organ systems can be viewed as one integrated system.

## LARYNGOPHARYNGITIS

To quote a colleague, Jacqueline Corey, "Although both rhinitis and asthma may occur without a recognized allergic mechanism, IgE mediated inflammation is the most common mechanism found in both diseases. However, there are no epidemiologic data on the existence and prevalence of allergic diseases affecting the larynx other than studies on anaphylaxis with laryngeal edema of allergic origin. By focusing on a rare manifestation of the allergic reaction, these studies are not representative of the true population incidence of allergic disease affecting the larynx" (2). Brodnitz comments in his *Allergy of the Larynx,* "Although a whole library could be filled with the writing on allergy in general and voluminous reports exist on all phases of allergy in the upper as well as in the lower respiratory tract, hardly anything could be found on specific involvement of the larynx" (3).

To this day, the true incidence of allergy affecting the laryngopharynx is unknown. The literature is spotted with reports on allergy statistics in which the larynx is only briefly discussed. There are no consistent statements of direct or indirect effects of allergy on the laryngopharynx from a symptom standpoint. In addition, there is no discussion of other factors that may contribute to the same set of symptoms, such as the presence or absence of laryngopharyngeal reflux, vocal nodules, postnasal drainage, cough variant asthma, and so forth. Not only are the numbers of physical examination reports relatively small, there is no uniformity in the details of the physical examination. Techniques of varying degrees of sensitivity and specificity have been used, including indirect laryngoscopy, fiberoptic laryngoscopy, and strobovideolaryngoscopy (4–7). It also is not clear that all of the reported cases are truly allergic or immunoglobulin E (IgE) mediated. This even includes the accounts of anaphylaxis, for anaphylactic-like or anaphylactoid reactions, including various forms of angioedema, are mediated by nonallergic mechanisms (8–11).

The allergy/allergy-like spectrum of laryngitis therefore can be examined in two groups. The first is a group of acute and severe forms of laryngitis, including anaphylaxis, oral

**S. J. Chadwick:** Section of Otolaryngology, Southern Illinois University School of Medicine, Springfield, Illinois.

allergy syndrome (OAS), and special comments on angioedema associated with drug interactions, particularly the reaction to angiotensin-converting enzyme (ACE) inhibitors and angiotensin II blockers. The second group includes "all the other" less severe, allergy-related laryngitides. Because the severe and acute forms of laryngitis involve edema of the laryngopharynx, some initial comments on anatomy are appropriate.

## Laryngopharyngeal Anatomy

Anatomically, the mucosa of the larynx and the vocal fold is a pseudostratified ciliated columnar epithelium, with the exception of the actual vibratory margin, which is a stratified squamous epithelium. Below this layer is a lamina propria, which is divided into three distinct layers. The most superficial layer consists of a very loose connective tissue with scant fibroblasts. The intermediate and deep layers combine together to form the vocal ligament. The intermediate layer consists of a larger quantity of fibroblasts with elastic fibers. The deepest layer consists of the highest concentration of fibroblasts along with collagen fibers. The thyroarytenoid muscle (i.e., the vocalis muscle) is the actual muscular entity of the vocal fold (Fig. 19.1). The region between the vocal ligament and the superficial layer of the lamina propria is called *Reinke's space.* Functionally, the covering of the vocal cord, consisting of the epithelium and the superficial layer of the lamina propria, readily vibrates and slides over the vocal ligament and vocalis muscle. This occurs during phonation, which, in essence, is effected by the negative pressure that occurs when tubal airflow is forced across the constric-

tion of the glottic chink. This process is called the *Bernoulli effect.* It is apparent that in times of swelling, such as with angioedema, Reinke's space is the most severely affected area in the larynx (6,12).

The pharynx is a megaphone-shaped structure extending in a broad-based fashion from the base of the skull superiorly to a more narrowed aperture at the level of the laryngeal cone and the esophageal introitus (Fig. 19.2). It has five orifices that integrate it with the rest of the aerodigestive tract, including the glottic chink of the larynx, the cricopharyngeal ingress to the esophagus, the oropharynx, two eustachian tube orifices, and two nasochoanal apertures. Regionally, the pharynx is subdivided into three areas, the nasopharynx, oropharynx, and hypopharynx.

The nasopharynx extends from the base of the skull to the level of the soft palate (Fig. 19.3). The American Joint Committee on Cancer divides the nasopharynx into three subdivisions: a superior-posterior wall, the lateral wall structures, and a more anterior and inferior pharyngeal wall (13). The superior-posterior wall extends from the level of the palate to the base of the skull and includes the bony structures of the spinal column and the base of the skull, the longus colli and capitis muscles, and the retropharyngeal connective tissue and fascial planes. The layer of fascia that envelopes the spinal column and paraspinous muscles is the prevertebral space, which consists of prevertebral and alar layers. The space actually proceeds on down to the diaphragm. The retropharyngeal space is anterior to the prevertebral space, but behind the pharyngeal wall. This extends from the base of the skull to the tracheal bifurcation. Because of this relationship with the tracheal bifurcation, and

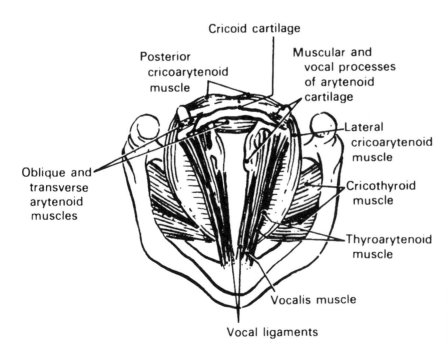

**FIG. 19.1.** Intrinsic muscles of the larynx, seen from above. (From Becker RF, Wilson JW, Gehweiler JA. *The anatomical basis of medical practice.* Baltimore: Williams & Wilkins, 1971, with permission.)

Space filled by
pharyngobasilar
fascia

Superior
constrictor

Stylopharyngeus

Middle constrictor

Inferior constrictor

Esophagus

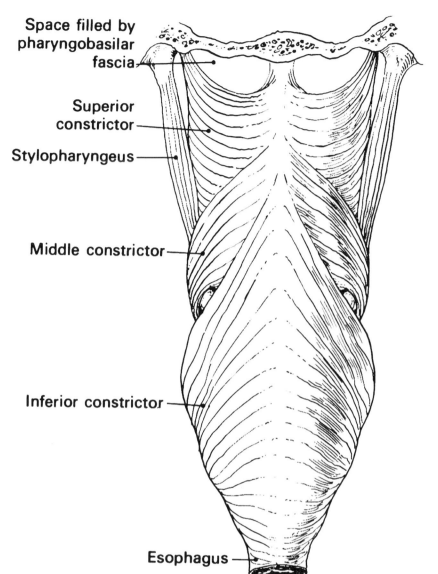

**FIG. 19.2.** The muscular cone of the pharynx, with the base of the skull superiorly and the esophagus inferiorly. (From Becker RF, Wilson JW, Gehweiler JA. *The anatomical basis of medical practice.* Baltimore: Williams & Wilkins, 1971, with permission.)

thus the mediastinum, this has often been called *the danger space,* usually in reference to spread of bacterial cellulitis. Of clinical relevance is the report by Altman et al. of angioedema presenting in the retropharyngeal space due to hereditary angioedema (HAE) (14). The lymphatic plexus in this space potentially drains the nasopharynx, paranasal sinuses, and posterior portion of the nose. The superior portion of the nasopharynx at the level of the choana is somewhat devoid of submucosal connective tissue. However, actual tissue depth here may vary with the amount of lymphoid (adenoid) tissue that may proliferate there. The lateral wall structures include the cartilaginous termination of the eustachian tube orifice or the torus tubarius. The posterior lateral pharyngeal recess, behind the torus, is called the *fossa of Rosenmüller.* The anterior-inferior wall extends

from the base of the skull to the junction of the soft palate and hard palate.

The oropharynx includes the base of the tongue anteriorly from the circumvallate papillae and, inferiorly and posterior, the lingual tonsils and the vallecula (Fig. 19.3). Superiorly, it includes the soft palate and uvula. Of clinical note, although uvular edema and inflammation may be a part of a more generalized pharyngeal process, acute isolated cases of angioedema of the uvula, with the exception of those triggered by HAE or some drug reactions, are relatively rare, but do occur with potentially fatal consequences. Isolated uvular edema was first reported by Quincke in 1882 (15). Further reports were made by Jarvis and Corey (16). Laterally, the oropharynx includes the pharyngeal walls containing the palatine tonsils and the tonsillar pillars (the pala-

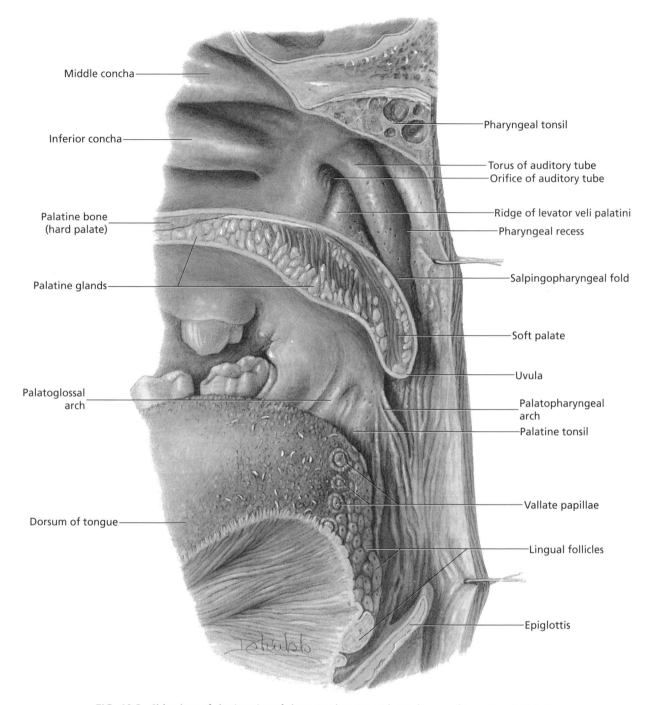

**FIG. 19.3.** Side view of the interior of the nasopharynx and oropharynx. (From Grant JCB. *An atlas of anatomy,* 6th ed. Baltimore: Williams & Wilkins, 1972, with permission.)

topharyngeus and palatoglossus muscles). The lateral wall also includes the superior and medial pharyngeal constrictors. At the junction of the superior and medial pharyngeal constrictures, near the level of the vallecula where the glossopharyngeal nerve and the styloid ligament pass from lateral to medial, is a "weak spot" that is one of the two primary sites for possible pharyngoceles. The parapharyngeal space, which is adjacent to the retropharyngeal space, also passes from this area, extending from the base of the skull superiorly to the hyoid bone inferiorly with its lateral borders being the mandible and the parotid gland. The peritonsillar space envelopes the peripalatine tonsillar tissue and is medial to the pharyngeal fascia, whereas the parapharyngeal space is more lateral to it. The posterior pharyngeal wall of the

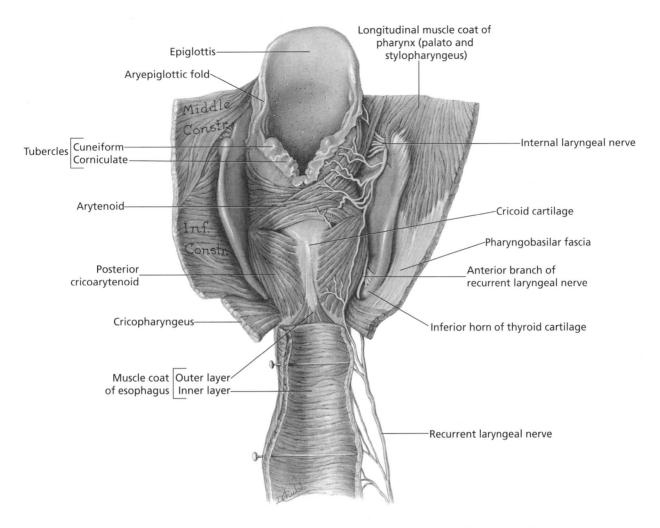

**FIG. 19.4.** Posterior view of the nerves and muscles of the hypopharynx. (From Grant JCB. *An atlas of anatomy,* 6th ed. Baltimore: Williams & Wilkins, 1972, with permission.)

oropharynx extends from the plane of the soft palate–hard palate junction to the pharyngoepiglottic folds and hyoid bone.

The hypopharynx extends from the introitus of the esophagus at the cricopharyngeal musculature to the pharyngoepiglottic folds (Fig. 19.4). Inferiorly, the hypopharynx includes the retrocricoid structures behind the larynx and the piriform sinuses along with the lateral pharyngeal wall. These structures, of course, cordon off the laryngeal cone. From a muscular standpoint, there is another weak area in the constrictor system at the junction of the inferior and medial pharyngeal constrictors at the level of the piriform sinus, where the superior laryngeal nerve and the superior laryngeal artery penetrate the thyrohyoid membrane. This is another site of dehiscence that is a potential location for pharyngocele formation. The submucosal, fascial, perimuscular connective tissue has cellular elements, lymphatic and vascular structures in the confines of well defined, con-

densed connective tissue or fascial planes. These expansile planes are subject to the effects of inflammatory and inflammatory-like responses, whether they be infectious, allergic, or otherwise immune-modulated. Familiarity with this anatomy not only is important in diagnosing and treating allergic and angioedematous reactions, but in dealing with infections of the neck (17–20).

## Severe Acute Laryngopharyngitis: Anaphylaxis

Death by Hymenoptera envenomation was first recorded well over 4,000 years ago (21). In 1914, Richet received a Nobel prize for his work on anaphylaxis (22). The term *anaphylaxis,* meaning "without protection," was introduced by Portier and Richet in 1902 for their initial trials with sea anemone toxin and the sensitization and provocation of the symptom complex of anaphylaxis in dogs (22). Since that time, the medical profession and the lay public have come to recognize the importance of anaphylaxis syndrome, and are able readily to identify a number of common and widely proclaimed inciting agents, such as aspirin and non-steroidal antiinflammatory drugs (23), penicillin (24), the horse serum used in numerous vaccines (25), more recently, latex (26), numerous other agents, including radiographic contrast media, and Hymenoptera venom. For most physicians and health care workers, anaphylaxis refers to an allergy-related type I Gell and Coombs IgE-mediated reaction, immediate in onset and extreme in consequence. In fact, however, other, non–IgE-mediated processes can trigger the mediator cascade. These processes may involve immune complexes, physical factors such as exercise, and complement activation, among others. These non–IgE-mediated reactions are collectively called *anaphylactoid reactions.* It has been suggested that both types of reactions be referred to as *anaphylaxis syndrome* or *anaphylactic response* (9) because the clinical presentation, course, and treatment are similar regardless of the nature of the initiating event. The actual list of known allergic and nonallergic triggers is beyond the scope of this chapter, but includes antibiotics and other drugs, hormones, enzymes and other proteins, tissue products, various venoms, allergen extracts, latex, anesthetic agents, foods, food additives, and radiocontrast media, to name a few broad categories.

Laryngopharyngeal involvement in anaphylaxis syndrome, especially in the moderate and severe forms, is not uncommon. Respiratory obstruction secondary to *laryngopharyngeal edema* along with status asthmaticus and cardiovascular collapse are the most common causes of death due to anaphylaxis. The clinician's attention should be stimulated when any of the common associated laryngopharyngeal symptoms such as voice change, hoarseness, dysphagia, globus, stridor, throat itching, or the patient's "sensation of impending doom" are part of the initial clinical presentation. Symptoms of anaphylaxis may be mild, moderate, or severe, and may be biphasic or protracted (20). In biphasic situations, the initial presentation may be followed in as early as 4 hours with another recrudescence of symptoms. In general, the earlier the onset of symptoms after the inciting exposure, the more severe the evolving syndrome.

Although literally any organ can be involved, the upper and lower respiratory tract, cardiovascular system, gastrointestinal tract, and the skin usually are affected. Initial symptoms may include a sense or "funny feeling" that something is wrong, gastrointestinal upset or the feeling of bladder urgency, itching and erythema or flushing, *voice change, itching in the throat, the need to clear the throat,* tachycardia, mild palpitations, coughing, and itching between the shoulder blades. Symptoms may progress to a more moderate stage, including urticaria and early angioedema, *hoarseness, dysphagia, frank globus sensation,* tightness in the chest with shortness of breath, possible audible wheezing, increased nausea and vomiting, diarrhea and abdominal cramping,

and increased tachycardia with headache. (Cessation of progression of symptoms may immediately define the ultimate degree of severity; however, the rapidity with which symptoms evolve and continue to progress prognosticates the more severe outcomes.) The most severe symptoms include cardiovascular decompensation with hypotension, arrhythmia, myocardial infarction, and cardiovascular collapse, further respiratory distress with progression to status asthmaticus and pulmonary obstruction, *stridor, loss of voice, and upper airway obstruction.* Sinonasal symptoms of varying degrees may be found at any stage throughout the process. Death can occur within a relatively short time (minutes), but also can occur in a delayed fashion even when the patient has seemingly been adequately resuscitated through the initial phase. This delayed effect is presumed due to early-stage organ damage with late organ dysfunction and lethal outcomes (27,28). Histopathologic studies in fatal cases involving airway obstruction have shown airway swelling involving a watery or thin fluid-type edema affecting mainly the lamina propria of the endolarynx, epiglottis, and hypopharynx with remarkably few inflammatory cells. Edematous involvement of the structures has been noted in over 65% of fatal cases (10,28–31).

A more in-depth consideration of the anaphylaxis syndrome, its incidence, pathophysiologic process, inciting agents, clinical presentations, and treatment is found in Chapter 7. Studies are needed to define further the pathophysiologic process of anaphylactic and anaphylactoid reactions at the immunochemical level. Understanding these mechanisms and the occasions under which they may arise can permit prophylaxis. Such studies also will allow the development of better treatment options, such as improved treatment of anaphylaxis in patients on β-blocking agents.

## Angioedema and Urticaria

Very few clinical situations demand the otolaryngologist's immediate attention as urgently as airway swelling. Anaphylaxis with angioedema of the laryngopharynx is perhaps the most clinically significant acute scenario. A spectrum of evolution of laryngopharyngeal symptoms with angioedema has been discussed. What the clinician must realize, however, is that there is a wide spectrum of non–anaphylactic-driven angioedema, with or without urticaria, with the potential for chronicity and recurrence. Episodes can be rapid and fulminant, as seen with anaphylaxis, or much slower in onset and less responsive to treatment and resolution. With a wide and varied etiologic differential, considerable research still needs to be done to define further and integrate the pathophysiologic mechanisms.

Urticaria and angioedema have similarities in their mechanisms, except the histologic location of the pathologic process differs, with angioedema involving deeper layers of the skin and internal organs. The etiologies also tend to be similar and the incidence is underestimated, with some reports indicating that up to 20% of Americans are affected at some time in their life (32–34). To recognize and treat the laryngopharyngeal and other presenting signs and symptoms of anaphylaxis, the clinician should have a firm basis from which to diagnose and treat other forms of angioedema with or without urticaria. The clinician must be aware of the breadth of the differential of etiologic factors to help with diagnostic questions that arise beyond dealing with the acute episodes.

Attempts have been made to divide angioedema into diagnostic groups (35). Landerman describes four such categories of angioedema: (a) HAE, (b) hereditary allergic angioedema, (c) nonhereditary allergic angioedema, and (d) idiopathic angioedema (36). Metzger provides a current appraisal of angioedema by categorizing on the basis of potential mechanisms of mast cell activation as well as on the basis of clinical etiology (37). He classifies the patterns of mast cell activation into five groups, including those of IgE immediate hypersensitivity, activation of the classic and the alternate pathways of complement, a direct activation of mast cell membrane, and the plasma-kinin generating system. Both the clinician who is confronted with angioedema and the otolaryngologist dealing with laryngopharyngeal and other head and neck manifestations of angioedema should be aware of the potential etiologic triggers for this process.

Metzger's classification of urticaria provides a good framework and should be familiar to clinicians (Table 19.1). One broad group of his classifications includes nonimmunologic etiologies. In this group is dermatographism with both the idiopathic and cutaneous mastocytosis forms. Adrenergic and physical urticaria also are nonimmunologic. The physical urticarias include forms generated by pressure, vibration, sunlight, cholinergic stimuli, cold, and local heat. The hereditary urticarias and angioedemas also are nonimmunologic. These are relatively rare conditions and include both primary and acquired angioedema, the syndrome of urticaria, deafness, and amyloidosis, familial localized heat urticaria, porphyria, papular urticaria, urticaria pigmentosa, and the C3b-inactivator deficiency. The miscellaneous nonimmunologic etiologies are very important to the clinician. This group includes infections, which can be bacterial, parasitic, fungal, and viral (including hepatitis and infectious mononucleosis) (38,39). Collagen vascular disease is another systemic group that includes Sjögren's syndrome, rheumatoid arthritis, and systemic lupus erythematosus (40). There also are reported cases of angioedema and urticaria associated with various neoplasia, including a variety of lymphoid and hematologic malignancies, and carcinomas of the rectum, lung, and colon (37). Obviously, this grouping of infection, collagen vascular disease, and neoplasia represents etiologies that the clinician would not want to overlook. Last, some forms of anaphylaxis such as recurrent idiopathic and exercise-induced anaphylaxis may not be truly IgE mediated.

The second broad grouping of urticarias by Metzger in-

### TABLE 19.1. METZGER'S CLASSIFICATION OF URTICARIA

**Nonimmunologic etiologies**
Dermatographism
  Idiopathic
  Cutaneous mastocytosis
Adrenergic urticaria
Physical urticaria
  Pressure
  Vibratory
  Solar
  Cholinergic
  Cold
  Heat
Hereditary urticaria angioedema
  Hereditary angioedema
  Syndrome of urticaria, deafness, and amyloidosis
  Familial localized heat urticaria
  Porphyria
  Papular urticaria
  Urticaria pigmentosa
  $C3b^-$ inactivator deficiency
Infectious
Collagen vascular diseases
Neoplastic

**Immunologic etiologies**
Foods
Drugs
Insect stings
Atopic reactions
Transfusion reactions
Autoimmune IgE
Anti-FceRI
Schnitzler's syndrome
Acquired C1 inhibitor deficiency
**Uncertain etiologies**
Aspirin
Opiates
Metabisulfites
Tartrazines
Idiopathic

cludes those of immunologic etiology, which includes foods, drugs, insect stings, atopy, transfusion reactions, and other rare entities such as autoimmune IgE or other anti-immunoglobulin syndromes, Schnitzler's syndrome, and acquired C1 inhibitor deficiency. He also gives a third grouping of identifiable agents of which the mechanisms are uncertain, such as aspirin, opiates, metabisulfites, and tartrazines. These last two broad groupings, immunologic and those of uncertain mechanisms, have etiologies that are very important to the otolaryngologist and allergist (37,41). These are all well referenced and further discussion of these disorders is beyond the scope of this chapter.

There is one last broad grouping of angioedema and urticaria, the idiopathic, for which a thorough evaluation has been made but no etiologic agent has been found. Unfortunately, especially for chronic urticaria, this tends to be a rather large group. One study indicated that precipitating causes are found only in up to 30% of the patients receiving a comprehensive evaluation (42). This fact should not deter the clinician from taking a responsible etiologic, diagnostic approach along with the course of treatment.

The otolaryngologist *will* come in contact with angioedema and urticaria. The angioedema at times will involve the laryngopharynx and it is important for the otolaryngologist to consider the various etiologies involved because some of them represent significant diseases.

## Angioedema: Angiotensin-converting Enzyme Inhibitors and Angiotensin II Blockers

Some increasingly common causes of angioedema particularly involving the oral cavity and the laryngopharynx are those associated with drugs. A few comments are appropriate regarding the ACE inhibitors (43–49). This problem is characterized by intermittent angioedema involving any of the facial, oral, hypopharyngeal, or laryngeal-related structures. The presentation of angioedema in patients can range from rare and insignificant to frequent and life threatening on the basis of airway obstruction. Such reactions are not exclusive to these drugs. However, because these drugs are used frequently in the management of hypertension and congestive heart failure, otolaryngologists are likely to be involved in the management of some of their adverse effects. In fact, over the last 2 years this author has personally managed almost two dozen cases requiring aggressive airway monitoring or intervention. Initial estimates of the incidence of this problem ranged from 0.1% to 0.5% of patients on these drugs. It was thought that reactions would occur within the first week of therapy. However, it became apparent that patients could be under therapy for a number of years before development of edematous reactions. With that thought in mind, the incidence is now thought to be approximately 1.2%. Episodes have been shown to become more frequent with recurrent exposure to the drug, and there is an increased incidence among African Americans. There also may be an increased incidence in patients with a history of idiopathic angioedema. ACE inhibitors were first introduced in the 1970s with captopril. In the 1980s, they also were associated with another frequent side effect, chronic cough, a problem for which otolaryngologists frequently are consulted. However, it was in 1980 that the first case of angioedema was reported with captopril. There also are some reports of a history of recent airway manipulation being a comorbid factor, with one report citing angioedema occurring during the time of oral surgery (49). A clear dose–response relationship has not been described.

The exact mechanism of the angioedema related to ACE inhibitors is not fully understood, but there is evidence that it probably is not IgE mediated. The pathogenesis is thought to involve increased levels of bradykinin, possibly associated with either kinase II inhibition, ACE deficiency, or problems with bradykinin metabolism. Kinase II inactivates bradykinin. ACE inhibitors block the action of kinase II. Spontaneous wheal-and-flare reactions to injected bradykinin have been shown to increase after oral ACE inhibitor use. Other mechanisms are thought to involve deficiencies in certain enzymes, particularly carboxypeptidase N, and complement components, particularly C1 esterase inhibitor and complement 4 (C4). When ACE is inhibited in patients with low levels of carboxypeptidase N, there may be lowered inactivation of bradykinin, possibly predisposing to the triggering of angioedema. Studies also have commented on the role of C1 esterase and C4 in the possible pathophysiologic process of patients with HAE (48).

A study by Warner et al. (46) examined angiotensin II receptor blockers as an alternative medication in patients with ACE inhibitor–reactive angioedema. The authors did a literature review and found that 32% of the patients who had angioedema induced by angiotensin II receptor blockers also had a prior history of ACE inhibitor–induced angioedema. This report is of significance principally for three reasons. First, it alerts clinicians to the fact that angiotensin II receptor blockers also may be of significance in creating potential airway problems. Second, it raises a question as to whether bradykinin is the only principle in the mechanism by which ACE inhibitors induce swelling. Warner et al. again raise the question of C1 esterase metabolism as being a part of the clinical pathophysiologic process of angioedema. Altman et al. also discussed angioedema of the retropharyngeal space in a patient with acquired hereditary angioneurotic edema and pharyngitis (14). Third, until the mechanisms of angioedema in patients treated with ACE inhibitors are worked out, Warner et al. recommend that angiotensin II receptor blockers should be used with *extreme* caution in patients with a prior history of angioedema.

Although treatment for ACE inhibitor–related angioedema may involve nothing more than discontinuance of the drug for milder cases such as minimal lip swelling, tongue or laryngopharyngeal edema requires an aggressive evaluation. In these more severe cases, the otolaryngologist must make a decision about whether to establish an airway with intubation (or, less likely, tracheotomy) or to monitor the airway aggressively in an intensive care setting. Because the mechanism may well be nonallergic and related to bradykinin metabolism, the response to epinephrine may not be as immediate or efficacious as with forms of allergic angioedema. Because the response to treatment is not necessarily as rapid as might be desired, there is a chance of significant progression of the edema before its eventual recession. This response echoes the need for very close airway monitoring and, when indicated, a more aggressive approach for securing an airway.

Despite this fact, epinephrine still should be used as part of the first-line treatment for angioedema. The mainstay of treatment may well be the use of *steroids,* which, of course, may require some time to exert clinical effect. Antihistamines and histamine type 2 receptor ($H_2$) blockers are other drugs to include in the regimen. Obviously, discontinuance of the precipitating medication is of utmost importance. In addition, switching types of ACE inhibitors in patients who have had adverse reactions with one ACE inhibitor is fraught with continued problems because angioedema is a class-wide phenomenon. Because steroids play a significant role in the treatment of this problem, airway management usually is critical up to 72 hours after treatment has been instituted. Unfortunately, angioedema has been reported to persist up to a week after stopping the drug. ACE inhibitors should be used with caution in all patients with a prior history of angioedema. Other oropharyngeal side effects from these drugs may include oral ulceration and glossitis.

Although the issue of ACE inhibitors and angiotensin II blockers presents a clinically significant and unique problem for the otolaryngologist, other drugs also can be associated with edema of the head and neck and, in particular, laryngopharyngeal edema. A review of medications used at the time of clinical presentation with inquiry into their side effects provides additional possibilities in the differential of acute airway obstruction.

Finally, there are reported cases of congenital ACE deficiency. In 1995, Sreeram and Corey (50) reported a case and review of angioedema of the upper airway associated with congenital ACE deficiency. They offer an excellent review of the renin–angiotensin–aldosterone system, comment on the coexistence of atopy in this patient, and discuss treatment issues in this setting. They advocate the judicious use of epinephrine and note that these patients respond poorly to steroids. With this in mind, and the experience of others who have treated angioedema related to the ACE inhibitors, until all the mechanisms have been thoroughly worked out, there will remain some degree of uncertainty on the exact drug regimen to undertake. With any medications given, there may be a critical and lengthy period until resolution is achieved. Proactive discretionary use of a regimen of epinephrine, steroids, antihistamines, and $H_2$ blockers, along with very cautious and close airway management, is recommended. For the rare condition of congenital ACE deficiency (to be considered as part of the differential for angioedema), Sreeram and Corey advocate the immediate use of self-administered epinephrine and proceeding to an emergency department for further evaluation and treatment as needed.

## Angioedema: Oral Allergy Syndrome

Sensitivities to food can cause laryngopharyngeal edema as well as edema of other head and neck and gastrointestinal mucosal structures. One particular syndrome that merits discussion is OAS. Pastorello notes that OAS implies a complex of clinical symptoms localized to the mucosa of the mouth and pharynx that occur with contact to a specific food (51–53). Allergies to fresh fruits and vegetables associated with different inhalant allergens, usually pollens, are the most frequent causes. The suspected relationship is a cross-reactivity between the inhalant and the food, with symptoms occurring when the food in question is ingested (54). This problem may be much more common than is currently appreciated. One study indicated that as many as 40% of people with various forms of pollenosis report adverse symptoms on eating vegetables or fruits (55). Another study has indicated that as many as 75% of patients allergic to birch pollen complain of symptoms with ingestion of apples (56).

Laryngopharyngeal edema occurs frequently with exposure to foods. Ortolani et al. in 1988 reported a series of 262 patients with OAS involving fresh fruits and vegetables in which 62 cases, or 26%, presented with laryngeal edema (53). In another series of 706 patients, Ortolani et al. found that 92 (13%) had had laryngeal edema, with a small number also demonstrating anaphylactic shock (57). The mucosa of the upper aerodigestive tract has a rather large concentration of mast cells, which in the case of IgE-mediated disease would provide an abundance of binding sites for specific IgE. Fortunately, not all reactions are as severe as laryngopharyngeal edema, with many of them involving only minor and brief symptomatology. For that reason, the true incidence of such cross-reactivity may be underestimated.

A key issue here is the cross-reactivity between an inhalant, usually a pollen, and a food, such as a fruit or vegetable. Although all of the details of cross-reactivity have not been worked out and are under further study, the concept of a cross-reactive epitope (antigen–antibody recognition site) provides a working model. Cross-reactive epitopes of two botanically unrelated species react with similar antibodies. For example, work has been done with silver birch and hazelnuts (58). Some birch pollen–sensitive people produce antibodies in response to birch pollen antigens. These people then react to the ingestion of hazelnut antigens because they are structurally similar to birch pollen antigens. The antibody recognition sites of these select birch pollen and hazelnut antigens (i.e., cross-reacting epitopes) are similar enough to cause formation of antibodies that subsequently elicit an allergic reaction when hazelnut is ingested by birch pollen–sensitive people. However, not all birch pollen–sensitive people have antibodies that will cross-react with hazelnut. Therefore, not every birch pollen–sensitive person will have an adverse reaction with the ingestion of hazelnut. A lengthy discussion on cross-reactivity is beyond the scope of this chapter; however, cross-reactivity may occur between similar botanical species such as within the variety of ragweeds or the species of grasses, or with botanically dissimilar entities such as foods and inhalants. Other terms given for this phenomenon are *concomitant allergy* or *cluster of hypersensitivity* (59). Other cross-reactive food combinations are described in Chapter 4, as well as in other sources (60).

These relationships have been studied by a number of methods, including radioallergosorbent test inhibition, crossedline immunoelectrophoresis technique, and sodium dodecyl sulfate-PAGE (polyacrylamide gel electrophoresis) and immunoblotting techniques, all of which have contributed to the evidence of cross-reactivity between some pollens and foods (51,58).

Diagnosis of OAS relies heavily on a complete and thorough history with a corroborating physical examination. Unfortunately, the efficacy of objective testing, using both in vivo and in vitro techniques, is somewhat in question. This issue centers on the suspected lability of the antigens involved (61). The processing of an antigen to produce extracts for skin testing or substrates for an in vitro test has been the suspected reason for the inconsistent results in the correlation of history and objective testing. Even the double-blind, placebo-controlled food challenge, often considered the gold standard of food testing, requires a lyophilization process in preparation of the food. Furthermore, there also is the problem with gastric acidity deactivating the allergens, thus lessening the validity of the test (58,60). Other methods have been reported with some degree of efficacy, including fresh extract in vitro and in vivo (prick + prick) methods (51,62,63), as well as some mononuclear cell histamine release assays. Therefore, positive objective studies that correlate with the history can be considered significant, whereas negative objective studies may indeed be false-negative results. Treatment of OAS would then involve avoidance of the food that provokes symptoms or at least avoidance of the food in the form that is known to cause the symptoms, because some provoking foods when cooked fail to evoke the response. The use of antihistamines may be of some help in curbing symptoms (64). In more severe forms, the clinician must provide patients with appropriate educational materials and a protocol of action for dealing with these severe, acute symptoms, including seeking and obtaining proper treatment for anaphylaxis when necessary. More work needs to be done on epitope–allergen identification, especially with fresh vegetables and fruits.

*Qod aliis cibus est aliis fuat acre benenum,* "What is food for some may be fierce poison for others."—Lucretius (65). A quote that is both literal and figurative.

## COMMON ALLERGIC MANIFESTATIONS OF THE LARYNGOPHARYNX

The paucity of information in the literature on allergic manifestations of the laryngopharynx has already been noted in this chapter. Other authors also have described this dilemma (66,67). The current interest in allergy and its role in respiratory disease is being driven by an increasing incidence of respiratory illnesses such as allergic rhinitis and asthma. Early reports by Alimov (4), Pang (68), and Duncan and Duncan (69) cite the incidence of allergy-related laryngitis

and throat problems and also discuss the association of laryngeal manifestations of allergy in sinonasal and asthmatic allergic patients. Alimov, in a 1968 report, cited 69 of 245 patients (28%) with acute or chronic laryngitis as having allergy as the underlying cause (4). Duncan and Duncan surveyed 680 patients treated for respiratory allergy, of which there were 261 complaints of pharynx-related symptomatology, including itching, irritation, soreness, burning and laryngitis (69). Of these 261 complaints, 245 (94%) improved with proper allergy-related therapy.

In another study, Pang identified the laryngopharynx as an integrated part of the upper and lower respiratory tract, being affected by allergy just as the sinonasal and pulmonary tract would be affected (68). His approach to the allergic patient included consideration of inhalants, foods, and chemical irritants using both a historical approach as well as multiple objective measures, including skin testing and provocation testing. Pang used indirect laryngoscopy in his examinations of the larynx. It was his belief that edema of the vocal cords was a key component of the allergic reaction. In anaphylaxis, the edema could involve the epiglottis, arytenoids, ventricles, false vocal cords, vocal cords, and the subglottic airway. In nonanaphylactic reactions, however, he noted edema of the larynx with a pale, glistening appearance to the vocal cords in which the contact surface of the cords were rather white and more glistening than normal. According to Pang, allergic edema was distinct from edema due to infection in which there also was a hyperemia. Pang also was one of the first researchers to discuss special problems in professional voice users, especially singers, who would complain of dysphonia with very minimal or subtle findings on indirect examination. His thoughts about vibration changes involving the vocal cords that are generated by this subtle edema are currently being confirmed. Pang believed that he could provoke changes in vocal cord symptoms and signs with provocation testing and also could resolve signs and symptoms with allergy management. He cited one patient who he thought had a laryngeal edematous reaction to a squash allergy that resolved promptly with elimination of the food (68).

Williams, in 1972, reported a series of 22 cases of allergic laryngitis caused by inhalants or foods using provocation techniques to verify the allergic nature of the laryngitis (70). In 1991, Sala et al. wrote about occupational laryngitis with immediate allergic or chemical hypersensitivity (67). They referred to a series by Yamaguchi et al. in 1971 on laryngoscopic findings of allergic rhinitis (71). In their series the diagnosis of laryngitis was made on the basis of erythema and swelling of the laryngeal and vocal cord mucosa on indirect laryngoscopy. The studies of Sala et al. also were performed on the basis of provocation. They looked at a number of factors, including age, sex, occupation, duration of exposure, causative agents, vocal cord status change with provocation, skin prick testing, specific IgE levels to the causative agent, personal and family history of atopy, and the existence of other allergic disease. Their conclusion was that, based on their study, *true* allergic laryngitis may be a rare entity. A critical analysis of the study regarding materials, methods, and conclusion suggests that Sala and colleagues' assertion may not be justified. What Sala et al. did, however, was to take a more organized approach to the subject, attempting to objectify its evaluation. In addition, they discussed the issue of speech abnormalities and the need for objective measures of voice for future studies (67).

Using his environmental control unit, Rea studied two patients with chronic dysphonia. He determined that laryngeal edema was due to the accumulation of a number of provoking agents that included a broad spectrum of foods, inhalants, and chemicals, suggesting that multiple inciting factors stimulated an allergic load phenomenon (8,11).

In 1998, Nito et al. looked at the effect of Japanese cedar pollen and pollution on laryngeal symptoms (5). They looked at sensitive patients in polluted and nonpolluted areas; at the same time, they conducted studies on sensitized rats, exposing some to pollutants and cedar antigen and others just to cedar antigen. They investigated the effect of these potential allergens on IgE levels and eosinophilia of the laryngeal tissue. Patients were objectively diagnosed on the basis of eosinophilia in the nasal secretions and specific serum IgE antibody for Japanese cedar pollen. Assessment of change in allergic status was made on the basis of symptoms, including nasal stuffiness, itching of the eyes, soreness of the throat, cough, sputum, hoarseness, and foreign body sensation in the larynx. Pollen counts were higher in the rural areas and pollution concentrations were higher in the urban industrial areas. They found that 40% to 70% of the patients with cedar pollenosis had laryngeal symptoms that occurred in parallel to seasonal changes in cedar pollen counts. They also found that the grades of eosinophilia in nasal and laryngeal mucosa of sensitized rats were higher than those in the mucosa of the control group. Furthermore, the specific serum IgE levels for Japanese cedar pollen were higher in the sensitized rats that were exposed to nitrogen dioxide versus the sensitized rats that were unexposed. They hypothesized that the exposure to the pollutant enhanced the rats' ability to produce specific IgE to the Japanese cedar pollen (5). More studies are needed to investigate the concept of allergic load and the possible synergy between pollutants and the allergic response.

> Excessive use of the voice, either in screaming or singing, when continued for a certain period, finally causes the temporary congestion which exists at the time, to assume the chronic state. In hucksters, for example, hoarseness is almost universal. . . . His [the singer's] efforts to produce as high a note as possible and give his voice a volume which it does not possess, strain the muscles and produce in them an inflammatory state which soon becomes chronic and extremely difficult to eradicate." *Diseases of the Nose and Throat,* 1886 (72).

The medical demands of the modern professional voice, the realization of a need for better diagnostic and treatment approaches, an evolved awareness of the complexities of multiple factors that affect laryngopharyngeal function, the increasing awareness of how the laryngopharynx integrates itself into the respiratory and upper gastrointestinal tract, and the evolution of more elegant and sophisticated diagnostic tools such as fiberoptic endoscopy and strobovideolaryngoscopy have provided a breakthrough in diagnosis and treatment and led to new directions in the management and research of laryngopharyngeal problems. A multidisciplinary approach to evaluation of voice and laryngeal problems now may include a comprehensive history, otolaryngologic consultation, acoustic analysis, strobovideolaryngoscopy, consideration for allergy testing, and other related consultations and procedures that might include pulmonary and gastroenterologic investigations (66,73). This multidisciplinary approach can serve as a general template for evaluation of virtually all laryngeal-related problems. The degree to which this template is expanded or contracted depends on the clinical situation of the patient on a case-by-case basis. For example, videolaryngoscopy has been used in cancer staging for lesions of the larynx and pharynx (74). In this situation, only a few components of this multidisciplinary evaluation may be needed.

Dixon used strobovideolaryngoscopy to evaluate patients with dysphonia and suspected delayed food allergy using provocation/neutralization techniques (7). Dixon previously noted that the vocal examination of voice professionals with conventional telescopic magnifying laryngoscopy would not show changes that could be picked up on strobovideolaryngoscopy with provocation/neutralization techniques (6). In intermittently dysphonic patients, he performed a double-blind intradermal provocation/neutralization skin test to food antigen using strobovideolaryngoscopy to document changes in the vocal cords and the quality of voice. He also obtained double-blind measurements of signs and symptoms, digital audio recordings of the voice for perceptual and acoustic analysis, and aerodynamic laryngeal airflow and resistance measurements. He concluded that the dysphonia was due to irregular glottic edge edema and thick mucus production. Although this study involved a double-blind protocol, statistical analysis was not conducted. Dixon called for further studies using such protocols to confirm the findings and carry on further research (7). This study, along with others (75,76), strongly suggested that consideration of allergic factors should be made in the evaluation of voice and other laryngeal problems.

Jackson-Menaldi et al. (66) looked at the role of allergy in voice patients. They took a multidisciplinary approach to their group of patients, including patient history, acoustic analysis, and strobovideolaryngoscopy. They also included allergy testing and studies for gastroesophageal reflux when appropriate. The authors realized that there are numerous conditions that could lead to changes in the larynx and the voice. They wanted to collect a set of signs that would help distinguish one diagnosis from another and give some credence that inhalant allergy does, indeed, have some affect on the larynx. Perennial allergens, especially dust mite, were the prevalent positives on skin testing (serial endpoint titration was the most common method used). Vocal assessment indicated that all of their subjects had evidence of vocal abuse or misuse. Fifteen of the 17 patients had documented allergy, and only 2 could be documented to have gastroesophageal reflux–laryngopharyngeal reflux problems. Strobovideolaryngoscopic findings indicated the presence of vocal fold edema corroborated by changes in phase closure, amplitude, and supraglottal activity. The authors also noted an increase of mucus and discussed possible contributions by the upper and lower respiratory tract. They also argued that standard pulmonary function studies may not be adequate to evaluate patients with subtle lower airway dysfunction. Although their numbers were relatively small, they believed that allergic reactions involving the larynx do exist and found vocal fold edema in 100% of their allergic patients. Jackson-Menaldi et al. argued that an allergy evaluation was appropriate in patients who present with patterns of vocal abuse and misuse (66).

With a better understanding of gastroesophageal reflux and an appreciation of the roles and relationships of the upper and lower respiratory tract, a multidisciplinary approach to the larynx holds a key to research in the role of allergy in laryngopharyngeal problems.

## THE INTEGRATED RESPIRATORY TRACT

As stated in the introduction, other juxtaposed organs can have an affect on the laryngopharynx. Sinonasal, asthmatic, and similar conditions are important, and in evaluating patients with laryngopharyngeal symptoms, an inquiry into an allergy history is essential. The coexistence of upper and lower respiratory tract inflammatory conditions has been well appreciated. There is mounting evidence that these conditions may be a continuum of inflammation, in which the laryngopharynx is not only included, but may play an integrating role.

> Division of the airway into an upper and lower part is neither anatomically nor physiologically correct. The airway is a single integrated system (77).
>
> As our understanding of the role of inflammation and airway disease evolves, the classical perspective that allergic rhinitis and asthma are distinct entities is being displaced by the increasing evidence that they are a manifestation of a continuous inflammation within one common airway (78).

Exploring these notions and how the laryngopharynx may play a role involves looking at models of how the nervous system affects the respiratory tract and investigating the biology of inflammation.

As long ago as the second century, Galen noted a relationship between inflammatory nasal conditions and asthma and described how treating the nose helped the lower respiratory tract symptoms (79,80). Interest in this relationship began to emerge in the early 20th century with further clinical observation and some initial experimental trials (81–84). Causally and clinically, the association between rhinitis, sinusitis, and asthma has been well documented (77,85). As much as 90% of all patients with asthma have rhinitis (86). Fifteen to 30% of patients with allergic rhinitis will at some time in their life experience hyperreactive lower respiratory tract symptoms (87). Series have been cited showing a significant relationship between abnormal sinus radiographs and the coexistence of asthma (88–97). Medical and surgical management of rhinitis and sinusitis have also been shown to improve the severity of asthma and positively influence its treatment (81,91,98–106). How these relationships are driven and where the laryngopharynx plays a role requires a look at neuroanatomy and inflammation itself. A review of the neurologic anatomic relationships in the laryngopharynx and how they may relate to the sinonasal and pulmonary system is appropriate at this time.

The *pharyngeal plexus* (Fig. 19.4) is a composite of neural fibers from many different sources, including the glossopharyngeal, vagus, hypoglossus, superior laryngeal, and sympathetic nerves. The glossopharyngeal nerve sends three or four pharyngeal branches that join with the vagus and the sympathetic nerves at the level of the medial pharyngeal constrictor to form the pharyngeal plexus. These elements penetrate through the muscular layer and innervate the mucosa. Other branches to the area include motor branches to the stylopharyngeus as well as tonsillar and lingual branches. The vagus nerve has a superior and inferior ganglion at the level of the brain stem. Branches from the superior part of the inferior ganglion containing sensory fibers meld with motor fibers from the spinal accessory nerve and make their way to join the glossopharyngeal sympathetics in the superior laryngeal nerve to form the pharyngeal plexus. Besides muscular and mucosal innervation, most of the soft palate and the carotid body also are innervated. The superior laryngeal nerve arises from the inferior end of the inferior ganglion and eventually branches into an external and internal branch. It is the external branch that contributes fibers to the pharyngeal plexus and communicates with the superior sympathetic cardiac nerve. Fibers from the hypoglossus communicate with the vagus nerve in a band of tissue at the level of the inferior ganglion. As this tissue lines around the occipital artery, it communicates by several filaments with the pharyngeal plexus. One to six filaments from the sympathetic ganglion communicate with the pharyngeal branches of the other nerves to form the plexus. These filaments form both the lateral wall as well as the posterior wall plexus, and connect with the superior laryngeal nerve directly. This complex, varied, and intricate networking of neural elements with a wide diversity of generalized and specific motor, sensory, sympathetic, and parasympathetic functions lays the basic groundwork for theories on neural reflex response and is a model for explaining various relationships of inflammation in the respiratory tract (107).

In the early 20th century, cellular biology did not have any clear neural reflex models to explain the rhinosinobronchial relationships. Perhaps one of the earliest attempts to elucidate their relationship was the 1919 hypothesis of Sluder of a sinonasal-bronchial reflex consisting of a trigeminal afferent–vagal efferent neural arc (84). More recently, Slavin elaborated on this subject by suggesting a trigeminal–brain stem–parasympathetic (vagal to bronchial) circuit (96,108,109). Although some allergen-, irritant-, and vasomotor stimuli–related studies have supported this reflex (82,83,110–114), the lack of studies that demonstrate a clear proof of mechanism as well as studies unable to replicate these results have led to a questioning of the existence of this arc (77,80,85,115). In response to these negatives, other studies suggest that the existence of a reflex arc acting to a dedicated response may be too simplistic. Still others suggest that a critical threshold of respiratory inflammation may need to be surpassed before the reflex is triggered (77).

Studies with allergic (77,85,116) and nonallergic (117) stimuli to the *pharynx,* rather than to the nose, have demonstrated reflex bronchial constriction (pharyngobronchial reflex). These observations also suggest that inflammatory changes of the upper respiratory tract are associated with pulmonary functional changes of the lower respiratory tract. Although reports have debated whether the lower respiratory tract can be soiled with inflammatory secretions from the upper respiratory tract (118–120), and although the normal clearance of secretions from the lower respiratory tract is into the pharynx by ciliary activity, it is attractive to think that reflex activity stimulated by secretions in an inflamed pharynx adds to clinical asthmatic activity. Thus, the laryngopharynx may well integrate the upper and lower respiratory tract on a neurologic as well as an anatomic basis, especially during times of allergic and nonallergic inflammation (77,85).

The aforementioned studies led to an important area of research, that of respiratory tract inflammation. The study of respiratory inflammation is central in the concept of an integrated respiratory tract. In the final quarter of the 20th century, and now into the 21st, the literature has demonstrated increased attention to inflammatory injury, repair, and remodeling. This research has examined the interaction of inflammatory cells (especially neutrophils, mast cells, eosinophils, lymphocytes), proinflammatory proteins, cytokines, chemokines, adhesion molecules, and the like (121). The literature tends to suggest the concept, especially in allergic inflammation, of one common inflammatory response in an integrated respiratory tract, the model of which includes:

1. Evidence of epithelial damage and mucosal responses in the nose and sinuses similar to those in the bronchial tree in patients with sinusitis or rhinitis and asthma, including eosinophilic infiltrates, deposition of major basic protein, and epithelial histologic changes (desquamation of superficial columnar epithelium) (77,106, 122–124).

2. Activated T cells pervading sinus, bronchial tissue, and peripheral blood at times of allergic stress. This motivates eosinophil activation through cytokine and adhesion molecule signaling (125–127).

A discussion of neural reflexes, the biology of inflammation, and their integration in the respiratory tract can be found in two excellent works by Herwitz (77) and de Benedictis and Bush (85). A paraphrase of DeBenedictis's summary of the inflammatory pathways follows. Central to the epithelial injury and response of the respiratory tract (rhinitis, sinusitis, asthma) to allergens and microbes (viral, bacterial) is an eosinophil-driven inflammation. This injury leads to:

1. Mediator release and increased secretions with progressing bronchial reactivity through direct soilage stimulating pulmonary and pharyngobronchial reflexes.

2. Nasal obstruction that, with further or secondary bacterial infection, leads to more inflammation and increased bronchial reactivity secondary to mouth breathing (128) (dryness–reflex bronchial reactivity) or sinonasal reflex bronchial reactivity

3. Which now in a circular fashion leads to further epithelial damage and repair.

In this model of a single inflammatory response in an integrated respiratory tract with the larynx and pharynx at the center, the clinician must consider gastroenterologic and pulmonary aspects of the patient presenting with laryngopharyngeal symptomatology.

## GASTROESOPHAGEAL REFLUX

Gastric disturbances, especially caused by debauchery, are frequent causes of chronic laryngitis as evidenced by the hoarseness of drunkards (72).

As noted in the multidisciplinary approach to laryngeal voice problems, the upper gastrointestinal tract can play a role in the genesis of symptoms, mimicking allergic disease of the laryngopharynx and the remainder of the respiratory tract. Therefore, a review of the gastrointestinal system is appropriate, especially with regard to gastroesophageal reflux disease (GERD) and its relationship to laryngopharyngeal reflux (LPR; i.e., gastroesophageal reflux with otolaryngic symptoms). Although some controversy still exists, and more studies are needed, evidence from prospective studies and consensus reports confirms the role of gastroesophageal reflux in the pathogenesis of extraesophageal symptoms and diseases. These conditions include (129–135):

1. Dysphonia, hoarseness
2. Muscle tension or hyperfunctional symptoms—pitch breaks, cracks, vocal fatigue
3. Excessive mucus and symptoms of postnasal drainage, excessive throat clearing, globus
4. Dysphagia, odynophagia
5. Chronic cough
6. Chronic and intermittent laryngitis with or without subglottic or posterior glottic stenosis
7. Hypertrophic mucosal disorders such as vocal nodules, polypoid degeneration, contact ulcers and granulomas, and trauma such as endotracheal intubation injury or arytenoid fixation
8. Miscellaneous disorders, including neoplasia, laryngospasm, and laryngomalacia

The importance of food and inhalant allergy in GERD currently is not well understood. Sufficient studies to confirm a direct affect of allergy in the pathogenesis of GERD or LPR do not exist, although a recent study by Mishra et al. suggests such a relationship (136). However, the evaluation and treatment of upper respiratory tract allergy in patients with symptoms associated with possible reflux always is included.

Koufman enumerates four general reasons for the misdiagnosis or undertreatment of GERD and LPR:

1. Patients with LPR *usually* deny heartburn.
2. On physical examination, laryngeal findings of GERD/LPR vary and edema often is missed.
3. Tests for LPR lack sensitivity and specificity.
4. Traditional treatment for GERD may not be sufficient for LPR, or the diagnosis of GERD/LPR is not made or the condition is thought not to be a problem (128).

Although heartburn has traditionally been associated with GERD and esophagitis, there is mounting evidence that LPR is different from GERD, often presenting with hoarseness or voice change without heartburn or esophagitis (129,131,137,138). One series demonstrated that only 4% of patients with LPR reported heartburn (139). In addition, although heartburn is a feature of most patients with GERD, it is not necessarily a symptom of some patients with esophagitis (129,137,140). It is possible for a patient to have both GERD and LPR. Patients with LPR have been found to have a high incidence of normal results on esophageal manometry (normal lower esophageal sphincter function), acid perfusion tests, and esophagoscopy even, with a large percentage of abnormal single-probe esophageal pH studies (141). Esophagitis, on the other hand, can be found in almost all patients with GERD. The development of double- and triple-probe pH monitoring allows a high degree of sensitivity and specificity in detecting abnormal pH patterns and LPR (139,140). Patients with suspected

gastroesophageal reflux and otolaryngic symptoms can now be separated from patients with GERD [esophagitis] on the basis of this study. With the emergence of proton pump inhibitors and their success in treating reflux disease, it became possible to confirm clinical observations (129).

Improved diagnostic techniques in laryngopharyngeal reflux have also provided further confirmation of physical findings that distinguish patients with GERD from those with LPR. These findings include erythema, often splotchy, of the hypopharynx, arytenoid, and posterior laryngeal commissure as well as mild edema with or without hypervascularity of the vocal cords. Reinke's edema also is seen either as a generalized vocal cord edema or a subglottic edema often comparable with a sulcus vocalis. The advent of strobovideolaryngoscopy demonstrates these findings with greater ease and sensitivity. With a proper history, an increased level of suspicion, physical findings to corroborate the history, and studies that may include a barium swallow, double- or triple-probe pH monitoring, and esophagoscopy, a diagnosis can be made and treatment initiated. If studies are not possible, then empiric treatment can be undertaken. The success of treatment with or without studies can presumptively confirm the diagnosis.

Treatment for LPR and GERD may be as simple as an antireflux regimen with changes in lifestyle and behavior modification, including:

1. Elevation of the head of the bed on 6- to 8-inch shock blocks or the use of a wedge for waterbeds
2. Not eating 3 hours before bedtime
3. Avoiding specific foods known to increase acidity or have an affect on lower esophageal sphincter tone such as citric juices, nuts, mints, chocolate, fatty foods, spicy foods, caffeine, and so forth
4. Not wearing binding clothing
5. Losing weight
6. Judicious use of antacids either at bedtime or 1 to 3 hours after meals

Some patients may require the addition of an $H_2$ blocker either twice a day or just at bedtime. Acid production at nighttime is a histamine-related phenomenon. More severe cases may require the addition of a proton pump inhibitor, which usually is given once daily in the morning before eating with or without an $H_2$ blocker at night. There is evidence that patients with LPR require a more aggressive approach in dealing with reflux, particularly in the use of proton pump inhibitors. Some advocate that higher doses of proton pump inhibitors over longer periods of time, up to 4 to 6 months, are needed to treat patients with LPR adequately and successfully.

Last, another presenting problem that links the upper gastrointestinal tract with the respiratory system is chronic cough. Chronic cough is one of the most common presenting symptoms in outpatient medicine and is a very common complaint in the general otolaryngology practice

(142–146). Gastroesophageal reflux (GERD or LPR), chronic rhinitis, and a hyperreactive lower respiratory tract are the mainstays of chronic cough diagnostic protocols.

In conclusion, gastroesophageal reflux in otolaryngic patients can be associated with many of the symptom complexes that otolaryngologists evaluate on a daily basis. Many of these presentations are laryngopharyngeal and sinonasal and, therefore, can fall into a differential diagnosis with allergic disease. Recognizing this relationship is essential. Patients with LPR can require more advanced technology in corroborating the diagnosis, possibly through strobovideolaryngoscopy and multiple-probe pH-metry studies. A more aggressive and prolonged treatment regimen also may be indicated for successfully treating LPR. Although foods that may be implicated in LPR syndromes may not provoke IgE-mediated responses, avoidance and proactive medical management still are in order.

## ADENOTONSILLAR DISEASE AND THE ALLERGIC PATIENT

> The change from [tonsillotomy to tonsillectomy] is one of the greatest of the advances that have been made in recent years in surgery of the nose and throat. Nevertheless, it has met with great opposition in certain quarters, largely because of the mystery that appears to surround the question of function of the organs . . . . That the tonsils are important physiological tissues during childhood; that they should never be removed without adequate cause; but that when such cause exists, their function is either permanently impaired or is easily taken up by other lymphoid tissues. There should, therefore, be no hesitation on that score, to totally removing diseased tonsils (147).

This quote is from Dr. Harry A. Barnes's 1914 book, *The Tonsils.* These comments from the early 20th century evoke questions and controversies about the treatment of tonsil and adenoid disease that are still relevant today. There are several questions that still are not fully understood:

1. What is the function of the palatine tonsils and adenoids?
2. In an adenotonsillectomized state, can this function be taken over by other functional elements of the body?
3. Is there a potential harm to health in doing a tonsillectomy or adenoidectomy?
4. Will adenotonsillectomy promote the emergence or amplification of respiratory tract allergy or asthma?
5. Should respiratory tract allergy be aggressively treated before adenotonsillectomy?
6. What, then, are the proper indications for adenotonsillectomy?

The tonsillar, adenoidal, and other lymphoid tissue in Waldeyer's ring constitute a portion of the mucosa-associated lymphoid tissue. As such, they act as a peripheral lymphatic organ, not dissimilar to the peripheral lymph node

in function (148–150). This lymphoid tissue is rich in B cells, yet low in both T cells and monocytes, with concentrations of T cells being approximately 40% by volume, as opposed to plasma T-cell concentrations of 70%. Tonsil and adenoid tissues, sometimes called *antigen traps,* are thought to be responsible for antibody (immunoglobulin) formation, distribution, and secretion. There are processing cells for clonal proliferation and isotype switching, in addition to proinflammatory proteins of T-cell origin such as lymphokines. Local processing of antigens is favored because of endothelial-covered channels contiguous with the airway, as opposed to lymph nodes, which depend on afferent lymphatics (151–159). There is very little in the literature, however, about IgE formation as a result of nonmicroorganism antigenic stimulation. With the involution of tonsil and adenoid tissue beginning at approximately 10 years of age, it is generally thought that the most active time for immune function is between the ages of 3 and 10 years (152).

Variations in function and morphologic character can be seen in different age groups and also different disease orders (160–165). Bussi et al. examined the distinction between chronic and recurrent tonsillitis in adults and children from the standpoint of early-, intermediate-, and late-stage responses to inflammation (165). Knowing that bacteria and viruses can stimulate tonsillar mononuclear cells and giving a challenging battery of monoclonal antibodies specific for antigens associated with these stages, they suggested that recurrent infectious tonsillitis in adults is truly a chronic infection–stimulated process. In children, however, it tends to act more like a chronic inflammatory state with secondary tonsillar hypertrophy (166). These findings would take into account differences in the immune system of adults versus children (mainly a maturation process), similarities in bacteria cultured from patients with a diagnosis of recurrent tonsillitis versus tonsillar hypertrophy, and host environmental factors, including allergic disease (167–173). Although it is intuitively likely that recurrent and chronic tonsillitis are different entities, immunologic markers differentiating the two have not been demonstrated (174). Richardson, in citing separate papers by Ogra and Siegel, states that tonsillectomy and adenoidectomy do not seem to cause any "significant immunologic consequence" in most people (151). These observations over the last 25 to 30 years give reason to calm earlier alarming suggestions that tonsillectomy removes a "lymphoid tissue barrier" and might predispose a patient to immunodeficiency and a higher incidence of related problems such as Hodgkin's disease (175).

Respiratory tract allergy and asthma must be discussed together in considering any effect of or relationship to adenotonsillectomy. As illustrated by the quote in Dr. Barnes's book, the dilemma with these two remains somewhat controversial today. To gain perspective on how this problem has evolved requires a look at earlier, often dichotomous, thinking and often unscientific conclusions based on non-validated observations. In 1952, Clein criticized the performance of tonsillectomy for allergic symptoms (176). Tonsillectomy was in fact being performed in an attempt to improve known allergic states (177,178). Of course, it is easy to see why outcomes were not satisfactory. Undiagnosed and untreated allergic states would tend to progress and give a false perspective that adenotonsillectomy was causative. No articles or studies contribute scientific evidence to the truth of these accusations.

Asthma is a disease of hyperreactive airways in which allergy is only one of many triggers. It is generally known that as many as 20% to 30% of patients with allergic rhinitis at some time experience some degree of hyperreactivity of the lower respiratory tract. This number probably is low, given our current conceptual models of a single integrated respiratory tract affected by both allergic rhinitis and asthma. It follows that a number of adenotonsillectomized patients who also have allergic rhinitis will at some time in their life have asthmatic symptoms. No one has unequivocally proven a causative relationship.

As of 1994, Griffin et al. reported that there were few papers in the literature regarding the relationship of adenotonsillar disease and the allergic state. They devised a study of 180 patients with 59 control subjects, which concluded that the prevalence of allergy in children with severe adenotonsillar disease is the same as that of age-matched control subjects. In addition, they noted that there is no relationship between the resolution of symptoms after tonsillectomy and the presence of allergy. The authors also found no increased prevalence in the development of asthma after tonsillectomy in the allergic child (177). They also recommended that residual symptomatology after tonsillectomy and adenoidectomy would then be appropriate to evaluate and treat for allergy. This concept is important for two reasons. First, it dispels the previous notion that an allergic patient undergoing tonsillectomy should be aggressively evaluated and treated before tonsillectomy on a routine basis (154). Even though Griffin and colleagues' study may be somewhat faulted for the use of invalidated questionnaires in the outcomes evaluation, and even though they did not examine food allergy (which has been reported to be associated with tonsil and adenoid hypertrophy) (172,173), the study was of clinical significance. Second, they tend to dispel a causal relationship between tonsillectomy and adenoidectomy and the evolution of asthma or worsening of the allergic state.

In 1989, Leher et al. (171) described 10 patients initially considered for tonsillectomy but first evaluated using in vitro testing for allergy and treated with immunotherapy. They found that with successful allergy management, none of the 10 patients required surgery. This study raises the issue of diagnostic acumen and a possible synergy between microbial and allergic inflammation. Bussi et al. suggest that tonsillitis in children may be more of an inflammatory response (165). Although this inflammation may be primarily microbial, it also is appreciated that an inflammatory

response to viral organisms in allergic people quite often is more severe. Feingold (179) also elaborates on a "copathogenicity" of primary bacterial pathogens with other bacteria whose role in the past has been underestimated, such as anaerobic bacteria. In examining this situation historically, the clinician must use diagnostic acumen to suspect and delineate the relative importance of allergic disease in patients who present with adenotonsillar disease. Certainly, medical or surgical management of adenotonsillar disease should include appropriate and timely treatment of the allergy-unstable patient. Although aggressive allergy management could be sufficient to change the overall clinical course and eliminate the need for aggressive measures such as surgery, it also may reduce the morbidity of surgery in those patients who require surgical and allergy management to achieve optimum outcomes. The timing of the allergy evaluation therefore remains a clinical decision.

In summarizing this dilemma, the tenets of Dr. Barnes's 1914 comment still hold true after all these years, " . . . that [tonsils and adenoids] should never be removed without adequate cause; but that when such cause exists, their function is either permanently impaired or is easily taken up by other lymphoid tissues" (158). Although there has been some variation in what are considered "good indications" over the years, most authors agree that tonsillectomy, with or without adenoidectomy, can be safely performed in the allergic patient.

Sound indications for tonsillectomy should include (180, 181):

1. Recurrent or chronic tonsillitis refractory to medical management—roughly five to seven cases in 1 year, four to five per year for 2 years, or three cases per year for 3 years or more. Special consideration is given to recalcitrant cases of lesser frequency that present difficulty in resolution or loss of significant work or school time. Consideration should also be given to the risk for development of allergy to antibiotics, adverse effects of antibiotics, and resistance of organisms in prolonged nonsurgical management options.
2. Deep neck-space cellulitis or abscess, including peritonsillar, parapharyngeal, and other infections such as retropharyngeal, parotid, or cervical carbunculated adenopathy abscesses.
3. Severe, incapacitating halitosis possibly due to chronic inspissated tonsillar debris and chronic tonsillitis when other sources for halitosis have been eliminated.
4. Suspicion of tonsillar or nasopharyngeal malignancy.
5. Airway obstruction, acute and chronic, refractory to medical management with or without evidence of sleep apnea or cor pulmonale.
6. Deglutition problems with or without failure to thrive based on tonsil and adenoid obstruction.
7. Maxillofacial maldevelopment due to tonsil or adenoid obstruction.

Adenoidectomy may be considered for the following:

1. Hypertrophy or chronic adenoiditis as a source for severe, unremitting chronic sinusitis, particularly in a child. Medical management and other forms of workup have been exhausted and as a possible alternative to sinus surgery in the child.
2. In conjunction with treatment of choanal atresia.
3. As an adjunct in the treatment of chronic, recurrent, refractory, recalcitrant eustachian tube dysfunction with evidence of chronic adenoiditis and eustachian tube effacement.
4. Trauma.

Other indications for tonsillectomy or adenoidectomy exist that depend on more unusual case scenarios. Further studies are indicated to help clarify some of these dilemmas and better understand the role of inflammation in the respiratory tract. Research is on the horizon for the understanding of inflammatory cells and mediators and their relationship to microorganisms, environmental factors, antigens, and other excitants of disease states. Studies must be done involving both normal people and patients with adenotonsillar hypertrophy, recurrent tonsillitis, and chronic tonsillitis (both allergic and nonallergic), with exploration of immune functional changes, and with medical and surgical management. Cellular and mediator studies are of the utmost importance. Measurement and monitoring of airway hyperreactivity, from onset and over a protracted period after treatment, is warranted.

## CONCLUSION

Because the laryngopharynx sits at the center of the respiratory system in continuity with the upper gastrointestinal tract, it is involved in a rather large differential of presenting complaints commonly seen in an otolaryngology practice. Allergy may play a role in many of these problems either directly or indirectly. In addition, there are many other nonallergic conditions that may aggravate the allergic situation. As Hollender suggested in the introductory quote, and as echoed into the current multidisciplinary approach to laryngopharyngeal problems, the clinician must have the diagnostic acumen to consider the differential diagnoses and how they may integrate into the current presenting problem. Allergic disease is an important consideration in laryngopharyngeal disease.

## ACKNOWLEDGMENTS

I thank Mrs. Karen Stoner, Chief Librarian of the Decatur Memorial Foundation Library, for her untiring energy and invaluable assistance with research. I thank my transcriptionists, Julie Causey and Susan Dunham, for their patience and good nature. I thank my wife, Melinda, and my son, Nicholson, for their patience and understanding. Finally, I would like to dedicate these words to the memory of my parents, Bernice and Charles, and my father-in-law, Gale Hedrick, all of whom departed during the writing of this chapter. They will be missed.

## REFERENCES

1. Hollender AR, ed. *The pharynx: basic aspects in clinical problems.* Chicago: Yearbook, 1953:44.
2. Corey JP. Allergy for the laryngologist. *Otol Clin North Am* 1998;31:189–205.
3. Brodnitz FS. Allergy of the larynx. *Otol Clin North Am* 1971; IV:579–582.
4. Alimov AL. The clinical symptomatology in the diagnosis of allergy in acute and chronic laryngitis. *Otol Rhinol Laryngol* 1968;30:71–75.
5. Nito K, et al. Laryngeal symptoms in patients exposed to japanese cedar pollen: allergic reactions and environmental pollution. *Eur Arch Otorhinolaryngol* 1999;256:209–211.
6. Dixon HS. Allergy in laryngeal disease. *Otol Clin North Am* 1992;25:239–249.
7. Dixon HS. Dysphonia and delayed food allergy: a provocation/neutralization study with strobovideolaryngoscopy. *Otolaryngol Head Neck Surg* 1999;121:418–429.
8. Rea WJ. Environmental aspects of ear, nose, and throat disease: part I. *Journal of Clinical Ecology in Otorhinolaryngology Allergy* 1979;41:41.
9. DeJarnatt AC, Grant AJ. Basic mechanisms of anaphylaxis and anaphylactoid reactions. *Immunol Allergy Clin North Am* 1992; 12:501–515.
10. Marquardt DL, Wasserman SI. Anaphylaxis. In: Middleton JE, Reed CE, Ellis EF, et al., eds. *Allergy principles and practice,* 4th ed. St. Louis: Mosby, 1993:1525–1536.
11. Rea WJ. Elimination of oral food challenge reaction by ingestion of food extracts: a double blind study. *Arch Otolaryngol* 1984; 110:248.
12. Hirano M. *Clinical examination of the voice.* New York: Springer-Verlag, 1981:5.
13. Fleming ID, et al., eds. Pharynx. In: *AJCC cancer staging manual.* Philadelphia: Lippincott–Raven, 1997:31–41.
14. Altman KW, et al. Angioedema presenting in the retropharyngeal space in an adult. *Am J Otolaryngol* 1999;20:136–138.
15. Quincke H. Über akutes und unschriebenes Hautodem. *Monatschr Prakt Dermatol* 1882;1:129–131.
16. Jarvis BL, Corey JP. Acute uvular edema. *Ear Nose Throat J* 1988;67:665–669.
17. Ferro PS, North IB. Roentgenological appearance of lesions of the larynx. *CRC Crit Rev Diagn Imaging* 1979;11:335–382.
18. Schuit KE. Infections of the head and neck. *Ped Clin N Amer* 1981;28:965–971.
19. van de Ven PM, Schutte HK. The pharyngocele: infrequently encountered and easily misdiagnosed. *J Laryngol Otol* 1995;109: 247–249.
20. Norris CW. Pharyngoceles of the hypopharynx. *Laryngoscope* 1979;89:1788–1807.
21. Shaffer AL. Anaphylaxis. *J Allergy Clin Immunol* 1985;75:227.
22. Vaughn WT. Steps in the development of our present understanding of clinical allergy: historical anaphylaxis. In: *Practice of allergy.* St. Louis: CV Mosby, 1939:11.
23. Stark BJ, Sullivan TJ. Biphasic and protracted anaphylaxis. *J Allergy Clin Immunol* 1986;78:76.

24. Waldbott GL. Anaphylactic death from penicillin. *JAMA* 1949; 139:526.
25. Lamson RW. Fatal anaphylaxis in sudden death associated with injection of foreign substances. *JAMA* 1924;82:109.
26. Slater JE. Rubber anaphylaxis. *N Engl J Med* 1989;320:1126.
27. Barnard AH. Studies of 4,000 hymenoptera sting deaths in the United States. *J Allergy Clin Immunol* 1973;52:259.
28. James LP, Austin KF. Fatal systemic anaphylaxis in man. *N Engl J Med* 1964;270:597.
29. Sheppe WN. Fatal anaphylaxis in man. *J Lab Clin Med* 1980; 16:372.
30. Zizmor J. Miscellaneous disorders of the larynx and pharynx. *Semin Roentgenol* 1974;9:24–31.
31. Bernstein AD, Robinson KE. Allergic edema of arytenoids in aryepiglottic folds. *NY State J Med* 1981;81:1359–1360.
32. Matthews KP. Urticaria and angioedema. *J Allergy Clin Immunol* 1983;25:11.
33. McKee WD. The incidence and familial occurrence of allergy. *J Allergy* 1966;38:226.
34. Swinny B. The atopic factor in urticaria. *South Med J* 1941;34: 855.
35. Kaplan AP. Urticaria and angioedema. In: Middleton JE, Reed CE, Ellis EF, et al., eds. *Allergy principles and practice,* 4th ed, vol 2. St. Louis: CV Mosby, 1993:1553.
36. Landerman NA. Hereditary angioneurotic edema. *J Allergy Clin Immunol* 1962;33:316–329.
37. Metzger WJ. Urticaria, angioedema, and hereditary angioedema. In: Patterson et al., eds. *Allergic diseases: diagnosis and management,* 5th ed. Philadelphia: Lippincott–Raven, 1997: 265.
38. Lokshin NA, Hurley H. Urticaria as a sign of viral hepatitis. *Arch Dermatol* 1972;105:105.
39. Cadresiodry SC, Reynolds JS. Acute urticaria in infectious mononucleosis. *Ann Allergy* 1969;27:182.
40. Soterna S, et al. The complement system in necrotizing angitis of the skin: analysis of complement component activities in serum of patients with concomitant collagen/vascular diseases. *J Invest Dermatol* 1974;63:219.
41. Thompson T, Frable MAS. Drug-induced, life-threatening angioedema revisited. *Laryngoscope* 1993;103:10–12.
42. Green GR, et al. Etiology and pathogenesis of chronic urticaria. *Ann Allergy* 1965;23:30.
43. Agostoni A, et al. Angioedema due to angiotensin-converting enzyme inhibitors. *Immunopharmacology* 1999;44:21–25.
44. Blais C, et al. Serum metabolism of bradykinin and Des-Arg⁹-Bradykinin in patients with angiotensin-converting enzyme inhibitor–associated angioedema. *Immunopharmacology* 1999;43: 293–302.
45. Werber J, Pincus R. Oropharyngeal angioedema associated with the use of angiotensin-converting enzyme inhibitors. *Otolaryngol Head Neck Surg* 1989;101:96–98.
46. Warner KK, et al. Angiotensin II receptor blockers in patients with ACE inhibitor–induced angioedema. *Ann Pharmacother* 2000;34:526–528.
47. Pylypchuk GB. Ace inhibitor versus angiotensin II blocker–induced cough and angioedema. *Ann Pharmacother* 1998;32: 1060–1066.
48. Sigler C, et al. Examination of baseline levels of carboxypeptidase N and complement components as potential predictors of angioedema associated with the use of angiotensin-converting enzyme inhibitor. *Arch Dermatol* 1997;133:972–975.
49. Seymour RA, et al. Angiotensin converting enzyme (ACE) inhibitors and their implications for the dental surgeon. *Br Dent J* 1997;183:214–218.
50. Sreeram AB, Corey JP. Congenital angiotensin-converting enzyme deficiency presenting as recurrent angioedema of upper airway in adult life. *Otolaryngol Head Neck Surg* 1995;112: 421–423.
51. Pastorello EA, et al. Mechanisms in adverse reactions to foods: the mouth and pharynx. *Allergy* 1995;50:41–44.
52. Amlot PL, et al. Oral allergy syndrome [OAS]: symptoms of IgE mediated hypersensitivity to foods. *Clin Allergy* 1987;17: 33–42.
53. Ortolani C, et al. The oral allergy syndrome. *Ann Allergy* 1988; 61:47.
54. Alaberse RC, et al. Immunoglobulin E antibodies that cross-react with vegetable foods, pollen, and Hymenoptera venom. *J Allergy Clin Immunol* 1981;68:356–364.
55. Bircher AJ, et al. IgE to food allergens are highly prevalent in patients allergic to pollens, with and without symptoms of food allergy. *Clin Exp Allergy* 1994;24:367.
56. Ebner C, et al. Common epitopes of birch, pollen, and apples: studies by Western and Northern blot. *J Allergy Clin Immunol* 1991;88:588.
57. Ortolani C, et al. IgE mediated allergy from vegetable allergens. *Ann Allergy* 1993;71:470.
58. Andersen KE, Lowenstein H. An investigation of the possible immunologic relationship between allergen extracts from birch pollen, hazelnut, potato, and apple. *Contact Dermatitis* 1978; 4:73–79.
59. Eriksson NE. Clustering of food stuffs in food hypersensitivity and inquiry study in pollen-allergic patients. *J Allergol Immunol Pathol* 1984;12:28.
60. Pastorello EA, Ortolani C. Oral allergy syndrome. In: Metcalfe DD, et al., eds. *Food allergy: adverse reactions to foods and food additives,* 2nd ed. Oxford: Blackwell Science, 1997:221–223.
61. Björkstén F, et al. Extraction and properties of apple antigens. *Allergy* 1980;35:671–677.
62. Dreborg S, Foucard T. Allergy to apple, carrot, and potato in children with birch pollen allergy. *J Allergy* 1983;38:167.
63. Lahti A, Hannuksela M. Hypersensitivity to apple and carrot can be reliably detected with fresh material. *Allergy* 1978;33: 143.
64. Bindslev-Jensen C. Oral allergy syndrome: the affect of astemizole. *Allergy* 1991;46:610–613.
65. Vaughn WT. *The story of allergy.* New York: Blue Ribbon Books, 1943:13.
66. Jackson-Menaldi CA, et al. Allergies and vocal fold edema: a preliminary report. *J Voice* 1999;13:113–122.
67. Sala E, et. al. Occupational laryngitis with immediate allergic or immediate-type specific chemical hypersensitivity. *Clin Otol Laryngol* 1996;21:42–48.
68. Pang LQ. Allergy of the larynx, trachea, and bronchial tree. Symposium on allergy and otolaryngology. *Otol Laryngol Clin North Am* 1974;7:719–734.
69. Duncan RB, Duncan TD. Otolaryngeal allergy in Wellington 1971–1975. *N Z Med J* 1977;85:45–48.
70. Williams RI. Allergic laryngitis. *Ann Otol* 1972;81:558–564.
71. Yamaguchi M, et al. Laryngoscopic findings in cases with laryngeal allergy. *J Jpn Bronchoesophagol Soc* 1991;42:259–263.
72. Sajous CE. *Lectures of the diseases of the nose and throat.* FA Davis. Philadelphia: ATT'Y Publishers, 1886:337–338.
73. Sataloff RT. *Professional voice: the science and art of clinical care,* 2nd ed. San Diego: Singular Publishing Group, 1997.
74. Bastian RW, Collins SL, et al. Indirect video-laryngoscopy versus direct endoscopy for larynx and pharynx cancer staging toward elimination of preliminary direct laryngoscopy. *Ann Otol Rhinol Laryngol* 1989;98:693–698.
75. Cohn J, Spiegel J, Sataloff R. Vocal disorders and the professional voice user: the allergist's role. *Ann Allergy Asthma Immunol* 1995;74:363–373.

76. Boon DR. The singing/acting voice in the mature adult: the three ages of voice. *J Voice* 1997;11(2):161–164.

77. Hurwitz B. Nasal pathophysiology impacts bronchial reactivity in asthmatic patients with allergic rhinitis. *J Asthma* 1997;34: 427–431.

78. Grossman J. One airway, one disease. *Chest* 1997;11 [Suppl]: 11S–16S.

79. Blanton PL, Biggs NL. Eighteen hundred years of controversy: the paranasal sinuses. *Am J Anat* 1969;124:135–147.

80. McFadden ER. Nasal sinus pulmonary reflexes in bronchial asthma. *J Allergy Clin Immunol* 1986;78:1–3.

81. Gottlieb MJ. Relation of intranasal disease and production of asthma. *JAMA* 1925;85:105–108.

82. Kratchmer I. Affect on respiration, blood pressure, and carotid pulse of various inhaled and insufflated vapors when stimulating one cranial nerve and various combinations of cranial nerves. *Am J Physiol* 1928;87:319–325.

83. Dixon WE, Brodie TG. Bronchial muscles, their innervation and the action of drugs on them. *J Physiol (Lond)* 1903;29: 93–97.

84. Sluder G. Asthma as a nasal reflex. *JAMA* 1919:73:589–591.

85. de Benedictis F, Bush A. Rhinosinusitis and asthma: epiphenomenon or causal association? *Chest* 1999;115:550–556.

86. Smith JM. Epidemiology and natural history of asthma, allergic rhinitis, and atopic dermatitis (eczema). In: Middleton JE, Reed CE, Ellis EF, et al., eds. *Allergy principles and practice,* 2nd ed. St. Louis: Mosby, 1983:771–803.

87. Braman SS, et al. Airway hyperresponsiveness in allergic rhinitis: a risk factor for asthma. *Chest* 1987;91:671–674.

88. Lusk RP, Stankiewicz JA. Pediatric rhinosinusitis. *Otolaryngol Head Neck Surg* 1997;116[Suppl]:S53–S57.

89. Gungor A, Corey JP. Pediatric sinusitis: a literature review with emphasis on the role of allergy. *Otolaryngol Head Neck Surg* 1997;116: 4–15.

90. Rachelefsky GS, et al. Sinus disease in children with respiratory allergy. *J Allergy Clin Immunol* 1978;61:310–314.

91. Slavin RG, et al. Sinusitis and bronchial asthma. *J Allergy Clin Immunol* 1980;66:250–257.

92. Abinoff AD, et al. Chronic sinusitis in childhood asthma: correlation of symptoms, x-ray, cultures, and response to treatment. *Pediatr Res* 1983;17:373.

93. Schwartz HJ, et al. Occult sinus abnormalities in the asthmatic patient. *Arch Intern Med* 1987;147:2194–2196.

94. Zimmerman B, et al. Prevalence of abnormalities found by sinus x-rays in childhood asthma: lack of relation to severity of asthma. *J Allergy Clin Immunol* 1987;80:268–273.

95. Nguyen KL, et al. Chronic sinusitis among pediatric patients with chronic respiratory complaints. *J Allergy Clin Immunol* 1993;92:824–830.

96. Slavin RG. Asthma and sinusitis. *Clin Immunol* 1992;90: 534–537.

97. Brown JA. Sinobronchial reflex asthma and sinusitis. *J S C Med Assoc* 1992;88:340–343.

98. Senior BA, Kennedy DW. Management of sinusitis in the asthmatic patient. *Ann Allergy Asthma Immunol* 1996;77:6–15.

99. Friedman R, et al. Asthma and bacterial sinusitis in children. *J Allergy Clin Immunol* 1984;74:185–189.

100. Manning SC, et al. Results of endoscopic sinus surgery in pediatric patients with chronic sinusitis and asthma. *Arch Otolaryngol Head Neck Surg* 1994;120:1142–1145.

101. Koren J, et al. Nasal beclomethasone prevents the seasonal increase in bronchial responsiveness in patients with allergic rhinitis and asthma. *J Allergy Clin Immunol* 1992;90:250–256.

102. Watson WTA, et al. Treatment of allergic rhinitis with intranasal corticosteroids in patients with mild asthma: effect on lower airway responsiveness. *J Allergy Clin Immunol* 1993;91:97–101.

103. Oliveria CAA, et al. Improvement of bronchial hyper-responsiveness in asthmatic children treated for concomitant sinusitis. *Ann Allergy Asthma Immunol* 1997;79:70–74.

104. Fokkens W, et al. The interaction between upper and lower airways and allergic rhinitis. *The nose 2000 and beyond: International Rhinologic Society programs and abstracts.* Biennial Meeting of the International Rhinologic Society, Washington, DC, Sep. 21–25, 2000. Washington, DC: A-158(abs.).

105. Hoehne JH, Reed CE. Where is the allergic reaction in ragweed asthma? *J Allergy Clin Immunol* 1971;48:36–39.

106. Ingram JM, et al. Eosinophilic cat ionic protein and serum and nasal washings from wheezing infants in children. *J Pediatr* 1995;127(4)558–564.

107. Gray H. *Anatomy of the human body,* 28th ed. Philadelphia: Lea & Febiger, 1970.

108. Slavin RG. Relationship of nasal disease and sinusitis to bronchial asthma. *Ann Allergy* 1982;49:76–79.

109. Slavin RG. Sinopulmonary relationships. *Am J Otolaryngol* 1994;15:18–25.

110. Kaufman J, Wright GW. The affect of nasal and nasopharyngeal irritation on airway resistance in man. *Am Rev Respir Dis* 1969; 100:626–630.

111. Bucca C, et al. Extrathoracic and intrathoracic airway responsiveness and sinusitis. *J Allergy Clin Immunol* 1995;95:52–59.

112. Nolte D, Berger D. Vagal bronchial constriction in asthmatic patients by nasal irritation. *Eur J Respir Dis* 1983;64[Suppl 128]: 110–114.

113. Togawak T, Ogura JH. Physiologic relationships between nasal breathing and pulmonary function. *Laryngoscope* 1966;76: 30–63.

114. Benchev R. The influence of the surgical treatment of nasal polyposis on coexisting bronchial asthma. *The nose 2000 and beyond: International Rhinologic Society programs and abstracts.* Biennial Meeting of the International Rhinologic Society, Washington, DC, Sep. 21–25, 2000. Washington, DC: A-187(abs.).

115. Rosenberg GL, et al. Inhalational challenge with ragweed pollen and ragweed-sensitive asthmatics. *J Allergy Clin Immunol* 1983; 71:302–310.

116. Irvin CG. Sinusitis and asthma: an animal model. *J Allergy Clin Immunol* 1992;90:521–533.

117. Voegels R, et al. Can endoscopic nasal surgery improve asthma symptoms? *The nose 2000 and beyond: International Rhinologic Society programs and abstracts.* Biennial Meeting of the International Rhinologic Society, Washington, DC, Sep. 21–25, 2000. Washington, DC: A-30(abs.).

118. Pierce AK, Sanford JP. Aerobic gram-negative bacillary pneumonias. *Am Rev Respir Dis* 1974;110:647–658.

119. Bardin PG, et al. Absence of pulmonary aspiration of sinus contents in patients with asthma and sinusitis. *J Allergy Clin Immunol* 1990;86:82–88.

120. Baraniuk JN. Pathogenesis of allergic rhinitis. *J Allergy Clin Immunol* 1997;96[Suppl]:S763–S772.

121. Harlan SL, et al. A clinical and pathologic study of chronic sinusitis: the role of the eosinophil. *J Allergy Clin Immunol* 1988; 81:867–875.

122. Juntunen K, et al. Caldwell-Luc operation in the treatment of childhood bronchial asthma. *Laryngoscope* 1984;94:249–251.

123. Littell NT, et al. Changes in airway resistance following nasal provocation. *Am Rev Respir Dis* 1990;141:580–583.

124. Small P, Bisken N. The affects of allergen-induced nasal provocation on pulmonary function in patients with perennial allergic rhinitis. *Am J Rhinol* 1989;3:17–20.

125. Hamilos DL, et al. Evidence for distinct cytokine expression in allergic versus non-allergic chronic sinusitis. *J Allergy Clin Immunol* 1995;96:537–544.

126. al Ghamdi K, et al. IL-4 and IL-13 expression in chronic sinusitis: relationship with cellular infiltrate and affect of topical corticosteroid treatment. *J Otolaryngol* 1997;26:160–166.

127. Demoly P, et al. Assessment of inflammation in non-infectious chronic maxillary sinusitis. *J Allergy Clin Immunol* 1994;94:95–108.

128. Koufman JA. Reflux and voice disorders. In: Korovin SK, et al., eds. *Diagnosis and treatment of voice disorders.* New York: Igaku-Shoin, 1995.

129. Hogan WJ. Spectrum of supra-esophageal complications of gastroesophageal reflux disease. *Am J Med* 1997;103(5A):77S–83S.

130. Koufman JA. The otolaryngologic manifestations of gastroesophageal reflux disease: a clinical investigation of 225 patients using ambulatory 24-hour pH monitoring and an experimental investigation of the role of acid and pepcid in the development of laryngeal injury. *Laryngoscope* 1991;101[Suppl 53]:1–78.

131. Bortolotti M. Laryngospasm and reflex central apnea caused by aspiration of reflux, gastric contents in adults. *Gut* 1989;30:233–238.

132. Campbell AH. Brief upper airway (laryngeal) dysfunction. *Aust N Z J Med* 1990;20:663–668.

133. Hanson DG, Jiang JJ. Diagnosis and management of chronic laryngitis associated with reflux. *Am J Med* 2000;108(4A):112S–119S.

134. Koufman JA, Cummins MM. The prevalence and spectrum in reflux and laryngology: a prospective study of 132 consecutive patients with laryngeal and voice disorders. In: *Nature of reflux and laryngeal and voice disorders.* Winston-Salem, NC: Center for Voice Disorders of Wake Forest University, 1–10.

135. Ossakow SJ. Esophageal and reflux and dysmotility as the basis for persistent cervical symptoms. *Ann Otol Rhinol Laryngol* 1987;96:387–392.

136. Mishra A, Hogan SP, Brandt EB, et al. An etiological role for aeroallergens and eosinophils in experimental esophagitis. *J Clin Invest* 2001;107:83–90.

137. Toohill RJ. Pharyngeal, laryngeal and tracheal bronchial manifestations of gastroesophageal reflux. In: *Proceedings of the XXIV World Congress of Otolaryngology Head and Neck Surgery.* Berkeley, CA: Kugler and Ghendini, 1995.

138. Loughlin CJ, Koufman JA. Paroxysmal laryngospasm secondary to gastroesophageal reflux. Winston-Salem, NC: Center for Voice Disorders of Wake Forest University, 1–6. *Laryngoscope* 1996;106:1502–1505.

139. Wiener GJ, et al. Is hoarseness an atypical manifestation of gastroesophageal reflux (GERD)? An ambulatory 24-hour pH study. *Gastroenterology* 1986;90A:1691(abstr).

140. Irwin RS, et al. Chronic cough: spectrum and frequency of causes, key components of the diagnostic evaluation and outcome of specific therapy. *Am Rev Respir Dis* 1990;141:640–647.

141. Irwin RS, Madison JM. Anatomical diagnostic protocol in evaluating chronic cough with specific reference to gastroesophageal reflux disease. *Am J Med* 2000;108(4A):126S–130S.

142. McGarvey LPA, et al. Evaluation and outcome of patients with chronic nonproductive cough using a comprehensive diagnostic protocol. *Thorax* 1998;53:738–743.

143. Palombini BC, et al. A pathologic triad in chronic cough: asthma, post nasal drip syndrome, and gastroesophageal reflux disease. *Chest* 1999;116:279–284.

144. O'Connell F. Management of persistent dry cough. *Thorax* 1995;53:123–124.

145. Carney IK, et al. A systematic evaluation of mechanisms in chronic cough. *Am J Respir Crit Care Med* 1997;156:211–216.

146. Barnes HA. *The tonsil.* St. Louis: CV Mosby, 1914:128.

147. Bachert C, Moller P. MALT (mucosa associated lymphoid tissue) der Nasenschleimhaut. *Laryngol Rhinol Otol* 1990;69:515–520.

148. Ge ZH, Lin ZQ, Wang RY. A study of lymphocytic subsets in human normal tonsil and lymph node. *Shih Yen Sheng Wu Hsueh Pao* 1989;22(1):75–85.

149. Matsuyama H, Yamanaka N. Immunological study on immunocompetent cells in palatine tonsil and pharyngeal tonsil: the qualitative study by image analyzer. *Nippon Jibiinkoka, Gakkai Kaiho* 1989;92:2064–2079.

150. Hans-Peter Z, Franz-Xaver B. Immunological aspects of tonsils and tonsillitis. *Acta Otolaryngol Suppl (Stockh)* 1988;454:70–74.

151. Richardson MA. Sore throat, tonsillitis, and adenoiditis in otolaryngology for the internist. *Med Clin North Am* 1999;83:76–84.

152. Moraga FA, et al. Immunologic aspects of tonsils. *Ann Otol Rhinol Laryngol* 1975;84[Suppl 19]:37.

153. Ying M-D. Immunologic basis for indications for tonsillectomy and adenoidectomy. *Acta Otolaryngol Suppl (Stockh)* 1988;454:279–285.

154. Ivarsson M, Lundberg C. Nasopharyngeal tonsils, vision of surface secretions with immunocytes, a property additional to antigen processing. *Ann Otol Rhinol Laryngol* 2000;109:99–105.

155. Winther B, Innes DJ. The human adenoid: a morphologic study. *Arch Otolaryngol Head Neck Surg* 1994;120:144–149.

156. Korsrud FR. Immune systems of human nasopharyngeal and palatine tonsils; histomorphometry of lymphoid components and quantification of immunoglobulin-producing cells in health and disease. *Clin Exp Immunol* 1980;39:361–370.

157. Parry ME. The specialized structure of crypt epithelium in human palatine tonsil and its functional significance. *J Anat* 1994;1985:111–127.

158. Forsgren J, et al. In situ analysis of the immune micro-environment of the adenoid in children with and without secretory otitis media. *Ann Otol Rhinol Laryngol* 1995;104:189–196.

159. Burnstein JM, et al. Are thymus-derived lymphocytes [T-cells] defective in nasopharyngeal and palatine tonsils in children? *Otolaryngol Head Neck Surg* 1993;109:693–700.

160. Brodsky L, et al. The immunology of tonsils in children: the effect of bacterial load on the presence of B- and T-cell subsets. *Laryngoscope* 1998;98:93–98.

161. Kawaguchi T. Gamma delta T-cells in palatine tonsil: immunohistological and functional study. *Nippon Jibiinkoka Gakkai Kaiho* 1993;96:810–817.

162. Ryan Y, et al. Immunohistological identification of the activated lymphocytes in human palatine tonsil. *Nippon Jibiinkoka Gakkai Kaiho* 1989;92:1958–1963.

163. Harada K. Histopathological study of human palatine tonsils: especially age change. *Nippon Jibiinkoka Gakkai Kaiho* 1989;92:1049–1064.

164. Klmel'nitshaia NM. Morphological characteristics and function of the tonsil as an organ of immunogenesis. *Arkh Patol* 1983;45:83–89.

165. Bussi M, et al. Expression of antigens associated with the individual stages of the inflammatory response in child and adult as a possible distinctive method for recurrent and chronic tonsillitis. *Int J Pediatr Otorhinolaryngol* 1996;35:243–250.

166. Astruc J, Toubin RM. Recurrent pharyngitis: indications for tonsillectomy. *Rev Prat* 1992;42:298–330.

167. Stjernquist-Desatnik A, et al. High recovery of *Hemophilus influenzae* and group A streptococcae in recurrent tonsillar infection or hypertrophy as compared with normal tonsils. *J Laryngol Otol* 1991;105:439–441.

168. Sugiyama M, et al. Immunological and biochemical properties of tonsillar lymphocytes. *Acta Otolaryngol (Stockh)* 1984;416:45–55.

169. Brodsky L, Loch RJ. Bacteriology and immunology of normal and diseased adenoids in children. *Arch Otolaryngol Head Neck Surg* 1993;119:821.

170. Aginer DC. Respiratory diseases in food allergy. *Ann Allergy* 1984;53:657–665.
171. Lehrer JF, et al. IgE determinations in the management of sinusitis and pharyngo-tonsillitis in an otolaryngology practice. In: Fadal, Nalebuff, eds. *RAST in clinical allergy.* Miami: Symposia Foundation, 1989:147–155.
172. Donn AS, Giles ML. Do children waiting for tonsillectomy grow out of their tonsillitis? *N Z Med J* 1991;104:161–162.
173. Ohta N, et al. Neutrophil-activating activity in tonsillar cells from patients with tonsillitis. *Acta Otolaryngol (Stockh)* 1993; 511:214–217.
174. Koch RJ, Brodsky L. Effect of specific bacteria on lymphocyte proliferation and disease in non-diseased tonsils. *Laryngoscope* 1993;103:1020–1026.
175. Vianna NJ, et al. Tonsillectomy and Hodgkin's disease: the lymphoid tissue barrier. *Lancet 1* 1971;431.

176. Clein NW. Influence of tonsillectomy and adenoidectomy in children with special reference to the allergic implications on respiratory symptoms. *Ann Allergy* 1952;21:568–573.
177. Griffin JL, et al. Prevalence of IgE mediated hypersensitivity in children with adenotonsillar disease. *Arch Otolaryngol Head Neck Surg* 1994;120:150–153.
178. Neele HB III, McDonald TJ. Tonsillectomy and adenoidectomy—are there any indications? *Postgrad Med* 1981;70(3): 107–112.
179. Feingold SM. Role of anaerobic bacteria in infections of tonsils and adenoids. In: Bluestone CS, Stool SE, McKenna MA, eds. *Pediatric otolaryngology.* Philadelphia: WB Saunders, 1995.
180. Feron B, Strezlow V. Pediatric adenoidectomy and tonsillectomy: personal viewpoints. *J Otolaryngol* 1979;8:40–48.
181. Paradise LJ. Tonsillectomy and adenoidectomy. *Pediatr Otolaryngol* 1983;11:992–1004.

# ASTHMA DIAGNOSIS AND MANAGEMENT

## BRUCE R. GORDON

Asthma is a chronic inflammatory disease of the lower respiratory tract that is triggered by exposure to allergens and other airway irritants. Because the inflammatory process is highly variable, asthma is a disorder with many possible presentations. It therefore may proceed for years without clinical recognition, and may challenge the most astute diagnostician. Because asthma is a common disease, it is important to be able to suspect, diagnose, and treat asthma. Asthma is one of the important diseases in the differential diagnosis of respiratory complaints, and is a frequent comorbid condition that may complicate the treatment of other medical or surgical problems. Also, the understanding of asthma's pathophysiologic process has changed in recent years, and with a new appreciation of the role of chronic allergic inflammation, there have been radical changes in recommendations for optimum asthma treatment. This discussion reviews the current understanding of asthma, and summarizes diagnosis and treatment guidelines that can assist clinicians in effectively managing their asthmatic patients.

## PATHOPHYSIOLOGY

Asthma is a chronic inflammatory disease of the lower respiratory tract (1) that is triggered by exposure to allergens or other airway irritants. This inflammation results in airway hyperresponsiveness (2), bronchial muscle spasm, mucous gland hypersecretion, and mucosal edema, which combine to increase the work of breathing and to create symptoms such as cough, wheezing, chest pain or tightness, and respiratory distress. The obstruction to airflow that occurs during asthmatic inflammation is potentially reversible, a factor that usually distinguishes asthma from chronic obstructive pulmonary disease (COPD) (3). The inflammatory process

is highly variable, both from time to time in any individual, and from person to person, so that asthma is a disorder with many possible presentations and with drastic differences in severity. Wheezing asthma, or asthma requiring hospital treatment, usually is obvious, whereas asthma masquerading as COPD, easy fatigability, intermittent asthma, exercise-induced asthma, or cough variant asthma may proceed for years without clinical recognition.

## PREVALENCE

Asthma is the most common serious chronic disease in most industrialized nations (4). It is also the most common potentially serious illness to complicate pregnancy (5). Estimates of the current asthma prevalence in the United States range from 12 to 14.6 million persons (6,7). The incidence of asthma in children appears to be increasing, and because long-term studies have shown persistence of symptomatic asthma as children age, it is likely that the future prevalence of asthma will be even greater (6). Asthma has risen to become the sixth most common diagnosis for office medical visits, and the fourth most common reason for repeat visits (7). Since the 1970s, the overall mortality rate due to asthma also has been steadily increasing worldwide, growing by 40% in the United States between 1982 and the end of 1991 (8). In the United States, there are approximately 4,000 to 5,000 cases of fatal asthma each year (9). Self-reported asthma increased by 42% during the same period, to almost 5% of the population. Asthma morbidity and hospitalization rates also are increasing. However, the data are not precise because of difficulties identifying all affected patients and in classifying pulmonary disorders as asthmatic (3).

## VARIABILITY OF ASTHMA EXPRESSION

The phenotypic expression of asthma appears to be controlled by multiple genes (10), which may help to explain the variable nature of this disease. Most asthmatic patients

B. R. Gordon: Department of Otology and Laryngology, Harvard University, Cambridge; Associate Surgeon, Massachusetts Eye and Ear Infirmary, Boston; Chief of Otolaryngology, Cape Cod Hospital, Hyannis, Massachusetts.

are now known to be allergic (11,12), so that the old distinction between intrinsic and extrinsic asthma no longer pertains. However, the reverse is not true because asthma is present only in a fraction of allergic persons—for example, in up to 11% of people with allergic rhinitis (13). How the various genetic and environmental factors that are active in asthma interact to produce clinical illness in any individual remains largely unknown. In the near future, genome analysis should illuminate this issue. At present, it is known that only 26% of children in families with one asthmatic parent become asthmatic during childhood (10). However, there is no question that environmental triggers are of major importance. For example, approximately two thirds of asthmatic patients in the United States live in areas with significant smog (8), and it is known that the oxidant chemical pollutants in both indoor and outdoor air cause lung inflammation and act as priming agents for subsequent allergen exposure (14,15). Many other nonallergic environmental factors are known to trigger or exacerbate asthma, including viral infections (16), bacterial infections (17,18), exercise (19), stress (20), cold air, gastroesophageal reflux, sinusitis, exposure to certain drugs and chemicals, and endocrine dysfunction (9). Allergic asthma triggers include the full range of inhalant (21,22), food (23), and chemical (24,25) allergens. Finally, nutrition, especially antioxidant status, significantly influences allergic disease severity (26–28). The clinical variability of asthma thus may depend on how many of these factors are simultaneously or sequentially interacting with the unique genetic makeup of each individual.

## CLINICAL DIAGNOSIS

Asthma is diagnosed primarily by clinical suspicion, noting a history of typical episodic symptoms and triggering patterns. Anyone with unexplained wheezing, frequent coughing, or dyspnea, especially when associated with recognized asthma triggers, should be suspected of having asthma. Confirmation of asthma depends on the combined use of physical examination, pulmonary function testing (PFT), and, when indicated, radiologic examination, as well as on a successful response to asthma management.

Chest auscultation may detect typical expiratory wheezes or decreased breath sounds, but often cough is the only audible symptom. The asthmatic cough usually is dry and may sound like a barking seal. Asthmatic sputum, when produced, is clear and tenacious. Although asthmatic mucus sometimes is lightly colored, dark, opaque, or bloody mucus should raise suspicion of infection or malignancy. Discovery of a past personal or family history of allergy, especially of asthma, hay fever, serous otitis, eczema, or migraine, suggests that atopy may be present, and increases the chances for asthma to be present. Current evidence for allergy also should be sought. For example, eczema, old tympanic membrane scars, enlarged or inflamed turbinates, pharyngeal bands, allergic eyelid edema, conjunctival edema, or lower lid discoloration may be found. Laryngeal evaluation also should be done to evaluate possible gastroesophageal reflux.

## ASSESSMENT OF SEVERITY

Once asthma is suspected, assessment of the possible severity of disease is important. Episodes of prior emergency department or hospital care for respiratory problems, including multiple episodes of croup as a child or multiple episodes of systemic corticosteroid therapy, are significant indicators of possibly severe asthma. On the other hand, infrequent symptoms associated primarily with infections or exercise normally identifies mild asthma. The frequency and severity of symptoms have particular value in classifying patients (Table 20.1). For example, daily to weekly wheezing, nighttime awakening or arising more than once a week with symptoms, or daily to weekly limitation of home or sporting activities usually indicates moderate to severe asthma (29). Daily use of β-adrenergic agonist bronchodilators also is a sign of at least moderate asthma (30). This clinical evaluation should yield a rough risk assessment, and this will, in turn, dictate the speed and depth of subsequent evaluation.

### Pulmonary Function Testing

In all cases, PFTs should be the next step (3). Spirometry done before and after bronchodilator use gives objective

**TABLE 20.1. CLASSIFICATION OF CHRONIC ASTHMA SEVERITY**[a]

| Classification | Day Symptoms | Night Symptoms | Lung Function | β-Agonist Use |
|---|---|---|---|---|
| Mild intermittent | <2 wk | ≤2 mo | $FEV_1$, PF ≥ 80% | Rare |
| Mild persistent | <1 d | >2 mo | $FEV_1$, PF ≥ 80% | Occasional |
| Moderate Persistent | >1 d | >1 wk | $FEV_1$, PF 61%–79% | Daily |
| Severe persistent | Continual | Frequent | $FEV_1$, PF ≤ 60% | More than one canister/month |

$FEV_1$, forced expiratory volume in 1 second; PF, peak flow.
[a]Modified from 1997 Revised U.S. Guidelines.

data to establish the diagnosis of reversible obstructive lung disease. PFTs also allow the objective assessment of disease severity. This should match the clinical severity assessment, and if it does not, special care in the subsequent evaluation is warranted. PFTs also should be used to measure the response to therapy, and are used to adjust objectively the intensity of antiinflammatory treatment. The 1-second forced expiratory volume ($FEV_1$) is the measurement most often used for severity assessment. Less than a 20% decrease from normal indicates mild asthma, a drop of 20% to 40% is moderate asthma, and a greater than 40% decline is severe asthma (31). In some cases, initial PFT results may be normal, or there may be no bronchodilator effect, yet provocative PFTs using a graded methacholine inhalation challenge yield positive results. Finally, PFTs may sometimes detect other lung diseases, such as pneumonitis, COPD, or a fixed airway obstruction. In these cases, in addition to simple spirometry, helium dilution, carbon monoxide diffusion, and other tests may be necessary (32). For accuracy, office spirometers need regular calibration, and spirometric technicians need to coach patients carefully so that reliable PFTs are recorded (33). Knowledgeable technicians can perform PFTs on cooperative young children, most adults, and, with appropriate adapters, patients with tracheotomy or laryngectomy.

Graphing spirometric flow–volume curves gives a visually distinctive pattern to different pulmonary diseases, and makes office use of PFTs both easy and clinically valuable (Fig. 20.1). Rate of airflow in liters per second is graphed on the vertical axis, and volume of exhaled or inhaled air in liters is graphed on the horizontal axis. Both the vital capacity and the peak expiratory flow can be read from the graph. Asthma usually is easily recognized because the exhaled flow–volume curve is reduced compared with age-, sex-, and height-adjusted normal data, the downslope becomes concave in shape, and use of a bronchodilator partially or completely reverses the curve to normal. However, lack of rapid reversibility does not exclude asthma because long-standing inflammation may require months of treatment before improvement is measurable (32).

Methacholine challenge may be helpful in these cases of apparently irreversible obstruction. During a methacholine challenge, progressively more concentrated nebulized solutions of methacholine, a cholinergic agonist, are inhaled. In patients with reactive airways, eventually a dose is reached that produces greater than a 20% drop in the $FEV_1$, which is a positive result. Persons with nonreactive airways have minimal or no reaction to the highest dose of methacholine. If the $FEV_1$ is greater than 60% of predicted, a methacholine challenge may be safely performed, and if it shows a further drop in $FEV_1$, then asthma, rather than COPD, is the probable diagnosis (34). If PFTs are done on a patient with mild asthma when there are no symptoms, the flow–volume curve may be normal. In this situation, provocation with methacholine usually produces a greater than 20% drop in $FEV_1$, which is diagnostic of asthma (34).

Pulmonary function tests also are very useful for ongoing monitoring of asthma control. Sequential PFTs can show whether the current therapy is effectively controlling both the inflammatory and bronchospastic components. PFTs also can be used during an exacerbation to help decide how aggressive the therapy change must be. Graded methacholine challenges also may be useful in monitoring therapy. One study compared monitoring with added measurement of lung hyperresponsiveness, as assessed by methacholine challenge, to monitoring with only symptoms, peak flows (PFs), PFTs every 3 months, and β-agonist use (35,36). Patients treated with the added information of methacholine challenges did better clinically, and had much more improvement of subepithelial inflammation in lung biopsies. This may indicate that methacholine sensitivity is an easily measured surrogate marker for the degree of lung inflammation.

## Peak Flow Measurements

For home monitoring, a hand-held PF meter should be prescribed for all patients with moderate to severe asthma. In most asthmatic patients, PF records are more reliable in detecting problems than are subjective sensations of dyspnea. PF meters can give variable results if patients are not carefully instructed in correct technique, and if they do not make the measurements at the same time each day. The normal diurnal cycle of lung function has a maximum at approximately 2 to 4 P.M., and a minimum at approximately

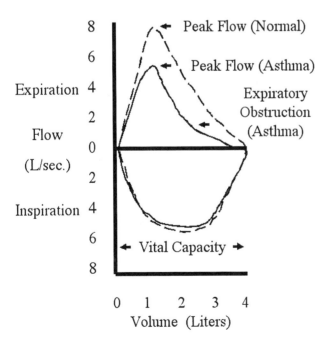

**FIG. 20.1.** Pulmonary function tests, normal compared with moderate asthma.

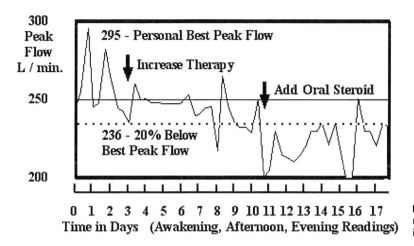

**FIG. 20.2.** Peak flow record in uncontrolled, moderately severe asthma. Low peak flow values indicate risk for pulmonary failure.

2 to 4 A.M., with the amplitude (variation in PF from peak to trough) being greater for more severe categories of asthma (37). However, asthma attacks that are precipitated by viral infections show reduced PF variation, so that variability is not always a good clinical indicator. Recording PF on arising, before use of inhalers, gives consistent results near the low end of a patient's PF range (37). If patients check and record their PF on a regular schedule, gradual declines in lung function can become apparent to visual inspection of the record, long before symptoms develop (Fig. 20.2). Then, early intervention may prevent an asthma attack from ever developing. This is important because prevention of an imminent attack is relatively easy, but treatment of an established attack takes much longer to achieve results, is much more expensive, and runs a risk of hospitalization and serious complications.

There is a lot of variation in PF values, both as measured by different devices and in individual variation from person to person. However, each person, by repeatedly using a specific device, will be able to establish a consistent, narrow upper range of PF values. Most young, healthy people have a personal best PF of up to 600 to 700 L/minute. Middle-aged patients with asthma often have maximum morning PF values of 400 to 500 L/minute, so that a drop of 20% to approximately 320 to 400 L/minute is enough to raise concern and to recommend an increase in therapy. A drop of 50% or more, to 200 to 250 L/minute, is a severe change, warrants aggressive management that usually involves the use of oral corticosteroids, and often precipitates an emergency department visit (see later). Patients whose personal best PF values are already in this low range must be very carefully followed because a drop of less than 50% in their PF may rapidly become life threatening. In general, PF values less than 200 L/minute indicate severe, dangerous levels of pulmonary impairment. In the actual PF record example shown in Fig. 20.2, the downward trend is of great concern because the flow values already are low.

## Other Examinations

In most cases of asthma, history, examination, PFTs, and PF records are sufficient information on which to base clinical management. However, when there is a history of tobacco use, exposure to tuberculosis or environmental risk factors, unusual symptoms, or failure to respond to treatment, radiologic studies and bronchoscopy may be needed. Computed tomography has been shown to be significantly more sensitive than plain chest radiographs, and should be considered for high-risk cases. Even in definite cases of asthma, lung cancer, tuberculosis, asbestosis, and other diseases also may be present, and timely consultations with pulmonologists and other specialists can be important. Pulmonology consultations also are helpful for sharing the management of patients with moderately severe and severe asthma because pulmonologists' experience with managing hospital treatment of these patients complements the outpatient allergy management skills of otolaryngic allergists.

## STRATEGY FOR ASTHMA MANAGEMENT

### Treatment Guidelines

Guidelines for asthma diagnosis and management were developed by the British, and were published in 1990 (38, 39). Shortly thereafter, the U.S. National Heart, Lung, and Blood Institute published similar guidelines (40). These guidelines all emphasize three basic components in an integrated strategy for asthma control: environmental control, antiinflammatory therapy, and education. Furthermore, because asthma is now recognized as a chronic allergic inflammatory disease, antiinflammatory treatment is indicated in all but the mildest asthma. This is a significant change in therapeutic emphasis, with bronchodilator treatment no longer considered to be adequate for more than symptomatic use. Furthermore, increasing evidence is appearing to show that uncontrolled asthma produces subbasement membrane fibrosis and permanent reduction in lung function. This makes complete control of the inflammation imperative. A flow chart of the U.S. guidelines has been published (41).

A second, updated set of U.S. guidelines was published in 1997 (30), followed in 1998 by new British guidelines (42). The updated British guidelines propose five modifications to the original strategy. Emphasis now is placed on gaining rapid initial control of asthma with adequate doses of corticosteroids, and then backing off to a maintenance level. Long acting β-agonists now are more readily recommended as adjunctive therapy. Inhaled corticosteroids now are acceptable as a choice for children younger than 5 years of age. New inhaler devices and spacers are easier to use and more efficient, so that nebulizers now usually are considered unnecessary (43,44). Finally, patient education and self-management plans have been reemphasized (45). The updated U.S. guidelines agree with the emphasis on education and added long-acting β-agonists, and also advocate increased use of anticholinergic inhalers and leukotriene modifiers. Also, new PF cutoff values are proposed as a guide to care (30), and assessment and monitoring have been added as a fourth component in asthma management (see earlier). A flow chart of the revised U.S. guidelines also has been published (30). The revised classification of asthma severity is summarized in Table 20.1.

## Environmental Controls

Prevention of exposure to antigens and irritants can be very effective because the elimination of incitants prevents lung inflammation from occurring, but it is often difficult to implement fully (40). However, any achievable measures that reduce exposure to allergens or pollutants are very beneficial. For example, simple enclosure of the mattress with a zippered casing can reduce dust mite exposure by 99% (46). Air cleaners remain controversial because controlled studies have in general failed to show significant effects (47), yet many patients report clear benefit from their use. In cases of extreme sensitivity, even the control of sources of indoor combustion from fireplaces and gas appliances may be required (48). In general, the more severely affected the person, the greater the potential benefits that can accrue from thorough investigation of incitants and institution of effective environmental controls (49).

## Antiinflammatory Therapy

Properly administered antiinflammatory treatment can effectively control asthma in almost all patients. Two general types of antiinflammatory treatment are available, pharmacologic and immunotherapeutic. Some form of antiinflammatory therapy is indicated for all patients with moderate or severe asthma, and also is useful for mild asthma (31).

This antiinflammatory treatment imperative evolved during the 1990s, during which it became evident that the irreversibility of chronic asthma is due to uncontrolled chronic inflammation, and that bronchodilator treatment does not affect the underlying pathologic process (40). The most contentious issue to date has been at what level of symptoms to begin antiinflammatory treatment. As more supportive research has been completed, experts are recommending treatment for less and less severe categories of symptoms. There now even is evidence that antiinflammatory therapy should be started for any sign of airway inflammation, including exercise-induced symptoms (50).

Three antiinflammatory inhaled drugs are available: cromolyn, nedocromil, and several varieties of glucocorticoids. The oral leukotriene modifiers also are antiinflammatory and are useful for all categories of asthma. Mild to moderate asthma often can be managed with leukotriene modifiers or with inhaled cromolyn or nedocromil, whereas moderate and severe asthma normally requires inhaled steroid use. Until recently, children younger than 5 years of age usually were managed without inhaled steroids, but now this is an option. Severe asthma cases also may require systemic steroid treatment, either intermittent during attacks or as continuous therapy.

Immunotherapy can be used as the sole antiinflammatory therapy in mild asthma, but is more commonly used as adjunctive therapy, along with pharmacotherapy, for any severity of asthma. In more severe asthma cases, immunotherapy is used as a steroid-sparing treatment, and may be able to reduce or eliminate the need for systemic steroid treatment. The addition of active immunotherapy to the asthma treatment regimen may be one of the reasons why better asthma management occurs when patients are treated by allergists compared with nonspecialists (51).

## Education and Self-management

This is the fourth crucial component in asthma control. Without enlisting the patient and their family in their own therapy, and educating them adequately, asthma control is neither easily achieved nor maintained. For example, at least half of patients do not follow physicians' office instructions (31), but a family education program can improve compliance enough to decrease emergency department visits and hospitalizations significantly (52). Education also can improve the use of inhalers, increase environmental controls, increase activity, decrease symptoms, and help patients and families adjust to their illness. In some cases, education reduces treatment costs (53). Education can be especially effective in teaching patients how to monitor and respond to their asthma, such as by initiating a regular program of home PF monitoring (54). Ongoing physician education and review of these home monitoring records is a very effective way to improve asthma control in motivated patients.

Principles of patient education and sample home instructions have been reviewed (7,55).

There are 12 essential areas of knowledge that must be imparted to patients:

1. What asthma is, how it affects the lungs, and how the lungs are irreversibly damaged if the inflammation is not controlled
2. The available means to improve asthmatic inflammation by environmental controls, antioxidant nutrients, immunotherapy, and antiinflammatory medications
3. How to do a home and work environmental cleanup, and smoking cessation advice/support
4. Nutritional counseling about diet and supplements
5. Allergy education, including inhalant, food, and chemical exposures and control measures
6. The difference between antiinflammatory and symptom-relieving medicines, and why both are needed
7. If long-acting β-agonists are used, an explanation of why they cannot be used for rapid symptom relief, and why antiinflammatory medicine still must be used with a long-acting bronchodilator
8. Correct use of inhalers, spacers, and mouth rinsing
9. Use of a PF meter and how to keep a PF and symptom diary
10. Warning symptoms, important changes in PF, and an action plan for when to call the office or go to the emergency department
11. A management plan, including normal treatment, treatment for an exacerbation, and expected monitoring and follow-up
12. A plan for exercise, sports, school, and work activities

Verbal discussions should be supplemented with written material to read at home, and reinforced during every visit by appropriate questions and by diary review.

A typical emergency action plan for acute asthma attacks consists of three steps (56). First, evaluate symptoms and PF diary. If symptomatic and PF is greater than 20% below the personal best, start treatment. Second, use a short-acting β-agonist or ipratropium every 20 minutes for three doses, and then check symptoms and PF again. Third, decide on extent of further treatment. If improvement is complete, continue regular maintenance therapy and observe closely for further problems. If recovery is partial, and PF is better than 50% of personal best, call office for advice. If there is little recovery, or PF is decreased more than 50% from personal best, go to the emergency department. If symptoms are very severe, or PF is below 200 L/minute, call 911 for ambulance transport.

## PHARMACOTHERAPY

### Role of Drug Therapy

Pharmacotherapy is an important part of asthma treatment, but if used without patient education, environmental con-

trol measures, regular monitoring, and periodic physician contact, results of medications alone seldom are satisfactory. Asthma currently can be effectively treated, singly, or in combination, by either systemic or topical use of eight classes of drugs: mucolytics, anticholinergic agents, antihistamines, theophylline, β-agonists, mast cell stabilizers, leukotriene modifiers, and corticosteroids. A variety of other treatments, including antioxidant vitamins (26), magnesium (57), other nutrients, various immunosuppressants (58,59), and anti-immunoglobulin E (IgE) (60) have been reported to have activity. Drugs capable of blocking leukotrienes, either during synthesis (61) or at receptor sites (62), have very useful antiinflammatory activity (63). Farther in the future, there is potential for other agents based on selective antagonists for cytokines, adhesion molecules, platelet activating factor, bradykinin, and other inflammatory mediators.

## Mucolytics

Mucolytic, expectorant, or mucokinetic agents are useful as adjunctive agents to thin the excessively viscid mucus component of asthma. Some agents can be applied topically, as in steam inhalation, or by inhalation of the substituted amino acid *N*-acetylcysteine [(NAC) Mucomyst; Bristol-Myers Squibb, Princeton, NJ]], which has long been used by inhalation (64). NAC, purchased over the counter or in health food stores, also is orally effective. Related, parenterally administered mercaptans also have been postulated to have a direct antiallergic effect through the in vivo denaturation of IgE molecules (65). Finally, two other agents, iodides and guaifenesin, are available only in oral form. Potassium iodide, calcium iodide, and iodinated glycerol are effective in asthma treatment (66), but normally are indicated only for short-term use. At present, iodides seldom are used. Guaifenesin often is used for long-term therapy, but there is no convincing objective evidence of efficacy (66).

## Anticholinergic Agents

Anticholinergic agents have been found to be effective treatment, but administration by oral and transdermal routes often produces unacceptable cardiac, central nervous system, ophthalmic (67), and antisecretory side effects. Glycopyrrolate (Robinul; Wyeth-Ayerst, Philadelphia, PA) and ipratropium (Atrovent; Boehringer Mannheim, Gaithersburg, MD) are more effective than atropine (68). Direct inhalation by nebulizer or inhaler decreases secretions and bronchodilates, with few side effects (68). These drugs are poorly absorbed, producing blood levels that usually are too low to cause anticholinergic side effects (69). The degree of response to anticholinergics is variable, so these drugs have been considered to be secondary agents, for use when other drugs are not well tolerated or not fully effective (68).

However, many patients respond well, and the bronchodilation attained usually is synergistic with that from β-agonists (70). Also, in asthma emergency treatment, ipratropium (71) always should be tried because anticholinergic bronchodilation is not blocked by β-blockers (70), and inhaled anticholinergics are low in toxicity. More severely obstructed patients benefit the most, and there is a reduced risk of hospitalization (72).

## Antihistamines

Although type 1 ($H_1$), type 2 ($H_2$), and other histamine receptors all are present in the lung, only $H_1$ antihistamines appear to have a significant clinical effect on bronchial hyperreactivity or chronic asthma symptoms (73). $H_2$ antihistamines do have a role in treatment of reflux, which often is an exacerbating factor in asthma, and also are used during emergency treatment of anaphylaxis. $H_3$ antihistamines are in clinical trials, and their role in asthma is still uncertain (74). $H_1$ antihistamines are generally useful to reduce all allergic symptoms, but were not officially recommended for asthma treatment until 1993 because of concerns for causing overdrying and formation of mucus plugs (75). Although effective for both prophylactic and symptomatic therapy, classic orally administered $H_1$ antihistamines often produce unacceptable anticholinergic or central nervous system side effects. In addition, constant use of these drugs frequently leads to tolerance.

The development of nonsedating antihistamines that have little central nervous system penetration (76) or anticholinergic activity has been a significant therapeutic advance. These new drugs have high-affinity binding to histamine receptors, producing potent clinical effects and eliminating drug tolerance (77,78). Further, the lack of anticholinergic activity allows these drugs to be used in asthma treatment without any concern that mucus plugs will form. A number of these drugs, including cetirizine, desloratadine, ebastine, fexofenadine, loratadine, mequitazine, mizolastine, noberastine, and norastemizole, have active metabolites with long enough elimination half-lives to allow once-daily dosing (79–84). Because there is increased asthma severity during the night and on awakening (80), nighttime use of these long-acting drugs is especially helpful. Many of these new antihistamines also have additional antiallergic and antiinflammatory actions, which may extend the drug's activity beyond blockade of the immediate allergic reaction to ameliorate the late-phase reaction as well (84–86). For example, cetirizine inhibits monocyte and T-lymphocyte chemotaxis (87), and has been shown to improve pulmonary function (88). Because of these added properties, the second-generation antihistamines also are not necessarily equivalent in their therapeutic effects, either to classic antihistamines or to each other. They also are not necessarily equivalent in their side effects. Cetirizine, loratadine, and fexofenadine, in contrast to older drugs, have been shown

not to alter cardiac conduction at usual clinical doses (89–91). Cetirizine and doxylamine, in contrast to loratadine and hydroxyzine, do not promote tumor growth in mice (92,93).

In addition to the four currently approved agents, cetirizine, fexofenadine, loratadine, and acrivastine (94–101), a few antihistamines are under U.S. Food and Drug Administration review, including norastemizole and desloratadine. Ketotifen, available abroad, is significantly sedating, but also has useful antiinflammatory activity (102). Like anticholinergic drugs and mucolytics, antihistamines are considered as secondary antiasthma drugs, useful in certain patients, especially when other drugs are not satisfactory (85). A major argument against newer antihistamines is their price, which is more than tenfold greater than first-generation $H_1$ antihistamines. However, the nonsedating $H_1$ drugs have superior side effect profiles (94). Because of low toxicity and possible benefit, a trial of several antihistamines is warranted in all asthmatic patients.

## Theophylline

Since 1937, intravenous theophylline has been used for emergency asthma treatment, and oral therapy has been used for chronic asthma (103). However, several more recent controlled trials have shown little efficacy of theophylline in the emergency treatment of bronchospasm, and greater toxicity than competing therapies (68,104–106). Despite these reports, theophylline does decrease asthma symptoms, especially nocturnal dyspnea (103), and also may decrease corticosteroid needs (107). Theophylline has multiple modes of action, and has been found to have significant antiinflammatory activity at lower serum levels, where toxicity is minimal (108,109). Because theophylline clearance is variable, and maintaining an appropriate serum level is important in preventing side effects (107), monitoring of theophylline levels is recommended (68). The exact place of theophylline in asthma treatment is currently in flux. Formerly a first-line agent, it has recently been deemphasized, but is still useful, especially in difficult-to-control asthma or when nocturnal symptoms are prominent. A trial of theophylline should be considered as a possible means to decrease systemic steroid use.

## β-Adrenergic Agonists

Ephedrine has been used since ancient times, and chemically similar inhaled β-adrenergic agonists are still the drugs of choice for rapid control of bronchoconstriction that is mediated by smooth muscle contraction. Acting by stimulating $\beta_2$ receptors (68), they have a rapid, predictable onset, are more potent than anticholinergic drugs or theophylline, and usually are well tolerated (68,110). The primary side effects, which may limit β-agonist use, are tremor and cardiac excitability. Older β-agonists, such as epinephrine, isoproterenol, and metaproterenol, are less $\beta_2$ selective, and thus more likely to cause side effects (107). Available short-acting $\beta_2$-selective agonists include albuterol, bitolterol, pirbuterol, and terbutaline. Inhalation of these drugs decreases systemic side effects, but oral use may be beneficial in children who have not been able to learn to use metered-dose inhalers (110).

In 1994, a slow-onset, long-duration, selective $\beta$-agonist, salmeterol (Serevent; GlaxoWellcome, Research Triangle Park, NC) was introduced in the United States (111), and a similar drug, formoterol, is available abroad and likely to be licensed in the United States soon. Unlike other $\beta$-agonists, the long-acting drugs are not useful for relief of acute asthma symptoms, but are very useful for prolonged symptom suppression, especially for nocturnal asthma. Both of these drugs are highly $\beta_2$ selective, more so than albuterol (112). When first introduced, many experts recommended salmeterol only for patients who were regularly using inhaled corticosteroids (107). The 1997 U.S. guidelines now permit salmeterol to be added to the treatment of patients with moderate asthma before raising their inhaled steroid dose. There is one significant precaution to the use of long-acting $\beta$-agonists. Because salmeterol works so effectively to reduce bronchospasm, patients who use it twice daily may become lulled into a false sense of security, and discontinue their maintenance inhaled steroids. For this reason, some physicians prescribe long-acting $\beta$-agonists only for night use.

Whether $\beta$-agonists should be used on a regular schedule or only on an as-needed basis was previously controversial (107,110). In numerous studies, increased use of $\beta$-agonists has been correlated with increased risk of death from asthma. In the province of Saskatchewan, use of more than 1.4 canisters of $\beta$-agonist per month was the threshold for increased risk, and the higher the use above that point, the higher the risk (110). The central issue is whether the correlation actually reflects adverse physiologic effects from the drug, or whether increased drug use is a marker for more severe asthma, which naturally has a higher death rate. This issue has been reviewed (107,113,114). In New Zealand, changes in asthma deaths appear to have been correlated with use of fenoterol, a very long-duration, nonselective $\beta$-agonist that was never available in the United States. In this case, it is suspected that the excess mortality was due to direct effects the drug, and not to insufficient use of antiinflammatory agents or to poor education and medical supervision (107,115). Salmeterol has been investigated and has been found not to cause excess mortality (116). Because of this controversy, the most conservative practice is always to institute antiinflammatory therapy if short-duration $\beta$-agonist use exceeds three times weekly (31), or one canister per month (68). Furthermore, patients who are using a long-duration drug, such as salmeterol, should be warned to use one of the rapid-acting $\beta$-agonists, rather than salmeterol, for relief of acute symptoms (107).

## β-Adrenergic Antagonists (β-Blockers)

Drug interactions may complicate treatment of asthma, especially during $\beta$-agonist treatment of status asthmaticus or anaphylaxis. $\beta$-Adrenergic antagonists (117) are the class of interfering drug most likely to be encountered, but other drugs also may be of concern, especially in elderly patients (118). $\beta$-Blockade has three major types of adverse effects during asthma treatment. First, $\beta$-blockade is proallergic because it both blocks smooth muscle relaxation and amplifies the production of anaphylactic mediators (117), thus increasing the severity of asthma, or any allergic reaction (119). Second, $\beta$-blockade increases the dose of $\beta$-agonist required to overcome the block and produce bronchodilation. Third, $\beta$-blockade may cause hypertensive crisis because of unopposed $\alpha$-adrenergic effects, which occur if epinephrine is used to treat the asthma (119). $\beta_1$-Selective $\beta$-blockers have relatively less bronchoconstricting effect than desirable cardiac effects (mediated by $\beta_1$ receptors), and theoretically should be less likely to cause harm when used in allergic persons. However, the effects of $\beta$-blockers on mediator production are nonselective, and thus even $\beta_1$-selective drugs are proallergic (118). Consequently, use of $\beta$-antagonists in patients with asthma is not recommended unless there is no good alternative treatment.

## Mast Cell Stabilizers

There are only two clinically useful drugs that are primarily mast cell stabilizers, although both corticosteroids and some of the antihistamines also may produce some of their antiallergic activity by cell stabilization. The first drug in this class, cromolyn, or sodium cromoglycate, was introduced in the mid-1970s, almost simultaneously with the introduction of inhaled corticosteroids (120). Cromolyn has been found to be effective and extremely safe for allergic therapy, but is limited by being essentially nonabsorbed and thus restricted to topical treatment. Cromolyn also is most effective when used every 6 hours, so that compliance is an issue. Cromolyn is available in an inhaled form, Intal (Medeva Pharmaceuticals, Rochester, NY), and an oral form, Gastrocrom (Medeva), which may block the effects of allergic foods that can trigger asthma (121). In treatment of allergic rhinitis, cromolyn has been found to be comparable in efficacy with oral doses of nonsedating antihistamines (122), and the combination of cromolyn and an antihistamine is more effective than either drug used alone (123). However, cromolyn is less effective than intranasal corticosteroids in control of most rhinitis symptoms (124,125). The experience with mast cell stabilizers in asthma therapy parallels their use in rhinitis. Cromolyn is an effective antiinflammatory agent for exercise-induced asthma or mild chronic asthma (31,107). When used to treat exercise-induced asthma, the combination of cromolyn and $\beta$-agonist is superior to either drug alone (126).

A second drug, chemically unrelated to cromolyn but with a similar pharmacologic activity profile and similar receptor sites, was subsequently found. This drug, nedocromil (Tilade; Medeva), differs from cromolyn in having slightly greater oral absorption, but is available only in an inhaled formulation. By in vitro tests, nedocromil is approximately tenfold more potent on a molar basis than cromolyn, whereas in animal studies the two drugs are equally effective when applied topically, but nedocromil has a longer duration of action (127). The only side effect of nedocromil is a metallic, bitter taste that some patients find unacceptable. Nedocromil, like cromolyn, is an effective antiinflammatory agent for exercise-induced asthma or mild chronic asthma. It is as effective as beclomethasone in mild asthma (128), but is less effective than corticosteroids in moderate or severe asthma (107). Nedocromil appears both to prevent granulocyte mediator release and reduce local irritative axon reflexes by blocking membrane chloride channels (128).

If administered before allergen challenge, both mast cell stabilizers inhibit both the immediate and late-phase allergic reactions. However, neither drug can prevent the late-phase reaction if given after the immediate reaction has begun (129). The action of mast cell stabilizers differs from that of corticosteroids in two ways. First, mast cell stabilizers effectively prevent the immediate reaction, whereas corticosteroids, even when used for prolonged periods, have only a weak effect on the immediate reaction (130). Second, unlike mast cell stabilizers, corticosteroids significantly attenuate the late-phase reaction if given during or after the immediate reaction (129). Both mast cell stabilizers and corticosteroids are most effective when used before allergen challenge (129,131). Mast cell stabilizers are most useful as an alternative to corticosteroids in mild or moderate asthma, and also are used as adjunctive therapy in difficult-to-control asthma. Both cromolyn and nedocromil have been shown significantly to improve daytime symptom control when added to a regimen of inhaled bronchodilators and corticosteroids (132). Furthermore, adding nedocromil also improves nighttime symptom control and allows the dose of inhaled steroid to be reduced (128,133).

## Leukotriene Modifiers

The antileukotriene drugs are the first new class of agents approved for the treatment of asthma in more than 20 years. Leukotrienes are locally released, potent mediators of late-phase allergic reactions that act by binding to membrane and nuclear receptors (134). Because leukotrienes are proinflammatory, it was believed that leukotriene modifiers would be effective in asthma control. Two kinds of antileukotriene drugs were developed. Leukotriene biosynthesis occurs through the action of arachidonate 5-lipoxygenase, which catalyzes the initial steps in the multistep conversion of arachidonic acid to cysteinyl leukotrienes. Leukotriene-modifying drugs either prevent leukotrienes from binding to and activating lung receptors (receptor antagonists) or inhibit arachidonate 5-lipoxygenase, and thus leukotriene synthesis (synthesis inhibitors).

Antileukotriene drugs block the late-phase reaction, and therefore are especially beneficial when used regularly for chronic asthma (135), but they also prevent bronchoconstriction from being triggered by cold air, exercise, allergens, aspirin, or sulfur dioxide. Except for aspirin sensitivity, where the antileukotrienes are almost uniformly effective, individual responses to these drugs are variable (136). The effectiveness of these drugs in most patients is intermediate between cromolyn and high-dose inhaled corticosteroids. In general, synthesis inhibitors are more effective than receptor antagonists. Animal studies also demonstrate benefits when leukotriene antagonists are used before anaphylaxis (74) or β-blockade (137). Because oral leukotriene antagonists have a rapid onset of action (138), some emergency physicians are now including them as part of standard therapy for acute asthma.

At present, there are three available receptor antagonists, montelukast (Singulair; Merck & Co., West Point, PA), zafirlukast (Accolate; Zeneca Pharmaceuticals, Wilmington, DE), and in Japan, pranlukast. There is also a single available synthesis inhibitor, zileuton (Zyflo; Abbott Laboratories, Abbott Park, IL). The first several years' experience with antileukotriene drugs showed limited toxicity, but as the number of treated cases increased, two problems emerged. The first was hepatotoxicity. Several prospective antileukotriene drugs were canceled during development owing to liver toxicity. After release, zileuton was found to have approximately a 2% incidence of significant liver injury, so that mandatory aminotransferase monitoring is necessary when using this drug (138). To date, there have been few reports of hepatic injury with the receptor antagonists, but at four times the recommended dose, zafirlukast appears rarely to cause serum aminotransferase elevation (138).

The second concern is a possible link to Churg-Strauss syndrome (CSS), an eosinophilic vasculitis. All three receptor antagonists, as well as high-dose inhaled steroids, have been temporally linked with recognition of CSS (139–141). It had been thought that the syndrome was unmasked as systemic steroids were tapered, and that leukotriene modifiers were not causative. But one case has now been reported where CSS arose in a patient taking only montelukast (142). Therefore, patients using these drugs should be observed for systemic symptoms that might herald onset of this syndrome. One of the most useful warnings of possible CSS is the onset of severe or recurrent sinusitis, often requiring surgical drainage (143). Accompanying systemic symptoms often include arthralgias, myalgias, neuropathy, malaise, weight loss, fever, and palpable purpura. Diagnostic clues to CSS consist of persistent eosinophilia, especially more than $1.5 \times 10^9$ cells/L, chest radiographic findings of transient infiltrates or cardiomegaly, microscopic hematuria, and, in the absence of infection, elevated erythrocyte sedimentation rate and C-reactive protein (143). There may also be a positive anti-neutrophil cytoplasmic antibody test result, with perinuclear staining, but this is not always present, and is not required for diagnosis.

Leukotriene modifiers are most useful as once-daily, easy-to-use, high-compliance agents for mild to moderate asthma. They will probably have their greatest use as an alternative to low-dose inhaled corticosteroids in children and teenagers. However, it remains to be seen if the long-term effectiveness of leukotriene modifiers will be as good as that from inhaled corticosteroids. They also are becoming very useful as additional drugs for severe asthma and difficult-to-control cases (144), and may allow reductions in corticosteroid doses. In fact, it is in this role, as a steroid-sparing treatment, that leukotriene-associated CSS is most likely to be identified (143).

## Corticosteroids

Corticosteroids are the most effective class of drugs for control of asthma. In addition to decreasing inflammatory airway edema, corticosteroids potentiate the effect of β-agonists on smooth muscle relaxation, decrease β-agonist tachyphylaxis, and decrease mucus production (68). In treatment of acute asthma attacks, corticosteroids decrease immediate mortality, hospital admissions, and risk of relapse within 10 days of treatment (68). Corticosteroids primarily block late-phase reactions, and although their effects begin immediately, they do not become maximally effective for several days after treatment begins. This gradual effect on late-phase inflammation appears to be due to inhibition of interleukin-4 expression (131) as well as suppression of the conversion of arachidonic acid into prostaglandins and leukotrienes (31). Other studies suggest that there may be additional corticosteroid effects, including even some effects on early-phase reactions (130).

The use of inhaled corticosteroids to treat allergic inflammation dates from the introduction of beclomethasone in 1974, and has been viewed as the most important advance in allergy treatment since the discovery of antihistamines (145). Before topical steroids, glucocorticoids could be administered only systemically, with significant long-term risks (145,146). Possible steroid side effects are protean: osteoporosis with fractures, glucose intolerance, infections, gastric ulcers and gastrointestinal bleeding, cataracts, glaucoma, and accelerated arteriosclerosis, among many. There is a direct dose–risk relationship with long-term oral steroid use, with detectable increases in risk even for very low doses, such as 5 mg/day of prednisone (146). Because of this, since the earliest days of corticosteroid use in the 1950s, there have been attempts to use these drugs topically rather than systemically. Early attempts at topical treatment failed be-

cause of insufficient potency, or from high systemic absorption and adrenal suppression, or because of poor delivery methods, problems that were overcome by Brostoff and Czarny's work in 1968 (147). Fortuitously, highly potent corticosteroids appear to be even more effective when administered topically, rather than orally (147,148).

Although physician acceptance initially was slow, inhaled corticosteroids have gradually become accepted as primary treatment for serious asthma. Topical steroids now are advocated for even mild asthma, although this remains contentious because the long-term risk–benefit analysis has not been established for mild asthma. Because mild asthma is diagnosed in approximately two thirds of all asthmatic patients, the long-term safety, potential benefits, and treatment cost of using inhaled corticosteroids in these cases is of major importance (149). Particularly critical to resolving this issue is the current lack of knowledge regarding whether patients with untreated mild asthma have any natural progression of their disease or ever sustain irreversible obstruction. There is early research to support this concern (50). However, there is no question that inhaled corticosteroids are both safe and effective for moderate or severe asthma, and that they do ameliorate the natural progression of the disease (149). In fact, physician reluctance to use adequate doses of corticosteroids currently causes significant preventable disability and decreased quality of life, whereas steroid-induced side effects are rarely observed (150).

Five different strategies for using corticosteroids in asthma can be formulated (31,150). First, for outpatient treatment of acute asthma exacerbations, short-term oral corticosteroids for up to 10 days are appropriate (107), and simultaneous consideration should be given to adding or increasing inhaled corticosteroids. Second, for emergency department or inpatient treatment of acute severe asthma, short-term intravenous corticosteroids are used (151), followed by tapering outpatient oral treatment and maintenance inhaled therapy. Third, inhaled corticosteroids, at standard doses, are appropriate maintenance therapy for moderate or severe asthma. Fourth, if asthma control is not achieved, inhaled corticosteroid doses should be increased to a high-dose regimen. Finally, in difficult cases, long-term maintenance oral corticosteroid therapy, using a short-duration drug such as prednisone or prednisolone, can be added to inhaled corticosteroids. When regular use of oral steroids is necessary, the use of alternate-day morning dosing can significantly decrease the incidence of corticosteroid side effects (107,150).

With over 20 years of clinical use in the United States, topical inhaled glucocorticoids have shown few major side effects. Problems with throat irritation, hoarseness, and cough have been decreased by developing improved formulations or dispensers, and by providing more patient education to encourage throat rinsing after inhaler use. Local fungal infections may occur in the oral cavity or larynx (150), but usually clear with short-term antifungal therapy. Occasionally, inhaled steroids may trigger contact allergy (152). Available drugs differ mainly in degree of absorption into the systemic circulation, speed of metabolic inactivation, inhaler design (ease of use and inhalation efficiency), and in frequency of dosing required to maintain efficacy. Inhaler design is very important because corticosteroids administered in powdered form may have better lung deposition, stay on the mucosa longer, and are more slowly absorbed, so effectiveness is increased and the systemic effect is lessened (153).

Of the available drugs, flunisolide has a narrow safety margin (154) but does not ordinarily cause systemic effects. Only inhaled dexamethasone regularly caused significant hypothalamic–pituitary–adrenal axis suppression (124, 148,155), and it has been withdrawn from the U.S. market. Beclomethasone dipropionate is the only available drug that lacks first-pass hepatic inactivation. Beclomethasone dipropionate is approximately half as potent as dexamethasone, and is rapidly hydrolyzed in tissues to the 17-monopropionate, which is 13 times more potent than dexamethasone, and ultimately to beclomethasone, which has approximately 75% the activity of dexamethasone (156). The more recently developed topical corticosteroids have been designed to have low systemic bioavailability. They are highly lipophilic and consequently poorly absorbed from the gastrointestinal tract, but also undergo rapid first-pass metabolism (except for beclomethasone) to inactive metabolites (157). High lipophilicity also ensures prolonged retention at the desired site of action in the respiratory mucosa. Corticosteroid systemic bioavailability is the total amount of the drug that becomes systemically available after direct absorption from the lung or nose, added to that remaining after gastrointestinal absorption and first-pass metabolism of the swallowed fraction of the dose. Steroids administered orally, nasally, intramuscularly, or to skin enter the venous circulation and are affected by hepatic metabolism. Systemic bioavailability is markedly reduced for recently developed corticosteroids that do exhibit efficient first-pass hepatic inactivation. However, this mechanism is circumvented for steroids given intravenously or inhaled. Inhaled steroids are absorbed topically into the pulmonary mucosa, and then transported by the pulmonary artery to the left ventricle and on to the systemic circulation.

When used in recommended doses for normal pulmonary inhalation, significant systemic absorption and steroid side effects seldom have been observed with the newer agents (150,158,159). However, even with low-dose intranasal steroid use (160), a few cases of posterior subcapsular cataracts have been noted, and measurable growth retardation may occur in children (161). There also are single case reports of detectable adrenal suppression from intranasal beclomethasone (162,163) and fluticasone (164), and measurable changes in daily serum and urinary cortisol levels

**TABLE 20.2. COMPARISON OF DAILY DOSES OF INHALED CORTICOSTEROIDS**

| Drug/Strength (μg/Puff) | Low Dose (Puffs/Day) | Medium Dose (Puffs/Day) | High Dose (Puffs/Day) |
|---|---|---|---|
| Beclomethasone | | | |
| 42 | 4–12 | 12–20 | >20 |
| 84 | 2–6 | 6–10 | >10 |
| Flunisolide | | | |
| 250 | 2–4 | 4–8 | >8 |
| Triamcinolone | | | |
| 100 | 4–10 | 10–20 | >20 |
| Fluticasone | | | |
| 44 | 2–4 | — | — |
| 110 | 2 | 2–6 | >6 |
| 220 | — | 1–2 | >3 |
| Budesonide | | | |
| 200 | 1–2 | 2–3 | >3 |

with both fluticasone and budesonide (165). Furthermore, in circulating lymphocytes, specific glucocorticoid receptor–regulated genes show measurable changes in levels of messenger RNA transcription during intranasal treatment with fluticasone or budesonide (165). Pulmonary doses of inhaled corticosteroids are higher than nasal doses, but clinically apparent, steroid-induced side effects still are very uncommon (150,166), although dose-related mild suppression of bone metabolism, of unknown clinical relevance, may be detected (31,167). Temporary mild growth retardation may be seen in children in the first year of use, but does not continue to occur after the second year, and final adult height appears unaffected (107). In a large study group on budesonide followed over 13 years, catch-up growth to normal adult height was documented (168). Whether these changes may eventually increase osteoporosis is not known (167), although 6- and 10-year studies suggest not (169, 170). Bone density testing should be considered for patients who are on very–long-term treatment with either inhaled or oral corticosteroids (171). Rarely, significant adrenal suppression can occur with usual pulmonary doses, and with progressively higher-dose pulmonary treatment, toxicity may ultimately approach that of chronic oral steroid use (167). Comparative daily doses of available inhaled corticosteroids for low-, medium-, and high-dose treatment are shown in Table 20.2 (172).

## Recommendations for Use of Inhaled Corticosteroids

Unfortunately, few objective data on relative drug potencies and risks in humans are available to allow detailed comparison of the available topical corticosteroids (167). Also of concern is the fact that significant differences in patient susceptibility to steroid-induced side effects have been observed (167). Finally, the potential for complications from very long periods (>30 years) of topical corticosteroid use is not known. Taken together, all of these observations indicate the need for thoughtful use of corticosteroids. There are six aspects to this intelligent use of topical steroids. First, adhere to proper indications and doses, using published guidelines for asthma treatment (7,30,38–42,55,173,174). Second, use the lowest possible dose of steroids that can completely control the asthma (by symptoms and by PFTs), in topical form whenever possible (175,176). Third, use all possible measures to reduce unwanted corticosteroid absorption, for example, by use of solid or powder formulations, spacers, and mouth rinsing to minimize swallowing of inhaled steroids (177). Fourth, preferentially use corticosteroids with high levels of first-pass hepatic metabolism into inactive compounds. Fifth, add all reasonable treatments, such as immunotherapy and adjunctive drugs (178), as steroid-sparing measures. Last, periodically reevaluate each patient's condition for possible reduction of corticosteroids. After prolonged corticosteroid therapy, in some cases it is possible simply to discontinue treatment with no clinical worsening (179). In other cases, corticosteroids may be replaced with a mast cell stabilizer. Or, the corticosteroid dose may be reduced by addition of a mast cell stabilizer (128,180), theophylline, antihistamine, leukotriene modifier, or immunotherapy, or by successful efforts at environmental control measures and nutritional management (see Chapter 27).

## IMMUNOTHERAPY

Immunotherapy has been used for asthma since 1918, and has always been controversial for this indication (181). Before the introduction of corticosteroids, immunotherapy was the only available antiinflammatory treatment for asthma, and was widely practiced. Immunotherapy is clinically effective for asthma (182); however, an asthma diagnosis is the single greatest risk factor for immunotherapy reactions (181). Since the advent of effective drug treatments, the risk–benefit analysis for immunotherapy has been reevaluated, and in some areas, particularly in Scandinavia and the United Kingdom, concern over possible anaphylaxis risk has led to a marked decrease in immunotherapy. In the rest of the world and the United States, immunotherapy use continues (183). Available data strongly indicate that asthmatic patients are at increased risk of undergoing anaphylaxis compared with other patients with allergy treated with immunotherapy (184). On the other hand, a meta-analysis (185) reviewing 20 placebo-controlled, randomized, double-blind studies of immunotherapy for asthma found that there is significant improvement with immunotherapy. Positive effects are found for symptomatic improvement, reduced medication use, reduced bronchial hy-

perreactivity, and improvement in FEV$_1$. Use of well standardized extracts (182) and cautious immunotherapy (see Chapter 12) reduces the risk of reactions. Immunotherapy therefore should be considered for use in asthmatic patients (186), especially in moderate or severe cases, as a means of reducing the need for corticosteroid therapy, and in mild cases because of the ease of compliance or because of patient preference for an alternative to pharmacotherapy.

## Clinical Example

An example follows of the use of immunotherapy during combined therapy of asthma. A 52-year-old nonsmoking school music teacher was first seen in November, 1996 with complaints of frequent episodes of bronchitis and sinusitis, and recent shortness of breath and night awakenings. She had a 15-year history of chronic fatigue, chronic obstructive rhinitis, cough, and episodic conjunctivitis, usually triggered by mold or dust exposure. In the past month, she had had two courses of antibiotics, and had been treated with a β-agonist inhaler, intranasal steroids, and inhaled steroids, but was currently off of all medications. She was feeling better, she believed, because she had been out of school for the Thanksgiving vacation. There was a positive family history of allergies, but not asthma. The review of systems was negative, and she specifically denied acid reflux. She worked in a moldy, dusty school basement, but had a dry, clean home without pets. The physical examination showed allergic shiners, turbinate edema but no sinusitis, no laryngeal evidence of reflux, and normal lungs. She was given prescriptions for cromolyn ophthalmic solution and a second-generation antihistamine, and reinstructed in proper use of her β-agonist inhaler. Blood was drawn for in vitro allergy testing, and PFTs were scheduled. Her initial PFT (Fig. 20.3A) surprisingly showed severe obstruction with little bronchodilator effect, and her in vitro test was positive only to the two dust mites (class 2).

The next office visit was used entirely for education (see earlier). She was reinstructed in maintenance use of inhaled steroids, and begun on a medium dose, with spacer. Pharmacologic doses of vitamins C and E, a multiple vitamin with minerals, and NAC were started. Because of her history of mold sensitivity and multiple equivocal in vitro test results, skin endpoint titration (SET) tests were scheduled. SET was positive to three foods: corn, milk, and cane sugar, and to cat, dog, all three grass families, ragweed, lamb's quarters, *Candida,* and 11 inhalant molds. Milk and cane sugar were strong positives (dilution 4 or 5), whereas the rest endpointed only on dilution 2. A rotation diet was initiated, and inhalant immunotherapy was begun using a cautious advancement schedule.

Over the next 4 years, there was steady progress in symptom relief, gradual reduction in the frequency of infections, and steady improvement in PFTs. She had no problems

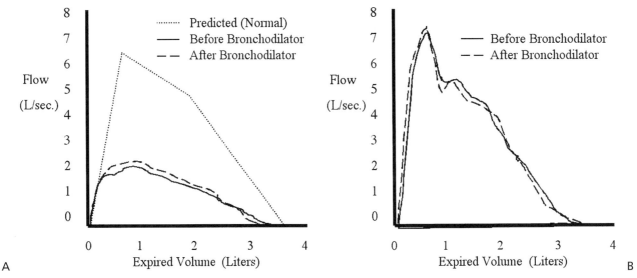

**FIG. 20.3. A:** Pulmonary function at diagnosis: severe asthma with cough, fatigue, progressive dyspnea, and night awakening. **B:** Normal pulmonary function after 4 years of combined therapy with environmental controls, nutrition, immunotherapy, and pharmacotherapy.

with immunotherapy, and reached maintenance doses within 6 months. By June 1997 her fatigue had lifted, and she felt well. In 1998, reflux developed that was treated medically. In 1999, after persistent efforts, her classroom was moved out of the basement. In 2000, she was switched to a solid inhaled steroid, and the dose was decreased to two puffs daily. Four years after beginning treatment, her PFT was normal (Fig. 20.3B). In this case, long-standing, severe asthma was completely controlled by a combination of environmental controls, immunotherapy, nutrition, and appropriate pharmacotherapy.

## TREATMENT DURING PREGNANCY

Asthma is the most common potentially serious illness to complicate pregnancy (5), and it increases the risk of perinatal complications (187). However, if asthma is well controlled, the outcomes are no different than those of nonasthmatic pregnancies. A combined position statement on the use of medications in pregnancy was published by the American College of Allergy, Asthma, and Immunology and the American College of Obstetricians and Gynecologists (187). This report summarizes the available data regarding safety, in animals and humans, for each of the major antiasthmatic drugs except theophylline, and makes recommendations for treatment of asthma of different degrees of severity. Other reports raise the possibility that theophylline is a first-

trimester teratogen (188,189). These combined recommendations are summarized in Table 20.3. Before using any of these drugs in pregnancy, the full text of these references should be consulted. It also is advisable to consult with the gynecologist managing any pregnant asthmatic patient so that a joint treatment plan can be agreed on.

## CONCLUSION

Asthma is an increasingly common disease worldwide, and occurs frequently in all age groups in the allergic patient population. Because unrecognized asthma is an important source of patient morbidity and is a potential risk during medical and surgical treatment, all clinicians should be familiar with this disease. Asthma diagnosis relies primarily on clinical suspicion when patients have wheezing, dyspnea, chest discomfort, or cough. Appropriate use of PFTs and other objective monitoring, environmental control measures, antiinflammatory therapy, nutritional management, and patient education is critical to successful intervention. Rational use of pharmacotherapy and immunotherapy entails knowledge of indications, side effects, limitations, and useful combinations of treatments. Finally, timely consultation with other specialists may be essential for developing an optimum treatment plan for each patient, and for anticipating and treating possible complications of therapy.

## TABLE 20.3. SUMMARY OF RECOMMENDATIONS FOR ASTHMA TREATMENT DURING PREGNANCY

| Medication | Comments |
| --- | --- |
| **Not usually recommended** | |
| Nedocromil | Insufficient data |
| Pseudoephedrine | Low risk of gastroschisis |
| Leukotriene inhibitors | Zileuton—adverse effects in animals |
| Initiate immunotherapy | Do not normally begin immunotherapy during pregnancy |
| **Recommended with restrictions** | |
| Long-acting β-agonists | Salmeterol—use if essential and known to be effective |
| Ipratropium | Probably safe, use if short-acting β-agonists not adequate |
| Nasal corticosteroids | Probably safe, use if needed and known to be effective |
| Antihistamines, nonsedating | Loratadine or cetirizine, after first trimester, use if alternatives too sedating |
| Leukotriene antagonists | Montelukast or zafirlukast—use if essential and known to be effective |
| Theophylline | Suspected teratogen in first trimester, probably safe thereafter |
| Oral corticosteroids | Suspected teratogen in first trimester, use only if life-saving or no safe alternative |
| **Recommended** | |
| Environmental controls | Very important |
| Smoking cessation | Very important |
| Continue immunotherapy | Continue immunotherapy (if not having systemic reactions) |
| Short-acting β-agonists | Albuterol, metaproterenol, terbutaline—safe |
| Antihistamines, sedating | Chlorpheniramine, tripelennamine—safe |
| Cromolyn | Safe |
| Inhaled corticosteroids | Budesonide preferred, beclomethasone acceptable |
| Oral corticosteroids | After first trimester, benefits outweigh risks for severe asthma |

For details, see Dombrowski et al. (187), Stenius-Aatniala et al. (188), and Park et al. (189).

## ACKNOWLEDGMENTS

The author thanks June L. Bianchi, Beverly J. Flynn, Phyllis J. Foley, Sally C. Schumann, librarians, Nancy E. Frazier, former head librarian (deceased), and Jeanie M. Vander Pyl, head librarian, Cape Cod Hospital Medical Library, for their expertise in medical literature research.

## REFERENCES

1. Laitinen A, Laitinen LA. Pathology of asthma. *Allergy Proc* 1994; 15:323–328.
2. Brusasco V, Crimi E, Gianiorio P, et al. Allergen-induced increase in airway responsiveness and inflammation in mild asthma. *J Appl Physiol* 1990;69:2209–2214.
3. Subramanian D, Guntupalli KK. Diagnosing obstructive lung disease. *Postgrad Med* 1994;95:69–85.
4. Weiss KB, Gergen PJ, Hodgson TA. An economic evaluation of asthma in the United States. *N Engl J Med* 1992;326:862–866.
5. Schatz M. Asthma and pregnancy: background, recommendations, and issues: introduction to the workshop. *J Allergy Clin Immunol* 1999;103:S329.
6. Godden DJ, Ross S, Abdalla M, et al. Outcome of wheeze in childhood. *Am J Respir Crit Care Med* 1994;149:106–112.
7. Autio L, Rosenow D. Effectively managing asthma in young and middle adulthood. *Nurse Pract* 1999;24:100–111.
8. Centers for Disease Control and Prevention, Air Pollution and Respiratory Health Branch. Asthma—United States, 1982–1992. *MMWR Morb Mortal Wkly Rep* 1995;43: 952–955.
9. Busse W, Banks-Schlegel SP, Larsen GL. Childhood- versus adult-onset asthma. *Am J Respir Crit Care Med* 1995;151: 1635–1639.
10. Meyers DA. Approaches to genetic studies of asthma. *Am J Respir Crit Care Med* 1994;150:S91–S93.
11. Burrows B, Martinez FD, Halonen M, et al. Association of asthma with serum IgE levels and skin-test reactivity to allergens. *N Engl J Med* 1989;320:271–277.
12. Corne J, Smith S, Schreiber J, et al. Prevalence of atopy in asthma. *Lancet* 1994;344:344–345.
13. Broder I, Higgins MW, Mathews KP, et al. Epidemiology of asthma and allergic rhinitis in a total community: Tecumseh, Michigan. *J Allergy Clin Immunol* 1974;54:100–110.
14. Tunnicliffe WS, Burge PS, Ayres JG. Effect of domestic concentrations of nitrogen dioxide on airway responses to inhaled allergen in asthmatic patients. *Lancet* 1994;344:1733–1736.
15. Peden DB, Setzer RW Jr, Devlin RB. Ozone exposure has both a priming effect on allergen-induced responses and an intrinsic inflammatory action in the nasal airways of perennially allergic asthmatics. *Am J Respir Crit Care Med* 1995;151:1336–1345.
16. Hogg JC. Adenoviral infection and childhood asthma. *Am J Respir Crit Care Med* 1994;150:2–3.
17. Forteza R, Lauredo IT, Burch R, et al. Extracellular metabolites of *Pseudomonas aeruginosa* produce bronchoconstriction by different mechanisms. *Am J Respir Crit Care Med* 1994;149: 687–693.
18. Emre U, Sokolovskaya N, Roblin PM, et al. Detection of anti-*Chlamydia pneumoniae* IgE in children with reactive airway disease. *J Infect Dis* 1995;172:265–267.
19. Beck KC, Offord KP, Scanlon PD. Bronchoconstriction occurring during exercise in asthmatic subjects. *Am J Respir Crit Care Med* 1994;149:352–357.
20. Busse WW, Kiecolt-Glaser JK, Coe C, et al. Stress and asthma. *Am J Respir Crit Care Med* 1995;151:249–252.
21. Sporik R, Ingram JM, Price W, et al. Association of asthma with serum IgE and skin test reactivity to allergens among children living at high altitude. *Am J Respir Crit Care Med* 1995; 151:1388–1392.
22. Targonski PV, Persky VW, Ramekrishnan V. Effect of environmental molds on risk of death from asthma during the pollen season. *J Allergy Clin Immunol* 1995;95:955–961.
23. James JM, Bernhisel-Broadbent J, et al. Respiratory reactions provoked by double blind food challenges in children. *Am J Respir Crit Care Med* 1994;149:59–64.

24. Vandenplas O, Delwiche JP, Evrard G, et al. Prevalence of occupational asthma due to latex among hospital personnel. *Am J Respir Crit Care Med* 1995;151:54–60.

25. Deschamps D, Questel F, Baud FJ, et al. Persistent asthma after acute inhalation of organophosphate insecticide. *Lancet* 1994; 344:1712.

26. Britton JR, Pavord ID, Richards KA, et al. Dietary antioxidant vitamin intake and lung function in the general population. *Am J Respir Crit Care Med* 1995;151:1383–1387.

27. Gordon BR. Update on the importance of nutrition in allergy management. *Curr Opin Otolaryngol Head Neck Surg* 1998;6: 67–69.

28. Gordon BR. The importance of nutrition in allergy management. *Curr Opin Otolaryngol Head Neck Surg* 1997;5:53–54.

29. Rosier MJ, Bishop J, Nolan T, et al. Measurement of functional severity of asthma in children. *Am J Respir Crit Care Med* 1994; 149:1434–1441.

30. Emond SD, Camargo CA, Nowak RM. 1997 National Asthma Education and Prevention Program guidelines: a practical summary for emergency physicians. *Ann Emerg Med* 1998;31: 579–589.

31. Sheffer AL. Management of the adult asthma patient. *Allergy Proc* 1995;16:1–4.

32. Enright P, Scanlon PD. Why and how to use office spirometry. *Contemp Int Med* 1993;5:14–29.

33. Crapo RO. Pulmonary function testing. *N Engl J Med* 1994; 331:25–30.

34. Woolcock AJ, Reddel H, Trevillion L. Assessment of airway responsiveness as a guide to diagnosis, prognosis, and therapy in asthma. *Allergy Proc* 1995;16:23–26.

35. Sont JK. How do we monitor asthma control? *Allergy* 1999; 49[Suppl 54]:68–73.

36. Sont JK, Willems LN, Bel EH, et al. Clinical control and histo-pathologic outcome of asthma when using airway hyperrespon-siveness as an additional guide to long-term treatment. *Am J Respir Crit Care Med* 1999;159:1043–1051.

37. Reddel H, Jenkins C, Woolcock A. Diurnal variability: time to change asthma guidelines? *BMJ* 1999;319:45–47.

38. British Thoracic Society. Guidelines for management of asthma in adults: I. chronic persistent asthma. Statement by the British Thoracic Society, Research Unit of the Royal College of Physicians of London, King's Fund Centre, National Asthma Campaign. *BMJ* 1990;301:651–653.

39. British Thoracic Society. Guidelines for management of asthma in adults: II. acute severe asthma. Statement by the British Thoracic Society, Research Unit of the Royal College of Physicians of London, King's Fund Centre, National Asthma Campaign. *BMJ* 1990;301:797–800.

40. Sheffer AL. Guidelines for the diagnosis and management of asthma. *J Allergy Clin Immunol* 1991;88:425–533.

41. Lemanske RF. A review of the current guidelines for allergic rhinitis and asthma. *J Allergy Clin Immunol* 1998;101: S392–S396.

42. Partridge MR, Harrison BD, Rudolph M, et al. The British asthma guidelines: their production, dissemination, and imple-mentation.. *Respir Med* 1998;92:1046–1052.

43. O'Callaghan C, Barry PW. Asthma drug delivery devices for children. *BMJ* 2000;320:664.

44. Newhouse M. Asthma therapy in children: nebulizers or me-tered dose inhalers with holding chambers? Reply. *J Pediatr* 2000;137:139–141.

45. Keeley D, Rees J. New guidelines on asthma management. *BMJ* 1997;314:315–316.

46. Fernandez-Caldas E, Fox RW. Environmental control of indoor air pollution. *Med Clin North Am* 1992;76:935–952.

47. Thien FCK, Leung RCC, Czarny D, et al. Indoor allergens and IgE-mediated respiratory illness. *Immunol Allergy Clin North Am* 1994;14:567–590.

48. Rea WJ. *Chemical sensitivity.* Boca Raton, FL: CRC Press, 1994: 706–707.

49. Call RS, Ward G, Jackson S, et al. Investigating severe and fatal asthma. *J Allergy Clin Immunol* 1994;94:1065–1072.

50. Laitinen LA, Altraja A, Karjalainen EM, et al. Early interven-tions in asthma with inhaled corticosteroids. *J Allergy Clin Immunol* 2000;105:S582–S585.

51. Vollmer WM, O'Hollaren M, Ettinger KM, et al. Specialty differences in the management of asthma: a cross-sectional as-sessment of allergists' patients and generalists' patients in a large HMO. *Arch Intern Med* 1997;157:1201–1208.

52. Clark NM, Feldman CH, Evans D, et al. The impact of health education on frequency and cost of health care use by low in-come children with asthma. *J Allergy Clin Immunol* 1986;78: 108–115.

53. Krahn M. Issues in the cost-effectiveness of asthma education. *Chest* 1994;106:264S–269S.

54. Li JTC. Do peak flow meters lead to better asthma control? *J Respir Dis* 1995;16:381–398.

55. Mellins RB, Evans D, Clark N, et al. Developing and communi-cating a long-term treatment plan for asthma. *Am Fam Physician* 2000;61:2419–2434.

56. Wise RA, Liu MC. Obstructive airways diseases: asthma and chronic obstructive pulmonary disease. In: Barker LR, Burton JR, Zieve PD, eds. *Principles of ambulatory medicine,* 5th ed. Baltimore: Williams & Wilkins, 1999:677–706.

57. Britton J, Pavord I, Richards K, et al. Dietary magnesium, lung function, wheezing, and airway hyperreactivity in a random adult population sample. *Lancet* 1994;344:357–362.

58. Paterson JW, Lulich KM, Goldie RG. Pharmacology of asthma treatment: an overview. *Med J Aust* 1995;162:42–43.

59. Fukuda T. Immunosuppressive agents and asthma. *Clin Rev Allergy* 1994;12:95–108.

60. Barnes PJ. Anti-IgE therapy in asthma: rationale and therapeutic potential *Int Arch Allergy Immunol* 2000;123:196–204.

61. Knapp HR. Reduced allergen-induced nasal congestion and leu-kotriene synthesis with an orally active 5-lipoxygenase inhibitor. *N Engl J Med* 1990;323:1745–1748.

62. Donnelly AL, Glass M, Minkwitz MC, et al. The leukotriene D4-receptor antagonist ICI 204,219, relieves symptoms of acute seasonal allergic rhinitis. *Am J Respir Crit Care Med* 1995;151: 1734–1739.

63. Taniguchi Y, Tamura G, Honma M, et al. The effect of an oral leukotriene antagonist, ONO-1078, on allergen-induced immediate bronchoconstriction in asthmatic subjects. *J Allergy Clin Immunol* 1993;92:507–512.

64. Millman M, Grundon W. Use of acetylcysteine in bronchial asthma and emphysema. *J Asthma Res* 1969;6:199–209.

65. Kisil FT, Sehon AH, Hollinger HZ. In vitro and in vivo inacti-vation of reagins with mercaptans. *Clin Allergy* 1971;1: 387–397.

66. Bone RC. Managing mucus secretions in patients with asthma or COPD. *J Respir Dis* 1990;11:240–259.

67. Berdy GJ, Berdy SS, Odin LS, et al. Angle closure glaucoma precipitated by aerosolized atropine. *Arch Intern Med* 1991;151: 1658–1660.

68. Corbridge TC, Hall JB. The assessment and management of adults with status asthmaticus. *Am J Respir Crit Care Med* 1995; 151:1296–1316.

69. Wood CC, Fireman P, Grossman J, et al. Product characteristics and pharmacokinetics of intranasal ipratropium bromide. *J Al-lergy Clin Immunol* 1995;95:1111–1116.

70. Beakes DE. The use of anticholinergics in asthma. *J Asthma* 1997;34:357–368.

71. Polosa R, Phillips GD, Rajakulasingham K, et al. The effect of inhaled ipratropium bromide alone and in combination with oral terfenadine on bronchoconstriction provoked by adenosine 5′-monophosphate and histamine in asthma. *J Allergy Clin Immunol* 1991;87:939–946.
72. Stoodley RG, Aaron SD, Dales RE. The role of ipratropium bromide in the emergency management of acute asthma exacerbation: a meta-analysis of randomized clinical trials. *Ann Emerg Med* 1999;34:8–18.
73. Holgate ST. Antihistamines in the treatment of asthma. *Clin Rev Allergy* 1994;12:65–78.
74. Chrusch C, Sharma S, Unruh H, et al. Histamine H3 receptor blockade improves cardiac function in canine anaphylaxis. *Am J Respir Crit Care Med* 1999;160:1142–1149.
75. Weintraub M. Letter to the editor. *N Engl J Med* 1994;331:1019.
76. Marzanatti M, Monopoli A, Trampus M, et al. Effects of nonsedating histamine H1-antagonists on EEG activity and behavior in the cat. *Pharmacol Biochem Behav* 1989;32:861–866.
77. Simons FER, Simons KJ. H$_1$ receptor antagonist treatment of chronic rhinitis. *J Allergy Clin Immunol* 1988;81:975–980.
78. Tarnasky PR, VanArsdel PP Jr. Antihistamine therapy in allergic rhinitis. *J Fam Pract* 1990;30:71–80.
79. Cua-Lim F. An evaluation of the efficacy and safety of loratadine syrup vs. astemizole syrup in perennial allergic rhinitis. *Immunol Allergy Pract* 1991;13:47–53.
80. Knight A, Drouin MA, Yang WH, et al. Clinical evaluation of the efficacy and safety of noberastine, a new H1 antagonist, in seasonal allergic rhinitis: a placebo-controlled, dose-response study. *J Allergy Clin Immunol* 1991;88:926–934.
81. Smolensky MH, Reinberg A, Labrecque G. Twenty-four hour pattern in symptom intensity of viral and allergic rhinitis: treatment implications. *J Allergy Clin Immunol* 1995;95:1084–1096.
82. Pariente-Khayat A, Rey E, Dubois MC, et al. Pharmacokinetics of cetirizine in 2- to 6-year-old children. *Int J Clin Pharmacol Ther* 1995;33:340–344.
83. Simons FE, Simons KJ. Clinical pharmacology of new histamine H1 receptor antagonists. *Clin Pharmacokinet* 1999;36:329–352.
84. Henz BM. The pharmacologic profile of desloratadine: a review. *Allergy* 2001;56[Suppl 65]:7–13.
85. Holgate ST, Finnerty JP. Antihistamines in asthma. *J Allergy Clin Immunol* 1989;83:537–547.
86. Rafferty P, Holgate ST. Histamine and its antagonists in asthma. *J Allergy Clin Immunol* 1989;84:144–151.
87. Jinquan T, Reimert CM, Deleuran B, et al. Cetirizine inhibits the in vitro and ex vivo chemotactic response of T lymphocytes and monocytes. *J Allergy Clin Immunol* 1995;95:979–986.
88. Spector SL, Nicodemus CF, Corren J, et al. Comparison of the bronchodilatory effects of cetirizine, albuterol, and both together versus placebo in patients with mild-to-moderate asthma. *J Allergy Clin Immunol* 1995;96:174–181.
89. Zechnich AD, Hedges JR, Eiselt-Proteau D, et al. Possible interactions with terfenadine or astemizole. *West J Med* 1994;160:321–325.
90. Darrow WR. *Important diagnostic information.* Letter to U.S. physicians from Schering-Plough Research Institute, Kenilworth, NJ, July 1, 1994.
91. Pratt CM, Mason J, Russell T, et al. Cardiovascular safety of fexofenadine HCl. *Am J Cardiol* 1999;83:1451–1454.
92. Brandes LJ, Warrington RC, Arron RJ, et al. Enhanced cancer growth in mice administered daily human-equivalent doses of some H1-antihistamines: predictive in vitro correlates. *J Natl Cancer Inst* 1994;86:770–775.
93. Weed DL. Between science and technology: the case of antihistamines and cancer. *J Natl Cancer Inst* 1994;86:740–741.
94. Abramowicz M. Acrivastine/pseudoephedrine (Semprex-D) for seasonal allergic rhinitis. *Med Lett* 1994;36:78–80.
95. Girard JP, Sommacal-Schopf D, Bigliardi P, et al. Double-blind comparison of astemizole, terfenadine, and placebo in hay fever with special regard to onset of action. *J Int Med Res* 1985;13:102–108.
96. Kaliner M, Check WA. Non-sedating antihistamines. *Allergy Proc* 1988;9:649–663.
97. Salomonsson P, Gottberg L, Heilborn H, et al. Efficacy of an oral antihistamine, astemizole, as compared to a nasal steroid spray in hay fever. *Allergy* 1988;43:214–218.
98. Rohr AS. Non-sedating antihistamines: a selective review of terfenadine, astemizole, cetirizine, and loratadine. *Immunol Allergy Pract* 1989;11:334–337.
99. Barenholtz HA, McLeod DC. Loratadine: a nonsedating antihistamine with once-daily dosing. *Ann Pharmacol* 1989;23:445–450.
100. Mann KV, Crowe JP, Tietze KJ. Nonsedating histamine H$_1$-receptor antagonists. *Clin Pharm* 1989;8:331–344.
101. Juhlin L, Arendt C. Treatment of chronic urticaria with cetirizine dihydrochloride a non-sedating antihistamine. *Br J Dermatol* 1988;119:67–72.
102. Reid JJ. Double-blind trial of ketotifen in childhood chronic cough and wheeze. *Immunol Allergy Pract* 1989;11:143–149.
103. Banner AS. Theophylline: should we discard an old friend ? *Lancet* 1994;343:618.
104. Littenberg B. Aminophylline treatment in severe, acute asthma: a meta-analysis. *JAMA* 1988;259:1678–1684.
105. Self TH, Abou-Shala N, Burns R, et al. Inhaled albuterol and oral prednisone therapy in hospitalized adult asthmatics: does aminophylline add any benefit? *Chest* 1990;98:1317–1321.
106. Strauss RE, Wertheim DL, Bonagura VR, et al. Aminophylline therapy does not improve outcome and increases adverse effects in children hospitalized with acute asthmatic exacerbations. *Pediatrics* 1994;93:205–210.
107. Abramowicz M. Drugs for asthma. *Med Lett* 1995;37:1–4.
108. Sullivan P, Bekir S, Jaffar Z, et al. Anti-inflammatory effects of low-dose oral theophylline in atopic asthma. *Lancet* 1994;343:1006–1008.
109. Kidney J, Dominguez M, Taylor PM, et al. Immunomodulation by theophylline in asthma: demonstration by withdrawal of therapy. *Am J Respir Crit Care Med* 1995;151:1907–1914.
110. Nelson HS. Beta-adrenergic bronchodilators. *N Engl J Med* 1995;333:499–506.
111. Abramowicz M. Salmeterol. *Med Lett* 1994;36:37–39.
112. Roux FJ, Grandordy B, Douglas JS. Functional and binding characteristics of long-acting beta2-agonists in lung and heart. *Am J Respir Crit Care Med* 1996;153:1489–1495.
113. Barrett TE, Strom BL. Inhaled beta-adrenergic receptor agonists in asthma: more harm than good? *Am J Respir Crit Care Med* 1995;151:574–577.
114. van Schayck CP, Cloosterman SG, Hofland ID, et al. How detrimental is chronic use of bronchodilators in asthma and chronic obstructive pulmonary disease? *Am J Respir Crit Care Med* 1995;151:1317–1319.
115. Beasley R, Burgess C, Crane J, et al. A review of the studies of the asthma mortality epidemic in New Zealand. *Allergy Proc* 1995;16:27–32.
116. Williams C, Crossland L, Finnerty J, et al. Case-control study of salmeterol and near-fatal attacks of asthma. *Thorax* 1998;53:7–13.
117. Toogood JH. Risk of anaphylaxis in patients receiving beta-blocker drugs. *J Allergy Clin Immunol* 1988;81:1–5.

118. Anderson CJ, Bardana EJ. Asthma in the elderly: interactions to be wary of. *J Respir Dis* 1995;16:965–976.

119. Hepner MJ, Ownby DR, Anderson JA, et al. Risk of systemic reactions in patients taking beta-blocker drugs receiving allergen immunotherapy injections. *J Allergy Clin Immunol* 1990;86:407–411.

120. Price HV. Cromolyn sodium: post-market surveillance. *Immunol Allergy Pract* 1986;8:89–96.

121. Pelikan Z, Pelikan-Filipek M. Effects of oral cromolyn on the nasal response due to foods. *Arch Otolaryngol Head Neck Surg* 1989;115:1238–1243.

122. Orgel HA, Meltzer EO, Kemp JP, et al. Comparison of intranasal cromolyn sodium, 4%, and oral terfenadine for allergic rhinitis: symptoms, nasal cytology, nasal ciliary clearance, and rhinomanometry. *Ann Allergy* 1991;66:237–244.

123. Lindsay-Miller ACM, Chambers A. Group comparative trial of cromolyn sodium and terfenadine in the treatment of seasonal allergic rhinitis. *Ann Allergy* 1987;58:28–32.

124. Wilson JA, Walker SR. A clinical study of the prophylactic use of betamethasone valerate and sodium cromoglycate in the treatment of seasonal allergic rhinitis. *J Laryngol Otol* 1976;90:201–206.

125. Bousquet J, Chanal I, Alquie MC, et al. Prevention of pollen rhinitis symptoms: comparison of fluticasone propionate aqueous nasal spray and disodium cromoglycate aqueous nasal spray: a multicenter, double-blind, double-dummy, parallel-group study. *Allergy* 1993;48:327–333.

126. McFadden ER Jr, Gilbert IA. Exercise-induced asthma. *N Engl J Med* 1994;330:1362–1367.

127. Thomson NC. Nedocromil sodium: an overview. *Respir Med* 1989;83:269–276.

128. Barnes PJ, Holgate ST, Laitinen LA, et al. Asthma mechanisms, determinants of severity and treatment: the role of nedocromil sodium. *Clin Exp Allergy* 1995;25:771–787.

129. Crimi E, Violante B, Pellegrino R, et al. Effect of multiple doses of nedocromil sodium given after allergen inhalation in asthma. *J Allergy Clin Immunol* 1993;92:777–783.

130. Naclario RM, Baroody FM, Kagey-Sobotka A, et al. Basophils and eosinophils in allergic rhinitis. *J Allergy Clin Immunol* 1994;94:1303–1309.

131. Bradding P, Feather IH, Wilson S, et al. Cytokine immunoreactivity in seasonal rhinitis: regulation by a topical corticosteroid. *Am J Respir Crit Care Med* 1995;151:1900–1906.

132. Drazen JM, Israel E. Treating mild asthma: when are inhaled steroids indicated? *N Engl J Med* 1994;331:737–739.

133. Lal S, Dorow PD, Venho KK, et al. Nedocromil sodium is more effective than cromolyn sodium for the treatment of chronic reversible obstructive airway disease. *Chest* 1993;104:438–447.

134. Steinhilber D. 5-Lipoxygenase: a target for anti-inflammatory drugs revisited. *Curr Med Chem* 1999;6:71–85.

135. Laviolette M, Malmstrom K, Lu S, et al. Montelukast added to inhaled beclomethasone in treatment of asthma. *Am J Respir Crit Care Med* 1999;160:1862–1868.

136. Smith LJ. A risk-benefit assessment of anti-leukotrienes in asthma. *Drug Saf* 1998;19:205–218.

137. Fujimura M, Abo M, Kamio Y, et al. Effect of leukotriene and thromboxane antagonist on propranolol-induced bronchoconstriction. *Am J Respir Crit Care Med* 1999;160:2100–2103.

138. Barnes NC. Effects of anti-leukotrienes in the treatment of asthma. *Am J Respir Crit Care Med* 2000;161:S73–S76.

139. Baba K, Niwa S, Yagi T, et al. Churg-Strauss syndrome during corticosteroid tapering in a patient with bronchial asthma receiving pranlukast. *Arerugi* 2000;49:512–515.

140. Wechsler ME, Pauwels RA, Drazen JM. Leukotriene modifiers and Churg-Strauss syndrome: adverse effect or response to corticosteroid withdrawal? *Drug Saf* 1999;21:241–251.

141. Wechsler ME, Finn D, Gunawardena D, et al. Churg-Strauss syndrome in patients receiving montelukast as treatment for asthma. *Chest* 2000;117:708–713.

142. Tuggey JM, Hosker HS. Churg-Strauss syndrome associated with montelukast therapy. *Thorax* 2000;55:805–806.

143. D'Cruz DP, Barnes NC, Lockwood CM. Difficult asthma or Churg-Strauss syndrome? *BMJ* 1999;318:475–476.

144. Christian Virchow J, Prasse A, Naya I, et al. Zafirlukast improves asthma control in patients receiving high-dose inhaled corticosteroids. *Am J Respir Crit Care Med* 2000;162:578–585.

145. Mygind N. Pharmacological management of perennial rhinitis. *Rhinology* 1991;11[Suppl]:21–26.

146. Saag KG, Koehnke R, Caldwell JR, et al. Low dose long-term corticosteroid therapy in rheumatoid arthritis: an analysis of serious adverse events. *Am J Med* 1994;96:115–123.

147. Christy NP. Pituitary-adrenal function during corticosteroid therapy: learning to live with uncertainty. *N Engl J Med* 1992;326:266–267.

148. Brostoff J, Czarny D. Effect of intranasal betamethasone-17-valerate on allergic rhinitis and adrenal function. *J Allergy* 1969;44:77–81.

149. Siegel S. Topical intranasal corticosteroid therapy in rhinitis. *J Allergy Clin Immunol* 1988;81:984–991.

150. Shapiro G. Childhood asthma. *Allergy Proc* 1995;16:5–11.

151. Manthous CA. Management of severe exacerbations of asthma. *Am J Med* 1995;99:298–308.

152. Peris-Tortajada A, Giner A, Perez C, et al. Contact allergy to topical budesonide. *J Allergy Clin Immunol* 1991;87:597–598.

153. Agertoft L, Pedersen S. Importance of the inhalation device on the effect of budesonide. *Arch Dis Child* 1993;69:130–133.

154. Sipila P, Sorri M, Ojala K, et al. Comparative trial of flunisolide and beclomethasone dipropionate nasal sprays in patients with seasonal allergic rhinitis. *Allergy* 1983;38:303–307.

155. Busse W, Randlev B, Sedgwick J. The effect of azelastine on neutrophil and eosinophil generation of superoxide. *J Allergy Clin Immunol* 1989;83:400–405.

156. Wurthwein G, Rohdewald P. Activation of beclomethasone dipropionate by hydrolysis to beclomethasone-17-monopropionate. *Biopharm Drug Dispos* 1990;11:381–394.

157. Dushay ME, Johnson CE. Management of allergic rhinitis: focus on intranasal agents. *Pharmacotherapy* 1989;9:338–350.

158. Stead RJ, Cooke NJ. Adverse effects of inhaled corticosteroids. *BMJ* 1989;298:403–404.

159. Goldstein DE, Konig P. Effect of inhaled beclomethasone dipropionate on hypothalamic–pituitary–adrenal axis function in children with asthma. *Pediatrics* 1983;72:60–64.

160. Fraunfelder FT, Meyer SM. Posterior subcapsular cataracts associated with nasal or inhalation corticosteroids. *Am J Ophthalmol* 1990;109:489–490.

161. Wolthers OD, Pedersen S. Short-term growth in children with allergic rhinitis treated with oral antihistamine, depot and intranasal glucocorticoids. *Acta Paediatr* 1993;82:635–640.

162. Sorkin S, Warren D. Probable adrenal suppression from intranasal beclomethasone. *J Fam Pract* 1986;22:449–450.

163. Czarny D, Brostoff J. Effect of intranasal betamethasone-17-valerate on perennial rhinitis and adrenal function. *Lancet* 1968:188–190.

164. Grossman J, Banov C, Bronsky EA, et al. Fluticasone propionate aqueous nasal spray is safe and effective for children with seasonal allergic rhinitis. *Pediatrics* 1993;92:594–599.

165. Knutsson U, Stierna P, Marcus C, et al. Effects of intranasal glucocorticoids on endogenous glucocorticoid peripheral and central function. *J Endocrinol* 1995;144:301–310.

166. Agertoft L, Larsen FE, Pedersen S. Posterior subcapsular cataracts, bruises and hoarseness in children with asthma receiving

long-term treatment with inhaled budesonide. *Eur Respir J* 1998;12:130–135.

167. Kamada AK. Therapeutic controversies in the treatment of asthma. *Ann Pharmacother* 1994;28:904–914.

168. Agertoft L, Pedersen S. Effect of long-term treatment with inhaled budesonide on adult height in children with asthma. *N Engl J Med* 2000;343:1064–1069.

169. Toogood JH, Baskerville JC, Markov AE, et al. Bone mineral density and the risk of fracture in patients receiving long-term inhaled steroid therapy for asthma. *J Allergy Clin Immunol* 1995; 96:157–166.

170. Agertoft L, Pedersen S. Bone mineral density in children with asthma receiving long-term treatment with inhaled budesonide. *Am J Respir Crit Care Med* 1998;157:178–183.

171. Toogood JH, Hodsman AB, Fraher LJ, et al. Serum osteocalcin and procollagen as markers for the risk of osteoporotic fracture in corticosteroid-treated asthmatic adults. *J Allergy Clin Immunol* 1999;104:769–774.

172. Staton GW Jr, Ingram RH Jr. Asthma. In: Dale DC, Federman DD, eds. *Scientific American medicine.* New York: WebMD Corporation, 2000;14,II:1–16.

173. National Heart, Lung, and Blood Institute. International consensus report on diagnosis and treatment of asthma. *Eur Respir J* 1992;5:601–641.

174. Hargreave FE, Dolovich J, Newhouse MT. The assessment and treatment of asthma: a conference report. *J Allergy Clin Immunol* 1990;85:1098–1111.

175. Hanania NA, Chapman KR, Kesten S. Adverse effects of inhaled corticosteroids. *Am J Med* 1995;98:196–208.

176. Barnes PJ, Pedersen S. Efficacy and safety of inhaled corticosteroids in asthma. *Am Rev Respir Dis* 1993;148:S1–S26.

177. Barnes PJ. Inhaled glucocorticoids for asthma. *N Engl J Med* 1995;332:868–875.

178. Helms PJ. Corticosteroid-sparing options in the treatment of childhood asthma. *Drugs* 2000;59[Suppl 1]:15–22.

179. van Schayck CP, van den Broek PJ, den Otter JJ, et al. Periodic treatment regimens with inhaled steroids in asthma or chronic obstructive pulmonary disease: is it possible? *JAMA* 1995;274: 161–164.

180. Svendsen UG, Jorgensen H. Inhaled nedocromil sodium as additional treatment to high dose inhaled corticosteroids in the management of bronchial asthma. *Eur Respir J* 1991;4: 992–999.

181. Hurst DS, Gordon BR, Fornadley JA, et al. Safety of home based and office allergy immunotherapy: a multicenter prospective study. *Otolaryngol Head Neck Surg* 1999;121:553–561.

182. Bosquet J. Specific immunotherapy in asthma. *Allergy* 1999;54: 37–38.

183. Bosquet J, Michel FB. Specific immunotherapy in asthma. *Allergy Proc* 1994;15:329–333.

184. Bousquet J, Hejjaoui A, Dhivert H, et al. Immunotherapy with a standardized *Dermatophagoides pteronyssinus* extract: III. systemic reactions during the rush protocol in patients suffering from asthma. *J Allergy Clin Immunol* 1989;83:797–802.

185. Abramson MJ, Puv RM, Weiner JM. Is allergen immunotherapy effective in asthma? *Am J Respir Crit Care Med* 1995;151: 969–974.

186. Craig T, Sawyer AM, Fornadley JA. Use of immunotherapy in a primary care office. *Am Fam Physician* 1998;57:1888–1894; 1897–1898.

187. Dombrowski MP, Huff R, Lipkowitz M, et al. Position statement: the use of newer asthma and allergy medications during pregnancy. *Ann Allergy Asthma Immunol* 2000;84:475–480.

188. Stenius-Aarniala B, Riikonen S, Teramo K. Slow-release theophylline in pregnant asthmatics. *Chest* 1995;107:642–647.

189. Park JM, Schmer V, Myers TL. Cardiovascular anomalies associated with prenatal exposure to theophylline. *South Med J* 1990;83:1487–1488.

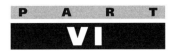

# RELATED ALLERGIC DISEASES

# OCULAR ALLERGY

**MARK B. ABELSON**
**MATTHEW J. CHAPIN**
**ELIZABETH R. SANDMAN**

Ocular allergy is one of the most frequent complaints heard by ophthalmologists and optometrists, affecting an estimated 20% of the general population. Over 50 million people have the most common form, allergic conjunctivitis. The prevalence of allergy in developed countries is increasing, and with a large sum being spent on allergy-related medications, visits to clinicians, and lost days of work, the importance of appropriate diagnosis and treatment is clearly evident. Clinicians are confronted with how to alleviate the clinical and economic impact of allergy. This chapter discusses the relevant pathophysiologic processes and mechanisms of ocular allergy, which will serve as a foundation for proper differential diagnosis and ultimately matching the right treatment to the patient's specific allergic disease.

The general category of ocular allergy includes two types, acute and chronic. Approximately 95% of ocular allergy sufferers have the acute form of the disease, either seasonal or perennial allergic conjunctivitis. Seasonal allergic conjunctivitis encompasses the episodic form of the disease that affects people sensitive to pollens such as grass, ragweed, or trees. Perennial allergic conjunctivitis includes those panseasonal sensitivities to allergens such as animal dander or hair, mold, or dust mites. Most topical antiallergy medications have been developed to treat acute ocular allergy. Although less frequent, the other chronic allergic disease are associated with more severe signs and symptoms, often resulting in some visual impairment. The chronic forms of ocular allergy include vernal keratoconjunctivitis (VKC), atopic keratoconjunctivitis (AKC), and allergic giant papillary conjunctivitis (GPC), which collectively account for the remaining 5% of ocular allergy.

**M. B. Abelson:** Associate Clinical Professor of Ophthalmology, Harvard Medical School; Senior Scientist, Schepens Eye Research Institute, Boston, Massachusetts.
**M. J. Chapin:** Ophthalmic Research Associates, Inc., North Andover, Massachusetts.
**E. R. Sandman:** Clinical Research Associate, Ophthalmic Research Associates, Inc., North Andover, Massachusetts.

## PATHOPHYSIOLOGY OF THE ALLERGIC REACTION

The eye has certain defenses, both specific and nonspecific, that protect the ocular surface. Eyebrows and eyelashes protect the ocular surface from large particles. The tear film is an antigen diluent, eyewash, and barrier. Tears contain specific immunoglobulin E (IgE) molecules that inhibit antigen penetration into the conjunctiva by intercepting and binding to them. When these defenses are compromised, antigens are able to bind to the IgE on the surface of the conjunctival mast cells, triggering the sequence of events that results in ocular allergy. In fact, however, allergy itself is a localized protective response that serves to destroy, dilute, or isolate both the injurious agent and the injured tissue (1).

Factors involved in the diathesis of ocular allergy include environmental conditions, genetic predisposition, exposure to medication and cosmetics, and chronic irritation induced by ocular mechanical devices. Environmental factors such as indigenous pollens, type of climate, geographic location, and stress all affect the incidence of ocular allergy. Allergens continuously bombard the ocular surface, but the severity of the bombardment varies across pollination periods in seasonal allergic conjunctivitis and exposure to antigen in the home or work environment in perennial allergic conjunctivitis. Climatic conditions also can exacerbate or alleviate ocular allergy by affecting both the concentration of airborne allergens and the barrier function of the ocular surface. The genetic factor of ocular allergy is well recognized. Researchers do not know which genes are responsible for allergen sensitivity; however, the probability of allergy developing in a child increases fourfold if one parent is atopic, and by tenfold if both parents are affected. Certain active drugs (e.g., systemic antihistamines), drug vehicles, or cosmetic agents can serve as sensitizing agents or immune modulators by either affecting the normal defense in the eye (destabilizing the tear film, thereby making ocular tissue more exposed to allergen penetration) or by nonspecifically stimulating mast cell activation. Ocular devices such as contact lenses can act as mechanical stimulators in immune reactions.

The Gell and Coombs classification of antigenic responses has been used to divide the immune response into four types (I, II, III, and IV). This classification has proved to be helpful in understanding the disease processes. Type I reactions result from the release of pharmacologically active substances from IgE-sensitized basophils and mast cells. The type II response is usually mediated by cytotoxic antibodies resulting from the activation of complement by IgG or IgM antibodies. Type III reactions result from deposition of soluble circulating antigen–antibody complexes. Type IV reactions are cell mediated, and involve sensitized lymphocytes (T cells). Although some form of eye disease represents each of these types, ocular allergy usually involves either type I or type IV hypersensitivity reactions. Distinguishing between the reactions is important because as more selective therapies become available, proper distinction and identification of the allergic disease process in a patient will be necessary.

## Sensitization

The allergic reaction requires that the person first become sensitized to a specific antigen. On initial exposure to an antigen, a macrophage or dendritic cell [antigen-presenting cells (APC)] encounters, engulfs, and processes the antigen. This processing forms cell surface proteins, binding to T helper lymphocytes (Th cells) specific for the antigen, forming a major histocompatability complex (MHC). This binding stimulates the APC and Th cell to secrete factors [interleukin (IL)-1, IL-2, respectively] that further stimulate the Th cell to proliferate and mature, and stimulate antigen-specific B cells to differentiate and proliferate. The mature Th cells travel through the bloodstream, ultimately arriving in the substantia propria in the conjunctiva, where they await cell-mediated cytotoxic reactions. Mature B cells travel to the lacrimal gland, accessory lacrimal glands, and the conjunctiva, where they produce specific antibody (IgE) (2). Once sensitization has occurred, the immune system reacts quickly and powerfully to repeated antigen exposure, producing the typical type I hypersensitivity reaction.

The type I allergic reaction is a complex deluge of reactions that is dominated by the mast cell. The human eye has over 50 million mast cells, each of which can have up to a half million surface IgE molecules (3). Antigen penetrates the tear film, reaching the mast cells of the conjunctiva. The free antigen then binds to IgE molecules on the surface of the mast cell, cross-linking IgE molecules in pairs. The binding induces serine esterase to initiate a change in the Fc receptor, the IgE receptor found on mast cells and basophils, resulting in the phosphorylation of phospholipase C by protein tyrosine kinase (4). Phospholipase breaks down the cellular membrane, and initiates other second messenger molecules to activate the release of intracellular calcium stores. The increased transients of calcium induce granules containing preformed inflammatory mediators to fuse with the cellular membrane and be exocytosed. These proinflammatory substances include histamine, tryptase, chymase, eosinophil chemotactic factor (ECP), neutrophil chemotactic factor (NCF), platelet-activating factor (PAF), interleukins, tumor necrosis factor (TNF), and heparin (5). The free calcium also activates phospholipase $A_2$, which cleaves arachidonic acid from membrane phospholipids to form other inflammatory mediators.

## The Allergic Response

Histamine is the primary mediator in allergy. Histamine is a preformed biogenic amine stored and release by mast cells and basophils. It acts directly on nerve endings, smooth muscle, and blood vessels to produce the characteristic itching, redness, and chemosis found in allergy. To date, three different histamine receptor subtypes have been identified: $H_1$, $H_2$, and $H_3$. Both $H_1$ and $H_2$ receptors have been identified in ocular tissue. $H_1$ receptor activation results in itching (1) and redness (3), whereas $H_2$ receptor activation leads to redness (4). The redness is caused by vasodilation, whereas chemosis and lid swelling are caused by exudation of plasma through gaps between vascular endothelium of postcapillary venules, mediated by the $H_1$ receptor (6). Histamine also inhibits the production of immunoglobulins, downmodulates lymphocyte production, and enhances natural killer cell activity and fibroblast proliferation (7). Histamine levels are regulated by the enzyme histaminase, which breaks down histamine (8)

Two mast cell subtypes have been described: T mast cells, which contain tryptase, and TC mast cells, which contain tryptase and chymase (2). Tryptase and chymase are preformed serine endoproteases stored in mast cells. Because tryptase is unique to mast cells, it is an excellent marker for them (2,9). Tryptase has the ability to potentiate the effect of histamine, activate eosinophils and mast cells, and attract eosinophils and neutrophils. It also has the ability to degrade neuropeptides such as vasoactive intestinal peptide (VIP), peptide histidine-methionine, and calcitonin gene-related peptide. VIP is a prominent bronchodilator, and it is postulated that the destruction of VIP by tryptase results in the increased bronchomotor tone and bronchial hyperresponsiveness (10) of asthma. The exact role of tryptase in ocular inflammation is not fully understood. The presence of chymase has not yet been demonstrated in the eye, although its presence is suggested by the large number of conjunctival mast cells of the TC phenotype.

Heparin forms complexes with proteases and is released with degranulation of mast cells. Heparin has been shown to have antiinflammatory properties (5), but there are only preliminary reports on the use of heparin in ocular allergy (11). Heparin may serve as an endogenous mediator in a negative feedback loop regulating the release of proinflammatory mediators from the mast cell.

Platelet-activating factor is derived from membrane phospholipids after the action of phospholipase $A_2$ (12). PAF is released from most bone marrow–derived inflammatory cells, including macrophages, eosinophils, neutrophils, basophils, monocytes, and mast cells. PAF is the most potent eosinophil chemotactic factor (13). Histologically, PAF is chemotactic for conjunctival neutrophils and eosinophils, degranulates eosinophils, and produces dramatic intravascular margination in the conjunctiva (14).

As stated previously, phospholipase $A_2$ metabolizes membrane phospholipids, resulting in the release of arachidonic acid. Arachidonic acid then serves as a substrate for either cyclooxygenase or lipoxygenase. The cyclooxygenase produces prostaglandins (PG) and thromboxanes. Some of the effects attributed to these products are bronchospasm, coronary and pulmonary vasoconstriction, neutrophil chemoattraction, and augmentation of basophil histamine release ($PGF_{2\alpha}$, $PGD_2$) (15,16), pulmonary vasodilation and inhibition of platelet aggregation ($PGI_2$) (17), inhibition of macrophage spreading and surface adherence (18), and bronchodilation ($PGE_2$) (19). $PGE_1$ and $PGE_2$ produce vasodilation (20) and erythema (21). Prostaglandins also can potentiate edema, enhance pain and fever caused by inflammatory stimuli, and sensitize nerve endings to other agents that induce pain (22). $PGE_1$, $PGE_2$, $PGF_{2\alpha}$, and $PGD_2$ have all been isolated from ocular tissue and aqueous humor (23), but $PGD_2$ is the main prostaglandin produced by human mast cells in vitro (24,25) and in vivo (26,27). After topical application to guinea pig or human eyes, $PGD_2$ results in redness, conjunctival chemosis, tenacious mucus discharge, and eosinophilic infiltrate (28). Studies suggest that certain prostaglandins also may have antiinflammatory actions. Thus, prostaglandins also may play a role in the negative feedback system that defines the allergic response as self-limiting (29).

Thromboxane $A_2$ ($TXA_2$) and hydroxyheptadecatrienoic acid (HHT) are the other products of the cyclooxygenase pathway. $TXA_2$ is a potent vasoconstrictor (30), platelet aggregator (31), and bronchoconstrictor (9). These actions suggest that $TXA_2$ plays a role in bronchial asthma. The role of $TXA_2$ in ocular allergy is unclear. HHT serves as a chemotactic factor for human granulocytes (32).

Leukotrienes (LT) are products of arachidonic acid metabolism through the lipoxygenase pathway. The initial product, $LTA_4$, can be converted to $LTB_4$ or $LTC_4$, $LTD_4$, and $LTE_4$. $LTC_4$, $LTD_4$, and $LTE_4$ have been identified in tears after allergen challenge (33). $LTB_4$ is probably the best-studied leukotriene involved in ocular inflammation. $LTB_4$ is produced predominantly by eosinophils and basophils, but also by neutrophils, macrophages, and monocytes. It acts as a potent neutrophil chemotactic agent, and has been found in ocular tissue in rabbits and primates (33), as well as in tears after conjunctival allergen challenge. Applica-

tion of $LTB_4$ topically to human conjunctiva did not produce vasodilation, but biopsy revealed polymorphonuclear leukocyte infiltrates, and the subject reported migraine headaches lasting for more than 2 weeks (author's unpublished observation). Both $PGE_2$ and $PGD_2$ act synergistically with $LTB_4$ to enhance vascular permeability, resulting in edema formation, subsequent neutrophil infiltration, and mast cell degranulation. Topical application of $LTC_4$ elicited no observable effect in rabbits or humans (34). These finding suggest that leukotrienes have little role in ocular allergies, although they may play a role in potentiating inflammatory mechanisms that have already started.

In addition to leukotrienes, the lipoxygenase arm of arachidonic acid metabolism also produces hydroperoxyeicosatetraenoic acid (HPETE) and hydroxyeicosatetraenoic acid (HETE) (35). Topical ocular application of HPETE and HETE to rabbit and human eyes had no visible effect on the conjunctiva (author's unpublished data). HPETE and HETE are known to be potent mucus-stimulating mediators in the lung (36), and it is possible that such a role may exist in the eye. The role of HPETE and HETE in ocular allergy remains undefined, although two HETE subtypes (HETE 1 and HETE 2) have been identified in tears of patients with VKC, pemphigoid, or rosacea (37). Thus, a role in ocular inflammation seems probable.

Cytokines are a group of proteins that serve as communication conduits between various groups of immune cells (e.g., macrophages, mast cells, lymphocytes, eosinophils). IL-1 and IL-2, mentioned previously, play a role in activation of APC and T cells. IL-3 is produced by immunologically stimulated lymphocytes and supports the growth of a cell type resembling basophils or mast cells (38). IL-8 is a chemoattractant for neutrophils. TNF, another cytokine produced by mast cells, upregulates conjunctival mast cell surface receptors for adhesion molecules [e.g. intracellular adhesion molecule-1 (ICAM-1)], and stimulates mast cell histamine release (39). Interferon-$\gamma$ (IFN-$\gamma$) is produced by T cells and enhances activity of macrophages and increases MHC expression. T cells secrete IL-3 and IL-5, which in turn activate and recruit eosinophils; IL-4 also is secreted by Th cells, and enables the maturation of T cells and B cells and induces B cells to produce IgE. Mast cells also release IL-5, which in turn activates eosinophils. IL-6 also stimulates T- and B-cell formation (40). There also are interleukins that act in a negative feedback loop to regulate the proinflammatory interleukins. IL-12 and IFN-$\gamma$ both are natural inhibitors of IL-4 and Th2 cell differentiation, and they may modulate the inflammatory process. Other cytokines include granulocyte–macrophage-colony stimulating factor (GM-CSF), which helps mast cells proliferate (41), and transforming growth factor-$\beta$, which is chemoattractive for monocytes and macrophages.

Once recruited, the eosinophil contains a number of toxic proteins that are released in the eye and are responsible for tissue destruction. These include eosinophil-derived major basic protein (EMBP), major cationic protein, eosinophil-derived neurotoxin, and eosinophil-derived peroxidase. EMBP is the main toxic protein in the eosinophil and produces mast cell degranulation and epithelial damage (42). Eosinophil-derived peroxidase is toxic by enhancing peroxide levels (43).

Adhesion molecules represent another class of proteins that play a role in the inflammatory process. Adhesion molecules are membrane-bound proteins that allow cells to interact with one another. TNF, interleukins, antigen, histamine, leukotrienes, peroxide, and IFN may all serve as stimuli for adhesion molecules (44). There are several groups of adhesion molecules. The integrins include ICAM-1 (CD54). ICAM-1 is normally expressed on endothelium, but can be induced on other tissues by cytokines. Although ICAM-1 is not found in normal eyes, ICAM-1 expression was noted on conjunctival epithelium after antigen challenge (45). Many of the new antihistamines have been shown to reduce ICAM-1 in both eye and nasal allergy models (46,47). Selectins are another group of adhesion molecules and include ICAM-3, vascular cell adhesion molecule-1, and endothelium–leukocyte adhesion molecule-1 (E-selectin).

Chemokines are small proteins that combine with G-protein–coupled receptors expressed on certain leukocytes. Chemokines are secreted by endothelial cells and leukocytes and function to convert selectins into integrins, which leads to extravasation of cells into the tissues. Eotaxin, monocyte chemotactic protein-3, and "regulated on activation, normal T-cell expressed and secreted" (RANTES) are key types of chemokines that are released by airway epithelium and skin keratinocytes. One study shows that human conjunctival epithelial cells were capable of producing RANTES in response to inflammatory stimuli, suggesting that RANTES may play a role in recruiting inflammatory cells such as eosinophils and T lymphocytes toward the ocular surface (48).

Allergen challenges in the eye reveal both an early-phase response (0 to 60 minutes) and a late-phase response (4 to 24 hours). In severe forms of allergic reactions, conjunctival scrapings during the early phase may reveal increased numbers of neutrophils and eosinophils. Several authors have described varying types of late-phase reactions in the eye. An antigen challenge study demonstrated the presence of neutrophils within 20 minutes, eosinophils at 6 hours, and neutrophils, lymphocytes, and eosinophils at 12 to 24 hours after challenge (49). Degranulation occurs after the recruitment of these cells, propagating the allergic response. A second peak of histamine occurs, and the release of chemotactic factors during the early phase makes eosinophils and the eosinophil-derived toxins prevalent in the conjunctiva. Tryptase is not found during the late-phase reaction, thus supporting the findings showing that after nasal challenge, mast cells are not found (or are not degranulated) in the late-phase reaction (50). Although late-phase reactions have

been seen clinically in the nose and lung, and late-phase mediators are present in tears, the clinical features of the late-phase reaction in the eye have been witnessed only at the highest antigen doses (51). However, late-phase reactions probably contribute to the mechanism by which mild, self-limiting allergic disease becomes a chronic inflammatory disease such as VKC.

## Genetics of Allergy

Current allergy research has investigated the idea of genetic predisposition to antigen sensitivity. Genetic influences probably do exist, as suggested by clustering of allergic diseases in twins and families (52). The expression of genes of inflammatory proteins, such as cytokines, enzymes, receptors, and adhesion molecules, is modulated by transcription factors, which are proteins that bind to the promoter regions of these genes and may be activated by inflammatory stimuli, such as cytokines (53). Several transcription factors are involved in inflammation, including nuclear factor-κB, activator protein-1, nuclear factor of activated T-cells (NFAT), cyclic adenosine monophosphate (cAMP) response element–binding protein, and signal transducer and activator of transcription factors (STAT). These transcription factors coordinate the expression of multiple inflammatory genes in asthma. It is unclear whether similar mechanisms exist in ocular allergy, although it seems likely. The expression or suppression of transcription factors, cytokines, and chemokines may be genetically responsible for allergy (54). For example, studies on cytokine signal transduction have clarified the mechanism by which IL-4 exerts its functions. Two cytoplasmic proteins, STAT6 and IL-4–induced phosphotyrosine substrate/insulin receptor substrate-2, are activated in IL-4 signal transduction (55).

Studies have suggested that genes in the cytokine gene cluster on chromosome 5 (including IL-3, IL-4, IL-5, IL-9, and IL-13) (56), chromosome 11 (the β chain of the high-affinity IgE receptor), chromosome 16 (the IL-4 receptor), and chromosome 12 (stem cell factor, IFN-γ, insulin growth factor, and STAT6) may contribute to asthma and allergy development. In addition, data support involvement of genes in antigen presentation (MHC class II genes) and T-cell responses (the T-cell receptor α chain). Finally, disease-contributing alleles may be present on genes for the β-adrenergic receptor, 5-lipoxygenase, and LTC$_4$ synthase (57).

## CLASSIFICATION OF OCULAR ALLERGY

There are five main forms of ocular allergy: seasonal or perennial allergic conjunctivitis, VKC, AKC, GPC, and drug-induced allergic conjunctivitis (DIAC).

## Seasonal/Perennial Allergic Conjunctivitis

Seasonal and perennial allergic conjunctivitis are the most common forms of ocular allergy. Degranulation of the mast cells by antigens, and the subsequent release of proinflammatory substances mentioned previously, remains at the center of this reaction. Seasonal allergens include tree pollens (early spring), grasses (May through July), and weed (ragweed) pollen (August through October), and outdoor molds include *Cladosporium, Alternaria, Epicoccum,* and Basidiomycetes, although mold aerospora vary widely according to geographic location. The perennial allergens are house dust mites (*Dermatophagoides farinae* and *Dermatophagoides pteronyssinus*), indoor molds [largely *Aspergillus* (*Aspergillus flavus* and *Aspergillus fumigatus*) and *Penicillium* species], and animal danders (most often cat and dog).

### Clinical Presentation

The hallmark of allergic conjunctivitis is itching. Patients also may complain of tearing, burning, redness, and pressure behind the eyes and ears. The eye examination may reveal conjunctival hyperemia, chemosis (which may be visible only by slit-lamp examination), and lid or periorbital swelling (Fig. 21.1). Itching is the key symptom of seasonal and perennial allergic conjunctivitis. Often the conjunctiva appears milky or pale pink as a result of edema and dilatation of blood vessels. In the acute reaction, patients may exhibit a clear to white discharge. In chronic allergy, however, a mucopurulent, thick, or stringy exudates is more common. Also frequently present are "allergic shiners," a hyperpigmented periorbital coloring thought to be secondary to impaired venous return in the skin and subcutaneous tissue (58), and Dennie's lines, prominent folds on the lower eyelid.

The timing and duration of these signs and symptoms depend largely on the allergen, whether perennial or seasonal. Patients may have relief or exacerbations during particular seasons and exposures. In addition, different climates can exacerbate symptoms. Dry, warm climates tend to worsen symptoms, whereas cooler, wet climates tend to lessen symptoms.

When diagnosing the condition, medical histories are invaluable tools because a past or family history of allergic conjunctivitis is a strong indicator of the disease. Also important is the patient's personal or family history of atopy (allergies, asthma, eczema). Findings suggestive of allergic conjunctivitis include early age at onset, bilateral involvement, itching, and recurrence of the other symptoms. Corneal involvement is rare in acute allergic conjunctivitis, other than the occasional dellen adjacent to an area of extensive chemosis. The presence of discharge, follicles, cobbles, or keratitis is inconsistent with a sole diagnosis of allergic conjunctivitis.

Differential diagnosis from dry eye, blepharitis, and bacterial conjunctivitis can be difficult at times. Both allergic conjunctivitis and dry eye may produce intermittent conjunctival redness and burning. Ocular allergic symptoms usually do not include foreign body sensation, a symptom of dry eye. Patients with dry eye may be more prone to allergy as a result of a decreased ability of the tear film to dilute and wash allergens. Rose Bengal staining, meniscus height, tear breakup time, and Schirmer's testing, diagnostic tools for dry eye, should be used to differentiate properly between these two diseases. Systemic antihistamines taken for allergies may cause ocular dryness (59). Blepharitis, inspissation of the meibomian glands, and inflammation of the lid margin may be associated with staphylococcal infection, with the primary differentiating sign being scaly or flaky lid margins (60). Bacterial conjunctivitis tends to be

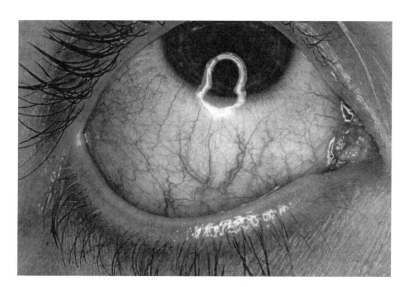

**FIG. 21.1.** Acute allergic conjunctivitis. Conjunctival hyperemia and chemosis are evident. Hyperemia and swelling of the lids may be present. Itching is the key symptom.

worse on wakening, with matting of the eyelashes and lids. Discharge in bacterial conjunctivitis can range from serous to purulent, and culture is positive.

Several tests can be performed for allergic conjunctivitis: conjunctival scrapings, tear levels of specific IgE, allergy skin testing, and ocular antigen challenge (61). Although 45% of allergic patients may have eosinophils (62) and neutrophils (63) present in scrapings, the absence of eosinophils in conjunctival scrapings does not rule out a diagnosis of allergic conjunctivitis because these cells may be located deeper in the conjunctiva (62). Tear levels of IgE can be measured by radioallergosorbent testing (64), and tear levels of tryptase also can be measured to indicate the degranulation of mast cells. Although conjunctival antigen challenge is used mostly for experimental purposes, nearly 85% of patients with allergic conjunctivitis respond when challenged with an allergen to which the person is sensitive. A positive challenge is one in which itching results in 3 to 5 minutes and redness within 20 minutes postchallenge (61). The author has found an 80% concordance between skin tests and ocular antigen challenge.

## Vernal Keratoconjunctivitis

Vernal keratoconjunctivitis is a severe, bilateral, inflammatory disease of the conjunctiva, and if it is left untreated, permanent impairment of vision can ensue. VKC is seen most often in patients between the ages of 3 and 20 years. The disease occurs more frequently in boys until the age of puberty; by 20 years of age, both sexes are affected equally (65). Although a family history of atopic disease correlates with VKC, suggesting a hereditary predisposition, other factors such as climate, season, and allergen exposure affect the likelihood and severity of the disease. Seasonal exacerbation is characteristic, although in very temperate climates, clinical signs may be nearly perennial. VKC has an increased incidence in hot, dry environments (66,67).

### Clinical Presentation

A cobblestone pattern of giant papillae on the upper tarsal conjunctiva is the classic sign of VKC (Fig. 21.2). Very rarely are the cobblestones found on the lower plate. Bulbar conjunctival cobblestones, papules, or follicles are almost never observed. The cobblestones are large, polygonal, and flat topped, and are seen without the aid of a slit lamp. The papillae usually are between 1 and 8 mm in diameter and rarely are evenly distributed. Each papilla has a central core of blood vessels. Fluorescein stains the tops of the papillae (67). Copious, tenacious, elastic, ropey discharge often lays between the papillae, forming a pseudomembrane (Maxwell-Lyons sign) (68–70). The ropy, thick strands of mucus differ from the mucus and lid crusting of bacterial conjunctivitis or the thinner strands seen in dry eye. The mucus of allergic conjunctivitis also is different in that it consists of

thin, short strands or small globules mostly localized over the medial canthal area. The cobblestones are higher and wider than those of GPC or viral conjunctivitis, and are more variable in shape than the homogeneous cobbles in GPC or viral conjunctivitis.

Mild to moderate chemosis, sometimes visible only with a slit lamp, with only slight separation of the conjunctiva from the episclera, is commonly seen in VKC, rather than the ballooning chemosis of acute conjunctivitis. Bulbar conjunctival vasodilation is diffuse and presents as pink, rather than red.

Because the enlarged papillae increase the bulk of the upper tarsus, ptosis also may develop. Horner-Trantas dots are chalk-white, raised superficial infiltrates straddling the limbus with no specific meridional predilection, unlike immune marginal infiltrates. Gelatinous, translucent, globular nodules or deposits at the limbus vary greatly in size and shape. Thickening, broadening, and opacification of the limbal conjunctiva also are seen. The gelatinous nodules of VKC are vascular and respond rapidly to steroids, differentiating them from other limbal tumors.

Diffuse keratitis is the most frequent corneal finding. These points of keratitis can break down, uniting into one single erosion. The margins of this erosion are raised and can collect cellular debris and mucus, seen as a white fibrin coating known as *shield ulcers*. These ulcers usually are found in younger patients and inhibit healing of the erosion, leaving a permanent gray subepithelial opacity. The shield shape of the ulcer in VKC differs from that of other corneal ulcers in the absence of surrounding haze, iritis, and purulent discharge.

The commonly found symptoms include persistent itching, photophobia, irritation, foreign body sensation, burning, tearing, mucus discharge, and pain (71). Although itching is the common symptom of all ocular allergic disease, the itching of VKC is of greater intensity. The itching and the absence of pearly follicles and pretragal nodes differentiate VKC from chlamydial conjunctivitis.

### Pathology of Vernal Keratoconjunctivitis

A type I reaction underlies VKC. Elevated histamine levels in the tears and findings of degranulated mast cells in the substantia propria and conjunctival epithelium point to a mast cell–mediated process. Approximately 80% of conjunctival mast cells degranulate (70), supported by an abnormal elevation of tear tryptase (72). Correspondingly, IgE levels in tears (73) and serum (74) are elevated. Histamine has been identified in tears but has not been found to be consistently higher in tears of allergic compared with normal subjects (75) These levels were, however, found to be consistently elevated in tears of patients with active VKC (16 ng/mL) (76,77). The increase in histamine probably is due to the extensive mast cell degranulation demonstrated in patients with VKC by light and electron microscopy (78).

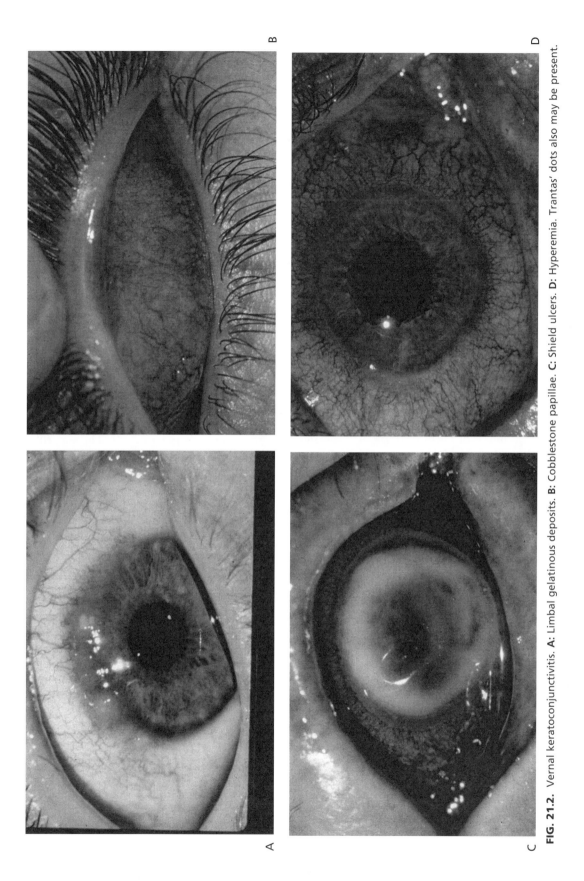

**FIG. 21.2.** Vernal keratoconjunctivitis. **A:** Limbal gelatinous deposits. **B:** Cobblestone papillae. **C:** Shield ulcers. **D:** Hyperemia. Trantas' dots also may be present.

Another factor is that histaminase activity is reported to be lower in patients with VKC, thus affecting the ability to regulate histamine levels (79). In addition, patients with VKC have four times as many mast cells in their conjunctiva than normal individuals (80), and the location of these mast cells is more superficial than in the normal conjunctiva (81). Such patients therefore are at greater risk for antigenic attack. Similarly, eosinophils are found in higher numbers and more superficially.

Mast cells, eosinophils, basophils, neutrophils, macrophages, and lymphocytes are all present in the conjunctival epithelium (82), and the epithelium thickens in VKC. This is important in that the normal epithelium contains neutrophils and lymphocytes, but not the other cells. The substantia propria has a proliferation of mast cells, eosinophils, and basophils, but it lacks lymphocytes (73). The finding of lymphocytes in VKC suggests that a type I reaction is not the only allergic reaction in this disorder, and that VKC may have a type IV component. Most lymphocytes found in the conjunctiva of VKC are Th cells, releasing IL-4 to stimulate B cells.

This influx of cells contributes to many of the findings of VKC. Each papilla contains plasma cells, eosinophils, mast cells, and lymphocytes. The Horner-Trantas dots are composed largely of eosinophils and cellular debris, but they also may contain neutrophils and lymphocytes. The mucus strands in VKC are alkaline and contain inflammatory cells, specifically eosinophils, contributing to the different consistency compared with mucus of other allergic disorders. Tear EMBP is thought to be linked to the corneal ulcers of VKC (83), and the plaque in the ulcer has been shown to contain eosinophils (84). Serum ECP also was found to be elevated (85). EMBP also may contribute to sustained mast cell degranulation and thus the severe and protracted allergic process associated with this condition (86). Increased expression of adhesion molecules also may play an important role in the pathogenesis of VKC (87).

## Atopic Keratoconjunctivitis

Atopic keratoconjunctivitis is a chronic type of ocular allergy that is associated with atopic dermatitis (Fig. 21.3). AKC is rare, affecting less than 1% of the population; however, approximately one fourth of patients with atopic dermatitis also may have AKC (88,89). Defining characteristics of AKC include atopic dermatitis of the eyelids as well as papillary conjunctivitis, disruption of the corneal epithelium, and, in severe cases, conjunctival and corneal scarring. The incidence of AKC peaks between the ages of 30 and 50 years (90). Emerging in the second and third decades, AKC may persist into the eighth decade (91) and then spontaneously resolve. It is a bilateral, perennial affliction (92) with occasional exacerbation during the winter.

### Clinical Presentation

A full medical history should be taken, paying special attention to personal and family history of other atopic disorders. A patient who does not have another family member with an atopic disorder is unlikely to have AKC. The nonocular signs of AKC begin in childhood, and the ocular signs commonly begin in adulthood. Asthma, eczema, allergic rhinitis, and migraine headaches are common nonocular indicators of AKC. Ocular signs and symptoms include constant inflammation, although environmental airborne allergens may cause exacerbations. Laboratory test for elevated tear and serum specific IgE also can aid in diagnosis.

Patients regularly complain of moderate to severe itching, burning, photophobia, and blurred vision. Tearing and a mucopurulent, thick, ropy, white mucus discharge also

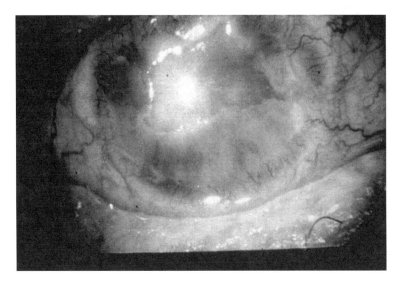

**FIG. 21.3.** Atopic keratoconjunctivitis (AKC). Corneal scarring, suppurative keratitis, and keratoconus usually lead to vision loss in patients with AKC. Trantas' dots, cysts, gelatinous infiltration, punctate epithelial keratopathy, and intraepithelial microcysts also are present. Smaller papillae on the lower tarsal conjunctiva, as opposed to the upper, differentiate AKC from vernal keratoconjunctivitis. The presence of severe itching and indurations of the lids is indicative of AKC and separates it from blepharitis.

can be present (93). Indurated lid margins that are thickened and scaly are seen. Other exudative, vesicular, or crusted lesions may be observed on other parts of the body as part of the atopic dermatitis complex. Maceration of the inner or outer canthi may be observed, and punctual stenosis can occur. The conjunctiva may be pale compared with other ocular allergic reactions, and there may be limbal redness. Chemosis may occur in the palpebral and bulbar conjunctiva. The inferior conjunctiva also show some papillary hypertrophy. Conjunctival scarring, which may lead to fornix shrinkage (94), also may be present.

Corneal involvement in AKC can be vision threatening. Corneal scarring, suppurative keratitis (95), and keratoconus (96) usually lead to vision loss in patients with AKC. Trantas' dots, cysts, gelatinous infiltration, punctate epithelial keratopathy, and intraepithelial microcysts (97) are additional signs of AKC. Ulcers are ovoid, with horizontal positioning and irregular edges. The cornea is subject to pannus and, in more severe cases, these corneal ulcers may become hazy and vascularize. Cataracts, posterior polar or anterior subscapular, form in 8% to 10% of patients with atopic dermatitis (98).

The severity of symptoms can differentiate AKC from other allergic disorders. The location of smaller papillae on the lower tarsal conjunctiva instead of the upper differentiates AKC from VKC. AKC usually lacks the seasonal exacerbations seen with VKC. The presence of severe itching and indurations of the lids is indicative of AKC and separates it from blepharitis.

### Pathology of Atopic Keratoconjunctivitis

Atopic keratoconjunctivitis is thought to involve both a type I and a type IV hypersensitivity reaction (92). Mast cell (99), lymphocyte, eosinophil, and basophil levels all are elevated in the conjunctiva. Mast cells and eosinophils are especially concentrated in the subepithelial tissue. There is pronounced degranulation of eosinophils and neutrophils. Mast cells hyperplasia has been suggested as the cause of the conjunctival papillae and scarring. Mast cell degranulation may release tryptase to stimulate collagenases and heparin to effect fibrinogenesis (100). Degranulation of eosinophils leaves deposits of toxic proteins, and the influx of basophils and neutrophils potentiates the reaction. In addition, Langerhans cell levels are escalated in the substantia propria and the epithelium (100). Because these cells act as APCs, IgE tear levels (95) and serum levels also are increased.

Goblet cells proliferate and mast cells and eosinophils invade the epithelium. B cells produce abnormally high levels of IgE. AKC seems to be caused by sustained T-cell and mast cell activation, controlling the IgE response and the release of cytokines, which in turn recruit more neutrophils, eosinophils, and macrophages.

Inherent feedback systems that are supposed to regulate the allergic reaction may be impaired in AKC, leading to continuous T-cell activation. The inflammatory process normally is regulated internally by a negative feedback system. The interaction of histamine with mast cell surface histamine receptors elevates cAMP concentrations, thereby "turning off" the mast cell (101). The second messengers, cAMP and cyclic guanosine monophosphate (cGMP), further control mediator release from mast cells and basophils (101). Increasing levels of cAMP block mediator release; increasing levels of cGMP stimulate mediator release. Prostaglandins act by way of adenyl cyclase to increase cAMP. Phosphodiesterase degrades cAMP, and therefore phosphodiesterase inhibitors can increase cAMP levels. A higher level of phosphodiesterase activity has been found in patients with AKC. A close correlation exists between phosphodiesterase activity and leukocyte histamine release, as well as between IgE production by B cells and interleukin activity.

## Giant Papillary Conjunctivitis

Giant papillary conjunctivitis is associated with the presence of contact lenses, surgical sutures, and ocular prostheses. GPC is characterized by itching, tearing, mucus discharge, and papillae on the upper palpebral conjunctiva (Fig. 21.4). The condition can be unilateral when sutures or external devices are used, but usually is bilateral. Ocular device hygiene often is compromised in patients with GPC, so GPC occurs more often in children, whose cleaning regimens may not be as strict as those of adults. In most cases of contact lens–related GPC, trauma is related to the shape of the lens edge or the lens material, two factors that can be remedied by the use of a different lens type. There is a high incidence of a history of atopy in patients with GPC. Removal of the offending suture or device usually resolves the papillae and symptoms of GPC.

### Clinical Presentation

The standard sign of GPC is the presence of enlarged papillae (diameter ≥0.3 mm) on the upper conjunctiva. The number of papillae varies from one papilla to several covering the entire upper tarsal surface (102). The top of each papilla is flat, with its vascularization radiating from a central vessel. Fluorescein staining is useful in identifying papillae smaller than 0.5 mm in diameter, and it may aid the clinician in seeing the flat tops of the papillae. The papillae in soft contact lens–related GPC usually appear in the upper zone of the tarsus, proceeding from there to the lid margin. When other external devices or sutures are the cause of the inflammation, papillae location depends on the location of the device.

Mucus vesicles in nongoblet epithelial cells of the conjunctiva contribute to an increase in the production of mucus. Redness and mucus discharge are signs that can be reversed by removing the device.

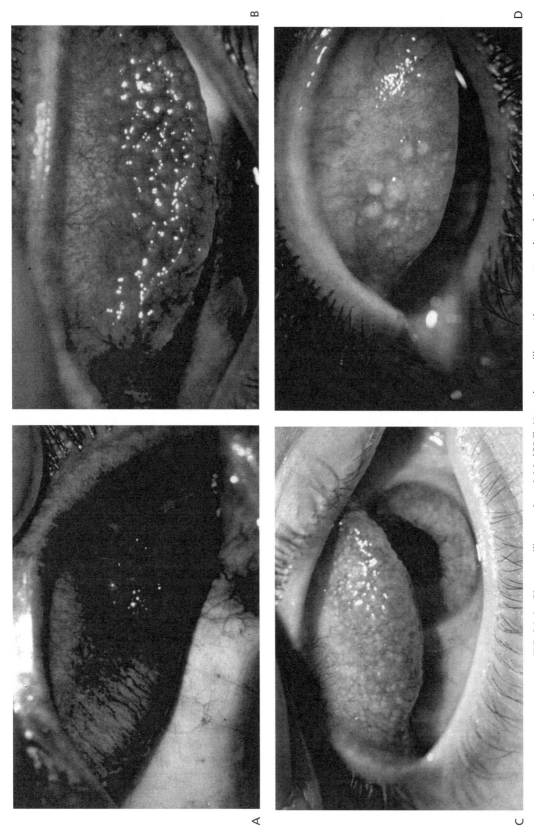

**FIG. 21.4.** Giant papillary conjunctivitis (GPC). Note the papillae on the upper tarsal conjunctiva. **A, D:** Suture-induced GPC. **C:** Contact lens–induced GPC. The papillae may be translucent in the early stages of the disease but become more opaque as the disease progresses. The papillae resolve with the removal of the foreign object (e.g., contact lens, suture, prosthesis).

In contact lens–related GPC, discomfort can range from minimal discomfort on insertion and removal of a lens to the complete intolerance of a lens. In this form of GPC, mild lens intolerance can progress to foreign body sensation, more severe lens intolerance, and pruritus. Hyperemia and mucus strands may be present on the upper tarsus, and a milky discharge may cover the papillae. Conjunctival thickening occurs and the conjunctiva may appear opaque at advanced stages. Trantas' dots (103), ptosis (104), and limbal infiltrates also may occur in GPC.

### Pathology of Giant Papillary Conjunctivitis

Patients with GPC have decreased concentrations of lactoferrin, a degradative enzyme found in tears (105). This decrease may be responsible for lack of control over inflammation or bacterial binding to the contact lens surface. One study has shown an increase in eosinophil degranulation with increased levels of EMBP, contributing to inflammation and collagen deposits (103). Another study showed increased levels in tears of the mediator, $LTC_4$ (106). Adhesion molecules also may play a large role in GPC. ICAM-1 and E-selectin are expressed in higher proportion in the conjunctiva of GPC, attracting neutrophils, macrophages, and lymphocytes.

Neutrophil and mast cell levels are found in GPC, with approximately 30% mast cell degranulation (80). Eosinophils and basophils are present in the substantia propria, although in lower levels than in VKC (73). Histamine levels are not increased significantly, but the presence of the inflammatory cells is an indication that the contact lens edge probably causes chronic inflammatory response. The trauma itself also may contribute to GPC. There also is a T-cell infiltration in GPC.

Meibomian gland dysfunction is a concern in GPC. The gland secretions, which are essential to proper tear functioning by delaying evaporation, tend to be more viscous in patients with GPC (107). With improper tear functioning, the eye has increased difficulty in removing airborne antigens and the chemicals present in lens cleaning solutions from the contact lens and the ocular surface.

## Drug-induced Allergic Conjunctivitis

Drug-induced allergic conjunctivitis is a type IV delayed hypersensitivity reaction induced by certain medications or chemicals. Resolution of these conditions depends on discontinuing the use of the offending agent. The allergic reaction requires repeated exposure to the sensitizing agent, and thus DIAC can occur within a few days of taking a medication, or it could take several years for sensitization of the immune system to occur.

The condition usually is mild and the symptoms reversible. DIAC can be treated pharmacologically, but the use of the causative medication should be discouraged.

### Clinical Presentation

The signs and symptoms of DIAC vary among patients. Sensitivity, frequency of the use of the medication, and concentration of the medication all play significant roles in this reaction. Conjunctival itching and redness, however, are present in all cases. The inferior half of the conjunctiva is preferentially chemotic and red (Fig. 21.5). Eyelid swelling also may occur, most frequently in the lower lid because of medication pooling. Excess pooling and subsequent runoff also may cause dermatitis of the lower lid and the surrounding area. In addition to redness, the conjunctival tissue response to toxic agents may result in follicular or papillary excrescences. Conjunctival scrapings reveal mononuclear cells, neutrophils, and mucus. Eosinophils usually are absent.

The clinician must correctly diagnose DIAC because failure to recognize it may lead to continuation of the symptoms, whereas misdiagnosis can lead to the discontinuation of an effective medication. Further complicating proper diagnosis is the confusion that can arise between DIAC and allergic conjunctivitis, especially because allergic patients are predisposed to DIAC. Infectious conjunctivitis, folliculosis, and dry eye also can complicate proper diagnosis, and patients with these conditions also may be predisposed to DIAC.

A medical history aids in identifying the offending agent. If the patient is currently using only one topical ophthalmic preparation, and the symptoms worsen immediately after use, diagnosis can be quite simple. However, when patients use several topical medications, the task of identifying the causative agent is more complicated. By removing each agent for a period, the clinician can use the process of elimination to determine the cause of the allergic reaction. For confirmation, the clinician can reintroduce the offending agent to reproduce the reaction.

## CURRENTLY APPROVED TREATMENTS

Depending on the severity of the disease and symptoms, several treatment plans can be formulated. Cold compresses and sterile irrigations (including artificial tears) are useful to relieve itching in mild reactions. These function by diluting and washing away diluent from the conjunctiva. For allergic reactions that do not respond to this treatment, pharmacologic agents are necessary.

## Topical Antihistamines

Topical antihistamines are probably the largest drug class used to treat ocular allergy. Antihistamines in general have gone through several evolutions. The first histamine receptor blockers were nonselective agents and had comparatively weak receptor affinity. As drug development progressed, $H_1$

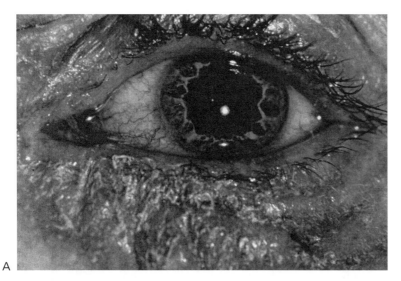

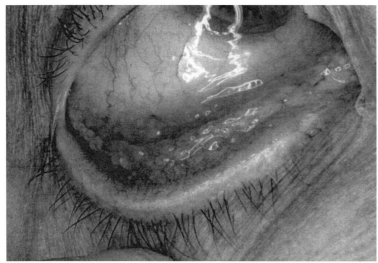

**FIG. 21.5.** Drug-induced allergic conjunctivitis. **A:** Neomycin allergy. **B:** Inferior follicular response to a topical drug. Note the hyperemia and edema of the inferior conjunctiva. Such follicles resolve on discontinuation of the drug.

antagonists were manufactured that were more selective and had a higher receptor affinity, leading to greater efficacy and longer duration of action. Antihistamines do not affect the release of histamine itself.

Antihistamines bind competitively and reversibly to histamine receptors located on nerves and blood vessels. They reduce itching, redness, and the transudation of fluid from the blood vessels into local tissue, reducing swelling and chemosis. Because of this action on histamine receptors, antihistamines can be used to treat an ongoing allergic reaction. In addition to treating allergic conjunctivitis, topical antihistamines frequently are used to treat the chronic forms of ocular allergy, including VKC and AKC. In these cases, the drug is used every 3 to 4 hours as needed, up to four times a day.

A multitude of topical antihistamines currently are on the market. It may be a challenge for the clinician to sift through these many options to determine those that will be most efficacious for his or her patients. Available topical antihistamines include olopatadine (Patanol; Alcon Laboratories, Fort Worth, TX), ketotifen (Zaditor; CIBA Vision, Duluth, GA), levocabastine (Livostin; CIBA Vision), emedastine (Emadine; Alcon Laboratories), and azelastine (Optivor; Bausch and Lomb/Muro-Asta Medica, Tampa, FL). Olopatadine, ketotifen, and azelastine are considered dual-action drugs, and have modes of action in addition to their antihistaminic properties. These three drugs are discussed in a later section.

Levocabastine hydrochloride 0.05% ophthalmic suspension (Livostin) is an older selective $H_1$ antagonist. It is indicated for the treatment of seasonal allergic conjunctivitis, with dosing four times a day. In preclinical and clinical trials, it was shown to be effective in reducing the chief sign and symptom of ocular allergy, redness and itching, as well as reducing chemosis and lid swelling (108,109).

Emedastine difumarate 0.05% ophthalmic solution

(Emadine) is a newer, more potent H$_1$ blocker that has been shown preclinically to be extremely effective in blocking histamine (110). Emedastine is equipotent to ketotifen and more potent than brompheniramine, clemastine, pyrilamine, levocabastine, pheniramine, diphenhydramine, and antazoline, 30 minutes postdosing (110). In the human antigen challenge model, emedastine was effective in reducing the signs and symptoms of allergic conjunctivitis and was superior to levocabastine for itching, redness, chemosis, and lid swelling (111), and to ketorolac for itching and redness (112). Emedastine provides clinically significant relief within minutes of instillation and lasts for at least 4 hours. It is indicated for the temporary relief of the signs and symptoms of allergic conjunctivitis in patients 3 years of age and older, and can be used as needed up to four times a day.

Systemic antihistamines, although indicated for patients presenting with multiple allergic conditions, including rhinitis and allergic asthma, are not ideal for the treatment of the ocular component of allergy. In fact, they should not be used at all in the absence of a systemic component. Systemic antihistamines are associated with more side effects, and may contribute to a decreased tear film. This drying effect may exacerbate ocular allergy by minimizing the barrier and diluent effect of the tear film.

## Topical Antihistamine/Vasoconstrictors

Antihistamine/vasoconstrictor combinations are available as over-the-counter medications for ocular allergy. Pheniramine and antazoline have been shown to inhibit ocular itching significantly. However, these agents are available only in combination with α-adrenergic agents as vasoconstrictors. The combination offers relief from both itching and redness. Sensitization and rebound congestion can occur with prolonged use of any decongestant.

There are a variety of medication combinations that fall into this class. Common combinations include pheniramine/naphazoline and antazoline/naphazoline. These combinations are marketed under a number of trade names, including Naphcon-A (pheniramine 0.3%/naphazoline 0.025%; Alcon Laboratories), Opcon-A (pheniramine 0.315%/naphazoline 0.02675%; Bausch and Lomb), and Visine-A (pheniramine 0.3%/naphazoline 0.025%; Pfizer, New York, NY), and Vasocon-A (antazoline 0.5%/naphazoline 0.05%; CIBA Vision).

In a study comparing Naphcon-A with its components, Naphcon-A performed as well as or better than pheniramine alone or naphazoline alone. In particular, Naphcon-A reduced redness better than naphazoline and was as effective as pheniramine at reducing itching (113). A similar study was done with Vasocon-A (114). The results of this study indicated that the combination of naphazoline and antazoline was more effective in inhibiting redness than naphazoline and more effective in inhibiting itching than antazoline. Although patients may prefer one of these preparations over the other in terms of comfort, the efficacy of these drugs has been shown to be similar (115). All of these medications are approved for use in children older than 6 years of age and for up to four times a day.

## Topical Mast Cell Stabilizers

Compounds that alter the function of the mast cell are potential agents for modulating the allergic response. These agents are particularly suitable for patients with chronic allergies. If compliance with the treatment regimen is followed before exposure to antigens, this treatment modality decreases the mast cell response and thus prevents the signs and symptoms of allergy.

There are several different pharmacologic classes of such agents: traditional mast cell stabilizers, dual-action compounds, steroids, and immunomodulating agents. The possible mechanism of action for these agents involves decreasing calcium influx into the cytoplasm (either by decreasing the influx from the extracellular space or decreasing the release of calcium from intracellular stores). A decrease in calcium influx in turn decreases the secretion of preformed mediators from intracellular stores. This is reported to be the mechanism of action of traditional mast cell stabilizers such as cromolyn, lodoxamide, nedocromil, and pemirolast. The traditional mast cell stabilizers are described here, and the other classes in later sections.

Pure mast cell stabilizers are preventive medications in that they cannot reduce histamine-related signs and symptoms after histamine has been released from the mast cell. Because of this property, mast cell stabilizers are not used to treat ongoing allergic reactions, but require a loading phase. In fact, it may require up to a 1-week loading period to obtain relief. Because these drugs do not have any antihistaminic or antiinflammatory properties, they can be used concomitantly with other allergy medications.

There are a number of mast cell stabilizers approved by the U.S. Food and Drug Administration (FDA), including Alamast (pemirolast potassium 0.1%; Santen, Napa, CA), Crolom (cromolyn sodium 4%; Bausch & Lomb), Alomide (lodoxamide tromethamine 0.1%, Alcon Laboratories), and Alocril (nedocromil sodium 2%; Allergan, Inc., Irvine, CA).

Cromolyn sodium has been available since the 1970s. It has been proven useful in allergic conjunctivitis, VKC, AKC, and GPC (116,117). Cromolyn also may be effective in inhibiting the chemotaxis, activation, degranulation, and cytotoxicity of neutrophils, eosinophils, and monocytes. It can be used in adults and children up to six times a day as necessary.

Lodoxamide tromethamine has a mechanism of action similar to cromolyn. Several clinical studies have found lodoxamide to be an effective mast cell stabilizer in various models of ocular allergy (118,119), and to be superior to cromolyn in reducing the signs and symptoms of VKC (120). This may be linked to decreased T-cell accumulation with lodoxamide compared with cromolyn (121). Lodoxamide also significantly reduces the number of eosinophils and neutrophils in VKC (122). It is approved for patients older than 2 years of age and for four-times-daily dosing.

Pemirolast potassium is a newer mast cell stabilizer added to the ocular allergy arsenal. Preclinical studies support the mast cell–stabilizing component of pemirolast, and show that it may prevent the activation of membrane phospholipase (123). In addition to its mast cell–stabilizing properties, pemirolast reduces degranulation and chemotaxis of eosinophils, thereby reducing release of $LTC_4$ and ECP from eosinophils (124). In a 120-subject, modified environmental model of allergic conjunctivitis, pemirolast was shown to be effective when used four times daily. Pemirolast has been approved for the prevention of itchy eyes due to allergic conjunctivitis and is used twice a day.

Nedocromil is another recently approved mast cell stabilizer, and one that has been used traditionally to treat asthma. As with the other drugs, nedocromil is effective for treating seasonal allergic conjunctivitis (125,126), VKC, and GPC (127). One study showed similar efficacy between nedocromil and cromolyn in allergic conjunctivitis (128), whereas another showed nedocromil to be superior in VKC (129). Nedocromil also is used twice daily.

Protein kinase plays a major role in mast cell degranulation and is one of the earliest signaling responses after antigen-induced cross-linking of IgE molecules. In animal models of asthma, inhibitors of the protein tyrosine kinase pathway blocked the release of histamine and leukotrienes from lung mast cells (130). Janus kinase 3 (JAK3), a member of the Janus family of protein-tyrosine kinases, is expressed in mast cells, and its enzymatic activity is enhanced by IgE receptor/FcεRI cross-linking. Inhibition of JAK3 with WHI-P131 [4-(4′-Hydroxyphenyl)-amino-6,7,-dimethoxyquinazoline HCl] blocked phospholipase C activation, calcium mobilization, activation of microtubule-associated protein kinase after IgE receptor/FcεRI cross-linking, and subsequent mast cell degranulation (131). Further, WHI-P131 blocked the release of leukotrienes and subsequent recruitment of eosinophils (132).

The pharmacologic mechanisms of action of the aforementioned drugs illuminate the central role of the mast cell in allergy. Modulation of specific kinases can lead to inhibition of surface receptor expression and altered calcium transients, stabilization of membrane phospholipids, control of the transcription of proinflammatory mediators, and regulation of the nitric oxide pathway, all potential targets for new-generation mast cell stabilizers that can be developed for providing relief to patients with chronic allergy.

## Topical Antihistamine/Mast Cell Stabilizers

Recently developed drugs such as olopatadine, ketotifen, and azelastine have multiple modes of action. In addition to their potent antihistaminic pharmacologic effects, they have mast cell–stabilizing properties. This action may be due in part to an effect on calcium transients, activity at the surface of the phospholipid cellular membrane (126, 128), or an effect on the nitric oxide pathway, which also has been found to play a role in the degranulation of mast cells (127,128).

This class of drugs is the newest addition to the pharmacologic armamentarium used by clinicians for ocular allergy treatment, and contains three members, Patanol (olopatadine 0.1%; Alcon Laboratories), Zaditor (ketotifen fumarate 0.025%; CIBA Vision), and Optivor (azelastine; Bausch & Lomb). These medications in general are superior to mast cell stabilizers because they do not require a loading phase, and they show improvement over traditional antihistamines because they prevent further mast cell degranulation, thereby halting additional histamine release. They therefore have optimal times of onset and durations of action.

Olopatadine was shown in standard screening models to have both antihistaminic and mast cell–stabilizing activity. In preclinical studies, olopatadine inhibited release of histamine (133), tryptase, $PGD_2$ (134), IL-6 and IL-8 (135), and TNF (136). Olopatadine also reduced expression of ICAM-1 and E-selectin (137). Olopatadine was shown to have high affinity for $H_1$ receptors, superior to that of levocabastine, antazoline, pheniramine, and ketotifen. In this study, olopatadine inhibited histamine-induced phosphoinositide turnover in human ocular cells, which may relate to its mechanism of action.

Olopatadine, dosed twice a day, has been evaluated in many clinical trials. In the antigen challenge model, olopatadine demonstrated rapid onset of action within minutes and a duration of action of at least 8 hours (138,139). Itching was significantly reduced in these studies. It is indicated by the FDA for reducing redness. Olopatadine was found to be safe for adults and children 3 years of age and older. Olopatadine has demonstrated superior patient comfort compared with other ocular allergy medications (140), and was found to be superior to ketorolac (141), nedocromil, ketotifen (142), and oral loratadine (143) in antigen challenge studies.

Ketotifen has been shown to inhibit eosinophil chemotaxis and function (144), and thus may lead to a decrease in the release of ECP. Ketotifen also prevents the release of other inflammatory mediators, including leukotrienes, PAF (144), adhesion molecules, and cytokines, including $LTC_4$ and $LTB_4$ (145) from mast cells (146), basophils, and neutrophils. Ketotifen was shown to be effective in reducing itching in pivotal clinical trials and is approved for twice-daily dosing.

Azelastine is a drug that was available only for rhinitis, but recently was approved for itching. Clinical studies have followed the course of inflammatory mediators and have shown that azelastine reduced inflammatory cell infiltration during both the early- and late-phase allergic reactions.

ICAM-1 on conjunctival epithelium also was downregulated with azelastine (147). Azelastine is effective compared with placebo (148), and in children at least 4 years of age (149), in both environmental and antigen challenge studies (150). Its duration of action was shown to be at least 8 hours. The most significant side effect with azelastine is an unpleasant taste after instillation.

## Nonsteroidal Antiinflammatory Drugs

Nonsteroidal antiinflammatory drugs (NSAIDs) block prostaglandin synthesis by inhibiting the activity of cyclooxygenase. Because of this action, NSAIDs have shown promise in the management of ocular allergy, although ketorolac 0.5% (Acular; Allergan) is the only NSAID currently approved by the FDA for allergy. The indication for ketorolac is relief of itch due to seasonal allergic conjunctivitis. In environmental studies, ketorolac was shown to be significantly better than placebo in reducing conjunctival inflammation, ocular itching, swollen eyes, discharge and tearing, foreign body sensation, and conjunctival redness (151,152). The recommended dose is 1 drop (0.25 mg) four times a day. Although not approved by the FDA, other NSAIDs, including diclofenac (153), flurbiprofen (154), aspirin, piroxicam, and indomethacin (155), have shown effectiveness in human and animal studies of allergic conjunctivitis.

Oral aspirin therapy has been shown to be useful in the relief of conjunctival and episcleral redness and in the resolution of keratitis and limbal infiltrates in VKC (156). Patients with VKC showed dramatic improvement after treatment with up to 1 g aspirin dosed daily for 6 weeks (157). Because of the relatively high dose required, the patient should be closely monitored and contraindications to aspirin therapy fully considered with the patient. Suprofen 1.0% also has proved to give relief to patients with VKC and GPC by suppressing papillae and discharge, when dosed four times daily for 4 weeks (158).

Because biotransformation of NSAIDs occurs primarily in the hepatic system, patients with underlying liver or kidney dysfunction are at significant risk for the development of a wide range of toxic effects. The most common undesirable effect with systemic NSAIDs is gastrointestinal irritation. NSAIDs also increase the bleeding time by inhibiting platelet production of thromboxane, another product of the cyclooxygenase pathway. Although topical NSAIDs appear to be significantly safer than oral NSAIDs, the most significant topical side effect is discomfort on instillation of the drop, which cannot be overlooked because comfort clearly is directly related to patient compliance. NSAIDs also have been shown to reduce the breakdown of the blood–aqueous barrier, an indication of inflammation, to a greater extent than steroids.

The NSAIDs available in ophthalmic preparations act by blocking both the cyclooxygenase-1 (COX-1) and cyclooxygenase-2 (COX-2) enzyme subtypes. When multiple isomers of the cyclooxygenase enzyme were identified, doors were opened for more selective antiinflammatory agents. Specifically, a new generation of NSAIDs has been described that selectively target the inducible form of COX-2. This isoform of the enzyme is expressed at sites of inflammation, which has led to the speculation that its inhibition could provide all the benefits of current NSAIDs but without their major side effects in the gastrointestinal system, which are due to inhibition of COX-1. Although COX-2 inhibitors such as celecoxib (Celebrex; Searle, Chicago, IL) and rofecoxib (Vioxx; Merck, West Point, PA), indicated for the signs and symptoms of osteoarthritis and management of acute pain, appear to be no more efficacious than conventional NSAIDs, they offer superior safety profiles. One study showed that after dental surgery, rofecoxib had superior analgesic effects compared with celecoxib regarding overall analgesic effect, time of onset, peak analgesic relief, and duration of effect. In this study, the efficacy of rofecoxib was similar to that of ibuprofen, but with a longer duration of action (159). Another study showed that in patients with osteoarthritis, rofecoxib 25 mg/day was as effective as diclofenac 50 mg three times a day, ibuprofen 800 mg three times a day, and nabumetone 1,500 mg once daily (160). Meloxicam (Mobic; Boehringer Ingelheim Pharmaceuticals, Ridgefield, CT) is another COX-2 inhibitor (161) that was recently approved by the FDA as an oral agent, and flosulide (162) is currently in the approval process. Questions concerning the role of COX-2 in maintaining homeostasis in organs and small blood vessels, and the role of COX-1 in inflammation, remain to be answered. Because COX-1 is constitutively expressed in tissues and is involved in the synthesis of prostaglandins required for the mediation and modulation of normal physiologic function, and COX-2 is rapidly induced by cytokines, growth factors, and bacterial endotoxins, we may see highly selective COX-2 inhibitors developed for the eye.

## Corticosteroids

Steroids have long been the most widely used antiinflammatory agents. Steroids work at two levels, molecular and cellular, which results in inhibition of all the cardinal signs of inflammation, such as pain, redness, edema, and heat. This is achieved through inhibition of (a) leukocyte chemotaxis, (b) production of chemical mediators such as products of the arachidonic acid pathway, and (c) immunocompetent cell functions. Steroids reduce vascular permeability, stabilize membranes to reduce the degranulation of leukocytes, prevent adhesion of cells to vascular endothelium, thus inhibiting access to site of inflammation, suppress lymphocyte proliferation, which is involved in late-phase and chronic inflammation, reduce circulating leukocytes, depress bactericidal activity of monocytes, and inhibit production of arachidonic acid and subsequent synthesis of prostaglandins and leukotrienes by both the cyclooxygenase and lipoxygenase pathways.

Steroids pass through the target cell membranes and bind to steroid receptor proteins in the cytoplasm. The steroid–receptor complex is then carried into the cell nucleus, where it interacts with specific DNA sequences. Because of their action directly at the cell nucleus, steroids affect gene expression. Although steroids do not possess mast cell stabilizer properties *per se,* they may modulate the mast cell response by decreasing substances (e.g., GM-CSF, IL-3, ICAM-1, IL-4) that induce the proliferation and recruitment of other mast cells. Thus, steroids may have an effect on subsequent allergic responses after an initial challenge. Because of their action on cellular chemotaxis, the corneal infiltrate disappears with the introduction of topical steroids.

The two strongest steroids available for ophthalmic use are prednisolone and dexamethasone. Although steroids remain the most potent antiinflammatory agents available for the eye, their side effects are well known. Ocular side effects with topical steroids include elevated intraocular pressure, leading to glaucoma; cataract formation; and, because steroids inhibit migration of leukocytes, which play a major role in host defense, increased secondary infections and inhibited corneal epithelial and stromal healing. Because of these effects, weaker steroids, termed *soft steroids,* have been developed that have minimal side effects. These soft steroids are quickly hydrolyzed in the anterior chamber of the eye to inactive metabolites. These drugs include loteprednol and rimexolone. Fluorometholone and medrysone are two other weaker steroids that have low corneal penetrability.

Loteprednol is available as 0.2% and 0.5% preparations. Loteprednol 0.2% (Alrex; Bausch & Lomb) is the only steroid currently approved for eye allergy; dosed four times a day, it was shown to reduce redness and itching in both an environmental (163) and an antigen challenge model (164) of allergic conjunctivitis. Loteprednol 0.5% is the only agent demonstrated to be effective in GPC (164).

Rimexolone has increased lipophilicity compared with other steroids, thus increasing its ability to penetrate ocular tissue and limiting its systemic absorption. Rimexolone has the antiinflammatory efficacy of 1.0% prednisolone, but has a safety profile comparable with that of fluorometholone (165). Rimexolone also may alleviate the signs and symptoms of allergic conjunctivitis.

Fluorometholone 0.1% (FML; Allergan) is another steroid that can be used to treat the chronic forms of ocular allergy. It comes in an ointment and in drop form. In a 1999 clinical study, fluorometholone significantly reduced the signs and symptoms of VKC, including watering, discharge, conjunctival redness, papillary hypertrophy, and Trantas' dots (166).

When using steroid therapy for ocular allergy, the minimal dose for the shortest time should be used. The therapeutic effects of the drug, as well as the potential side effects, should be monitored. Topical therapy should be tapered slowly over several days because abrupt discontinuation may be hazardous. Corticosteroids reduce the number of leukocytes in the blood. The proliferation of immature white blood cells that occurs after discontinuation can lead to the production of great quantities of antibodies to residual antigen in the tissue. This reaction is followed by a massive polymorphonuclear leukocytic reaction, which, if not interrupted, can lead to a serious necrotizing inflammatory reaction (167).

Steroids remain the central antiinflammatory therapy because they have such a widespread mechanism of action. Further, physicians are able to control the side effects by identifying risk factors, such as those for glaucoma and cataracts, and maintaining close follow-up with the patient. Triamcinolone acetonide (Azmacort; Rhone-Poulenc Rorer Pharmaceuticals, Collegeville, PA), fluticasone (Flonase; GlaxoWellcome, Research Triangle Park, NC), flunisolide (Nasalide; Dura Pharmaceuticals, San Diego, CA), mometasone (Nasonex; Schering-Plough, Kenilworth, NJ), budesonide (Pulmicort; AstraZeneca, Westborough, MA) are among the steroids that have been introduced to the asthma/rhinitis market. These steroids are more selective than prednisolone and dexamethasone, and may see their way to the ophthalmic market.

## PROMISING FUTURE TARGETS

The most recent research on ocular allergy has revealed a number of potential target sites for drug development. Although new, more selective drugs are being developed in the classes of dual-action antihistamines, mast cell stabilizers, steroids, and COX-2 inhibitors, there are several other possibilities, including leukotriene inhibitors, immunomodulators, and adhesion molecule blockers.

### Lipoxygenase Pathway Inhibition

Leukotrienes are an important target for future therapy. They play a significant role in asthma, causing potent contraction of bronchial smooth muscle, inducing edema by causing plasma leakage from blood vessels, and enhancing secretion of mucus. Leukotrienes can be inhibited either by blocking the action of lipoxygenase or by blocking leukotriene receptors. Various approaches can be used, including antagonism of 5-lipoxygenase activation protein (FLAP) or inhibition of the enzyme itself. FLAP antagonists (MK-886, MK-591) block the translocation of the enzyme to the cell membrane.

A number of antileukotriene agents have been developed for asthma, and three are approved by the FDA: zafirlukast (Accolate; AstraZeneca) and montelukast (Singulair; Merck), which act by inhibiting the receptors of $LTC_4$, $LTD_4$, and $LTE_4$, and zileuton (Zyflo; Abbott), which is a selective inhibitor of 5-lipoxygenase and thus inhibits $LTB_4$, $LTC_4$, $LTD_4$, and $LTE_4$ formation. C1-1004 is under development by Parke-Davis (Morris Plains, NJ; phase II as of late 1999) and is a 5-lipoxygenase and cyclooxygenase inhibitor. This compound may offer the efficacy of a steroid but with a better safety profile because the mechanism of action is not as wide. Bayer (West Haven, CT) is developing BAYx7195, another leukotriene receptor antagonist that is under phase II trials as of late 1999. Pranlukast (Ultair; SmithKline Beecham, Philadelphia, PA) also is in development for treatment of asthma, and may have additional properties of inhibiting eosinophils and the release of ECP (168).

Because leukotriene antagonists affect a relatively smaller portion of the inflammatory process, the exact role of leukotriene inhibitors in the asthma algorithm is still being questioned. Leukotriene antagonists in general are not replacements for steroids in asthma, but instead are "steroid-sparing" drugs. Although these compounds are not available in ophthalmic preparations, they represent another direction the treatment of ocular allergy may take. Although their role in acute allergy may be limited, they may have a place in treating chronic allergy because leukotrienes may play a large role in the late-phase response. In these conditions, antileukotrienes may reduce the eosinophil- and T-cell–driven responses (169).

## Anti–Immunoglobulin E

Human IgE pentapeptide (HEPP), a synthetic antiallergic agent, is thought competitively to block the binding of IgE to cell receptors. One study of 50 patients showed that 0.5% HEPP was safe and effective in relieving the signs and symptoms of allergic conjunctivitis (170). Another strategy is the development of antibodies specific for IgE, thus blocking the allergic reaction where it begins. Clinical studies will show if this class of agents is effective. Olizumab/rhuMab-E25 and anti-IgE (Xolair) is a novel agent under development for the treatment of allergic rhinitis and asthma. Xolair is a recombinant humanized monoclonal antibody to IgE called E25 designed to act early in the allergy cascade. The product is being jointly developed by Genentech, Inc. (South San Francisco, CA), Novartis (East Hanover, NJ), and Tanox, Inc. (Houston, TX).

## Adhesion Molecule Blockers

The role of adhesion molecules in allergic disease has generated much research. Adhesion molecules located on the vascular endothelium are vital to the recruitment of eosinophils in the late-phase response. P-selectin glycoprotein ligand 1 (sPSGL-1), was evaluated in a mouse model of ocular allergy. sPSGL-1 inhibited eosinophil recruitment, tissue infiltration, and late-phase inflammation (171). Adhesion

molecule blockers specifically may play a large role in the treatment in VKC, AKC, and GPC (172,173).

## Immunomodulators

Immunomodulating agents include drugs such as cyclosporine and tacrolimus (FK-506). Although not currently available in topical formulation for ocular allergy, this pharmacologic class may affect mast cell proliferation and survival (174). Both cyclosporine and FK-506 have been shown to inhibit histamine release from mast cells (175). Calcineurin, a serine/threonine phosphatase thought to be a primary target of these drugs, plays a role in the FcεRI-mediated exocytosis of preformed mediators from the mast cell (176). Cyclosporine and FK-506 may reduce degranulation of mast cells through this mechanism. They also may act on various kinases (protein tyrosine kinase, protein kinase C, phosphatidylinositol 3-kinase), thus altering calcium transients and inhibiting degranulation and cytokine gene expression (177). NFAT is a transcription factor that plays a role in the production of the inflammatory cytokines TNF, IFN, and IL-2, IL-3, IL-4, IL-5, and IL-13 (178, 179). NFAT is regulated by calcineurin, and thus cyclosporine and FK-506 affect the release of these substances from T lymphocytes and mast cells, reduce eosinophil infiltration, and decrease cellular adhesion at the site of inflammation (179). Cyclosporine also alters cellular histamine content in the mast cell (175). Immunomodulators offer hope of a drug with an efficacy similar to that of steroids, but with a better safety profile, for the treatment of severe chronic allergy.

## CONCLUSION

It is clear from the wide variety of topical antiallergy medications that the clinician is faced with many choices. Because of the overlapping signs and symptoms of the various forms of ocular allergy and other external eye diseases, proper diagnosis cannot be overstressed. There may be a tendency to treat all ocular redness and irritation in the same manner, but by looking closely at the pathogenesis of the disease, it becomes evident that the different diseases often require different treatment modalities. As new therapies become available that have specific targets in the allergy pathway, selection of the proper drug will become more important.

## REFERENCES

1. Weston JH, Udell IJ, Abelson MB. H1 receptors in the human ocular surface. *Invest Ophthalmol Vis Sci* 1981;20[Suppl]:32(abstr).
2. Schwartz LB. Mediators of human mast cells and human mast cell subsets. *Ann Allergy* 1987;58:226.
3. Abelson MB, Allansmith MR. Histamine and the eye. In: Sil-

verstein AM, O'Connor GF, eds. *Immunology and immunopathology of the eye.* New York: Masson, 1979.

4. Abelson MB, Udell IJ. H2 receptors in the human ocular surface. *Arch Ophthalmol* 1981;99:302.

5. Cahoalon L, Lider O, Schor H, et al. Heparin disaccharides inhibit tumor necrosis factor: production by macrophages and arrest immune inflammation in rodents. *Int Immunol* 1997;9:1517–1522.

6. Smith JA, Mansfield LE, deShazo R, et al. An evaluation of the pharmacologic inhibition of the immediate and late cutaneous effects to allergen. *J Allergy Clin Immunol* 1980;65:118.

7. Leonardi A, Radice M, Fregona IA, et al. Histamine effects on conjunctival fibroblasts from patients with vernal conjunctivitis. *Exp Eye Res* 1999;68:739–746.

8. Berdy GJ, Levene RB, Bateman ST, et al. Identification of histaminase activity in human tears after conjunctival antigen challenge. *Invest Ophthalmol Vis Sci* 1990;31[Suppl]:65(abstr).

9. Reiss J, Abelson MB, George MA, et al. Allergic conjunctivitis. In: Pepose J, Holland G, Wilhelmus K, eds. *Ocular infection and immunity.* Boston: Mosby, 1996:347.

10. Tam EK, Caughey GH. Degradation of airway neuropeptides by human lung tryptase. *Am J Respir Cell Mol Biol* 1990;3:27.

11. Anderson W, Chan CC, Nussenblatt RB, et al. Topical heparin inhibits compound 48/80 induced allergic conjunctivitis. *Invest Ophthalmol Vis Sci* 1994;35:1291.

12. Benveniste J, Chignard M, le Couedic JP, et al. Biosynthesis of platelet-activating factor (PAF-acether): II. involvement of phospholipase A2 in the formation of PAF-acether and lyso-PAF-acether from rabbit platelets. *Thromb Res* 1982;25:375.

13. Tamura N, Agrawal D, Suliman FA, et al. Effects of platelet-activating factor on the chemotaxis of normodense eosinophils from normal subjects. *Biochem Biophys Res Commun* 1986;142:638.

14. George MA, Smith LM, Berdy GJ, et al. Platelet activating factor induced inflammation following topical ocular challenge. *Invest Ophthalmol Vis Sci* 1990;31[Suppl]:63(abstr).

15. Wasserman M. Bronchopulmonary responses to prostaglandin F2 alpha, histamine, and acetylcholine in the dog. *Eur J Pharmacol* 1975;32:146.

16. Wasserman MA, DuCharme DW, Griffin RL, et al. Bronchopulmonary and cardiovascular effects of prostaglandin D2 in the dog. *Prostaglandins* 1977;13:255.

17. Szczeklik A, Gryglewski RJ, Nizankowska E, et al. Pulmonary and anti-platelet effects of intravenous and inhaled prostacyclin in man. *Prostaglandins* 1978;16:651.

18. Cantarow WD, Cheung HT, Sundharadas G. Effects of prostaglandins on the spreading, adhesion, and migration of mouse peritoneal macrophages. *Prostaglandins* 1978;16:39.

19. Mathe AA, Hedqvist P. Effect of prostaglandins F2 alpha and E2 on airway conductance in healthy subjects and asthmatic patients. *Am Rev Respir Dis* 1975;111:313.

20. Solomon LM, Juhlin L, Kirschenbaum MB. Prostaglandin on cutaneous vasculature. *J Invest Dermatol* 1968;51:280.

21. Crounkhorn P, Willis AL. Interaction between prostaglandins E and F given intradermally in the rat. *Br J Pharmacol* 1971;41:507.

22. Ferreira SH. Prostaglandins, aspirin-like drugs and analgesia. *Nature New Biol* 1972;240:200.

23. Leopold IH. Advances in ocular therapy: noncorticosteroid antiinflammatory agents. *Am J Ophthalmol* 1974;78:759–773.

24. Lewis RA, Holgate ST, Roberts LJ Jr, et al. Preferential generation of prostaglandin D2 by rat and human mast cells. In: Becker EL, Simon AS, Austen KF, eds. *Biochemistry of the Acute Allergic Reactions, Fourth International Symposium.* New York: Alan R. Liss, 1981:239–254.

25. Lewis RA, Soter NA, Diamond PT, et al. Prostaglandin D2

generation after activation of rat and human mast cells with anti-IgE. *J Immunol* 1982;129:1627.

26. Roberts LJ Jr, Sweetman BJ, Lewis RA, et al. Increased production of prostaglandin D2 in patients with systemic mastocytosis. *N Engl J Med* 1980;303:1400.

27. Roberts LJ Jr, Sweetman BJ, Lewis RA, et al. Markedly increased synthesis of prostaglandin D2 in systemic mastocytosis. *Trans Am Assoc Physicians* 1980;93:141.

28. Abelson MB, Madiwale NA, Weston JH. The role of prostaglandin D2 in allergic ocular disease. In: O'Connor GR, Chandler JW, eds. *Third International Symposium of the Immunology and Immunopathology of the Eye.* New York: Masson & Masson, 1985:163–166.

29. Bhattacherjee P. The role of arachidonate metabolism in ocular inflammation. *Prog Clin Biol Res* 1989;312:211.

30. Ellis EA, Oilz O, Roberts LJ, et al. Coronary arterial smooth muscle contraction by a substance released from platelets: evidence that it is thromboxane A2. *Science* 1976;193:1135.

31. Hamberg M, Svensson J, Samuelsson B. Thromboxanes: a new group of biologically active compounds derived from prostaglandin endoperoxides. *Proc Natl Acad Sci USA* 1975;72:2994.

32. Goetzl EJ, Gorman RR. Chemotactic and chemokinetic stimulation of human eosinophil and neutrophil polymorphonuclear leukocytes by 12-L-hydroxy-5,8,10-heptadecatrienoic acid (HHT). *J Immunol* 1978;120:526.

33. Bisgard H, Ford-Hutchinson AW, Charleson S, et al. Production of leukotrienes in human skin and conjunctival mucosa after specific allergen challenge. *Allergy* 1985;40:417.

34. Weston JH, Abelson MB. Leukotriene C4 in rabbit and human eyes. *Invest Ophthalmol Vis Sci* 1981;26[Suppl]:191(abstr).

35. Udel IJ, Abelson MB. Chemical mediators of inflammation. *Int Ophthalmol Clin* 1983;23:15.

36. Lundgren JD, Shelhamer JH, Kalimer MA. The role of eicosanoids in respiratory mucus hypersecretion. *Ann Allergy* 1985;55:55.

37. Abelson MB. Lipoxygenase products in ocular inflammation. *Invest Ophthalmol Vis Sci* 1984;25[Suppl]:42(abstr).

38. Ihle JN, Pepersack L, Rebar L. Regulation of T cell differentiation: in vitro induction of 20 alpha-hydroxysteroid dehydrogenase in splenic lymphocytes is mediated by a unique lymphokine. *J Immunol* 1981;126:2184.

39. Brzezinska-Blaszczyk E, Forczmanski M, Pietrzak A. The action of tumor necrosis factor-alpha on rat mast cells. *J Interferon Cytokine Res* 2000;20:377–382.

40. MacLeod JDA, Anderson DF, Holgate ST, et al. Immunolocalization of mast cell cytokines to mast cells in normal and allergic conjunctiva. *Clin Exp Allergy* 1997;27:1328–1334

41. Zhang S, Anderson DF, Bradding P, et al. Human mast cells express stem cell factor. *J Pathol* 1998;186:59–66.

42. Udell IJ, Gleich GJ, Allansmith MR, et. al. Eosinophil granule major basic protein and Charcot-Leyden crystal protein in human tears. *Am J Ophthalmol* 1981;92:824–828.

43. Kay AB. Eosinophils as effector cells in immunity and allergic disorders. In: Korenblat P, Wedner H, eds. *Allergy, theory and practice,* 2nd ed. Philadelphia: WB Saunders, 1992.

44. Passalacqua G, Senna G, Dama A, et al. The relationship between clinical efficacy of specific immunotherapy and serum intercellular adhesion molecule-1 levels. *J Investig Allergol Clin Immunol* 1998;8:123–124.

45. Ciprandi G, Buscaglia S, Pesce GP, et al. Allergic subjects express intercellular adhesion molecule-1 (ICAM-1 or CD54) on epithelial cells of conjunctiva after antigen challenge. *J Allergy Clin Immunol* 1993;91:783–792.

46. Canonica GW, Ciprandi G, Passalacqua G, et al. Molecular events in allergic inflammation: experimental models and possible modulation. *Allergy* 1997;52[34 Suppl]:25–30.

47. Ciprandi G, Buscaglia S, Pesce G, et al. Cetirizine reduces inflammatory cell recruitment and ICAM-1 (or CD54) expression on conjunctival epithelium in both early- and late-phase reactions after allergen-specific challenge. *J Allergy Clin Immunol* 1995;95:612–621.

48. Fukagawa K, Saito H, Tsubota K, et al. RANTES production in a conjunctival epithelial cell line. *Cornea* 1997;16:564–570.

49. Bonini S, Bonini S, Berruto A, et al. Conjunctival provocation test as a model for the study of allergy and inflammation in humans. *Int Arch Allergy Appl Immunol* 1989;88:144–148.

50. Naclerio RM, Proud D, Toglas AG, et al. Inflammatory mediators in late antigen-induced rhinitis. *N Engl J Med* 1985;313:6.

51. Bonini S, Bonini S, Bucci MG, et al. Allergen dose response and late symptoms in a human model of ocular allergy. *J Allergy Clin Immunol* 1990;86:869–876.

52. Blumenthal M, Bonini S. Immunogenetics of specific immunoresponses to allergens in twins and families. In: Marsh DG, Blumenthal M, eds. *Genetic and environmental factors in clinical allergy.* Minneapolis, MN: University of Minnesota Press, 1990:132.

53. Barnes PJ, Adcock IM. Transcription factors and asthma. *Eur Respir J* 1998;12:221–234.

54. Romagnani S. The role of lymphocytes in allergic disease. *J Allergy Clin Immunol* 2000;105:399–408

55. Takeda K, Kishimoto T, Akira S. STAT6: its role in interleukin 4-mediated biological functions. *J Mol Med* 1997;75:317–326.

56. Van Lee Uwen BH, Martinson WE, Webb GC, et al .Molecular organization of the cytokine gene cluster, involving the human IL-3, IL-4, IL-5, and GM-CSF genes on human chromosome 5. *Blood* 1989;73:1142.

57. Borish L. Genetics of allergy and asthma. *Ann Allergy Asthma Immunol* 1999;82:413–424.

58. Friedlander MH. Conjunctivitis of allergic origin: clinical presentation and differential diagnosis. *Surg Ophthalmol* 1993;38[Suppl]:105–114.

59. Nevius JM, Abelson MB, Welch D. The ocular drying effects of oral antihistamines (loratadine) in the normal eye population: an evaluation. *Invest Ophthalmol Vis Sci* 1999;40[Suppl](abstr):24.

60. Smolin B, Okumoto M. Staphylococcal blepharitis. *Arch Ophthalmol* 1983;95:812–816.

61. Abelson MB, Chamber WA, Smith LM. Conjunctival allergen challenge: a clinical approach to studying allergic conjunctivitis. *Arch Ophthalmol* 1990;108:84–88.

62. Abelson MB, Udell, Weston JH. Conjunctival eosinophils in allergic ocular disease. *Arch Ophthalmol* 1983;101:631–633.

63. Bonini S, Bonini S, Vecchione A, et al. Inflammatory changes in conjunctival scrapings after allergen provocation in humans. *J Allergy Clin Immunol* 1988;82:462.

64. Butrus SI, Abelson MB. Laboratory evaluation of ocular allergy. *Int Ophthalmol Clin* 1988;28:324–328.

65. Neumann E, Gutmann MJ, Blumenkrantz N, et al. A review of 400 cases of vernal conjunctivitis. *Am J Ophthalmol* 1959;47:166.

66. Beigleman MN. *Vernal conjunctivitis.* Los Angeles: University of Southern California Press, 1950.

67. Allansmith MR, Frick OL. Antibodies to grass in vernal conjunctivitis. *Allergy* 1963;34:535.

68. Brody JM, Foster CS. Vernal conjunctivitis. In: Pepose JS, Holland GN, Wilhelmus KR, eds. *Ocular infection and immunity.* Boston: Mosby, 1996.

69. Friedlaender MH, Cameron JA. Ocular diseases with immunologic features. In: Friedlaender MH, ed. *Allergy and immunology of the eye.* Hagerstown, PA: Harper & Row, 1979.

70. Buckley RJ. Vernal keratopathy and its management. *Tran Ophthalmic Soc UK* 1981;101:234–238.

71. Abelson MB, Udell IJ, Allansmith MR, et al. Allergic and toxic reactions. In: Albert DM, Jackobie FA, eds. *Principles and practices of ophthalmology.* Philadelphia: WB Saunders, 1994.

72. Margrini L, Bonini S, Centrofanti M, et al. Tear tryptase levels and allergic conjunctivitis. *Allergy* 1996;51:577–581.

73. Allansmith MR, Baird RS, Greiner JV. Vernal conjunctivitis and contact lens associated giant papillary conjunctivitis compared and contrasted. *Am J Ophthalmol* 1979;87:544–555.

74. Leonardi A, Fregona IA, Gismondi M, et al. Correlation between conjunctival provocation test (CPT) and systemic allergometric tests in allergic conjunctivitis. *Eye* 1990;4:760–764.

75. Proud D, Sweet J, Stein P, et al. Inflammatory mediator release on conjunctival provocation of allergic subjects with allergen. *J Allergy Clin Immunol* 1990;85:896–905.

76. Abelson MB, Baird RS, Allansmith MR. Tear histamine levels in vernal conjunctivitis and other ocular inflammations. *Ophthalmology* 1980;87:812.

77. Abelson MB, Soter N, Simon M, et al. Histamine in human tears. *Am J Ophthalmol* 1977;85:417.

78. Allansmith MR, Baird RS, Greiner JV. Density of Goblet cells in vernal conjunctivitis and contact lens associated giant papillary conjunctivitis. *Arch Ophthalmol* 1981;99:884–885.

79. Abelson MB, Leonardi A, Smith LM, et al. Histaminase activity in vernal keratoconjunctivitis. *Ophthalmology* 1995;102:1958–1963.

80. Henriquez AS, Kenyon KR, Allansmith MR. Mast cell ultrastructure: comparison in contact lens–associated giant papillary conjunctivitis and vernal conjunctivitis. *Arch Ophthalmol* 1981;99:1266.

81. Allansmith MR, Baird RS, Greiner JV. Vernal conjunctivitis and contact-lens associated giant papillary conjunctivitis and vernal conjunctivitis. *Arch Ophthalmol* 1981;99:1266.

82. Bonini S, Magrini L, Rotiroti G, et al. The eosinophil and the eye. *Allergy* 1997;52[34 Suppl]:44–47.

83. Udell IJ, Gleich GJ, Allansmith MR, et al. Eosinophil granule major basic protein and Charcot-Leyden crystal protein in human tears. *Am J Ophthalmol* 1981;92:824–828.

84. Golubovic S, Parunovic A. Vernal conjunctivitis: a cause of corneal mucoid plaques. *Fortschr Ophthalmol* 1986;83:272.

85. Leonardi A, Borghesan F, Faggian D, et al. Tear and serum soluble leukocyte activation markers in conjunctival allergic diseases. *Am J Ophthalmol* 2000;129:151–158.

86. Trocme SD, Kephart G, Bourne WM, et al. Eosinophil major basic protein deposition in human corneal shield ulcers. *Invest Ophthalmol Vis Sci* 1992;33[Suppl]:94(abstr).

87. Abu el-Asrar AM, Geboes K, al-Kharashi S, et al. Adhesion molecules in vernal keratoconjunctivitis. *Br J Ophthalmol* 1997;81:1099–1106.

88. Donshik PC. Allergic conjunctivitis. *Int Ophthalmol Clin* 1988;28:294–302.

89. Braude LS, Chandler JW. Atopic corneal disease. *Int Ophthalmol Clin* 1984;24:145–156.

90. Ehlers AH, Donshik PC. Allergic ocular disorders: a spectrum of diseases. *CLAO J* 1992;18:117.

91. Foster CS, Calonge M. Atopic keratoconjunctivitis. *Ophthalmology* 1990;97:992–1000.

92. Allansmith MR, Abelson MB. Immunological diseases. In: Smolin G, Thorft RA, eds. *The cornea.* Boston: Little, Brown, 1983.

93. Garrity JA, Liesegang TJ. Ocular complications of atopic dermatitis. *Can J Ophthalmol* 1984;19:21–24.

94. Power WJ, Tugal-Tutkun I, Foster CS. Long-term follow up of patients with atopic keratoconjunctivitis. *Ophthalmology* 1988;105:637–642.

95. Tuft SJ, Kemeny DM, Dart JK, et al. Clinical features of atopic keratoconjunctivitis. *Ophthalmology* 1991;98:150–158.

96. Freidlaender MH. *Allergy and immunology of the eye.* San Francisco: Harper & Row, 1979.

97. Foster CS, Rice BA, Dutt JE. Immunopathology of atopic keratoconjunctivitis. *Ophthalmology* 1991;98:1190–1196.

98. Allansmith MR, Ross RN. Ocular allergy. *Clin Allergy* 1988;18:1–13.

99. Morgan SJ, Williams JH, Walls AF, et al. Mast cell hyperplasia in atopic keratoconjunctivitis. *Eye* 1991;5:729–735.

100. Soukiasian SH, Rice B, Foster CS, et al. The T cell receptor in normal and inflamed human conjunctiva. *Invest Ophthalmol Vis Sci* 1992;33:453–459.

101. Allansmith MR. *The eye and immunology.* St. Louis: CV Mosby, 1982.

102. Allansmith MR, Korb DR, Greiner JV, et al. Giant papillary conjunctivitis in contact lens wearers. *Am J Ophthalmol* 1977;83:697–708.

103. Trocme SD, Kephart GM, Allansmith MR, et al. Conjunctival deposition of eosinophil granule major basic protein in vernal keratoconjunctivitis and contact lens associated giant papillary conjunctivitis. *Am J Ophthalmol* 1989;108:57–63.

104. Luxenberg MN. Blepharoptosis associated with giant papillary conjunctivitis. *Arch Ophthalmol* 1986;104:1706.

105. Rapacz P, Tedesco J, Donshik PC, et al. Tear lysozyme and lactoferrin levels in giant papillary conjunctivitis and vernal conjunctivitis. *CLAO J* 1988;14:207–209.

106. Irkee MT, Orhan M, Erener U. Role of tear inflammatory mediators in contact lens-associated giant papillary conjunctivitis in soft contact lens wearers. *Ocul Immunol Inflamm* 1999;7:35–38.

107. Mathers WD, Billborough M. Meibomian gland dysfunction and giant papillary conjunctivitis. *Am J Ophthalmol* 1992;114:188–192.

108. Abelson MB, Smith LM. Levocabastine: evaluation in the histamine and compound 48/80 model of ocular allergy in humans. *Ophthalmology* 1988;95:1494.

109. Smith LM, Abelson MB, George MA, et al. A double-masked study on the effects of ophthalmic levocabastine vs. placebo on the signs and symptoms of allergic conjunctivitis. *Invest Ophthalmol Vis Sci* 1992;33[Suppl]:1297(abstr).

110. Yanni JM, Stephens DJ, Parnell DW, et al. Preclinical efficacy of emedastine, a potent, selective histamine H1 antagonist for topical ocular use. *J Ocul Pharmacol* 1994;10:665.

111. Secchi A, Leonardi A, Discepola M, et al. An efficacy and tolerance comparison of emedastine difumarate 0.05% and levocabastine hydrochloride 0.05%: reducing chemosis and eyelid swelling in subjects with seasonal allergic conjunctivitis: Emadine Study Group. *Acta Ophthalmol Scand Suppl* 2000;230:48–51.

112. Discepola M, Deschenes J, Abelson M. Comparison of the topical ocular antiallergic efficacy of emedastine 0.05% ophthalmic solution to ketorolac 0.5% ophthalmic solution in a clinical model of allergic conjunctivitis. *Acta Ophthalmol Scand Suppl* 1999;228:43–46.

113. Dockhorn RJ, Duckett TG. Comparison of Naphcon-A and its components (naphazoline and pheniramine) in a provocative model of allergic conjunctivitis. *Curr Eye Res* 1994;13:319–324.

114. Abelson MB, Paradis A, George MA, et al. Effects of Vasocon-A in the allergen challenge model of acute allergic conjunctivitis. *Arch Ophthalmol* 1990;108:520–524.

115. Lanier BQ, Tremblay N, Smith JP, et al. A double-masked comparison of ocular decongestants as therapy for allergic conjunctivitis. *Ann Allergy* 1983;50:174–177.

116. Foster CS. Evaluation of topical cromolyn sodium in the treatment of vernal conjunctivitis. *Ophthalmology* 1988;95:194.

117. Calonge M, Montero JA, Herreras JM, et al. Efficacy of nedocromil sodium and cromolyn sodium in an experimental model of ocular allergy. *Ann Allergy Asthma Immunol* 1996;77:124.

118. Bonini S, Schiavone M, Bonini S, et al. Efficacy of lodoxamide eye drops on mast cells and eosinophils after allergen challenge in allergic conjunctivitis. *Ophthalmology* 1997;104:849–853.

119. Ciprandi G, Buscaglia S, Catrullo A, et al. Antiallergic activity of topical lodoxamide on in vivo and in vitro models. *Allergy* 1996;51:946–951.

120. Caldwell DR, Verin P, Hartwich-Young R, et al. Efficacy and safety of lodoxamide 0.1% vs cromolyn sodium 4% in patients with vernal conjunctivitis. *Am J Ophthalmol* 1992;113:632.

121. Avunduk AM, Avunduk MC, Kapicioglu Z, et al. Mechanisms and comparison of anti-allergic efficacy of topical lodoxamide and cromolyn sodium treatment in vernal keratoconjunctivitis. *Ophthalmology* 2000;107:1333–1337.

122. Oguz H, Bitiren M, Aslan OS, et al. Efficacy of lodoxamide eye drops on tear fluid cytology of patients with vernal conjunctivitis. *Acta Med Okayama* 1999;53:123–126.

123. Fujimiya H, Nakashima S, Miyata H, et al. Effect of a novel antiallergic drug, pemirolast, on activation of rat peritoneal mast cells: inhibition of exocytotic response and membrane phospholipid turnover. *Int Arch Allergy Appl Immunol* 1991;96:62–67.

124. Kawashima T, Iwamoto I, Nakagawa N, et al. Inhibitory effect of pemirolast, a novel antiallergic drug, on leukotriene C4 and granule protein release from human eosinophils. *Int Arch Allergy Immunol* 1994;103:405–409.

125. Leino M, Carlson C, Jaanio E, et al. Double-blind group comparative study of 2% nedocromil sodium eye drops with placebo eye drops in the treatment of seasonal allergic conjunctivitis. *Ann Allergy* 1990;64:398–402.

126. Blumenthal M, Casale T, Dockhorn R, et al. Efficacy and safety of nedocromil sodium ophthalmic solution in the treatment of seasonal allergic conjunctivitis. *Am J Ophthalmol* 1992;113:56–63.

127. Bailey CS, Buckley RJ. Nedocromil sodium in contact-lens-associated papillary conjunctivitis. *Eye* 1993;7[Pt 3 Suppl]:29–33.

128. Leino M, Ennevaara K, Latvala AL, et al. Double-blind group comparative study of 2% nedocromil sodium eye drops with 2% sodium cromoglycate and placebo eye drops in the treatment of seasonal allergic conjunctivitis. *Clin Exp Allergy* 1992;22:929–932.

129. el Hennawi M. A double blind placebo controlled group comparative study of ophthalmic sodium cromoglycate and nedocromil sodium in the treatment of vernal keratoconjunctivitis. *Br J Ophthalmol* 1994;78:365–369.

130. Wong WS, Tsang F, Li H, et al. Effects of inhibitors of the tyrosine kinase signaling cascade on an in vitro model of allergic airways. *Asian Pac J Allergy Immunol* 1999;17:229–237.

131. Malaviya R, Zhu D, Dibirdik I, et al. Targeting Janus kinase 3 in mast cells prevents immediate hypersensitivity reactions and anaphylaxis. *J Biol Chem* 1999;17;274:27028–27038.

132. Malaviya R, Chen CL, Navara C, et al. Treatment of allergic asthma by targeting janus kinase 3-dependent leukotriene synthesis in mast cells with 4-(3′, 5′-dibromo-4′-hydroxyphenyl)amino-6,7-dimethoxyquinazoline (WHI-P97). *J Pharmacol Exp Ther* 2000;295:912–926.

133. Sharif NA, Xu SX, Yanni JM. Olopatadine (AL-4943A): ligand binding and functional studies on a novel, long acting H1-selective histamine antagonist and anti-allergic agent for use in allergic conjunctivitis. *J Ocul Pharmacol Ther* 1996;12:401–407.

134. Sharif NA, Xu SX, Miller ST, et al. Characterization of the ocular antiallergic and antihistaminic effects of olopatadine (AL-

4943A), a novel drug for treating ocular allergic diseases. *J Pharmacol Exp Ther* 1996;278:1252–1261.

135. Yanni JM, Weimer LK, Sharif NA, et al. Inhibition of histamine-induced human conjunctival epithelial cell responses by ocular allergy drugs. *Arch Ophthalmol* 1999;117:643–647.

136. Cook EB, Stahl JL, Barney NP, et al. Olopatadine inhibits TNF-alpha release from human conjunctival mast cells. *Ann Allergy Asthma Immunol* 2000;84:504–508.

137. Miki I, Kusano A, Ohta S, et al. Histamine enhanced the TNF-alpha–induced expression of E-selectin and ICAM-1 on vascular endothelial cells. *Cell Immunol* 1996;171:285–258.

138. Abelson MB, Spitalny L. Combined analysis of two studies using the conjunctival allergen challenge model to evaluate olopatadine hydrochloride, a new ophthalmic antiallergic agent with dual activity. *Am J Ophthalmol* 1998;125:797–804.

139. Abelson MB. Evaluation of olopatadine, a new ophthalmic antiallergic agent with dual activity, using the conjunctival allergen challenge model. *Ann Allergy Asthma Immunol* 1998;81:211–218.

140. Artal MN, Luna JD, Discepola M. A forced choice comfort study of olopatadine hydrochloride 0.1% versus ketotifen fumarate 0.05%. *Acta Ophthalmol Scand Suppl* 2000;230:64–65.

141. Deschenes J, Discepola M, Abelson M. Comparative evaluation of olopatadine ophthalmic solution (0.1%) versus ketorolac ophthalmic solution (0.5%) using the provocative antigen challenge model. *Acta Ophthalmol Scand Suppl* 1999;228:47–52.

142. Berdy GJ, Spangler DL, Bensch G, et al. A comparison of the relative efficacy and clinical performance of olopatadine hydrochloride 0.1% ophthalmic solution and ketotifen fumarate 0.025% ophthalmic solution in the conjunctival antigen challenge model. *Clin Ther* 2000;22:826–833.

143. Abelson MB, Welch DL. An evaluation of onset and duration of action of Patanol (olopatadine hydrochloride ophthalmic solution 0.1%) compared to Claritin (loratadine 10 mg) tablets in acute allergic conjunctivitis in the conjunctival allergen challenge model. *Acta Ophthalmol Scand Suppl* 2000;230:60–63.

144. Devillier P, Arnoux B, Lalau KC, et al. Inhibition of human and rabbit platelet activation by ketotifen. *Fundam Clin Pharmacol* 1990:4;1.

145. Fink A, Bibi H, Eliraz A, et al. Ketotifen, disodium cromoglycate, and verapamil inhibit leukotriene activity: determination by tube leukocyte adherence inhibition assay. *Ann Allergy* 1986:57;103.

146. Kimura M, Mitani H, Bandoh T, et al. Mast cell degranulation in rate mesenteric venule: effects of 1-NAME, methylene blue and ketotifen. *Pharmacol Res* 1999:39;397.

147. Ciprandi G, Buscaglia S, Catrullo A, et al. Azelastine eye drops reduce and prevent allergic conjunctival reaction and exert antiallergic activity. *Clin Exp Allergy* 1997;27:182–191.

148. Lenhard G, Mivsek-Music E, Perrin-Fayolle M, et al. Double-blind, randomised, placebo-controlled study of two concentrations of azelastine eye drops in seasonal allergic conjunctivitis or rhinoconjunctivitis. *Curr Med Res Opin* 1997;14:21–28.

149. Sabbah A, Marzetto M. Azelastine eye drops in the treatment of seasonal allergic conjunctivitis or rhinoconjunctivitis in young children. *Curr Med Res Opin* 1998;14:161–170.

150. Friedlaender MH, Harris J, LaVallee N, et al. Evaluation of the onset and duration of effect of Azelastine eye drops (0.05%) versus placebo in patients with allergic conjunctivitis using an allergen challenge model. *Ophthalmology* 2000;107:2152–2157.

151. Tinkelman D, Rupp G, Kaufman H, et al. Ketorolac tromethamine 0.5% ophthalmic solution in the treatment of seasonal allergic conjunctivitis: a placebo-controlled clinical trial. *Surv Ophthalmol* 1993;38[Suppl]:133.

152. Rooks WH, Maloney PJ, Shott LD, et al. Clinical evaluation of ketorolac tromethamine 0.5% ophthalmic solution for treatment of seasonal allergic conjunctivitis. *Surv Ophthalmol* 1993;38[Suppl]:141.

153. Tauber J, Abelson M, Ostrov C, et al. A multicenter comparison of diclofenac sodium 0.1% (DS) to ketorolac tromethamine 0.5% (KT) in patients with acute seasonal allergic conjunctivitis (SAC). *Invest Ophthalmol Vis Sci* 1994;35[Suppl]:180(abstr).

154. Bishop K, Abelson MB, Cheetham J, et al. Evaluation of flurbiprofen in the treatment of antigen-induced allergic conjunctivitis. *Invest Ophthalmol Vis Sci* 1990;31[Suppl]:487(abstr).

155. Abelson MB, Butrus SI, Kliman GH, et al. Topical arachidonic acid: a model for screening anti-inflammatory agents. *J Ocul Pharmacol* 1987;3:63.

156. Abelson MB, Butrus SI, Weston JH. Aspirin therapy in vernal conjunctivitis. *Am J Ophthalmol* 1983;95:502.

157. Meyer E, Kraus E, Zonis S. Efficacy of antiprostaglandin therapy in vernal conjunctivitis. *Br J Ophthalmol* 1987;71:497.

158. Notivol R, Martinez M, Bergamini MVW. Treatment of chronic bacterial conjunctivitis with a cyclooxygenase inhibitor or a corticosteroid. *Am J Ophthalmol* 1994;117:651.

159. Malmstrom K, Daniels S, Kotey P, et al. Comparison of rofecoxib and celecoxib, two cyclooxygenase-2 inhibitors, in postoperative dental pain: a randomized, placebo- and active-comparator-controlled clinical trial. *Clin Ther* 1999;21:1653–1663.

160. Cannon GW, Caldwell JR, Holt P, et al. Rofecoxib, a specific inhibitor of cyclooxygenase 2, with clinical efficacy comparable with that of diclofenac sodium: results of a one-year, randomized, clinical trial in patients with osteoarthritis of the knee and hip: Rofecoxib Phase III Protocol 035 Study Group. *Arthritis Rheum* 2000;43:978–987.

161. Yocum D, Fleischmann R, Dalgin P, et al. Safety and efficacy of meloxicam in the treatment of osteoarthritis: a 12-week, double-blind, multiple-dose, placebo-controlled trial. *Arch Intern Med* 2000;160:2947–2954.

162. Berg J, Fellier H, Christoph T, et al. Pharmacology of a selective cyclooxygenase-2 inhibitor, HN-56249: a novel compound exhibiting a marked preference for the human enzyme in intact cells. *Naunyn Schmiedebergs Arch Pharmacol* 2000;361:363–372.

163. Dell SJ, Lowry GM, Northcutt JA, et al. A randomized, double-masked, placebo-controlled parallel study of 0.2% loteprednol etabonate in patients with seasonal allergic conjunctivitis. *J Allergy Clin Immunol* 1998;102:251–255.

164. Abelson M, Howes J, George M. The conjunctival provocation test model of ocular allergy: utility for assessment of an ocular corticosteroid, loteprednol etabonate. *J Ocul Pharmacol Ther* 1998;14:533.

165. Bartlett JD, Howes JF, Chormley NR, et al. Safety and efficacy of loteprednol etabonate for treatment of papillae in contact lens associated giant papillary conjunctivitis. *Curr Eye Res* 1993;12:313.

166. Tabbara KF, al-Kharashi SA. Efficacy of nedocromil 2% versus fluorometholone 0.1%: a randomised, double masked trial comparing the effects on severe vernal keratoconjunctivitis. *Br J Ophthalmol* 1999;83(2):180–184.

167. Abelson MB, Schaefer K. Conjunctivitis of allergic origin: immunological mechanisms and current approaches to therapy. *Surv Ophthalmol* 1993;38:115.

168. Ishioka S, Hozawa S, Haruta Y, et al. Pranlukast, a cysteinyl leukotriene antagonist, reduces serum eosinophil cationic protein levels in patients with asthma. *Hiroshima J Med Sci* 1999;48:105–110.

169. Hojo M, Suzuki M, Maghni K, et al. Role of cysteinyl leukotrienes in CD4(+) T cell-driven late allergic airway responses. *J Pharmacol Exp Ther* 2000;293:410–416.

170. Floyd R, Kalpaxis J, Thayer T, et al. Double-blind comparison

of HEPP (IgE pentapeptide) 0.5% ophthalmic solution (H) and sodium cromoglycate ophthalmic solution, USP 4% (O) in patients having allergic conjunctivitis. *Invest Ophthalmol Vis Sci* 1998;29[Suppl]:24(abstr).

171. Strauss EC, Larson KA, Brenneise I, et al. Soluble P-selectin glycoprotein ligand 1 inhibits ocular inflammation in a murine model of allergy. *Invest Ophthalmol Vis Sci* 1999;40:1336.

172. Abu el-Asrar AM, Geboes K, al-Kharashi S, et al. Adhesion molecules in vernal keratoconjunctivitis. *Br J Ophthalmol* 1997; 81:1099–1106.

173. Hingorani M, Calder VL, Buckley RJ, et al. The role of conjunctival epithelial cells in chronic ocular allergic disease. *Exp Eye Res* 1998;67:491–500.

174. Ito F, Toyota N, Sakai H, et al. FK506 and cyclosporin A inhibit stem cell factor-dependent cell proliferation/survival, while inducing upregulation of c-kit expression in cells of the mast cell line MC/9. *Arch Dermatol Res* 1999;291:275.

175. Toyota N, Hasimoto Y, Matsuo S, et al. Effects of FK506 and cyclosporin A on proliferation, histamine release, and phenotype of murine mast cells. *Arch Dermatol Res* 1996;288:474–480.

176. Hultsch T, Brand P, Lohmann S, et al. Direct evidence that FK506 inhibition of FcεRI-mediated exocytosis from RBL mast cells involves calcineurin. *Arch Dermatol Res* 1998;290: 258–263.

177. Ishizuka T, Chayama K, Takeda K, et al. Mitogen-activated protein kinase activation through Fc epsilon receptor I and stem cell factor receptor is differentially regulated by phosphatidyl-inositol 3-kinase and calcineurin in mouse bone marrow-derived mast cells. *J Immunol* 1999;162:2087–2094.

178. Hatfield S, Roehm N. Cyclosporin and FK506 inhibition of murine mast cell cytokine production. *J Pharmacol Exp Ther* 1992;260:680–688.

179. Matsuda S, Koyasu S. Mechanisms of action of cyclosporin. *Immunopharmacology* 2000;47:119–125.

# LATEX HYPERSENSITIVITY

## KIM E. PERSHALL

In the final two decades of the 20th century, the human immunodeficiency virus (HIV) became a very significant new problem in medicine. Latex sensitivity may be regarded as a loud echo of the changes brought on by HIV precautions. It has resulted in a major new challenge for allergists, health care workers, industrial managers, and patients who are sensitive to this ubiquitous antigen in many indoor settings.

Natural rubber or latex is a product that is manufactured from the milky cytosol obtained from the rubber tree, or weeping wood tree *(Hevea brasiliensis)*. It is used in several forms, with industrial chemicals being added to give different properties to the final rubber product. Latex rubber has qualities of high tensile strength, elasticity, and deformability. For medical purposes, it has optimal tactile sensitivity and superior barrier qualities. No other product contains all of the qualities possessed by latex at a price that would be competitive with this remarkable natural substance.

## HISTORY OF LATEX ALLERGY

The initial description of allergic reactions to latex gloves appeared in the American literature in 1933 (1). Reports of reactions followed sporadically for four decades. The first report of contact urticaria related to rubber was in 1966 by Rhodes and Warner (2). In the late 1980s, reports of latex-associated anaphylaxis increased sharply after the Centers for Disease Control recommended use of universal precautions because of the risk of transmission of HIV (3). During this time, annual use of surgical gloves increased from 800 million to 20 billion (4).

The first death traced to anaphylaxis from latex exposure was reported by Slater in 1989 (5). The first reports of intraoperative latex anaphylaxis appeared a short time thereafter (6). A series of deaths related to latex balloons used for barium enema catheters was published by Ownby in 1991 (7). This led to the first change in material for a

K. E. Pershall: Private Practice, Lubbock, Texas.

medical device to protect patients from exposure to latex. As of August 1997, the U.S. Food and Drug Administration (FDA) had received reports of over 2,300 allergic reactions to latex in a medical setting, including 225 cases of anaphylaxis, 53 cardiac arrests, and 17 deaths (8). One of the deaths was that of a health care worker wearing latex gloves. According to one report on the incidence of latex allergy, reports to the FDA represent only 1% of the actual number of reactions (9).

## CLINICAL PRESENTATION OF REACTIONS TO LATEX

There are three categories into which latex sensitivity reactions can be divided.

### Irritant Contact Dermatitis

This is not an allergic reaction, but a local inflammatory reaction related to the latex chemicals, as well as other chemicals found in rubber, or related to surgical scrubbing. It is associated with skin breakdown, redness, and swelling. The loss of skin barrier integrity can lead to increased absorption of latex antigen and subsequent allergic sensitization, but serologic and skin testing are negative at this stage. Irritant contact dermatitis is the most frequent type of presentation, accounting for 80% of glove-related incidents (10). Treatment is avoidance of latex exposure while skin is inflamed. Some patients are able to tolerate subsequent latex exposure if they avoid the use of petroleum-based skin emollients, which have been reported to degrade latex and increase the chance of irritation.

### Type IV Delayed Hypersensitivity

This immune-mediated reaction manifests as a local eczematous reaction in an exposed area. Also called *T-cell—mediated contact dermatitis,* or *allergic contact dermatitis,* this is the reaction typically associated with a poison ivy exposure, and can occur in any area exposed to latex, with exposure to gloves being the best known example. Eighty-four percent of immune-mediated reactions to latex are type IV (11). Serologic and delayed skin test results may be positive, but negative tests do not mean that a sensitized person will not react on repeat exposure. A patch test can be helpful if the clinical history is uncertain. The treatment for acute symptoms is a topical steroid preparation, or oral steroids for severe cases, and contact should be avoided in the future.

## Type I Immediate Hypersensitivity

This is the least common, but most severe type of reaction that can occur after latex exposure. Symptoms of pruritus, nasal congestion, sneezing, and wheezing are most commonly reported. More severe reactions can lead to local or widespread urticaria, angioedema, severe asthma, and anaphylaxis. Either local skin or mucosal contact exposure, or respiratory exposure from airborne antigen, can progress to systemic anaphylaxis. Reactions of this type occur when antibodies of the immunoglobulin E (IgE) class are present when exposure to antigen occurs. A cascade of events starting with release of histamine, leukotrienes, and other mediators may progress to mucosal swelling with airway obstruction and bronchospasm. In severe cases, shock and death can result. Unless specifically noted, the remainder of this chapter refers to IgE-mediated type I reactions as *acute latex sensitivity*.

## POPULATIONS AT RISK

There is substantial variation in the reported prevalence of acute latex sensitivity, depending on the population studied and the criteria used to define the presence of allergy. At-risk populations are determined by the frequency of exposure to latex. A good demonstration of this effect was reported by Tarlo et al. (12), who found that the prevalence of positive skin tests to latex increased with duration of medical school training. The incidence was zero in the first 2 years, when students were not exposed, 6% in year 3, and 10% in year 4.

Several distinct at-risk populations are recognized.

## Patients with a History of Multiple Surgical Procedures

Any patient population undergoing frequent surgery is at high risk for acute latex sensitivity (13). The highest incidence for acute latex sensitivity has been consistently in the spina bifida population, with between 30% and 70% of this group of patients found to be latex sensitive (14). Patients with spina bifida frequently need procedures to close the spinal defect and shunt hydrocephalus. They also often require chronic latex bladder catheters. Screening for acute latex sensitivity by history and testing should be routine in this population, or in any patient with a history of frequent procedures.

## Health Care Workers

The trend in published studies shows progressively higher incidences of latex sensitivity in health care workers. At present, approximately 70% of acute latex sensitivity reports to the FDA involve health care workers (8). The incidence of this problem among health care professionals has varied greatly, depending on study methods and the intensity of exposure in a given setting. Percentages of incidence range from 2.9% in general populations of hospital workers (15) to 35% in atopic intensive care workers (16). Most studies of persons with regular, but not daily, latex exposure report incidences in the range of 5% to 15%. Other findings of note in health care workers include a female-to-male preponderance of 35% to 23% for atopy, and 16% to 8% for workers with acute latex sensitivity (15). In this study, the control group of atopic patients without health care jobs had a 3.7% incidence of acute latex sensitivity, so the problem increases markedly with increased intensity of occupational exposure. For example, one study of anesthesiologists (17) found an incidence of symptomatic sensitization of 2.4%, but 10.1% were sensitized and asymptomatic. Twenty-four percent of the anesthesiologists also had a history of irritant contact dermatitis.

## Non–Health Care Occupations with Latex Exposure

Industries such as rubber manufacturing, consumer goods, and automotive tire manufacturing may place workers into frequent contact with latex, but there are far fewer reports regarding these patients.

## Atopic People

When studied in comparison with control subjects, allergic people consistently have higher percentages of sensitivity to latex, so they may be considered an at-risk population. The general population has an incidence of acute latex sensitivity varying between less than 1% and 6.7% (18,19). This surprisingly high level of sensitization in the general population may be due to inhalation of the black particles derived from breakdown of automobile tires that are a component of air pollution.

## LATEX AS AN ANTIGEN

Natural rubber latex is primarily a product of the rubber tree *(H. brasiliensis),* although the desert shrub, guayule

*(Parthenium argentatum),* and the common ornamental rubber plant *(Ficus elasticus)* also contain similar polymers. The latex cytosol contains polyisoprenes, lipids, phospholipids, and proteins. During processing, a number of other chemicals may be added, depending on the properties desired in the final product. These may include ammonia, sodium sulfate, thiurams, thiocarbamates, mercapto compounds, thioureas, phenylenediamine, and sulfur (13). Some of these chemicals are capable of becoming haptenic allergens.

Latex proteins, including the two major *Hevea* proteins, hevein and rubber elongation factor, are the primary allergy-inducing components of natural latex. To date, 7 sensitizing proteins have been identified (13), but there are at least 240 potentially antigenic compounds in processed latex. The protein content of latex gloves can vary up to a 1,000-fold among different lots, and 3,000-fold among gloves from different manufacturers. The allergen content is highest in powdered gloves, and lowest in powderless gloves that undergo washing and chlorination. This variation in protein content is part of the reason the FDA has yet to approve a latex antigen for skin testing, and also means that office preparations of latex allergen made by grinding gloves are subject to similar wide variations in potency.

In addition to latex proteins and chemical haptens, cornstarch glove powder also is a significant factor in latex allergy. Cornstarch molecules easily adsorb latex antigens, forming particles 3 μm in diameter. These particles are an ideal size to become airborne during the donning of gloves. A 3-μm particle, the size of small mold spores, is not easily filtered by the nose, resulting in a direct latex transportation onto the lung mucosa by inhalation (20). This fact makes a workplace where powdered gloves are used a potentially hazardous environment for a sensitized person (21). The high incidence of sensitization in health care workers is very easy to understand given the daily exposure for this population and the ease with which latex may come into contact with a mucosal surface through these airborne particles (22).

## ROUTES OF EXPOSURE

Latex antigen can come into contact with essentially any part of the body because of the many ways in which latex is used in medical, occupational, and home settings. Appendix A lists common latex contacts. Skin contact from gloves is the most frequent type of exposure, but mucosal contact also is common from examination gloves and condoms. Respiratory exposure is a frequent source of exposure because of the mechanism of transport by glove powder. Additional means of exposure include parenteral injection from rubber seals in vials and syringes, ingestion, and wound inoculation. Because the sensitization rates for the general population are lower than for health care workers, it would seem that occupational glove exposure is the primary factor associated with sensitization. However, in taking a latex exposure history, condom or diaphragm use and contact from clothing, toys, or sporting gear should not be neglected.

Aerosolized latex can cause a variety of symptoms, including rhinitis, sneezing, itching of the nose and eyes, bronchospasm, and even anaphylaxis. A strong association has been demonstrated between the development of allergy symptoms in hospital workers and airborne latex allergen concentrations in their workplace (23). The threshold for development of IgE antibodies to latex is 0.6 ng/m$^3$. Allergen levels may be reduced by a factor of ten by eliminating powdered gloves in favor of low-allergen powderless gloves (24).

Exposure of patients by parenteral routes occurs because needles are passed through rubber stoppers to obtain medications that are subsequently injected intravenously. For latex-sensitive patients, parenteral medications should be withdrawn only from glass ampoules or vials with silicone stoppers. Wound inoculation is another concern. One known case of anaphylaxis occurred in a patient who had undergone an extremity procedure and mounted a latex reaction when the tourniquet was let down, allowing antigen to be systemically absorbed.

Caring for patients with known acute latex sensitivity requires careful consideration in the choice of all materials with which they will come into contact. For the highly sensitive patient, even a slight contact could produce a significant reaction. Less sensitive patients may tolerate nominal exposures. Occupational exposure issues are a major concern, with few existing guidelines to steer the decision-making process.

## GLOVE TECHNOLOGY AND MANUFACTURING STANDARDS

Latex is the most frequently used substance for gloves because it is the most economical material possessing all the desirable properties. No one substance replaces latex rubber in every situation. The available alternatives are elastryn, neoprene, nitrile, polyurethane, silicone rubber, tactylon, vinyl, and synthetic polyisoprene rubber. Each material varies in elasticity, barrier qualities, strength, and tactile properties. What may be useful in one setting may not be useful in another. Natural latex gloves may be the best alternative if barrier qualities are important. HIV does not penetrate the pores of latex, but can penetrate the pores of certain other materials. Thus, a particular alternative material may not be appropriate if viral contamination is a concern. Even for natural latex, FDA standards for surgical gloves allow a failure rate of 2.5 per 100 gloves for barrier defects. Therefore, under high-risk circumstances, double gloving is prudent.

There also is an FDA requirement for identification of the latex content of medical equipment, but there is no current requirement to quantify the latex allergen level in gloves. Also, gloves no longer may be labeled *hypoallergenic* according to 1998 FDA regulations (25). The allergenicity of gloves varies depending on the method of manufacture of the specific product. There is wide variation in antigenicity even among glove lots, and there is variation in the presence of processing chemicals that may be associated with irritant contact dermatitis or with allergic sensitization. Ammoniation lowers the protein content. Chlorination, used in processing powderless gloves, makes surface proteins insoluble and much less likely to become detached from the glove, giving powderless gloves a significant safety advantage over powdered gloves.

Glove powder poses yet another factor in sensitivity. Most glove powder is cornstarch, which contains corn proteins that are known antigens. Its role as a latex antigen dispersal agent was previously discussed. Other materials such as talc, calcium carbonate, and oat powder also have been used, but oat powder also is allergenic, and talc may be contaminated with asbestos. Corn starch powder can result in sensitization by aerosol route or by direct contact. It can be transferred from the hands of the glove wearer to objects touched, such as a telephone or a tool. One worker even was found to have sensitized other family members by transporting latex powder particles to their home (26).

Endotoxin from bacterial contamination of latex medical products is yet another potential problem. Endotoxins are lipopolysaccharides from the cell wall of gram-negative bacteria, and can be a trigger for irritant contact dermatitis. Endotoxin also is known to enhance hypersensitivity reactions, and thus could be a potential sensitizer in both type IV and type I reactions. The highest concentration of endotoxin is found on the interior of powdered, nonsterile gloves, and can easily become aerosolized when donning the gloves (27). Powderless gloves again are a safer alternative because washing gloves does not significantly alleviate the exposure.

## MAKING THE DIAGNOSIS OF LATEX HYPERSENSITIVITY

Taking a good latex exposure history is the starting point for any patient. Given the clinician's understanding of significant risk factors, patients at risk can be identified and decisions regarding confirmatory testing made. Patients who have had allergic reactions of unknown cause, and who have no obvious contact with latex, should be asked to investigate their home and workplace for possible exposures. A questionnaire, such as the one depicted in Table 22.1, can be useful in screening patients for acute latex sensitivity risk factors. Many of the questions have been previously discussed, and the remaining ones are reviewed in this section.

One factor that may be revealed by the questions is a possible latex–fruit hypersensitivity syndrome. This syndrome is due to cross-reactivity for shared proteins present in both latex and certain fruits, as shown by radioallergosorbent test inhibition studies. The fruits with a high degree of latex cross-reactivity are banana, avocado, kiwi, chestnut, and rose family fruits such as cherry and peach (14). It has been suggested that this cross-reactivity is related to lysozyme, which is present in both latex and avocado (14). Prophyllin is another potentially cross-reactive antigen present in both latex and certain fruits. However, because there are multiple antigens involved in both acute latex sensitivity and fruit allergy, the cross-reactivity is likely to involve a variety of antigens. A history for reactivity to these fruits suggests the possibility of acute latex sensitivity, and patients with acute latex sensitivity should be counseled to avoid exposure to these foods.

In addition to exposure to possible risk factors, latex-allergic patients also may exhibit characteristic symptoms. For patients with type IV delayed sensitivity, the presenting symptoms may lead to suspicion of the diagnosis, such as repeated skin reactions in latex-exposed areas (e.g., the hands of health care workers). Differentiating irritant contact dermatitis from true type IV sensitivity may require patch testing with pieces of gloves with and without powder, as well as other historic contactants. A patch from a nonlatex glove can be used as a control (28). Reactions may begin in from 12 to 96 hours. For patients in whom the history is less clear-cut, also applying a standard battery of contact allergy patch tests may be helpful.

For patients with a history suggestive of type I immediate hypersensitivity, confirmation testing is appropriate. Patients with definite type IV sensitivity also should be tested to see if they are sensitized and at risk for type I reactions. Unfortunately, there is no latex extract approved in the United States for skin testing, although there are latex extracts available in Europe. Most clinicians currently use chopped gloves to prepare an extract for prick testing, despite the known variability in antigenic content and the presence of other of chemicals. The development of latex extracts suitable for skin testing has been the subject of much research, and current efforts center on the use of latex cytosol (29). There are several latex extracts under FDA consideration, and it may eventually be necessary to test patients for several different latex preparations, depending on the type of exposure they have.

In vitro latex testing is available in four different assays that are compared in a 1999 multicenter study (30). These tests are the Alastat (Diagnostic Products Corp., Los Angeles), which was the first to be FDA approved, the Coated Allergen Particle test (Pharmacia & Upjohn, Kalamazoo, MI), Immunolite, and HY-TEC (Hycor, Garden Grove,

## TABLE 22.1. QUESTIONNAIRE FOR LATEX HYPERSENSITIVITY

| Name: | Sex: | M | F |
|---|---|---|---|
| Have you ever been told by a doctor that you are allergic to latex or rubber? | | No | Yes |
| Have you ever had | | | |
|   Hay fever or allergy? | | No | Yes |
|   Asthma? | | No | Yes |
|   Eczema, skin reactions, or hives? | | No | Yes |
|   Lip or tongue swelling? | | No | Yes |
| Do you react to any foods? | | No | Yes |
| Which ones? | | | |
| Have you had a reaction to any of the following foods? | | No | Yes |
|   Bananas   Avocados   Kiwi fruit   Chestnuts   Peaches   Cherries | | | |

How many times have you had surgery?

Types of surgery:

Have you ever been catheterized to urinate?    No    Yes    Once     More than once

Do you work with products that contain latex or rubber?    No    Yes

If yes, how often?    Daily    Weekly    Not very often

Do you often wear clothing or use products that contain latex or rubber?    No    Yes

If yes, how often?    Daily    Weekly

| Have you ever had a reaction to any of the following latex objects? | | | |
|---|---|---|---|
|   Toy balloons | | No | Yes |
|   Condoms or a diaphragm | | No | Yes |
|   Gloves, during a dental, rectal, or vaginal exam? | | No | Yes |
|   While wearing rubber gloves? | | No | Yes |

If you have ever had a latex reaction, what kind of symptoms did you have?
  Runny nose    Watery eyes    Wheezing    Shortness of breath
  Hives or itching  where?
  Lip, tongue, or throat swelling
  Severe reaction where you needed emergency treatment

CA). These tests vary in their regional availability and in technical difficulty for the laboratory. For the clinician working without an FDA-approved extract, and uncertain about the effectiveness of an office-prepared glove extract, in vitro tests can be very useful. Of significant concern, any latex in vitro test can have a false-negativity rate as high as 30% because the test may not be able to detect an antigen to which a specific patient may be sensitized. For this reason, positive in vitro tests are more useful than negative tests.

Latex challenge testing also has been used in the research setting by having patients repeatedly blow up and inhale from a latex balloon, or by testing airborne latex exposure in a testing booth. Either test could provoke a serious respiratory reaction.

At this time, there is no standard for management of patients based on an in vitro or skin test score, but people with a suggestive history and positive test results should be counseled regarding latex avoidance. People with a suggestive history and a negative test should be told that their allergy status is uncertain, and that they should be cautious about latex exposure because their history suggests potential for reaction.

## MANAGEMENT OF LATEX-SENSITIVE PATIENTS

For a latex-sensitive patient, environmental control is the only treatment. Determining what will be an acceptable level of avoidance varies with the severity of each individual patient's symptoms. Complete control of all latex contacts can be a daunting challenge, and can even end a career. Desensitization to latex has been reported, but cannot be recommended at this time except as part of a formal research study. Once an FDA-approved extract is available, this may become a useful clinical option.

In general, patients with irritant contact dermatitis have more options than patients with type IV sensitivity. Type

I reactors need to be even more strict in their avoidance measures, and may not even be able to work in an environment where powdered gloves are in use. Because latex is a ubiquitous substance, particularly in medical occupations, this can be very challenging. Subsequent sections address the issue of latex control in the health care facility.

For people who must wear gloves, the use of glove liners, powderless gloves, and avoidance of petroleum-based emollients may suffice. Use of topical or oral steroids to control hand eczema, or of antihistamines to control nasal or ocular symptoms, is of value, but should not be depended on to prevent progression of latex sensitization. Changing to nonlatex gloves may be appropriate for certain circumstances, such as using vinyl examination gloves for barrier protection when infectious material is not being handled. The June 1997 National Institute for Occupational Safety and Health (NIOSH) alert entitled *Preventing Allergic Reactions to Natural Rubber Latex in the Workplace* recommended the use of nonlatex gloves for all activities that do not involve contact with potentially infectious materials (31). Nonlatex gloves are especially helpful for patients who experience severe symptoms on respiratory exposure. Because nonlatex gloves can be expensive, latex-sensitive employees can find themselves at odds with management over the issue of nonlatex glove availability. Clinicians may be called on to assist with these decisions because use of resources may be a significant issue. Determining suitable alternatives for the patient and accurately assessing the type of reaction can be of great benefit to both employer and patient. Often, experimentation with various alternatives is warranted, provided the patient is not experiencing life-threatening anaphylaxis.

When highly sensitive patients do contact latex, their management becomes urgent or emergent. Acute type I reactions are treated based on the location, severity, rapidity of onset, and duration of symptoms. Mild reactions, particularly rhinitis and conjunctivitis, may be treated as any other IgE-mediated sensitivity, with antihistamines, decongestants, mast cell stabilizers, and topical or oral steroids. Urticaria and pruritus may respond better to complete blockade with antihistamines that block both type 1 ($H_1$) and type 2 ($H_2$) histamine receptors. Oral steroids should be used acutely whenever symptom severity or abruptness of onset raises concern about a possible subsequent late-phase reaction.

Any reaction involving the airway must be aggressively managed, using all previously mentioned forms of treatment, as well as inhaled bronchodilators, epinephrine, and, if indicated, oxygen and intubation or tracheotomy. If anaphylaxis develops, it should be treated using a previously selected protocol. The important difference between treating anaphylaxis due to latex and anaphylaxis due to inhalants or foods is that the latex source may still be present, and must be removed. This may mean moving the patient to an area with the cleanest air possible, and, because of aerosolized latex present in the air, that may not be indoors

in the treating medical facility. After successful treatment of the reaction, documentation of the details, including identification of the source of latex, is important and should become a part of the patient's permanent clinical record.

## MANAGEMENT OF HEALTH CARE WORKERS WITH ACUTE LATEX SENSITIVITY

Glove use is a ubiquitous latex exposure for health care workers, and management of the problem centers around glove use. There are other latex sources, but they are more easily avoided. Ideally, health care workers will have access to nonlatex gloves, but a variety of products are necessary because differing barrier qualities and tactile properties may favor selection of one product over another in a given situation. Working knowledge of the porosity of various materials, and the size of the infectious agents that must be excluded, is essential. Because latex has the smallest pore size and best resistance to viral penetration, high-quality powderless latex gloves are the safest and best choice for general use in medical facilities. Powdered gloves raise the latex concentration ten times above that of a room where powderless gloves are in use (24). Because some workers are not able to remain in areas where powdered gloves are in use, and because glove powder is a major means for producing new latex sensitivities, the goal should be to discourage, and then to eliminate powdered glove use. After glove powder is eliminated, environmental surfaces, including walls and ceilings, may need to be cleaned. The transport of latex particles on clothing is another concern that also is substantially eliminated by the change to powderless gloves. The complete NIOSH recommendations for latex control are listed in Appendix B.

For sensitized people who continue to react despite use of all practical precautions, difficult choices may have to be made. A change in work location may be a possibility, or changes in exposure may be accomplished by changing work shift hours. Each case comes down to whether a person can be accommodated cost effectively and safely in his or her work environment. Disability related to acute latex sensitivity is an increasingly important issue facing health care facilities and health care workers. For a discussion from the perspective of professionals struggling to maintain their careers, see articles by Greer (32) and Bartlett (33).

Each health care facility should develop its own latex control policy to protect both employees and patients. Appendix C lists sources of information helpful in developing latex policies. As physicians who may have input in health care facility decisions, our goal should be a policy of protecting everyone at risk for latex allergy. Latex control should incorporate physician, nursing, allied health, housekeeping, and administrative input. Important issues include glove selection and use, protocols for managing patients and employees with acute latex sensitivity, reporting reactions to latex, and educational programs for all people who are exposed to latex. An article by Kim et al. offers useful advice for developing these policies (34). For the individual physician's office, minor changes such as making available nonlatex gloves and a change to powderless gloves may be sufficient. However, if the physician has a practice with many high-risk or acutely sensitized patients, or one or more latex-sensitive employees, hospital-level precautions may be required.

## MANAGEMENT OF THE LATEX-SENSITIVE PATIENT IN A HEALTH CARE FACILITY

Taking a history for latex allergy must become a routine part of the medical interview when a patient will be cared for in a health care facility. Any patient who might be exposed to latex in the course of treatment or a procedure could potentially be injured by a latex reaction. For example, the reported incidence of latex anaphylaxis during general anesthesia increased from 0.5% in 1989 to 12.5% 2 years later (13). For patients with no prior history of atopy, the probability of reaction is low, but not zero, because of the substantial incidence of latex allergy in the general population (18,19).

Patients who have a history of a documented reaction or positive laboratory or skin test results must be managed with complete latex avoidance (13). Because latex is ubiquitous in the medical environment, latex control should be addressed by a multidisciplinary task force so that effective policies will be in place to protect patients.

Latex-sensitive patients should be treated carefully to minimize their exposure to latex. For patients on a medical ward, appropriate latex-free materials and an isolated, cleaned room are appropriate, with suitable signage to direct staff not to bring latex into the area. The patient also should be identified by a bracelet or other system. Patients who undergo procedures are a greater challenge because the routes of exposure are increased by the nature of invasive procedures.

Preparation of an operating room for a latex-sensitive patient should be the subject of a protocol at every facility. For facilities with a large population of latex-sensitized patients, maintaining a designated latex-free operating room may be possible. Before any planned procedure, all latex-containing materials should be removed from the room, and the floors, walls, ceilings, fixtures, and equipment cleaned. A latex-free anesthesia machine with disposable plastic tubing and mask should be brought in, and the room should be marked with appropriate signs to prevent reintroduction of latex into the area. Scheduling a latex-sensitive patient as the first case of the morning, when the operating and recovery area are cleanest and latex aerosol levels are at their lowest, is ideal. Use of air filtration devices in the operating room is also encouraged.

A latex-free supply cart should be in the room at all times, and should contain suitable materials to perform the tasks that the patient requires. Appendix D lists typical cart contents. Additional latex-free products could be kept in a designated area in central supply, with a list on the operating room cart of items that can be brought in, if needed. Because respiratory exposure poses a high risk, and powderless gloves decrease airborne latex levels so greatly, when infection protection is critical, only powderless latex gloves should be used by the scrub team and surgeons, and they should be completely covered by nonlatex gloves. All surgical instruments should be checked for rubber guards or protectors, and if found, those instruments should be rewashed and resterilized without the rubber. Finally, all applied or invasive monitors, devices, tubes, and catheters should be double checked to be certain they are not latex.

Allergy premedication of the latex-sensitive person has been debated in the anesthesia literature (13). The current prevailing thought is to avoid use of medication until there are signs of a reaction. Medications that might be useful, if pretreatment is the preferred option, are diphenhydramine or other $H_1$ antihistamines, ranitidine or other $H_2$ antihistamines, and steroids. There also is debate over whether a latex-sensitive patient may receive medication drawn from a vial with a rubber stopper (13). One patient was reported to have a reaction, and the only possible source was the rubber stopper of the medication vial. Other studies have shown no latex contamination until a stopper had been penetrated over 40 times. Prudence would dictate that medications preferentially be taken from glass ampoules or silicone-stoppered vials.

## CONCLUSION

Acute latex sensitivity is a condition with which every physician should be familiar. In the short space of a decade, it was transformed from a bit of esoterica, of interest to only a few allergists, to a problem that every health care facility must address with careful policy. Because the incidence of atopy in the general population is increasing, and latex products continue to proliferate, the problem is likely only to become one of greater importance in the coming years.

The reason for the emergence of latex sensitivity has been the subject of some speculation. Latex has excellent properties of strength, durability, elasticity, and deformability, and may be molded into many useful shapes. Alternative materials do not have this combination of properties, and almost always are more expensive to produce. Consequently, uses for latex have continued to expand, and most people in industrialized nations now come into regular contact with rubber products. Several authors have mentioned that the low quality of latex gloves used by medical and emergency personnel, at a time when gloves were in short supply, may have contributed to the current problem. Given the persisting rise in latex allergy, despite current high-quality gloves, this cannot be the only explanation. The recent increase in condom use certainly may have played a role, and the black particulate residue from automobile tires that is a universal component of air pollution may help explain why the general population also is becoming sensitized.

The one fact that is certain is that frequency of latex exposure strongly correlates with the incidence of sensitivity in a specific population. In view of this observation, attempting to decrease the amount of latex in all environments would be a logical preventive public health measure. Labeling of products containing latex is an another important issue that can be addressed by governments, and will assist those attempting to avoid latex exposure. Also, every medical or industrial facility where latex is used needs to consider plans to decrease latex exposure, and each will be faced with issues of compliance and cost. Exposure in the workplace will continue to be an issue for debate in the health care, legal, and insurance arenas.

Avoidance of latex exposure is, at present, still the only effective treatment for latex sensitivity. The lack of an approved extract for skin testing and possible desensitization, after years of attempts, continues to handicap the allergist seeking to confirm the diagnosis, and makes desensitization unavailable. Research in this area is essential until a satisfactory extract is available. It is likely that acute latex sensitivity will continue to be a problem confronting the clinician managing allergic patients.

## APPENDIX A. COMMON ITEMS THAT MIGHT CONTAIN LATEX

### Home Setting

    Automobile tires
    Condoms
    Toys
    Balloons
    Gloves
    Shoes
    Packaging material
    Home construction materials such as seals or thresholds
    Sporting and camping supplies

### Medical Setting

    Gloves, both sterile and examination
    Finger cots
    Intravenous supplies with latex injection ports
    Medication pumps
    Medication vials with rubber stoppers
    Respiratory equipment such as masks or bags, airways, or endotracheal tubes
    Catheters, both indwelling and condom style

    Surgical garb, such as disposable hats, masks, and shoe covers
    Dental dams, bite blocks, and teeth protectors
    Bulb syringe
    Tourniquets
    Stethoscope tubing
    Disposable syringe plunger
    Dressings
    Adhesive tape
    Blood pressure cuffs
    Electrode pads
    Heating pads

## APPENDIX B. NIOSH RECOMMENDATIONS FOR PREVENTING LATEX ALLERGY IN THE WORKPLACE

### Employers

Latex allergy can be prevented only if there are policies to protect personnel from undue latex exposures. NIOSH recommends that employers take the following steps to protect workers from latex exposure and allergy in the workplace:

1. Provide workers with nonlatex gloves to use when there is little potential for contact with infectious materials (for example, in the food service industry)
2. Appropriate barrier protection is necessary when handling infectious materials (CDC 1987). If latex gloves are chosen, provide reduced-protein, powder-free gloves to protect workers from infectious materials.
3. Ensure that workers use good housekeeping practices to remove latex-containing dust from the workplace.
4. Provide workers with education programs and training materials about latex allergy.
5. Periodically screen high-risk workers for latex allergy symptoms. Detecting symptoms early and removing symptomatic workers from latex exposure are essential for preventing long-term health effects.
6. Evaluate current prevention strategies whenever a worker is diagnosed with latex allergy.

### Workers

Workers should take the following steps to protect themselves from latex exposure and allergy in the workplace:

1. Use nonlatex gloves for activities that are not likely to involve contact with infectious materials (food preparation, routine housekeeping, maintenance, etc.)
2. Appropriate barrier protection is necessary when handling infectious materials. If you choose latex, use powder-free gloves with reduced protein content: Such gloves reduce exposures to latex protein and thus reduce the risk of latex allergy (although symptoms may still

occur in some workers). Latex gloves labeled as "hypoallergenic" do not reduce the risk of latex allergy. However, they may reduce reactions to chemical additives in the latex (allergic contact dermatitis).

3. Use appropriate work practices to reduce the chance of reactions to latex: When wearing latex gloves, do not use oil-based hand creams or lotions (which can cause glove deterioration) unless they have been shown to reduce latex-related problems and maintain glove barrier protection. After removing latex gloves, wash hands with a mild soap and dry thoroughly. Use good housekeeping practices to remove latex-containing dust from the workplace.

4. Take advantage of all latex allergy education and training programs: Become familiar with procedures for preventing latex allergy. Learn to recognize the symptoms of latex allergy: skin rashes; hives; flushing; itching; nasal, eye or sinus symptoms; asthma; and shock.

5. If you develop symptoms of latex allergy, avoid direct contact with latex gloves and other latex-containing products until you can see a physician experienced in treating latex allergy.

6. For individuals with latex allergy, consult your physician regarding the following precautions: Avoid contact with latex gloves and other latex-containing products. Avoid areas where you might inhale the powder from latex gloves worn by other workers. Tell your employer and health care providers (physicians, nurses, dentists, etc.) that you have latex allergy. Wear a medical alert bracelet.

7. Carefully follow your physician's instructions for dealing with allergic reactions to latex.

From Department of Health and Human Services (DHHS) National Institute of Occupational Safety and Health (NIOSH). *NIOSH alert: preventing allergic reactions to natural rubber latex.* DHHS (NIOSH) publication no. 97-135. Washington, DC: Department of Health and Human Services, 1997.

## APPENDIX C. SOURCES OF ASSISTANCE IN DEVELOPING YOUR OWN LATEX POLICY

U.S. Food and Drug Administration (FDA)
http://www.fda.gov/

National Institute for Occupational Safety and Health (NIOSH)
http://www.cdc.gov/niosh/homepage.html

Centers for Disease Control and Prevention (CDC)
http://www.cdc.gov

American Academy of Allergy, Asthma and Immunology (AAAAI)
http://www.allergy.mcg.edu/physicians/latex.html

American Academy of Dermatology (AAD)
http://www.aad.org

Spina Bifida Association of America
4590 MacArthur Blvd., N.W. Suite 250
Washington D.C. 20007-4226
800-621-3141
FAX 202-944-3295
Email: SBAA@SBAA.org
http://www.sbaa.org

A.L.E.R.T., Inc. (American Latex Allergy Association)
P.O. Box 13930
Milwaukee, WI 53213-0930
http://www.execpc.com/~alert

FLARE (Foundation for Latex Allergy Research & Education)
5100 E. Anaheim Road
Long Beach, CA 90815
Telephone: 310-597-4304
FAX: 310-494-0250
http://www.FLARE.org/

American Society of Anesthesiologists (ASA)
520 N. Northwest Highway
Park Ridge, IL 60068-2573
847-825-5586
FAX 847-825-1692
mail@ASAhq.org

## APPENDIX D. CONTENTS OF A LATEX-FREE CART

Nonlatex gloves, several styles and materials, sterile and exam
Latex-free intravenous (IV) tubing and syringes
Needles
Polyvinyl chloride (PVC) IV tubing
Stopcocks
Alcohol wipes
Latex-free tape and tourniquets
Thermometer—esophageal
Disposable blood pressure cuffs
Vinyl stethoscope
Sterile cast padding
Latex-free electrocardiograph electrodes
Latex-free room signs
Nonlatex ambu-bag and respiratory supplies
Nasal cannula and tubing
PVC endotracheal tubes and oral airways
Medications for emergency use in glass ampoules
Silicone Foley catheter
Epidural and spinal trays
PVC suction catheters
Anesthesia circuits with latex-free bag and tubing
Anesthesia medications in glass ampoules
Reference guide for latex-free materials
Policy manual for latex-sensitive patients

# REFERENCES

1. Downing J. Dermatitis from rubber gloves. *N Engl J Med* 1933; 208:196–198.
2. Rhodes EL, Warner J. Contact eczema follow up study. *Br J Dermatol* 1996;78:640–644.
3. Centers for Disease Control. Recommendations for prevention of HIV transmission in health care settings. *MMWR Morb Mortal Wkly Rep* 1987;36[Suppl 2S]:1S–18S.
4. Center for Devices and Radiological Health. *Medical glove powder report.* Washington, DC. 1997:15.
5. Slater JE. Rubber anaphylaxis. *N Engl J Med* 1989;320: 1126–1130.
6. Leynadier F, Pecquet C, Dry J. Anaphylaxis to latex during surgery. *Anaesthesia* 1989;44:547–550.
7. Ownby DR, Tomlanovich M, Sammons N, et al. Anaphylaxis associated with latex allergy during barium enema examinations. *AJR Am J Roentgenol* 1991;1566:903–908.
8. U.S. Food and Drug Administration. Mandatory reporting database. www.fda.gov. October 1997.
9. Levy DA. Report on the International Latex Conference: sensitivity to latex in medical devices. Baltimore, MD, Nov. 5–7. *Allergy* 1993:48[Suppl]:1–9.
10. Del Savio B, Sheretz EF. Is allergic contact dermatitis being overlooked? *Arch Fam Med* 1994;3:537–543.
11. Heese A, Von Hintzenstern J, Peters KP, et al. Allergic and irritant reactions to rubber gloves in medical health services: spectrum, diagnostic approach, and therapy. *J Am Acad Dermatol* 1991;25:831–839.
12. Tarlo SM, Sussman GL, Holness L. Latex sensitivity in dental staff. *J Allergy Clin Immunol* 1997;73:309–314.
13. American Society of Anesthesiologists. Natural rubber latex allergy: considerations for anesthesiologists. www.asahq.org/ProfInfo/latexallergy.html.
14. Eseverri JL, Botey J, et al. Prevalence of allergy to latex in the pediatric population. *Allergol Immunopathol (Madr)* 1999;27(3): 133–140.
15. Liss GM, Sussman GI, et al. Latex allergy: epidemiology study of 1,351 hospital workers. *Occup Environ Med* 1997;54:335–342.
16. Watts DN, Jacobs RR, et al. An evaluation of the prevalence of latex sensitivity among atopic and non-atopic intensive care workers. *Am J Ind Med* 1998;34:359–363.
17. Brown RH, Schauble JF, Hamilton JG. Prevalence of latex allergy among anesthesiologists. *Anesthesiology* 1998;89:292–299.
18. Moneret-Vautrin DA, Beaudouin E, Widmer S, et al. Prospective study of risk factors in natural rubber latex hypersensitivity. *J Allergy Clin Immunol* 1993;92:668–677.
19. Lebenbom-Mansour MH, Oesterle JR, Ownby DR, et al. The incidence of latex sensitivity in ambulatory patients: a correlation of historical factors with positive serum immunoglobulin E levels. *Anesth Analg* 1997;85:44–49.
20. Vandesplas O, Delwiche JP, Depelchin S, et al. Latex gloves with a lower protein content reduce bronchial reactions in subjects with occupational asthma. *Am J Respir Crit Care Med* 1995;151: 887–891.
21. Beezhold D, Beck WC. Surgical glove powders bind latex antigens. *Arch Surg* 1992;127:1354–1357.
22. Tomazic VJ, Shampaine EL, Lamanna A, et al. Cornstarch powder on latex products as an allergen carrier. *J Allergy Clin Immunol* 1994;93:751–758.
23. Baur X, Chen Z, Allmers H. Can a threshold limit for natural rubber latex airborne allergens be defined? *J Allergy Clin Immunol* 1998;101:24–27.
24. Heilman DK, Jones RT, Swanson MC, et al. A prospective, controlled study showing that rubber gloves are the major contributor to latex aeroallergen levels in the operating room. *J Allergy Clin Immunol* 1996;98:325–330.
25. Meyer KK, Beezhold DH. Latex allergy: how safe are your gloves? *Am J Respir Crit Care Med* 1997;82:13–15.
26. Karanathasis P, Cooper A, Zhou K, et al. Indirect latex contact causes urticaria/anaphylaxis. *Ann Allergy* 1993;71:526–528.
27. Williams PB, Halsey JF. Endotoxin as a factor in adverse reactions to latex gloves. *Ann Allergy Asthma Immunol* 1997;79:303–310.
28. Turjanmaa K, Reunala T, Rasanen L. Comparison of diagnostic methods in latex surgical glove contact urticaria. *Contact Dermatitis* 1988;19:241–247.
29. Hamilton RG, Adkinson NF Jr. Diagnosis of natural rubber latex allergy: multicenter latex skin testing efficacy study: Multicenter Latex Skin Testing Study Task Force. *J Allergy Clin Immunol* 1998;102:482–490.
30. Hamilton RG, Biagini RE, Krieg EF. Diagnostic performance of Food and Drug Administration–cleared serologic assays for natural rubber latex-specific IgE antibody: the Multi-Center Latex Skin Testing Study Task Force. *J Allergy Clin Immunol* 1999;103:925–930.
31. Department of Health and Human Services (DHHS), National Institute of Occupational Safety and Health (NIOSH). *NIOSH alert: preventing allergic reactions to natural rubber latex.* DHHS (NIOSH) publication no. 97-135. Washington, DC: U.S. Department of Health and Human Services, 1997.
32. Greer S. Living and working with latex allergies: personal perspectives from a nurse. *Semin Periop Nurs* 1998;7:254–255.
33. Bartlett J. Latex sensitivity: a public health care challenge. *J Community Health Nurs* 1998;15:193–204.
34. Kim KT, Graves PB, Safadi GS, et al. Implementation recommendations for making health care facilities latex safe. *AORN J* 1998;67:615–632.

# CHEMICAL TOXICITY AND CHEMICAL SENSITIVITY

## BRUCE R. GORDON

Practicing allergists are now seeing patients with chemical sensitivity symptoms much more frequently than in past decades. However, unlike patients seen in emergency departments or occupational medicine clinics, most patients with chemical sensitivity seen in the allergy office are not acutely ill, and the chemical origin of their symptoms is not always obvious. Recognition that chemical exposure is an issue requires specific questioning and testing and, above all, the suspicion that chemicals might be playing a role. This chapter focuses on what is known about the biochemistry and immunology of exogenous chemicals in the body, and how these processes can become pathologic and cause toxic or allergic chemical sensitivity (CS) symptoms. Also discussed is how extremely low levels of environmental chemicals may potentially cause multiple chemical sensitivities (MCS). Learning how to recognize, diagnose, and treat allergy patients who have had significant chemical exposure also is discussed.

## WHY CHEMICAL SENSITIVITY EXISTS

Metabolism has been shaped by the environment. Living things have always existed in a sea of chemicals. The Precambrian primordial ocean teemed with exotic chemicals synthesized by geologic and atmospheric processes. As life evolved in this chemical ocean, the need to use these environmental chemicals for food required organisms to develop a complex biochemistry. Ultimately, primitive cells internalized the ocean, its chemicals, and their reactions as internal bodily fluids, the cytoplasm. Internally, compartmentalized by cell membranes, the biochemical reactions evolved to greater efficiency and coordination, eventually developing feedback loops and homeostasis. Sequestration or elimination of useless or dangerous chemicals, disposal and detoxifi-

cation, was an inevitable consequence of this evolving metabolism. Later, mobile animals began to prey on small or sessile forms, and the prey responded by developing chemical defenses, modifying and expanding the types of chemicals their biochemistry could produce. Predators either learned to avoid eating these creatures or evolved means to detoxify them, starting an evolutionary struggle that continues to this day. For these reasons, foods are the most chemically complex substances to which living creatures are commonly exposed. For example, each species of food plant has been estimated to contain over 500,000 different biochemicals [1]. All of these ingested chemicals, some of them toxic, must be either metabolized, stored, or excreted. All living organisms today have inherited the necessary biochemical capability to deal with this enormous variety of natural environmental chemicals.

Technology, however, has changed the environment. For over a billion years, living creatures were able effectively to handle these natural chemicals, and life flourished. Even during the Pleistocene ice age, as primitive human technology released combustion products from smoky fires, these chemicals were not unique, and could be detoxified by living organisms. It is only with the industrial revolution of the past few centuries that both truly novel chemicals, and enormous quantities of previously rare chemicals, are now entering the environment, and straining the natural detoxifying systems of living creatures. Since the First World War, the pace of chemical industry has accelerated, so that at present, with over 35,000 chemicals already in common use, approximately 3,000 new chemicals are being introduced each year [2]. In just the United States, this amounts to over 500 billion pounds, or approximately 1 ton of chemicals produced per person per year. It is little wonder, then, that sensitivity to chemicals is becoming a significant medical problem.

These novel chemicals are known as *xenobiotics,* organic molecules that are foreign to the human body. Currently, the definition of a xenobiotic substance includes all foreign chemicals, whether organic, inorganic, or organometallic. Xenobiotics are of concern because people are increasingly

**B. R. Gordon:** Department of Otology and Laryngology, Harvard University, Cambridge; Associate Surgeon, Massachusetts Eye and Ear Infirmary, Boston; Chief of Otolaryngology, Cape Cod Hospital, Hyannis, Massachusetts.

**TABLE 23.1. OPPORTUNITIES FOR CHEMICAL CONTAMINATION OF FOOD**

Containers, cookware (oils, plastics, metals)
Pesticides, fungicides
Transportation, cooking (fuel exhausts)
Ripening agents
Waxing
Bleaching
Sweeteners, flavorings, colorings
Preservatives, antibiotics
Smoking, grilling, fat frying (free radicals)
Emulsifiers, thickeners
Foaming/antifoaming agents
Solvent extraction
Irradiation

Modified from Rea WJ. *Chemical sensitivity,* vol II: *Sources of total body load.* Boca Raton, FL: Lewis Publishers, 1994:601.

exposed to these molecules, and have no choice in the matter. Xenobiotics pervade our environment: they are detectable in all ecologic niches from the land to the sea, and from the poles to the tropics. They are transported by air and water, through food (Table 23.1), and by all mobile living things.

Although evolution has provided us with significant ability to detoxify and excrete substances that are nonnutritive and potentially harmful, this capacity is not infinite. Furthermore, detoxification has metabolic costs and consequences, and can lead to disease even when we are capable of carrying it out. Finally, some xenobiotics, particularly synthetic ones, are impervious to our attempts to detoxify or excrete them, and persist in the body. Some of these have known harmful effects, and some interact synergistically, causing harm at lower concentrations than a single chemical,

alone, is capable of. But most xenobiotics simply have not been studied, either singly or in combinations. It is unlikely that storage of even nonreactive xenobiotics will be entirely without consequences: many are stored in cell membranes, where they may influence such critical functions as membrane fluidity and permeability. The following discussion surveys the categories of xenobiotics to which we are normally exposed, and briefly summarizes common ways in which they are encountered.

## Inorganic and Organometallic Xenobiotics

One major inorganic xenobiotic source is smog. Because there is global air circulation, everyone ultimately is exposed to every airborne pollutant, but individual doses vary. For example, the global effect of increasing pollution due to the industrial revolution can be clearly seen in data from polar ice core analyses (3). Global wind circulation carries pollutants to the poles, where it precipitates with snow and becomes compacted into the ice (Fig. 23.1). In the example shown, before approximately 1940, lead was primarily released into the atmosphere by ore smelting in the northern hemisphere. After 1940, most of the atmospheric lead in both hemispheres was generated from leaded gasoline. Levels of lead in Antarctica since 1940 are approximately one tenth of those in Greenland because most lead use is in the northern hemisphere, and substantial amounts of lead particles precipitate before crossing the equator. Smog contains many other components: carbon monoxide, nitrogen oxides, sulfur oxides, ozone, and particulates such as diesel exhaust, smoke, and minerals. Carbon monoxide prevents oxygen transport by hemoglobin, but also inactivates the cytochrome oxidase detoxification system. Nitrogen oxides, sulfur oxides, and ozone consume antioxidants, thus deplet-

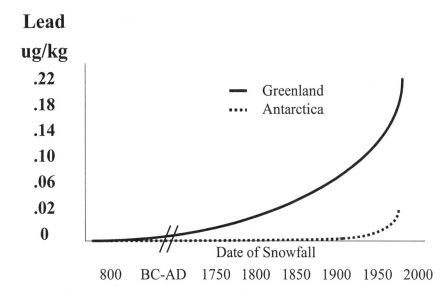

**FIG. 23.1.** Airborne lead pollution in polar ice caps.

ing glutathione and decreasing the ability to conjugate and excrete chemicals. These gases also are synergistic with allergens in causing respiratory tract inflammation. Ozone both is immunosuppressive and inactivates the mixed-function oxidase detoxification system. Particulates are very complex, but are known to contain potent carcinogens and to initiate respiratory inflammation. Recently, diesel exhaust particles also have been found to stimulate allergic hypersensitivity.

Halogens and halogen oxides are reactive, strong oxidizers found in air and water. Contact with halogens is ubiquitous because of their usefulness in water sterilization and in industry. Significant amounts of these elements often are inhaled because of outgassing from treated water (showers, pools, and hot tubs). Fluoride is a potent enzyme inhibitor, and all halogens are respiratory irritants and consume antioxidants. Halogens may react with organic compounds in water, forming toxic organochlorines and other similar molecules (see later). Detoxification capacity for halogens can be overwhelmed by significant or prolonged exposures.

Elemental metal and organometallic xenobiotics also are significant problems, particularly lead, which is widely distributed in air, soil, and the domestic environment. Lead, as well as other metals, also may be found in water, or can be bioconcentrated by the food chain, leading to substantial amounts in food. Lead inactivates many key enzymes, causing neurologic and hematologic injury. Lead, mercury, cadmium, and many other heavy metals share the ability to cause a major block in xenobiotic excretion by inhibition of glutathione recycling. Toxic metals also have individual inhibitory effects on specific enzymes and organs. Organic metals such as methyl mercury, butyl tin, and tetraethyl lead are especially hazardous because they are lipophilic, and very well absorbed.

## Organic Xenobiotics

Over 2 million organic compounds are currently known, and over 60,000 are produced on an industrial scale. Organic xenobiotics often are volatile, easily absorbed, and persistent in the body. There are two major routes of exposure: as volatile chemicals in the air, or as nonvolatile chemicals in water and food. In urban areas, quantities of volatile synthetic organic chemicals may equal or exceed levels of naturally occurring terpenes and methane. Even in rural areas, as much as 40% of the organic components of air are synthetic (Table 23.2). Although many volatile organic xenobiotics are present in low concentrations in outside air, because of their high lipid solubility, they are efficiently trapped in cell membranes on inhalation. In addition, these compounds often are present in considerably higher concentrations in indoor air, close to the source of evaporation or outgassing.

Nonvolatile xenobiotics include well known pollutants: pesticides like dichlorodiphenyltrichloroethane (DDT), and electrical insulators like polychlorinated biphenyls (PCBs).

### TABLE 23.2. MAJOR SOURCES OF OUTDOOR AIR POLLUTION, IN ORDER OF IMPORTANCE

**Synthetic**
1. Transportation (vehicles)
2. Fixed combustion sources (factories, power plants, homes)
3. Industrial processes (ore extraction, manufacturing)
4. Solid waste disposal
5. Chemical disposal
6. Agricultural spraying

**Both synthetic and natural**
7. Forest fires

**Natural**
8. Methane outgassing
9. Release of plant terpenes
10. Volcanoes

Modified from Rea WJ. *Chemical sensitivity*, vol II: *Sources of total body load.* Boca Raton, FL: Lewis Publishers, 1994:641.

These nonvolatile chemicals are concentrated in areas of use, like farms and industrial areas, but become incorporated into and are disseminated by the food chain. Because organic xenobiotics of all degrees of volatility are both plentiful and come into unavoidable contact with us, individual body burdens may be large enough to overload some individuals' detoxification systems.

Chemical industry is primarily based on extraction from fossil fuels, with some input from harvesting or farming of living plants. Petroleum, natural gas, and coal contain hundreds of hydrocarbons ranging in complexity from methane, to benzene, to giant polycyclic ring compounds found in tars. Small proportions of these petrochemicals, those that contain oxygen, sulfur, or nitrogen, normally are removed before use as either fuel or chemical feedstock. During the mining, drilling, transport, refining, and ultimate use of petrochemicals, significant quantities are released into the air. Even when venting and burning of undesired volatiles is prevented, and when care is taken to reduce evaporation and leakage, the sheer size of the petrochemical industry still guarantees that substantial amounts of petrochemicals will become airborne. Similar problems of escape into the environment exist for all of the industrial chemicals that are derived in enormous quantities from basic petrochemicals.

Petrochemicals containing only hydrogen and carbon are relatively nonreactive and are modified by manufacturers to increase their reactivity and hence their potential usefulness for synthesis of other compounds. Extracting hydrogen to make unsaturated molecules, or adding reactive functional groups like halogens, alcohols, and acids, produces a second, relatively small group, the industrial intermediate chemicals (Table 23.3). Examples are acetylene, methanol, acetic acid, and phthalic anhydride. These intermediates, like the primary petrochemicals, are produced in tens, hundreds, or

**TABLE 23.3. ORGANIC XENOBIOTIC CATEGORIES AND TYPICAL TOXIC BIOLOGIC EFFECTS**

| Category | Typical Examples | Major Biologic Effects |
|---|---|---|
| **Volatile aliphatic** | | |
| Hydrocarbons | Propane, n-hexane | Narcosis, irritant |
| Unsaturated | Ethylene, acetylene | Cross-linking |
| Amines | Hydrazine, butylamine | Narcosis, skin toxic |
| Oxygenated | Ethyl alcohol, formaldehyde | Narcosis, irritant, cross-linking |
| Chlorinated | Vinyl chloride | Narcosis, hepatotoxic, carcinogenic |
| Brominated | Bromoform | Hepatotoxic, spermicidal |
| **Volatile aromatic** | | |
| Hydrocarbons | Benzene, styrene | Narcosis, marrow toxic, carcinogenic, neurotoxic |
| Chlorinated | Hexachlorophene | Chloracne, neurotoxic, mutagenic, carcinogenic, immune suppressant |
| Oxygenated | Phthalates, phenol | Mutagenic, hepatotoxic, spermicidal |
| Nitrogenous | Aniline, toluidine | Mutagenic, carcinogenic |
| **Nonvolatile polyaromatic** | | |
| Hydrocarbons | Napthalene, benzopyrenes, | Carcinogenic |
| Halogenated | Polychlorinated biphenyls (PCBs), chlordane, dichlorodiphenyl-trichloroethane (DDT) | Alter hormone metabolism |
| Nitrogenous | Napthylamine, quinolines | Carcinogenic, hepatotoxic |
| **Other nonvolatile organics** | | |
| Detergents and glycols | Sodium dodecyl sulfate | Sensitizers |
| Polymers | Plastics, rubber, silicones | Release toxic or allergic monomers |

thousands of ton quantities, and also inevitably escape to the environment. Industrial intermediate chemicals ultimately are used to produce finished consumer products, including solvents, paints, rubbers, detergents, synthetic fibers, and various plastics. Many of these final products also are produced in huge quantities, and pollution from their manufacture occurs not only at the plant, but also by outgassing during transport, storage, and at the point of ultimate use (home, vehicle, or office). Because of outgassing, combined with tight, energy-efficient construction, indoor air often is more heavily polluted with chemicals than is outside air.

## MECHANISMS OF CHEMICAL INJURY

### Acute Poisoning

Approximately 3,000 of the millions of known chemicals are responsible for most of the acute reactions due to toxic overexposure (4). A few of these (ethanol, aspirin, acetaminophen) are common household products, whereas others (cyanides, chromates, organophosphate insecticides) usually are contacted in industrial or agricultural settings. Acute injury arises when the body has no effective defense because there has been no evolutionary exposure to the substance, such as in contact with corrosive white phosphorus. Much more commonly, however, injury occurs simply from the overwhelming of normal body defenses by the large quantity of chemical involved. For example, the small amounts of organic cyanides contained in fruits are easily detoxified, but being drenched with an industrial cyanide solution is beyond the capacity of human detoxifying systems to cope with. Similar examples are found with many common chemical poisons, from ethanol to organophosphate insecticides.

The type of acute chemical injury may range from gross tissue destruction by protein denaturation (phosphorus, acids, alkalis), to selective inactivation of key enzymes or structural components (organophosphate insecticides, heavy metals, cyanides). Activation of or injury to the immune system also may occur, such as in the anaphylactoid reactions that occur after exposure to certain drugs (radiocontrast agents, narcotics), or the cytolysis due to cell-specific toxins (pokeweed mitogen, chloramphenicol). One common form of injury, triggered by many chemicals, including acetaminophen, occurs from uncontrolled oxidation and free radical production. During this oxidative injury, reactive chemical intermediates are formed in a self-perpetuating chain reaction, some of which react immediately, chemically altering cellular macromolecules or causing cross-linking between macromolecules. Some of the reactive byproducts (epoxides and aldehydes) can even travel cellular distances before causing structural damage. The net results may impair cell function, cause mutations, or even prevent cell division. Altered cell immunogenicity also may result, leading to autoimmune disease. Chemical oxidative injury may involve any organ or tissue because detoxifying enzymes are widely distributed. However, oxidative injury most commonly causes hepatic dysfunction because of the high local concentration of detoxification enzymes and the consequent localization of free radical production.

## Role of Hepatic Metabolism

The liver is capable of detoxifying a very wide range of organic chemicals by biotransformation to less toxic substances that can be either metabolized or excreted (5). The principal mechanisms involve oxidation, reduction, hydrolysis, methylation, and conjugation with peptides, amino acids, sugars, or inorganic ions. Chemicals that can be acted on by the nonconjugation reactions usually are broken down into smaller compounds that can enter cellular metabolic pathways. When these reactions involve oxidation or reduction, the reactions are carefully compartmentalized in the hepatocyte, in close association with enzymes and cofactors capable of neutralizing reactive intermediates and quenching free radicals. Only when the chemical load exceeds the capacity of this protective system can toxicity occur. There is evidence that patients with CS may be deficient in some components of this protective system (6). Chemicals that can be conjugated usually are excreted in urine or bile. Some compounds, especially aromatic and halogenated hydrocarbons, are resistant to any detoxification mechanism, and accumulate in hydrophobic regions of the body, including cell membranes and fat storage cells, where their long-term effects are not well understood. Finally, and unfortunately, during these biotransformation reactions, some highly reactive chemical intermediates are formed that are carcinogens or mutagens (5) and may lead to potential delayed consequences for any survivor of an acute toxic chemical injury.

## Chronic Poisoning

Chronic chemical poisoning may take either of two forms: constant or repeated low-level exposure, or residual effects from chemicals stored in the body after an acute exposure episode. In either case, the total chemical load is less than what is required to produce acute toxicity. Probably many of the mechanisms are the same as in acute toxicity, but detoxification mechanisms are able to keep up with at least some of the chemical exposure, resulting in a state of com-

pensation. In the compensated state, reserves are depleted, toxic or carcinogenic byproducts may be generated, and resources are shifted to maintain the detoxification pathways, so that the organism is left less able to handle other stresses that may arise (7). There also may be adverse effects of chronic chemical exposure on particularly sensitive tissues, such as the triggering of autoimmune glomerulonephritis that may result from chronic mercury exposure (8). Other examples are central nervous system toxicity from styrene monomer (9), immune dysfunction from dioxin (9), and reproductive toxicity from 1,3-butadiene (9). Various organic solvents and organophosphate or chlorinated hydrocarbon pesticides also are known primarily to affect the central nervous system (10). Other chlorinated hydrocarbons primarily trigger the skin eruption, chloracne (11), whereas many types of chemicals are known to act on the cardiovascular system (12).

## Allergic Hypersensitivity to Chemicals

In atopic people, one of the most common results of chronic chemical exposure is the formation of protein-bound haptens, with the development of immunoglobulin E (IgE)-mediated immediate allergic sensitization. Small molecules, the size of pentapeptides or smaller, do not stimulate lymphocyte surface receptors. If, however, a small molecule is chemically bound to an immunogenic carrier molecule, then lymphocytes can be activated and can produce antibodies or sensitized cells that are capable of reacting with the free, non–carrier-bound small molecules (13). This is the mechanism behind most drug hypersensitivity reactions, but also accounts for reactions to many industrial chemicals such as mercury (14), natural latex rubber (15), and formaldehyde or glutaraldehyde (16). The ease with which a chemical causes sensitization is related to its chemical reactivity, or to the reactivity of its biotransformation metabolites with serum proteins (17,18). Sensitization to haptens happens frequently enough that from 2% to 15% of all recognized cases of acute allergic reactions are due to industrial chemicals (18). Some allergic reactions to chemicals are readily recognized, particularly when they cause skin rashes, such as reactions to latex or nickel. Many other chemical allergic reactions are difficult to identify, however, such as asthma due to toothpaste flavoring (19). Finally, in reactions due to exposure to complex mixtures (smoke), it may be almost impossible to identify the responsible chemical(s).

Delayed T-lymphocyte–mediated allergic reactions also may occur with chemical exposure. This is best known for the common isocyanate and anhydride plastic resins (20), metals such as nickel, and formaldehyde (18). Certain chemicals may induce both immediate and delayed reactions, and all four Gell and Coombs classes of hypersensitivity reactions to a chemical may coexist, just as in food sensitization. The existence of delayed hypersensitivity reactions to some chemicals raises the possibility that, like in delayed food reactions, it may be difficult both to recognize the condition as well as to identify the responsible chemical. The available evidence suggests that both immediate and delayed allergic reactions are common in atopic people exposed to chemicals.

## Immune System Toxicity

Chemicals can cause specific effects directly on the immune system (21). Generalized myelosuppression is known to occur from chronic solvent exposure (benzene), and also may occur due to lead, cadmium, and mercury. Halogenated aromatic hydrocarbons, such as dioxins and PCBs, polycyclic aromatic hydrocarbons (benzo[a]pyrene), mycotoxins, and organophosphate pesticides also damage immune cells (18). Immune activation effects also have been reported; for example, beryllium induces blastogenesis in T lymphocytes, whereas mercury causes B-lymphocyte activation and increased production of autoimmune antibodies (17). Trimellitic anhydride can chemically modify immunoglobulins, triggering production of anti-immunoglobulins (20). Finally, silica, silicone, paraffin, and several organic chemicals are known to trigger progressive systemic sclerosis or scleroderma-like diseases by chronic phagocytic activation (22).

Many other chemicals have been implicated in causing adverse immune effects, but in most cases the evidence is limited to case reports, and few or no controlled studies have been done. It remains to be established whether low-level exposures to environmental chemicals have significant immune effects on the general population (18). In animal studies, however, the immune system has been shown to be an extremely sensitive target for chemical injury, and it would be surprising if humans were not similarly affected. Some chemicals that have shown immunotoxic activity in animals are listed in Table 23.4 (18).

Immunotoxic chemicals ultimately alter the immune sur-

**TABLE 23.4. CHEMICALS KNOWN TO HAVE TOXIC EFFECTS ON THE IMMUNE SYSTEM IN ANIMALS**

Air pollutants (ozone, sulfur dioxide, nitrogen dioxide)
Aromatic amines (benzidine)
Aromatic hydrocarbons (benzene, toluene)
Diesel exhaust
Fungal mycotoxins
Halogenated aromatic hydrocarbons (dioxins, polychlorinated biphenyls)
Metals (lead, cadmium, arsenic, mercury)
Organometallics (tin, mercury)
Particulates (asbestos, silica)
Pesticides (organophosphates, chlordane)
Polycyclic aromatic hydrocarbons (benzo[a]pyrene, 3-methylcholanthrene)
Tobacco smoke

veillance and barrier functions between the organism and its environment. One important consequence of this damage is that other exogenous substances, such as allergens, toxins, or even pathogenic organisms, can then enter the body in greater quantities. This can in theory lead to frequent infections and, even more important, to a positive feedback loop and a vicious cycle of increasing illness.

## Synergism

Of even greater concern than the individual mechanisms of injury by single toxic chemicals is the recently demonstrated synergism that can be shown between different pollutants. For example, exposure to either photochemical smog (ozone) or to acidic aerosols (sulfur dioxide) markedly increases the susceptibility of allergic people to airborne pollens (23). Because most of the northern hemisphere is frequently exposed to significant levels of air pollution (23), chemical synergism may be one factor in the recent historic increase in asthma mortality rates. One possible mechanism is the production of cellular free radical injury by the pollutants, which exhausts containment mechanisms that normally would limit the extent of an allergic reaction. This direct chemical effect is similar to the well known priming effect, where exposure to one allergen increases sensitivity to a subsequent exposure to another allergen. Taken together with a decreased immune barrier (see earlier), the effects of chemical synergism and antigen priming help to explain both the often-observed phenomenon of extreme sensitivity to irritants (smoke, perfumes), and the cases of so-called universal reactors, people who are allergic to everything to which they are tested. Synergism may have even broader implications for chemical exposure because it also has been postulated to occur with environmental carcinogens and many other classes of toxic substances. One example of such chemical synergism is seen with diesel exhaust exposure.

## Diesel Particulates and Allergic Diseases

Peterson and Saxon (24) reviewed over 100 years of medical literature and clearly demonstrated dramatic, worldwide, long-term uptrends in symptomatic allergic rhinitis and asthma. Data from many countries and times are presented showing substantial and continuing increases over many decades. The parallel rise in air pollutants released by the industrial revolution and the increase in incidence of allergic diseases clearly indicates a possible causal link between the two. Other factors, such as decreasing exposure to bacterial illness (25), also may be factors in the increasing incidence of allergy, but the experimental evidence for chemicals is substantial, and both issues may be significant.

Peterson and Saxon (24) illustrate their thesis by choosing a single example, diesel exhaust particles, and reviewing the experimental data that suggest how exposure to this air pollutant can trigger allergy. Data from in vitro studies of isolated B lymphocytes show that the nonvolatile aromatic hydrocarbons in diesel exhaust are capable of binding to cell receptors and then preferentially augmenting IgE production during antigen stimulation. The same results occur during in vivo rodent studies, as well as in human studies. Furthermore, the effects of diesel exhaust are not limited to B cells; rather, most respiratory cells are similarly affected, causing measurable local tissue changes in production of many different cytokines. This is another plausible means by which chemicals can synergistically affect allergic disease severity.

## Individual Biochemical and Environmental Variability

In addition to global chemical exposure, individual factors, such as genetics, personal history of prior chemical exposure, and dietary preferences, also affect current susceptibility to chemical toxicity (6,26). Genetic factors now are suspected to lie behind susceptibility to both hydrocarbon-induced lung cancer and ethanol-induced hepatotoxicity or neurotoxicity, and it is likely that individual variation in levels of protective enzymes influences how a person handles any chemical exposure. Levels of dietary antioxidants, fats, minerals, and proteins are important in optimum function of the detoxification pathways, and these may vary widely depending on social status, ethnicity, and personal preference (see Chapter 27). Prior chemical exposure, from work, home, or leisure activity, is similarly variable and, depending on the specific chemicals involved, may lead to accumulation in the body and an increasing chemical burden. Obesity may be an added risk factor for CS because storage of chemicals increases at the expense of excretion. Older age may increase risk because of decreased renal function, whereas infants may have immature liver function and also be at increased risk. Concurrent diseases, altered hormone balance, and environmental or emotional stresses also are variables that may worsen CS. One of the strongest predictors of future CS among chemically exposed workers actually appears to be the presence of preexisting anxiety or autonomic symptoms (27). This finding has been ascribed to preexisting psychological factors in susceptible persons that lead to conditioned avoidance responses to chemical odors. However, because the autonomic nervous system is a known target tissue for chemical toxicity, the findings could equally well be explained as being due to early, unrecognized symptoms of chronic chemical toxicity.

## MULTIPLE CHEMICAL SENSITIVITIES

### History of Multiple Chemical Sensitivities

Acute and chronic chemical toxicity and chemical allergy are not controversial diagnoses, despite the infrequency with which these diagnoses are typically made in modern medicine. On the other hand, even the existence of the diagnosis of MCS is highly controversial. The modern concept of MCS was developed during the 1950s by Dr. Theron Randolph, based on his careful observations of chronically ill patients in Chicago (28). His teachings ultimately led to the development of the field of clinical ecology, now called *environmental medicine.* The key observation that Randolph made was that there were allergic patients who had variable symptoms that correlated with environmental chemical exposures, primarily with air pollution. The range of observed symptoms was extremely broad, ranging from typical allergy symptoms to musculoskeletal or nervous system problems. Some patients even became intoxicated, fatigued, or depressed, but all improved when returned to unpolluted towns upwind from industrial zones. Eventually, Randolph built an environmental unit where patients could be almost completely removed from chemicals, and in such an environment many of his chronic, most severely ill patients improved. He identified significant exposures from chemical contaminants in foods, water, air, and particularly in the outgassings of the indoor environment and vapors and combustion products from burning of fuels. However, he found that his observations were largely ignored by a nation infatuated with consumer goods and unwilling to alter their comfortable lifestyle, and by physicians who found it difficult to believe that minute exposures to chemicals could cause severe, multisystem illnesses.

## Definition of Multiple Chemical Sensitivities

Because many patients identified the source of their symptoms as arising from their work, specialists in occupational medicine also became involved in evaluation of MCS. The proposed working clinical case definition used in the Yale-New Haven Occupational Medicine Program is "Multiple chemical sensitivities (MCS) is an acquired disorder characterized by recurrent symptoms, referable to multiple organ systems, occurring in response to demonstrable exposure to many chemically unrelated compounds at doses far below those established in the general population to cause harmful effects. No single widely accepted test of physiologic function can be shown to correlate with symptoms" (29). A 1989 consensus conference of experts identified five key factors of MCS that have not changed with a decade of further research (30). These define MCS as (a) a chronic condition, (b) with symptoms that recur reproducibly, (c) in response to low levels of exposure, (d) to multiple unrelated chemicals, and (e) improve or resolve when incitants are removed. A sixth criterion has recently been proposed: that symptoms must occur in multiple organ systems.

The key concept in these definitions is that the exposures that trigger symptoms in patients with MCS are at levels far below those that cause symptoms in healthy people. This single fact, combined with the production of a myriad of symptoms by exposure to many different classes of chemicals, has made the MCS syndrome difficult to accept for many physicians and researchers. Some groups began to refer to MCS as *idiopathic environmental intolerances* (IEI) because of their belief that there is no credible evidence that chemical exposures are causally related to this syndrome (31). Despite this mental hurdle on the part of physicians, patients with MCS (or IEI) are undeniably sick, and can often date and place development of their symptoms to either a discrete past incident of chemical exposure or to a particular environment that they are exposed to. In this way, patients with MCS resemble patients with chronic fatigue. Patients with chronic fatigue and MCS also are alike in the extremely high coincidence of depression and allergies. The clinical problem of MCS is real, the association with environmental chemical exposure is real, and the required research, to understand why, is beginning to be reported.

## Prevalence of Multiple Chemical Sensitivities

A population survey in California (32) identified a large subpopulation of people who believed that they were adversely affected by chemicals. Overall, 16% of people surveyed reported allergy or unusual sensitivity to domestic chemicals, 12% were sensitive to more than one type of chemical, and 6.3% had physician-diagnosed environmental illness or MCS. CS also is from two to four times more common in U.S., Canadian, and United Kingdom veterans of the Gulf War than in nondeployed troops (30). A survey in North Carolina was even more worrisome. Meggs et al. (33) found that there was a significant crossover between people with allergies and those with CS, but there was not complete overlap of the groups. Approximately 35% of people surveyed had self-reported allergies, compared with approximately 33% with CS, yet only approximately half, or 17%, of the population believed that they had both allergy and CS (33). The perceived problem is huge because over half of the study population had either allergy or CS symptoms. The incidence of allergy in all of these groups probably is much higher than reported because many patients with perennial allergy are not aware of the origin of their symptoms.

## Psychiatric Theory

Although it is quite clear that many patients are complaining of MCS, physicians are not all in agreement over what to do about those complaints. There is a huge chasm between different groups of physicians in their interpretation of the likely pathophysiologic process of MCS. Many physicians believe the symptoms are completely psychiatric in origin, ascribing the syndrome to combinations of somatoform disorders, depression, and anxiety (34,35). There is some sup-

port for this view, including the finding of pseudoseizures, without electroencephalographic changes, that were provoked by chemical challenge tests in one patient with MCS (36). There also have been a few case reports of apparent cure of MCS by use of antidepressant drugs (37) or by psychotherapy (38). Finally, several small studies have shown that patients with MCS often react with typical symptoms of anxiety, hyperventilation, and panic when challenged with their triggering chemical (39), as well as with intravenous lactate (40) or with carbon dioxide inhalation (41), conditions that precipitate panic attacks in susceptible persons. However, in all of these studies, only very small numbers of patients were tested or treated.

## Neural Amplification Theory

On the other hand, there is a plausible theory to explain how neural amplification could occur in the olfactory–limbic system to produce the observed extreme sensitivity of patients with MCS (42,43). Supporting this theory are the findings of decreased performance on frontal lobe tasks in both patients with MCS and those with asthma (43), and decreased visual learning and memory in both chemically exposed patients and those with MCS (44). There are some supporting animal studies, but no human demonstrations of neural reinforcement or amplification of chemical cues.

## Chemical Causation Theory

Finally, there also is evidence to support the chemical causation theory. Foremost, there is a large body of repeated observations by many physicians over many years of patients with MCS improving after the institution of measures to restrict chemical exposure. These observations cannot be easily explained by either the psychiatric or neural amplification theories. Second, subtle immune derangements have been demonstrated in many patients with MCS, and measurable body burdens of many organic and inorganic chemicals have been repeatedly found. However, there is dispute over what is normal and what is not, so these studies have not proven definitive (35). Third, animal data support the idea that there can be orders-of-magnitude differences in the range of sensitivity of individuals to organic chemicals (45). Last, microscopic evidence has been found in the nasal mucosa that can be interpreted as showing a pathologic positive feedback loop of chemically induced inflammation (46,47). If this is a correct interpretation, chemicals may exert their damaging effects by disrupting the integrity of the nasal mucosal barrier and causing neurogenic inflammation. Therefore, chemical injury in MCS would be a situation analogous to that created by local anaphylaxis due to allergen exposure in either the gut or respiratory tract. What is fundamentally lacking to support the chemical causation theory, or any other theory, are data showing that substantial numbers of patients improve after being treated in a randomized outcome study.

For now, this debate has no scientific solution. Thus, the decision of how to evaluate and treat patients with MCS rests with each clinician. During the evaluation, it is important to be certain that a thorough medical examination and adequate laboratory testing are performed, so that the possibility of other serious illnesses can be excluded. For example, important illnesses that can masquerade as MCS include sleep apnea (48), mastocytosis (30), chemical toxicity from carbon monoxide, mercury, lead (49), or other neurotoxins, and simple anxiety or depression (50). An important part of this evaluation is an assessment of the total allergic load.

## TOTAL ALLERGIC LOAD

### Patient Load Assessment

Chemical sensitivity usually is not seen in isolation. Commonly, CS occurs in a person who already has symptoms of one or more allergic ailments. In these patients, CS must be considered together with the allergic problems because both problems are part of the total clinical picture. The concept of the total allergic load that affects a patient is an important part of clinical diagnosis, decision making, and treatment. A high total load total allergic load is a condition in which a patient is frequently contacting such large quantities of allergens that there always is a significant amount of allergic mediators circulating in his or her body. The addition of just a small allergen challenge, such as by inhaling a whiff of perfume or eating a small snack, is enough to raise the mediators to symptom-producing levels. Direct contributors to the total allergic load are drugs and additives, foods, inhalants, and chemical allergens. Illnesses or environmental stresses that increase allergen exposure, such as IgA deficiency or abnormal gastrointestinal permeability, or increase the response to allergens, such as diesel exhaust, contribute indirectly to the total load. Finally, the total load is heavily influenced by conditions that decrease the metabolic ability of the body to respond to the allergen challenge, especially by poor nutrition and toxic chemical exposure.

Assessment of the total allergic load should be performed during the initial patient interview (see Chapter 5). The possibility of an allergic etiology is obvious in many patients after the initial history and physical examination are obtained: either they have a significant personal or family history of allergic conditions, or enough physical findings are present to suggest allergy. In these patients, the number and severity of symptoms dictate how exhaustive the search must be for potential incitants. Normally, if patients are more than mildly symptomatic, inhalant, food, and dermatophyte allergy testing are warranted, and a drug and chemical exposure history should be taken to ensure that these possible significant exposures are not being overlooked. When deciding which allergens to test for, the total load concept should

be kept in mind because of the potential for poor allergy control, or outright failure of treatment, if major allergen or chemical contacts are not recognized.

## Screening Tests

In patients who have obvious allergies or chemical exposure, appropriate panels of tests should be ordered. In other patients, particularly those with multiple symptoms that are not clearly allergic or chemical exposure related, the presence or absence of allergy and chemical exposure needs to be established. This is a good place to use screening panels (either in vitro or skin) to evaluate inexpensively for inhalant and dermatophyte allergy (51), and a screening set of intradermal progressive food tests for common hidden foods in the patient's diet (52). Also, simple chemical allergy tests, such as in vitro tests for formaldehyde, latex, and suspected occupational exposures, should be obtained. Screening urine tests for chemical toxicity also are helpful (see later). If any of these screening test results are positive, then full inhalant, food, and chemical evaluation should be completed.

## Ingestant Contacts

Evaluation of an ingestant diary is necessary to check for suspect foods, food additives, and medications. Patients need to be instructed to write down absolutely everything they put into their mouth. In some patients, even minute amounts of food additives may be significant, and these are not likely to be discovered without use of a diary. For example, in one urticaria study, chemical food additives were found to be the triggering agent for 26% of patients (53). Inquiry should be made into the use of drugs, nonprescription medications, supplements, and herbs. Certain drugs, such as β-blockers and angiotensin-converting enzyme inhibitors, may exacerbate allergic symptoms and thus increase the effective total load. Drugs and supplements often contain yeast, corn, wheat, and other major food allergens, and botanical remedies may allergically cross-react with ragweed. Finally, some folk remedies may contain toxins or heavy metals.

## Environmental Contacts

Occupational, home, or recreational allergen and chemical exposures should be sought. Patients who exhibit symptoms from minor chemical exposure are among the most likely to be allergen overloaded. Because chemicals may stay in the body for life and continue to exert their effects, past exposure also is important. Sometimes, reviewing lists of categories of known occupational chemical allergens with the patient may trigger recognition (54). Also, because the skin is capable of allergen absorption, questions about contact exposures to chemicals and dusts should be included.

If a patient is on an allergy desensitization regimen and is having new problems, phenol allergy should be considered (see Chapter 12). Rarely, patients may become phenol sensitive and experience either local or systemic reactions. White collar office jobs are not free of potential occupational exposures because patients may be spending 8 hours a day in a closed building with high levels of outgassing chemicals, mold, bacteria, or dust (55,56). Therefore, the type of buildings in which people work or live may be as important as their actual jobs. Specifics of the home and work environments, including building age, heating, cooling, and cleaning systems, presence of a basement, new insulation, ventilation, presence of water leaks, moldy or musty smell, and chemical use or storage must be evaluated. The presence of many plastic or synthetic fixtures, such as in mobile homes, or recent remodeling or carpet installation usually is very significant. Periodic symptoms may lead to discovery of intermittent release of pollutants by a nearby industry. Recreational activities such as golf, painting, woodworking or metalworking, and restoring cars also can involve substantial chemical exposure. Metal allergy is another area often overlooked. Jewelry contact allergy normally is readily detected by the restricted location of the skin lesions; however, allergy due to ingestant or contactant metal exposure or to implanted metal alloy prostheses also occurs, and must be excluded by specific skin tests for the particular metals used (57). Implant sensitization is most likely with metal-to-metal articulation, rather than metal-to-plastic (58). Allergy to other implants and appliances, such as dentures, hearing aids, eyeglasses, plastic implants, and dental amalgams (8), also may be relevant to the total load.

## TESTING FOR CHEMICAL ILLNESS

### Before Testing for Chemical Sensitivity

When CS is clinically suspected, the first step in evaluation is *always* to take a complete history (59). Very often the history reveals a large exposure to a specific chemical or class of chemicals, thus suggesting what to test for. In evaluating chronic cases, specific questions must be asked because the person may not be thinking about exposure to termite-treated homes, fumigated vacation residences, time spent in mobile homes, chemicals used in hobbies or recreation, latex exposure, orthopedic or dental implants, nearby toxic waste sites, or industrial emissions in his or her area. The timing between exposure and seeing the physician also is crucial because, over time, metabolism, storage, and excretion change what chemicals can be detected and which tissues to examine. Finally, specific signs or symptoms may suggest what organ system tests would be most helpful. The selection of appropriate categories of tests is the first priority. There are three primary testing options: allergy tests, tests of detoxification capacity, and various types of chemical toxicity tests.

## Chemical Hypersensitivity Tests

Of the many possible methods that can be used for assisting in the diagnosis of possible chemical toxicity or hypersensitivity, those that are the easiest to perform in the typical office practice are tests for allergic hypersensitivity. Because the degree of a patient's sensitivity to a particular chemical usually is unknown, and because the population of sensitive people may react to a very wide range of possible chemical concentrations (60), testing a wide range of concentrations is required to minimize false-positive and false-negative results. In addition, beginning testing with very dilute chemicals is necessary to avoid irritant, toxic, or caustic skin reactions. Thus, the best diagnostic tests for chemical hypersensitivity are titration tests, either in vitro tests of specific anti-chemical IgE, in vitro histamine release tests, or skin endpoint titration (SET) according to the technique recommended by the American Academy of Otolaryngic Allergy (61). In vitro antibody tests, when available, are safe, relatively inexpensive, and very convenient, but are not 100% sensitive in identifying chemical allergens. Both IgE and IgG tests can be used. Positive IgE test results for a chemical indicate that it is acting as a hapten in a type I immediate hypersensitivity reaction, whereas positive IgG test results indicate the possibility of that chemical participating in a delayed hypersensitivity reaction. Positive IgG tests need clinical confirmation by a challenge test because IgG also may be normally produced after an exposure. Histamine release tests, performed on fresh blood cells, can be very helpful in evaluating difficult cases of suspected chemical allergy. In some cases, a sample of the suspect chemical also must be sent to the reference laboratory, along with a blood specimen. Always call the laboratory before requesting histamine release tests to learn about special shipping requirements and availability of the requested tests.

If in vitro test results are positive, they are extremely helpful. On the other hand, SET is extremely sensitive, but because of chemical skin irritation, may produce false-positive results. Skin patch testing with a range of concentrations of each chemical also may be used. For greatest accuracy, the skin must be reexamined periodically between 48 hours and several weeks after patch tests are applied (62). Patch testing is primarily useful in detecting delayed hypersensitivity reactions that can be missed with SET and in vitro tests. Finally, various types of challenge tests may be very helpful in diagnosis, especially for confirming negative in vitro test results or for evaluating possible false-positive skin test results. Challenge tests have the disadvantages of usually being time consuming, requiring specialized apparatus, and being potentially hazardous (63). However, ingestion challenge tests can be done in the typical office setting, and may be useful for testing of suspect drugs or food additives. Inhalation challenges with serial spirometric evaluation also can be done for airborne chemicals (64), or exposure may take place in an inert, airtight booth. For appropriate diagnosis in certain patients, several of these types of tests for allergic chemical hypersensitivity may need to be used.

## Measuring Detoxification Pathways

One approach to screening for nonallergic chemical toxicity is to measure directly the effectiveness of major detoxification pathways. Xenobiotics are transported to the liver, the body's primary detoxifying organ, and detoxification is carried out in two phases. Phase I adds functional groups through oxidation, reduction, or hydrolysis, using the cytochrome p450 mixed-function oxidase enzymes. This process increases the solubility of xenobiotic molecules and increases their chemical reactivity, preparing them for phase II reactions, which are intended to create excretable end products. Phase I reactions are necessary for detoxification, but the resulting production of reactive oxygen species, when of sufficient magnitude, can cause liver injury. When this occurs, elevated liver enzymes may be detected in serum, and D-glucaric acid levels rise in urine.

Phase II conjugation reactions add a hydrophilic molecule to the xenobiotic, converting lipophilic molecules into water-soluble ones. Major phase II pathways include glutathione, sulfate, glycine, and glucuronide conjugations. Individual xenobiotics may be processed by all pathways, but usually one or two predominate. A typical test of detoxification pathways measures excretion products from fixed doses of common drugs, such as aspirin, acetaminophen, and caffeine, and is capable of identifying significant abnormalities that would interfere with chemical excretion. An abnormal result of this test indicates the need for further evaluation because impaired or saturated xenobiotic excretion can lead to CS symptoms.

## Screening for Chemical Toxicity

When the history suggests direct chemical toxicity, two testing strategies may be used: first, direct chemical analysis of whatever tissue in which the suspect chemical is likely to be concentrated, and second, detection of metabolic or pathologic consequences of chemical toxicity. To do direct chemical analysis, the suspected class of chemicals must be known. Because it is expensive to conduct multiple chemical analyses, specific testing therefore must be narrowly targeted, and cannot be used if the type of chemical is unknown. Fortunately, under Occupational Safety and Health Administration (OSHA) rules, every company must have, on file, material safety data sheets (MSDS) for every chemical used, and these must be made available to employees on request. The MSDSs disclose the nature of any chemicals that a patient is known to be contacting.

On the other hand, the body has limited mechanisms for detoxification and excretion of chemicals, so that detection of the byproducts of chemical metabolism can be used both to screen for significant chemical exposure and to check for ineffective chemical detoxification. This approach often is productive, and is easily and relatively inexpensively accomplished by sending a 24-hour urine specimen to be analyzed for D-glucaric acid, an indicator of hepatic microsomal activation and thus of detoxification activity, and for conjugated mercapturic acids, which are the excretory conjugates of glutathione with xenobiotics. Either or both of these compounds usually are elevated in the urine when there has been significant organic chemical exposure. For example, measuring urinary mercapturic acids is a good method for detecting benzene (65) or acrylonitrile (66) exposure. Mercapturic acids are not always detected, however, because other conjugation or metabolic pathways may predominate in the excretion of certain chemicals. Monitoring levels of these metabolites, when present, also is a useful guide to the effectiveness of therapy.

## Direct Chemical Analysis

Testing by noninvasive or minimally invasive sampling may be the next diagnostic step, either to prove the etiology (e.g., for workmen's compensation claims) or to seek a diagnosis, if prior tests were still nondiagnostic. In a few cases, specific metabolic byproducts resulting from exposure to certain classes of chemicals can be easily analyzed. For example, clinically useful tests are available for the two most common classes of professionally applied insecticides. The acute effects of organophosphates (e.g., parathion, malathion, diazinon) can be detected by serial measurements of serum cholinesterase activity, which is available at any good clinical laboratory. The β-naphthol metabolites of carbamates (e.g., Sevin), as well as the nitrophenol metabolites of the organophosphates, are detectable in urine for a few days after exposure (67).

Total chronic body burdens of toxic heavy metals can be reliably assessed by hair analysis, but the harvesting procedure and the chemical analysis must both be done in a very specific manner to ensure reliability (68). For example, hair, urine, and blood mercury determinations have been found to be comparable methods when used to assess whether fish consumption or dental fillings are the major source of mercury accumulation in different populations (69–71). Urine analysis is a cheap, useful screen for heavy metal toxicity, but because it measures current excretion and not total body burden, it is best used for monitoring therapy rather than for diagnosis. Reference ranges for the urinary excretion of 25 trace elements by the U.S. population have been published (72). Because significant variation in urine element excretion occurs (73), 24-hour specimens should be tested. If heavy metal toxicity is suspected, and urinalysis is negative, blood or tissue analysis or postchelation urinalysis should be done (see later). Blood may be used for both heavy metal detection and for detection of organic chemicals (7). Although blood is convenient to obtain, blood analysis suffers from the fact that most xenobiotics are not concentrated in the blood; rather, many organic chemicals concentrate in the fat-rich tissues (fat, central nervous system, liver), and heavy metals gravitate toward specific tissues (e.g., lead to bones, cadmium to kidney). Some improvement in the detection of organic chemicals in blood is obtained from whole-blood or blood cell analysis, rather than serum analysis. Volatile chemicals often may be best detected by gas chromatography of exhaled air. This simple test has particular use for detection of low-level exposure to solvents such as benzene (74), but the necessary equipment is available only in sophisticated laboratories. A list of common industrial chemicals, the appropriate tissue to sample, and the population norms and toxic levels, is available (75).

## Enhanced Excretion

To prove a sequestered body burden exists in the face of apparently normal serum or urinary levels, chelation or other means of mobilization may be used. As an example, a specific chelating agent could be administered to extract a heavy metal from the tissues and allow subsequent detection of increased levels in serum or urine (76). This method is particularly useful for suspected chronic or past exposure to heavy metals. Recommended specific oral or intravenous chelators for different suspected toxic metals are listed in the current edition of the *Merck Manual of Diagnosis and Therapy* (77). Organic chemicals also can be mobilized from fat stores by weight loss or aerobic physical activity, and may then be more readily detected.

## Pathologic Examination

When signs or symptoms point to specific organ involvement, and other, less invasive tests have not been diagnostic, biopsy may be useful. Standard pathologic microscopic examination, aided by new monoclonal antibody reagents, can determine patterns of tissue injury and whether these support chemical injury. With newer microanalysis procedures, it also is feasible to perform elemental analysis (e.g., heavy metals) on core needle biopsy specimens, or chemical analysis (e.g., pesticides) on larger specimens. For example, the U.S. Environmental Protection Agency has been using subcutaneous fat biopsies to monitor environmental pollution (78). Because only a few laboratories are capable of these specialized analyses, patient biopsies should not be contemplated until an appropriate laboratory for the specific analysis required is located, and the pathologist agrees to cooperate with processing and forwarding the biopsy samples.

## Testing Facilities

The number of U.S. commercial laboratories that have the special expertise to analyze inorganic and organic chemicals in trace amounts is not large. There are more laboratories

**TABLE 23.5. COMMERCIAL LABORATORIES OFFERING CHEMICAL ALLERGY OR TOXICOLOGY SERVICES**

| | |
|---|---|
| **Accu-Chem Labs** <br> 990 North Bowser Road <br> Suite 800 <br> Richardson, TX 75081 | Phone: 972-234-5412 <br> Web site: www.accuchemlabs.com |
| **Doctor's Data** <br> P.O. Box 111 <br> West Chicago, IL 60186 | Phone: 800-323-2784 <br> Phone: 630-587-7860 <br> Fax: 630-377-8139 <br> Web site: www.doctorsdata.com |
| **Great Smokies Diagnostic Lab** <br> 63 Zillicoa Street <br> Asheville, NC 28801 | Phone: 800-522-4762 <br> Fax: 828-252-9303 <br> Web site: www.gsdl.com |
| **Laboratory Corp. of America** <br> 1447 York Court <br> Burlington, NC 27215 | Phone: 800-762-4344 <br> Phone: 336-584-5171 <br> Web site: www.labcorp.com |

with expertise in allergy testing, but not every laboratory is able to analyze specimens for every chemical. Therefore, physicians interested in quantitating either allergic or toxic chemical reactions need to become familiar with the tests available through several laboratories. When selecting laboratories, reputation and level of certification are both very important factors to consider. A third factor, especially important for physicians who do not often require chemical testing services, is the ready availability of expert advice to assist in selection and interpretation of the specific tests that will be most relevant in a particular case. Several laboratories that meet these criteria are listed in Table 23.5.

Additional information can be obtained from the U.S. Government National Toxicology Program at http://ntp-server.niehs.nih.gov/, or from a private listing of laboratories hosted at http://userzweb.lightspeed.net/~abarbour/labs.htm. There also is a national toxicology database maintained by the National Library of Medicine at http://toxnet.nlm.nih.gov/.

## TREATMENT OF CHEMICAL SENSITIVITY

Complete allergy treatment is based on a sequence of eight activities: (a) eliminate inciting substances, (b) reduce the allergic load, (c) rotate diet items and exclude severe reactors, (d) enhance chemical excretion, (e) supplement nutrition, (f) desensitize inhalants, (g) provide neutralization treatment of unavoidable food allergens, and (h) provide pharmacologic treatment of symptoms. Whenever practical, great efforts should be made to eliminate key incitants because this usually produces a rapid and profound symptom response. This could be as simple as enclosing the mattress or as difficult as draining, ventilating, and decontaminating the cellar. At the same time, efforts to clean up the overall allergic and chemical environment, and increase aerobic exercise, can decrease the allergic load and provide some leeway to protect against development of new symptoms. Dietary management is especially important because large quantities of allergens and chemicals can be ingested in food and water. A purified source of water must be ensured, and independent water testing may be needed to be certain of the quality. Organic foods are required for more severely affected patients, and should be encouraged, within budget limitations, for all patients. Nutritional supplements with antioxidants and cofactors to enhance detoxification and counter increased oxidant loads also are very helpful. All of these interventions can be started based just on taking a good history and doing basic testing for inhalant and food allergens. Last, pharmacologic treatment to relieve symptoms can be instituted, but is *not* a substitute for proper allergic evaluation and treatment. Most of these topics have been thoroughly covered in other chapters. Some specific comments relative to treating patients with CS, and a more detailed discussion of physical measures and nutritional means for treating patients with CS, are provided in the following sections.

## Pathologic Role of Oxidants in Allergy

Oxidants are reactive chemicals that can cause the functional destruction of critical cellular molecules such as lipids, proteins, and nucleic acids, leading to metabolic inefficiency, DNA mutations, and, ultimately, cell death (79). Free radicals and other oxidants are produced by normal cellular metabolism, such as during mitochondrial aerobic respiration, or hepatic microsomal detoxification. Large amounts of oxidants are generated by leukocytes during phagocytosis and degranulation, and important quantities of oxidants are produced during the spontaneous autooxidation of the polyunsaturated lipids in cell membranes and fat stores, or when iron stores exceed normal limits. Preformed oxidants also can enter the body by consumption of rancid foods, by inhalation of smog, tobacco smoke, or other combustion products, or by exposure to oxidant or toxic chemicals. Finally, it has been found that leukocytes activated during the allergic reaction (80) release significant amounts of oxidants.

Healthy, nutritionally normal cells possess sufficient capability to control and neutralize these sources of oxidants without incurring significant damage. However, cellular defenses can be stressed and finally overwhelmed when exposed to sufficiently large amounts of oxidants over a long enough time. Because all of these different sources of oxidants add together to determine the total personal oxidant load, any single source of oxidants may be small enough to be easily contained by cellular antioxidant defenses, yet the sum may be too great and lead to a pathologic state. This total oxidant load concept may be an explanation for the current worldwide increase in allergic diseases: the steadily increasing oxidant burden imposed by environmental pollutants may be enough to increase both the incidence of symptomatic allergies, and their severity (81). In fact, even small concentrations of atmospheric ozone have been found to be an important exacerbating factor in asthma (82). This is why allergy cannot be optimally treated without knowledge of CS and environmental pollution issues.

## Antioxidant Mechanisms and Required Nutritional Factors

Normal cells possess two basic antioxidant mechanisms: first, enzymes that can use specific reducing cofactors, and second, direct reaction of oxidants with small reducing molecules such as vitamin C or vitamin E (83). Enzymatic methods are especially important for protecting cell organelles from oxidants, and to function at maximum efficiency, they require adequate nutritional sources of high-quality protein, essential mineral cofactors such as iron, copper, zinc, magnesium, manganese, and molybdenum, and adequate amounts of B vitamin cofactors to act as reducing agents. Direct neutralization requires sufficient concentrations of vitamin C in the aqueous cell compartments and vitamin E in the lipid phases of the cell membranes to ensure that oxidants preferentially react with the vitamins instead of with cell components. Other plant-derived antioxidants, such as carotenoids, polyphenols, and flavonoids, also appear to have a direct protective role, but have not yet been well studied (79). Adequate antioxidant levels are maintained by a mechanism of antioxidant recycling through glutathione-dependent antioxidant enzymes, which require sulfur-containing amino acids, as well as selenium and B vitamins as cofactors. Some common toxins, such as lead, and most exogenous organic chemical pollutants increase the effective oxidant load by specifically inhibiting antioxidant enzymes, by preventing glutathione recycling, or by consuming glutathione and other cofactors, making them unavailable for recycling.

## Beneficial Role of Antioxidants in Allergy and Detoxification

Specific nutritional components do have effects on the treatment of allergic and chemically induced diseases (84,85). The major difficulty in assessing nutritional benefits is the great difficulty in controlling human behavior and diet for sufficiently long periods to allow observable effects. A second difficulty is that natural foods contain inconstant amounts of many component nutrients, so that intake of specific antioxidants may be highly variable, both among different people and in individuals, over time. A third difficulty is that in many diseases nutritional effects may be observed only if the intervention lasts for years or decades. Finally, chemical exposure varies widely, and in many cases the affected person has no knowledge of his or her exposure history. Despite these problems, epidemiologic studies have identified specific antioxidants as having potential benefits in several disease states. For example, vitamin C reduces cataracts and malignancies, vitamin E reduces coronary disease, and carotenoids reduce lipid peroxidation (79). There also is good evidence for the effects of either low cellular antioxidant levels or of increased oxidant exposures in causing a worsening of allergies. Further, vitamin C, selenium, and vitamin E levels appear to protect against allergic exacerbations (81,83), whereas high levels of iron or lead appear to increase the severity of allergies (83).

## Nutritional Recommendations

Epidemiologic and experimental studies have shown that oxidants are involved in both the pathogenesis and exacerbation of allergic and chemically induced diseases. However, consensus has not yet been reached, and the optimum dietary levels are not known for any of these substances. Because controlled long-term human dietary studies are exceedingly difficult to perform, authoritative antioxidant dose recommendations may not be available in the near future.

In lieu of specific knowledge, physicians should recommend that allergic patients and patients with CS consume a varied diet that includes a wide variety of organically grown vegetables, fruits, nuts, and other foods known to contain natural antioxidants (79), as well as enough high-quality protein to enable optimal antioxidant enzyme synthesis. In addition, use of vitamin and mineral supplements as insurance that sufficient quantities of critical B vitamin and mineral cofactors are ingested should be recommended, especially in the elderly, in growing children, and in anyone who may have increased metabolic needs. In the elderly, where both intestinal absorption and diet quality often are poor, deficiencies are very common and should be expected. Also, allergic patients who are following avoidance diets may inadvertently develop significant deficiencies. Iron supplements should *not* be used unless there is recently documented iron deficiency. Finally, use of pharmacologic amounts of individual antioxidants, especially vitamins C and E, should be considered in situations where the oxidant load is known to be either high or sustained (86), or in any cases of allergic disease that require more than occasional symptomatic treatment. For severely affected people, very large doses of supplemental nutrients may need to be given (Table 23.6). This is particularly the case when treating

**TABLE 23.6. IMPORTANT NUTRIENTS FOR DETOXIFICATION AND ALLERGY CONTROL**

| Nutrient | Risk of Deficiency | Suggested Daily Treatment Dose[a] |
|---|---|---|
| **Vitamins** | | |
| A | Common | 10,000 IU (as carotene) |
| B complex | Common | 5–100 mg, each vitamin |
| Folate | Common | 0.4–1 mg |
| C | Common | 4–20 g |
| E | Common | 200–1,400 IU |
| **Minerals**[b] | | |
| Copper | Common | 2–4 mg |
| Iron | Common | 10–100 mg |
| Magnesium | Common | 500–1,500 mg |
| Manganese | Rare | 3–5 mg |
| Molybdenum | Rare | 250 μg |
| Selenium | Common | 200–300 μg |
| Zinc | Common | 15–45 mg |
| **Amino acids** | | |
| Total protein | Rare | 55 g |
| Cysteine | ? | 0.5–4 g |
| Cystine | ? | 0.5–4 g |
| Glutathione | ? | 0.5–4 g |
| Methionine | Common | 0.5–3 g |
| Taurine | ? | 2 g |
| **Fatty acids** | | |
| Omega-3 | Common | 2–3 capsules flaxseed/fish oil |
| Omega-6 | Rare | 2–3 capsules evening primrose oil |
| **Antioxidants** | | |
| Carotenoids | Common | Eat a variety of vegetables and fruits |
| Polyphenols | ? | Eat a variety of vegetables and fruits |
| Flavonoids | ? | Eat a variety of vegetables and fruits |

[a]See Werbach (87,88) for discussion.
[b]Confirm deficiency before treatment.

severe asthma, chronic eczema or urticaria, and chronic fatigue syndrome, and, in conjunction with other therapies, for treatment of patients with CS and MCS. Because nutrients have potential toxicity as well as potential benefit, reference sources (87,88) should be consulted before recommending large doses of supplements. In particular, mineral levels should be determined before mineral supplementation.

## Physical Measures

Stored chemicals are mobilized by aerobic activity or by sauna treatment, and excreted in sweat and expired air (89). Most patients with CS can be treated by sauna or whirlpool therapy, except for very ill patients or those with significant cardiac disease (90). Precautions must be taken to prevent contamination of the sauna or tub by excreted chemicals. In the sauna, patients should sit on towels to absorb their sweat. In whirlpool baths, the water must be able to be drained and replaced. Regular aerobic physical activity also contributes significantly to chemical burden reduction and should be strongly encouraged.

## Search for Related Medical Conditions

Patients who have CS frequently have complicating medical conditions, especially hypofunction of one or more endocrine organs (91). Therefore, thyroid and adrenal status testing should be done as part of the usual medical evaluation of sick patients with CS, and when suggestive symptoms are present, other organs also should be evaluated. Endocrinology consultation should be considered for atypical or complex patients. CS often causes vascular symptoms, particularly hypothermia and peripheral vasospasm, that may be confused with hypothyroidism. Thyroid status must be measured (thyroid-stimulating hormone, thyroxine, free triiodothyronine, thyroid autoantibodies) because physical appearance is not a definitive indicator of true thyroid functioning. Mild reduction in cortisol production may occur, and substantial declines in dehydroepiandrosterone (DHEA) also may be seen. Both deficits lead to fatigue or poor energy reserves. Morning levels of cortisol and DHEA sulfate may be low, but if they are normal and poor adrenal reserve is still suspected, a corticotropin stimulation test can be used. Appropriate supplementation of low endocrine hormone levels may significantly improve fatigue and well-being in patients with CS, and improves the response to allergy immunotherapy.

## Begin Immunotherapy at Low Doses

Normally, allergy immunotherapy is the last intervention in patients with CS, after load reduction, nutritional management, endocrine supplementation, and physical measures. When initiating allergy immunotherapy in patients

with CS, inhalant desensitization should be started at neutralizing (endpoint) doses because these are, by definition, symptom-relieving doses. However, inhalant treatment should not be escalated until the allergic and chemical load has been substantially reduced, or symptoms frequently will provoked by treatment, and patients will be unable to advance. Once inhalant treatment has been successfully instituted, food neutralization for allergic foods that cannot easily be removed from the diet also may begin. Finally, if there are any chemicals that cannot be environmentally controlled, neutralization can be contemplated for those as well. Rea has found that most patients with CS cannot tolerate the concentrations of glycerin and phenol normally present in allergy immunotherapy treatment vials (92). Special precautions to prevent bacterial contamination are necessary if phenol-free solutions are used (see Chapter 12). Also, chemical solutions used for intradermal testing and neutralization treatment must be diluted sufficiently to prevent sloughing of the skin. According to Rea, sensitivity to terpenes, common petrochemicals, perfumes, various natural odors, and other chemicals can be successfully treated by neutralization therapy, when used in conjunction with the other measures for treating CS discussed previously.

## CONCLUSION

From the available data, it is reasonable to make a working model that persons with chemical toxicity, CS, and probably also MCS actually are suffering from complex, chemically induced derangements in their intermediary metabolism, structural damage to all macromolecular components of their cells, and consequent diffuse multisystem dysfunctioning. Much of this damage probably is mediated by free radicals generated during detoxification metabolism (58). It also is likely that all of these patients are deficient in multiple essential nutrients required for maximal detoxification and anabolic metabolism. Analysis of fat stores may yield abnormally elevated levels of nonpolar synthetic organic chemicals, and DNA analysis may detect cross-linking and excess numbers of point mutations. Subtle tests of the immune system also may show abnormalities in humoral, cell-mediated, or phagocytic functions. Endocrine functions can be deficient, and when present, contribute to feeling unwell. People with chemical exposure also may be clinically depressed, anxious, or both, and this also contributes to their symptoms. Both the hormonal and central nervous system abnormalities may actually be direct chemical effects, although this remains to be proven. Last, many, perhaps all, patients with CS and MCS will prove to be atopic, with demonstrable allergic sensitization to food and inhalant antigens.

Part of the CS problem is due to true allergy to chemical haptens, and another part arises because CS and allergy both generate excess oxidants. These patients labor under both a total allergic load and a total oxidant load, and both of these aspects of their disease process need to be addressed (93). Understanding how patients respond to the sum of all external and internal factors that affect their symptoms is vital to successful treatment of the more seriously ill patients. Complex patients require complex treatment regimens, and omission of any major factor from the treatment plan may produce therapeutic failure. Furthermore, failure to understand total allergic load can lead to allergen overdose during testing or treatment, with potentially serious anaphylactic consequences. Also, failure to appreciate all of the major allergen contacts, including chemicals, can lead to inadequate allergy therapy. Similarly, failure to understand total oxidant load can lead to inappropriate or ineffective treatment if nutritional management, environmental controls, and measures to reduce the body burden of chemicals are not put into place.

The problem of chemical pollution will continue to worsen as the earth's population continues to increase and people continue to demand improved living conditions. No matter how careful each person is, some personal absorption of chemical xenobiotics is inescapable. And, if people are not careful, or work or live in the wrong places, the exposure may be quite large. People are biochemically heterogeneous, and some are much better able than others to detoxify and excrete xenobiotics. Consequently, we can expect to see a spectrum of disease caused by xenobiotic exposure, ranging from apparent health, through mild, undiagnosed illness, to frank, serious disease. Even serious illness resulting from chemical exposure often is undiagnosed, or, more correctly, not completely diagnosed, because chemical toxicity seldom is included in the differential diagnosis. Finally, those who appear healthy really are not: at the very least, they are expending metabolic effort to detoxify xenobiotics, and thus have lower reserves available to deal with other environmental stressors.

Practicing allergists are left with a monumental challenge: caring for patients with CS and MCS on a daily basis. The working model of the pathophysiologic process of CS is used both for clinical care and to design and carry out clinical investigations that will advance our understanding of CS. Familiarity with the probable etiology and actual symptoms of CS will lead to improved ability to diagnose those patients who require treatment. Further clinical experience will then progress to development and testing of additional treatment methods, based on our improving understanding of the working model. Ultimately, by successfully doing all of this, it should be possible to bring the recognition, diagnosis, and treatment of CS into the mainstream of 21st century medical care.

## ACKNOWLEDGMENTS

The author thanks June L. Bianchi, Beverly J. Flynn, Phyllis J. Foley, Sally C. Schumann, librarians, Nancy E. Frazier, former head librarian (deceased), and Jeanie M. Vander Pyl, head librarian, Cape Cod Hospital Medical Library, for their expertise in medical literature research.

## REFERENCES

1. Morgan MRA, Fenwick GR. Natural foodborne toxicants. *Lancet* 1990;336:1492–1495.
2. Boyles JH Jr. Introduction to chemical-environmental allergy. In: Krause HF, ed. *Otolaryngic allergy and immunology.* Philadelphia: WB Saunders, 1989:263–267.
3. Murozumi M, Chow TJ, Patterson C. Chemical concentrations of pollutant aerosols, terrestrial dusts, and sea salts in Greenland and Antarctic snow strata. *Geochim Cosmochim Acta* 1969;33:1247–1294.
4. Poisoning. In: Beers MH, Berkow R, eds. *Merck manual of diagnosis and therapy,* 17th ed. Whitehouse Station, NJ: Merck & Co., 1999:2619–2644.
5. Pilsum JF. Metabolism of individual tissues. In: Devlin TM, ed. *Textbook of biochemistry.* New York: John Wiley & Sons, 1986:807–854.
6. Galland L. Biochemical abnormalities in patients with multiple chemical sensitivities. *Occup Med* 1987;2:713–720.
7. Rea WJ. Chemical hypersensitivity and the allergic response. *Ear Nose Throat J* 1988;67:50–56.
8. Hahn LJ, Kloiber R, Vimy MJ, et al. Dental "silver" tooth fillings: a source of mercury exposure revealed by whole-body image scan and tissue analysis. *Fed Am Soc Exp Biol J* 1989;3:2641–2646.
9. Division of Standards Development and Technology Transfer. Update: styrene, dioxin, and 1,3-butadiene in the workplace. *MMWR Morb Mortal Wkly Rep* 1984;33:179–180.
10. Andersen KE. Systemic toxicity from percutaneous absorption of industrial chemicals. In: Adams RM, ed. *Occupational skin disease.* Philadelphia: WB Saunders, 1990:73–88.
11. Zugerman C. Chloracne, chloracnegens, and other forms of environmental acne. In: Adams RM, ed. *Occupational skin disease.* Philadelphia: WB Saunders, 1990:127–135.
12. Rea WJ, Brown OD. Cardiovascular disease in response to chemicals and foods. In: Brostoff J, Challacombe SJ, ed. *Food allergy and intolerance.* London: Bailliere Tindall, 1987:737–753.
13. Belsito DV. Mechanisms of allergic contact dermatitis. *Immunol Allergy Clin North Am* 1989;9:579–595.
14. Vimy MJ, Lorscheider FL. Letter to the editor. *Am Ind Hyg Assoc J* 1988;49:A92–A93.
15. Turjanmaa K, Reunala T, Alenius H, et al. Allergens in latex surgical gloves and glove powder. *Lancet* 1990;336:1588.
16. Corrado OJ, Osman J, Davies RJ. Asthma and rhinitis after exposure to glutaraldehyde in endoscopy units. *Hum Toxicol* 1986;5:325–327.
17. Saxon A, Beall GN, Rohr AS, et al. Immediate hypersensitivity reactions to beta-lactam antibiotics. *Ann Intern Med* 1987;107:204–215.
18. Luster MI, Wierda D, Rosenthal GJ. Environmentally related disorders of the hematologic and immune systems. *Med Clin North Am* 1990;74:425–440.
19. Spurlock BW, Dailey TM. Shortness of (fresh) breath: toothpaste-induced bronchospasm. *N Engl J Med* 1990;323:1845–1846.
20. Zeiss CR. Reactive chemicals as inhalant allergens. *Immunol Allergy Clin North Am* 1989;9:235–244.
21. Levin AS, Byers VS. Environmental illness: a disorder of immune regulation. *Occup Med* 1987;2:669–681.
22. Zschunke E, Ziegler V, Haustein UF. Occupationally induced

connective tissue disorders. In: Adams RM, ed. *Occupational skin disease.* Philadelphia: WB Saunders, 1990:172–183.

23. Bates D. Ominous new data shows hazards of acid aerosols. *Respir News* 1990;10:1.

24. Peterson B, Saxon A. Global increases in allergic respiratory disease: the possible role of diesel exhaust particles. *Ann Allergy Asthma Immunol* 1996;77:263–268.

25. Strannegard O, Strannegard IL. The causes of the increasing prevalence of allergy: is atopy a microbial deprivation disorder? *Allergy* 2001;56:91–102.

26. Seba DB, Milam MJ, Laseter JL. Uptake, measurement, and elimination of synthetic chemicals by man. In: Brostoff J, Challacombe SJ, ed. *Food allergy and intolerance.* London: Bailliere Tindall, 1987:401–415.

27. Simon GE, Katon WJ, Sparks PJ. Allergic to life: psychological factors in environmental illness. *Am J Psychiatry* 1990;147:901–906.

28. Randolph TG. *Human ecology and susceptibility to the chemical environment.* Springfield, IL: Charles C Thomas, 1962.

29. Cullen MR. The worker with multiple chemical sensitivities: an overview. *Occup Med* 1987;2:655–661.

30. Anonymous. Multiple chemical sensitivity: a 1999 consensus. *Arch Environ Health* 1999;54:147–149.

31. AAAAI Board of Directors. Position statement: idiopathic environmental intolerances. *J Allergy Clin Immunol* 1999;103:36–40.

32. Kreutzer R, Neutra RR, Lashuay N. Prevalence of people reporting sensitivities to chemicals in a population-based survey. *Am J Epidemiol* 1999;150:1–12.

33. Meggs WJ, Dunn KA, Bloch RM, et al. Prevalence and nature of allergy and chemical sensitivity in a general population. *Arch Environ Health* 1996;51:275–282.

34. Brod BA. Multiple chemical sensitivities syndrome: a review. *Am J Contact Dermat* 1996;7:202–211.

35. Magill MK, Suruda A. Multiple chemical sensitivity syndrome. *Am Fam Physician* 1998;58:721–728.

36. Staudenmayer H, Kramer RE. Psychogenic chemical sensitivity: psychogenic pseudoseizures elicited by provocation challenges with fragrances. *J Psychosom Res* 1999;47:185–190.

37. Andine P, Ronnback L, Jarvholm B. Successful use of a selective serotonin reuptake inhibitor in a patient with multiple chemical sensitivities. *Acta Psychiatr Scand* 1997;96:82–83.

38. Haller E. Successful management of patients with "multiple chemical sensitivities" on an inpatient psychiatric unit. *J Clin Psychiatry* 1993;54:196–199.

39. Leznoff A. Provocative challenges in patients with multiple chemical sensitivity. *J Allergy Clin Immunol* 1997;99:438–442.

40. Binkley KE, Kutcher S. Panic response to sodium lactate infusion in patients with multiple chemical sensitivity syndrome. *J Allergy Clin Immunol* 1997;99:570–574.

41. Poonai N, Antony MM, Binkley KE, et al. Carbon dioxide inhalation challenges in idiopathic environmental intolerance. *J Allergy Clin Immunol* 2000;105:358–363.

42. Bell IR. Clinically relevant EEG studies and psychophysiological findings: possible neural mechanisms for multiple chemical sensitivity. *Toxicology* 1996;111:101–117.

43. Brown-DeGagne AM, McGlone J. Multiple chemical sensitivity: a test of the olfactory-limbic model. *J Occup Environ Med* 1999;41:366–377.

44. Bolla KI. Neurobehavioral performance in multiple chemical sensitivities. *Regul Toxicol Pharmacol* 1996;24:S52–S54.

45. MacPhail RC. Evolving concepts of chemical sensitivity. *Environ Health Perspect* 1997;105[Suppl 2]:455–456.

46. Meggs WJ. Hypothesis for induction and propagation of chemical sensitivity based on biopsy studies. *Environ Health Perspect* 1997;105[Suppl 2]:473–478.

47. Bascom R, Meggs WJ, Frampton M, et al. Neurogenic inflammation: with additional discussion of central and perceptual integration of nonneurogenic inflammation. *Environ Health Perspect* 1997;105[Suppl 2]:531–537.

48. Ross PM. Chemical sensitivity and fatigue syndromes from hypoxia/hypercapnia. *Med Hypotheses* 2000;54:734–738.

49. Hartman DE. Missed diagnoses and misdiagnoses of environmental toxicant exposure: the psychiatry of toxic exposure and multiple chemical sensitivity. *Psychiatr Clin North Am* 1998;21:659–670.

50. Levy F. Clinical features of multiple chemical sensitivity. *Scand J Work Environ Health* 1997;23[Suppl 3]:69–73.

51. King WP. Efficacy of a screening radioallergosorbent test. *Arch Otolaryngol* 1982;108:781–786.

52. King WP, Motes JM. The intracutaneous progressive dilution multi-food test. *Otolaryngol Head Neck Surg* 1991;104:235–238.

53. Malinin G, Kalimo K. The results of skin testing with food additives and the effect of an elimination diet in chronic and recurrent urticaria and recurrent angioedema. *Clin Exp Allergy* 1989;19:539–543.

54. Fisher AA. Contact urticaria due to occupational exposures. In: Adams RM, ed. *Occupational skin disease.* Philadelphia: WB Saunders, 1990:113–126.

55. Menzies D, Comtois P, Pasztor J, et al. Aeroallergens and work related respiratory symptoms among office workers. *J Allergy Clin Immunol* 1998;101:38–44.

56. Norback D, Walinder R, Wieslander G, et al. Indoor air pollutants in schools: nasal patency and biomarkers in nasal lavage. *Allergy* 2000;55:163–170.

57. Adachi A, Horikawa T, Takashima T, et al. Potential efficacy of low metal diets and dental metal elimination in the management of atopic dermatitis: an open clinical study. *J Dermatol* 1997;24:12–19.

58. Levine SA, Reinhardt JH. Biochemical-pathology initiated by free radicals, oxidant chemicals, and therapeutic drugs in the etiology of chemical hypersensitivity disease. *J Orthomol Psychiatry* 1983;12:166–183.

59. Sherman JD. *Chemical exposure and disease.* New York: Van Nostrand Reinhold, 1988:38–53.

60. Ashford NA, CS Miller. *Chemical exposures.* New York: Van Nostrand Reinhold, 1991:3–26.

61. Mabry RL, ed. *Skin endpoint titration.* New York: Thieme Medical, 1992.

62. Adams RM, Fischer T. Diagnostic patch testing. In: Adams RM, ed. *Occupational skin disease.* Philadelphia: WB Saunders, 1990:223–253.

63. King WP. Diagnostic and therapeutic techniques for chemical-environmental allergy and hypersensitivity. In: Krause HF, ed. *Otolaryngic allergy and immunology.* Philadelphia: WB Saunders, 1989:274–276.

64. Davies RJ, Blainey AD, Pepys J. Occupational asthma. In: Middleton E, Reed CE, Ellis EF, eds. *Allergy principles and practice,* 2nd ed. St. Louis: Mosby, 1983:1037–1066.

65. Kivisto H, Pekari K, Peltonen K, et al. Biological monitoring of exposure to benzene in the production of benzene and in a cokery. *Sci Total Environ* 1997;199:49–63.

66. Jakubowski M, Linhart I, Pielas G, et al. 2-Cyanoethylmercapturic acid (CEMA) in the urine as a possible indicator of exposure to acrylonitrile. *Br J Ind Med* 1987;44:834–840.

67. Arena JM. *Poisoning.* Springfield, IL: Charles C Thomas, 1986:174–221.

68. Seidel S, Kreutzer R, Smith D, et al. Assessment of commercial laboratories performing hair mineral analysis *JAMA* 2001;285:67–72.

69. Wilhelm M, Muller F, Idel H. Biological monitoring of mercury vapor exposure by scalp hair analysis in comparison to blood and urine. *Toxicol Lett* 1996;88:221–226.

70. Abe T, Ohtsuka R, Hongo T, et al. High hair and urinary mercury levels of fish eaters in the nonpolluted environment of Papua New Guinea. *Arch Environ Health* 1995;50:367–373.

71. Ahlqwist M, Bengtsson C, Lapidus L, et al. Concentrations of blood, serum, and urine components in relation to number of amalgam tooth fillings in Swedish women. *Community Dent Oral Epidemiol* 1995;23:217–221.

72. Komaromy-Hiller G, Ash KO, Costa R, et al. Comparison of representative ranges based on U.S. patient population and literature reference intervals for urinary trace elements. *Clin Chim Acta* 2000;296:71–90.

73. Medley DW, Kathren RL, Miller AG. Diurnal urinary volume and uranium output in uranium workers and unexposed controls. *Health Phys* 1994;67:122–130.

74. Blanke RV, Poklis A. Analytical/forensic toxicology. In: Amdur MO, Doull J, Klaassen CD, eds. *Toxicology.* New York: Pergamon Press, 1991:905–923.

75. Lauwerys RR. Occupational toxicology. In: Amdur MO, Doull J, Klaassen CD, eds. *Toxicology.* New York: Pergamon Press, 1991:947–969.

76. Torres-Alanis O, Garza-Ocanas L, Pineyro-Lopez A. Evaluation of urinary mercury excretion after administration of 2,3-dimercapto-1-propane sulfonic acid to occupationally exposed men. *J Toxicol Clin Toxicol* 1995;33:717–720.

77. Anonymous. Elimination of poisons. In: Beers MH, Berkow R, eds. *Merck manual of diagnosis and therapy,* 17th ed. Whitehouse Station, NJ: Merck & Co., 1999:2622.

78. Stanley JS. *Broad scan analysis of the FY82 National Human Adipose Tissue Survey specimens.* EPA publication 560/5-86-035. Washington, DC: Environmental Protection Agency, 1986.

79. Jacob RA, Burri BJ. Oxidative damage and defense. *Am J Clin Nutr* 1996;63:985S–990S.

80. Sanders SP, Zweier JL, Harrison SJ, et al. Spontaneous oxygen radical production at sites of antigen challenge in allergic subjects. *Am J Respir Crit Care Med* 1995;151:1725–1733.

81. Hatch GE. Asthma, inhaled oxidants, and dietary antioxidants. *Am J Clin Nutr* 1995;61:625S–630S.

82. Delfino RJ, Coate BD, Zeiger RS, et al. Daily asthma severity in relation to personal ozone exposure and outdoor fungal spores. *Am J Respir Crit Care Med* 1996;154:633–641.

83. Greene LS. Asthma and oxidant stress: nutritional, environmental, and genetic risk factors. *J Am Coll Nutr* 1995;14:317–324.

84. Gordon BR. Update on the importance of nutrition in allergy management. *Curr Opin Otolaryngol Head Neck Surg* 1998;6:67–69.

85. Gordon BR. The importance of nutrition in allergy management. *Curr Opin Otolaryngol Head Neck Surg* 1997;5:53–54.

86. Levine M, Dhariwal KR, Welch RW, et al. Determination of optimal vitamin C requirements in humans. *Am J Clin Nutr* 1995;62:1347S–1356S.

87. Werbach MR. *Foundations of nutritional medicine.* Tarzana, CA: Third Line Press, 1997.

88. Werbach MR. *Nutritional influences on illness,* 2nd ed. Tarzana, CA: Third Line Press, 1993.

89. Rea WJ. Thermal chamber depuration and physical therapy. In: *Chemical sensitivity.* Boca Raton, FL: CRC Press, 1997:2433–2479.

90. Hannuksela ML, Ellahham S. Benefits and risks of sauna bathing. *Am J Med* 2001;110:118–126.

91. Rea WJ. Endocrine treatment. In: *Chemical sensitivity.* Boca Raton, FL: CRC Press, 1997:2685–2713.

92. Rea WJ. Injection therapy, intradermal testing, and subcutaneous injection treatment. In: *Chemical sensitivity.* Boca Raton, FL: CRC Press, 1997:2481–2540.

93. Rea WJ. *Chemical sensitivity,* vol II: *Sources of total body load.* Boca Raton, FL: Lewis Publishers, 1994.

# ENT MANIFESTATIONS OF RHEUMATIC DISEASES

## RENEE Z. RINALDI
## MICHAEL H. WEISMAN

There are many rheumatologic diseases that have distinctive otolaryngic manifestations that must be considered in the differential diagnosis and management of patients with allergic illnesses. Categorizing these diseases by their most characteristic anatomic sites of involvement allows us to approach these illnesses in a systematic fashion.

## RHEUMATIC DISEASES AFFECTING THE NOSE AND NASAL PASSAGES

### Wegener's Granulomatosis

Wegener's granulomatosis (WG) is a form of systemic vasculitis primarily involving the respiratory tract and kidneys. Presenting complaints involving the upper respiratory tract are seen in greater than 90% of patients. WG should be considered when a patient displays a history of sinusitis and rhinitis that has not improved for several weeks and may be accompanied by a serosanguineous nasal discharge, epistaxis, crusting, obstruction, or associated pain over the dorsum of the nose and mucosal ulcerations. The unusual sign of nasal crusting should alert the clinician because it is uncommon in other rhinologic conditions (1). The patient may have accompanying systemic symptoms of weakness, malaise, night sweats, and arthralgias. On physical examination, diffuse crusting of the nose and nasopharynx is found. The underlying mucosa is very granular and friable. There may be septal perforations if the patient has been symptomatic for several months or more (2).

Other ear, nose, and throat (ENT) manifestations include hearing loss due to otitis media, or sensorineural hearing loss. In patients with more long-standing disease, saddle-nose deformity and tracheobronchial (subglottic) stenosis may develop.

In addition to upper respiratory tract involvement, there is pulmonary involvement in over 85% of patients. The patient may have symptoms of cough, dyspnea. pleuritic chest pain, or hemoptysis. The chest radiograph, even in some asymptomatic patients, may reveal infiltrates and nodules in the middle and lower lung, which may cavitate. There may be pleural effusions or lymphadenopathy in the hila or mediastinum, which can calcify. Pulmonary function tests show obstructive changes or decreased lung diffusing capacity for carbon monoxide and decreased lung volumes.

Patients with WG who have a limited form of the disease, defined as an absence of renal involvement, have only respiratory tract involvement, and those patients usually have a better prognosis. Patients with renal disease usually have a fulminant course that was associated with an 80% mortality rate at 1 year before the current therapeutic regimens were established. The renal pathologic finding is local segmental necrotizing glomerulonephritis (3).

The diagnosis of WG has traditionally relied on obtaining pathologic evidence of necrotizing granulomatous vasculitis on biopsy specimens. This may require open lung biopsy because upper airway pathologic findings usually are nonspecific or may reveal granulomatous changes without vasculitis. If there are signs of granular nasal mucosa, a nasal biopsy may yield diagnostic tissue, and is readily obtained under local anesthesia. Adequate tissue must be obtained; a punch biopsy from the ulcerated edge of a specimen often is inadequate. Biopsies from the paranasal sinuses usually have a higher diagnostic yield (1). Needle biopsy of lung tissue typically does not reveal the specific histologic findings of WG. Open lung biopsy often must be obtained because it has a greater than 90% diagnostic yield. Even after obtaining a large specimen from an open lung biopsy, the pathologist must examine the edge of the tissue surrounding the necrotic area to observe the specific histologic findings of WG.

Since the early 1980s, distinctive antibodies have been recognized in patients with WG, which may improve our ability to make an accurate diagnosis. Known as ANCA (anti-neutrophil cytoplasmic antibodies), these are serum

**R. Z. Rinaldi:** Department of Medicine, University of California—Los Angeles School of Medicine, Los Angeles, California.

**M. H. Weisman:** Department of Medicine, Division of Rheumatology, University of California at San Diego, La Jolla; and Division of Rheumatology, Cedars–Sinai Medical Center, Los Angeles, California.

antibodies that react with the cytoplasmic components of neutrophils. These can be identified by immunofluorescence, enzyme-linked immunosorbent assay (ELISA), or immunoblotting techniques. When the patient's serum is incubated with ethanol-fixed normal human neutrophils, two immunofluorescent patterns can be found in WG and related vasculitic syndromes (4). C-ANCA stains the cytoplasm diffusely, and the antibodies producing the pattern are directed primarily against a serine protease (i.e., proteinase-3) (5). P-ANCA, which localizes around the nuclear membrane during ethanol fixation, recognizes cytoplasmic myeloperoxidase (MPO). ELISA and immunoblotting techniques allow for direct identification of the MPO and proteinase-3 antibodies. This is important diagnostically because P-ANCA results may recognize antibodies directed against non-MPO antigens, such as elastase and lactoferrin, in a variety of nonvasculitic disorders (4) such as ulcerative colitis.

Almost all patients with otherwise typical active WG have a positive ANCA, and of these up to 95% are C-ANCA directed against proteinase-3. The remainder are P-ANCA antibodies primarily directed against MPO. Other ANCA-related illnesses include microscopic polyangiitis (where anti-MPO P-ANCA can be found in 40% to 80% of cases), idiopathic necrotizing glomerulonephritis (P-ANCA positive in 75% to 80%), and Churg-Strauss syndrome (variable reports of ANCA positivity). Although ANCA testing in some collected series of patients can be highly sensitive (73% for C-ANCA) and specific (95% for C-ANCA) for WG according to a large European collaborative study (6), its use as a sole agent to establish the diagnosis of WG without tissue biopsy remains controversial. Studies have shown that ANCA testing has a high positive predictive value in patients whose clinical presentations are most suggestive of this diagnosis. However, in patients with less typical symptoms (i.e., sinusitis alone), the sensitivity and specificity drop significantly. Because of the toxicity of the therapeutic agents used to treat WG, many rheumatologists prefer biopsy confirmation before proceeding with therapy—especially in cases without a classic presentation. Initial treatment of WG consists of high-dose oral steroids and oral cyclophosphamide (7).

Patients with WG often go for long periods without a specific diagnosis. This is because the clinical manifestations vary or are different over time, and there may be long intervals between flare-ups. Therefore, it is important to recognize the unique ENT features of the disease to avoid delays in diagnosis and, more important, to institute treatment in a timely manner.

## Churg-Strauss Syndrome

Churg Strauss syndrome is a form of vasculitis with allergic features, granulomatous infiltrates, and angiitis, in which characteristic ENT manifestations may occur. Patients with Churg-Strauss syndrome often display a prodromal phase of allergic rhinitis, nasal polyps, and asthma that persists for years before organ-threatening vasculitis develops. This may be followed by peripheral blood eosinophilia and clinicopathologic findings of eosinophilic infiltration of the lungs or gastrointestinal tract. Vasculitic lesions may develop as the asthma improves and include purpuric or ulcerating skin lesions, dyspnea and chest pain secondary to pulmonary lesions, peripheral neuropathy, especially mononeuritis multiplex, abdominal pain, abdominal mass or diarrhea, and mild glomerulonephritis. The diagnosis of Churg-Strauss syndrome can be confirmed from a biopsy of involved tissues. Pathologic examination shows angiitis and extramural necrotizing microgranulomas with eosinophils. Abdominal angiograms may show multiple arterial aneurysms along with tapered narrowing of vessels and vessel wall irregularities. An angiogram should be obtained if a biopsy site cannot be found, or if a blind biopsy is negative and the clinical suspicion is still present. Treatment consists of high-dose, daily prednisone with the addition of azathioprine or cyclophosphamide for refractory cases (7).

## Sarcoidosis

Sarcoidosis is a multisystem inflammatory disorder manifested by the formation of noncaseating granulomas that most commonly affects the lungs and lymph nodes.

The nasal lesions of sarcoidosis include crusting, epistaxis, and bilateral obstruction, and may be indistinguishable from WG. However, these lesions are very rare in sarcoidosis compared with their incidence in WG, and usually occur in a more benign clinical setting, where other features of sarcoidosis are present, such as hilar adenopathy, hypercalcemia, and elevated angiotensin-converting enzyme levels. Nasal mucosal biopsy shows typical noncaseating granulomas. Nasal lesions may be managed best with topical nasal corticosteroids, or with oral corticosteroids if needed to control systemic disease (8).

## Relapsing Polychondritis

In relapsing polychondritis, persistent or recurrent inflammation of the nasal cartilage may lead to nasal collapse and saddle-nose deformity (see later). Similar findings of chondritis leading to saddle-nose deformity may develop in patients with longstanding WG.

## MUCOSAL LESIONS

Mucosal lesions are seen in several rheumatic diseases, including systemic lupus erythematous (SLE), reactive arthritis (formerly known as *Reiter's syndrome*), WG, and Behçet's disease. Recurrent aphthous stomatitis (RAS), more usually known as *oral ulcerations* or *canker sores,* is an extremely common condition that can affect up to 20% of the general population (9) and must be differentiated from Behçet's disease or WG. RAS has been classified into simple and complex forms. In the simple forms, the patient has a few lesions that heal in 1 to 2 weeks and recur infrequently. In complex aphthosis, the patient has numerous, large or deep lesions that develop continuously and are very painful. In some of these patients, occasional genital aphthae may develop. Treatment options range from topical anesthetics, antihistamine rinses, and topical steroids, to systemic antihistamines or steroids.

## Systemic Lupus Erythematosus

Oral ulcerations are observed in 20% of patients with SLE and are included in the American College of Rheumatology criteria for diagnosis (3). They usually are painless, but not always. Occasionally, nasal ulcers and vaginal ulcers may be found. These lesions have a depressed surface filled with a yellow-white, fibrinous exudate surrounded by peripheral erythema. They can be difficult to differentiate clinically from RAS. When seen in the context of other characteristic features of SLE, such as photosensitive rashes, arthritis, renal disease, or pleuritis, the diagnosis of SLE is straightforward. The oral lesions of SLE usually demonstrate characteristic histopathologic findings of discord lupus and are repeatedly positive for immunoglobulin and complement deposition at the dermal–epidermal junction. The gingiva may appear red, edematous, friable, and eroded on clinical examination (10). Finally, vasculitis may (rarely) lead to nasal septal erosive lesions and perforation.

Other oral lesions found in SLE may resemble lichen planus or leukoplakia, which, again, may be differentiated from these conditions only by the clinical context in which they occur. Erosive and ulcerative lesions with patchy white keratotic margins may be seen that clinically (and histologically) resemble erosive lichen planus. They are painful lesions affecting the buccal mucosa, gingiva, and lateral tongue. The keratotic margins form delicate striae radiating away from the central ulcer. Leukoplakia-like lesions may appear as white patches that cannot be scraped off. These lesions may be thin and filmy or raised, white plaques that are irregularly shaped on the tongue or buccal mucosa, floor of the mouth, or lips. These lesions clinically and histologically resemble erosive lichen planus. Histologically, a perivascular lymphocytic infiltrate is seen in the deeper submucosal tissue (11).

## Behçet's Disease

Oral ulcerations usually are the initial manifestation of Behçet's disease. These lesions are painful shallow ulcers covered with a grayish-white pseudomembrane and have sharp, erythematous borders. They can occur as numerous crops of tiny, 2- to -3 mm, herpetiform ulcers, or as 1-cm or larger lesions. They may occur anywhere in the oral cavity and resolve after 1 to 3 weeks; larger lesions may heal with scarring. The characteristic association of these oral lesions with genital ulcers and ocular inflammation such as uveitis or iritis should lead to a suspicion of Behçet's disease. Male lesions are deeper and painful, occurring on the scrotum or penis, and heal with scarring. Female ulcers occur on the vulva premenstrually and are less painful. Oral and genital ulcerations are not specific for Behçet's disease and may be found in several other systemic diseases, as well as in patients with idiopathic RAS. These include ulcus vulvae acutum (severe oral and vulvar aphthae associated with infectious gastroenteritis), MAGIC syndrome (mouth and genital ulcers with inflamed cartilage), FAPA syndrome (fever, aphthosis, pharyngitis, and adenitis), and cyclic neutropenia (9). MAGIC syndrome is thought to be the confluence of Behçet's disease and relapsing polychondritis. Therapeutic modalities for Behçet's disease include steroids, thalidomide, azathioprine, and cyclosporine. Thalidomide has been shown to be effective in suppressing mucocutaneous lesions. Azathioprine and cyclosporine are used for eye involvement; cyclophosphamide is reserved for vasculitis and central nervous system involvement (12).

## Reactive Arthritis (Reiter's Syndrome)

In contrast to Behçet's disease, the oral ulcers found in this condition usually are painless and occur in a lingual or palatal distribution. The diagnosis should be suspected when oral ulcers are found in a patient with evidence of urethritis, conjunctivitis, or arthritis.

## Wegener's Granulomatosis

In WG, ulcerations of the nasal cavity, oral cavity, or sinuses may be the initial presentation of the disease, although in most cases, more diagnostic lesions soon develop in other organ systems.

## XEROSTOMIA: SJÖGREN'S SYNDROME

Xerostomia, or dry mouth, is a common symptom that can occur in a variety of clinical situations, including drug reactions (anticholinergic opiates), acute and chronic renal failure, after radiation therapy or chemotherapy, sarcoidosis, and lymphoma. When xerostomia occurs in conjunction with xerophthalmia, or dry eyes, a rheumatic etiology should be strongly considered.

Sjögren's syndrome is an autoimmune disease affecting primarily the lacrimal and salivary glands (as well as the other exocrine glands). Initially, the quality of tear content is affected; as the disease progresses, there is decreased lacrimal and salivary gland secretion. The presence of inflammatory arthritis in such patients in the absence of any other signs of other rheumatic diseases confirms the diagnosis of primary Sjögren's syndrome (3). Patients who have similar findings in the context of other autoimmune diseases are designated as having secondary Sjögren's syndrome, and these associated diseases include rheumatoid arthritis, SLE, scleroderma, polymyositis, chronic noninfectious hepatitis, cryoglobulinemia, vasculitis, and thyroiditis. Sjögren's syndrome has been described in patients with chronic hepatitis C infection.

Patients with xerostomia complain of difficulty with chewing and swallowing dry foods and foods sticking in the buccal surface. There may be a burning discomfort in the mouth and changes in the sense of taste. There is accelerated development of dental caries. The parotid and submandibular glands may become involved, with episodes of diffuse, nontender enlargement, either unilateral or bilateral. On physical examination, the oral surfaces tend to be dry; there may be oral ulcerations; and the tongue appears dry and red with atrophy of the papillae (3). Oral thrush commonly accompanies this condition.

The symptoms of xerophthalmia include dryness, which usually is interpreted by the patient as a sensation of sand or grittiness under the eyelids. Other symptoms include burning, decreased tearing, redness, itching, eye fatigue, and light sensitivity. The patient may note an accumulation of mucous thread strands at the inner canthus. Other exocrine glands may be involved. Dry nose, throat, and trachea may result from involvement of the mucous glands in the respiratory tract. The exocrine glands of the skin, external genitalia. and gastrointestinal tract may be affected, resulting in dry skin, esophageal mucosal atrophy, atrophic gastritis, and subclinical pancreatitis. The symptoms of Sjögren's syndrome may evolve slowly over 8 to 10 years before the full-blown syndrome is manifest. Although xerostomia can be measured by a variety of techniques, including salivary flow measurements, salivary scintigraphy, and parotid sialography, these techniques are not practical in clinical practice. Minor salivary gland biopsy usually is relied on for diagnosis. The lymphocytic infiltrate that damages salivary glandular tissue can be seen histologically as aggregates of lymphocytes with acinar atrophy and hypertrophy of ductal epithelial and myoepithelial cells. The focus score is a standardized and validated technique for diagnosis. Each "focus" consists of an aggregate of 50 lymphoid cells replacing acinar tissue. One focus per 4 mm$^2$ of glandular tissue is considered diagnostic (3). Biopsy of a minor salivary gland with analysis for focus score in the oral mucosa is a relatively noninvasive diagnostic technique that is popular in clinical practice.

Extraglandular involvement occurs in one half of the patients within 5 to 10 years of the diagnosis of primary Sjögren's syndrome, but is rare in secondary Sjögren's syndrome. Low-grade fevers, fatigue, subclinical diffuse interstitial lung disease, interstitial nephritis, and, more rarely, glomerulonephritis and renal tubular acidosis may occur. Vasculitis of the small or medium-sized vessels can involve virtually any organ. Subclinical thyroiditis occurs commonly. Laboratory studies help to identify patients with primary Sjögren's syndrome; these patients have a positive test for rheumatoid factor, hyperglobulinemia, and positive anti-SSA or anti-SSB antibodies.

Treatment of Sjögren's syndrome varies from symptomatic therapies to relieve xerostomia and xerophthalmia to steroids, antimalarial drugs, and immunosuppressive therapy for more advanced disease. Recent studies have shown that cholinergic agonists such as pilocarpine can significantly improve mouth dryness (Daiku Pharmaceuticals, personal communication).

## EARS: RELAPSING POLYCHONDRITIS

Inflammation of the cartilage of the outer ear is the hallmark of relapsing polychondritis and occurs in over 85% of patients. This is a relatively rare condition that is characterized by episodic inflammation of the cartilaginous structures of the ears, nose, and trachea. Recent studies have shown that immunologic mechanisms play a significant role in this disease. In one study, there was an increased incidence of human leukocyte antigen DR4 compared with healthy control subjects (13). Typical attacks involving the ear remit and recur unilaterally or bilaterally. The episodes persist for days to weeks. They involve cartilage of the pinna as erythematous or violaceous plaques, and the external auditory canal may become narrowed. If attacks are severe, the tissues may become ossified, leading to a cauliflower deformity (2). Inflammation of the nasal cartilage may lead to nasal collapse and saddle-nose deformity.

When the disease is fully expressed with multiple sites of cartilaginous inflammation, the diagnosis of relapsing polychondritis usually is obvious, and histologic confirmation rarely is necessary. However, at presentation, the findings may be limited to the ear alone, and may be confused with other conditions such as chondrodermatitis nodularis chronica helicis, an inflammatory nodular condition of the external ear (14).

Hearing loss may occur in 30% of patients because of conductive defects resulting from eustachian tube chondritis or sensorineural defects due to presumed vasculitis involving the internal auditory artery (15). Vestibular symptoms may accompany hearing loss due to vasculitis of the vestibular branch of the internal auditory artery. In some patients, a necrotizing glomerulonephritis develops, suggesting a widespread autoimmune disease. These patients are notoriously difficult to treat, have a poor prognosis, and require organic immunosuppressive management.

## LARYNX: RHEUMATOID ARTHRITIS

Laryngeal involvement may affect one third of patients with rheumatoid arthritis and cause symptoms of hoarseness, dyspnea, stridor, dysphagia, and a globus sensation (2). In early stages, there is active inflammation of the larynx characterized by tenderness and erythema. Late changes reveal ankylosis of the cricoarytenoid joint with normal laryngeal mucosa. Upper airway obstruction may develop acutely, manifested by stridor and respiratory distress; this may be a medical emergency.

## TRACHEA

### Relapsing Polychondritis

Tracheal stenosis occurs in 50% of cases of relapsing polychondritis. Symptoms include sore throat, hoarseness, dyspnea, cough, inspiratory stridor, and choking; these symptoms may be confused with those of bronchial asthma. There may be tracheal edema at first, resulting in scarring, which may lead to fibrotic subglottic stenosis or a dynamically collapsing, flaccid tracheobronchial tree. Vocal cord paralysis may complicate the clinical picture.

Magnetic resonance imaging sequences have been reported to be helpful in establishing the diagnosis when the larynx is the primary site of involvement and laryngoscopy and endoscopic biopsy have failed to establish the diagnosis (16). The most serious complication is airway obstruction, which may require tracheotomy or tracheal stenting. Patients therefore must be monitored carefully for early signs of respiratory compromise. Computed tomography scanning and bronchoscopy are not adequate to assess for impending upper airway obstruction. Pulmonary function tests, especially the flow volume loop during maximal inspiration and expiration, are sensitive tests for dynamic upper airway obstruction and should be monitored sequentially. Treatment includes intermittent high-dose steroid therapy, cytotoxic agents, or dapsone.

### Wegener's Granulomatosis

Laryngeal involvement may occur in approximately 8% to 15% of cases of WG, usually in the form of a subglottic mass or circumferential narrowing. Treatment with cyclophosphamide and steroids may be successful. Because of the potential for life-threatening upper airway obstruction, tracheostomy may be necessary while medical treatment is underway. If stenosis progresses despite medical treatment, tracheal dilation, stenting, or reconstruction may be necessary (11).

## VESTIBULAR SYSTEM: COGAN'S SYNDROME

This is a rare disorder consisting of interstitial keratitis, tinnitus, sensorineural hearing loss, and vertigo. Cogan's syndrome should be suspected when a young adult patient presents with eye inflammation and Ménière's disease–like episodes. Interstitial keratitis produces symptoms of blurred vision, pain, redness. and photophobia. There may be associated vasculitis of large, medium, or small arteries. Aortitis resulting in aortic insufficiency may be found. Treatment consists of topical and systemic corticosteroids and immunosuppressives for refractory cases (17).

## REFERENCES

1. Jones NS. Nasal manifestations of rheumatic diseases. *Ann Rheum Dis* 1999;58:589–590.
2. Gay RM, Ball CV. Vasculitis. In: Koopman WJ, ed. *Arthritis and allied conditions: a textbook of rheumatology,* vol 2. Baltimore: Williams & Wilkins, 1997:1491–1524.
3. Klippel JH, Weyand CM, et al. *Primer on the rheumatic diseases.* Atlanta: Arthritis Foundation, 1997.
4. Rose BD, et al. *Up-to-date in medicine,* 2000.
5. Langford CA. The diagnostic utility of c-ANCA in Wegener's granulomatosis. *Cleve Clin J Med* 1998;65:135–140.
6. Hagen EC, Daha MR, Hermans J, et al. Diagnostic value of standardized assays for anti-neutrophil cytoplasmic antibodies in idiopathic systemic vasculitis: EC/BCR Project for ANCA Assay Standardization. *Kidney Int* 1998;53:743–753.
7. St. Clair EW. Vasculitis. In: Weisman MH, Weinblatt ME, Louie JS. *Treatment of rheumatic diseases: a companion to Kelley's textbook of rheumatology,* 2nd ed. Philadelphia: WB Saunders, 2001.
8. Jones RE, Chatham WW. Update on sarcoidosis. *Curr Opin Rheumatol* 1999;11:83–87.
9. Rogers RS III. Recurrent aphthous stomatitis: clinical characteristics and associated systemic disorders. *Semin Cutan Med Surg* 1997;16:278–283.
10. Schur PH. *Systemic lupus erythematosus.* Orlando, FL: Grune & Stratton.
11. Cummings CW. *Otolaryngology: head and neck surgery.* St. Louis: Mosby, 1998.
12. Yazici H, Yurdakul S, Hamuryudan V. Behçet's syndrome. *Curr Opin Rheumatol* 1999;11:53–57.
13. Zeuner M, Straub RH, Rauh G, et al. Relapsing polychondritis: clinical and immunogenetic analysis of 62 patients. *J Rheumatol* 1997;24:96–101.
14. Zuber TJ, Jackson E. Chondrodermatitis nodularis chronica helicis. *Arch Fam Med* 1999;8:445–447.
15. Spraggs PD, Tostevin PM, Howard DJ. Management of laryngotracheobronchial sequelae and complications of relapsing polychondritis. *Laryngoscope* 1997;107:936–941.
16. Heman-Ackah YD, Remley KB, Goding GS Jr. A new role for magnetic resonance imaging in the diagnosis of laryngeal relapsing polychondritis. *Head Neck* 1999;21:484–489.
17. St. Clair EW, McCallum RM. Cogan's syndrome. *Curr Opin Rheumatol* 1999;11:47–52.

# CHRONIC FATIGUE SYNDROME

## ALAN B. MCDANIEL
## W. WHITNEY GABHART

Fatigue is a common and broad symptom of illness. Many patients with symptoms of fatigue frequently are difficult to diagnose accurately. Illnesses accompanied with inordinate fatigue can be traced to the 19th century, when DaCosta described severe exhaustion after acute gastroenteritis among veterans of the American Civil War (1).

The American neurologist George Beard introduced the term *neurasthenia* (2), which has been noted to demonstrate parallels to chronic fatigue syndrome (CFS) (3,4). Beard believed that the patient's bodily energy was depleted by stress, which dissipated force from critical homeostatic centers (5). Stress also exerts a direct effect on the adrenal glands (6), as we examine later.

A number of occurrences of vague, mysterious illnesses characterized by severe fatigue have been reported episodically, at intervals, and in scattered locations, described variously as "simulating poliomyelitis" (7,8), encephalomyelitis (9) and neuromyasthenia (10). The term *myalgic encephalitis* has been widely used by the British (11). Each of these names reveals the authors' impression that the ailment is somehow postinfectious. It therefore is understandable that the 1985 "outbreak" described around Incline Village at Lake Tahoe also would be attributed to a viral origin (12,13). In the latter episode, a plausible hypothesis had been offered, identifying the Epstein-Barr virus (EBV), which possesses extraordinary adaptations that enable it to enter and dwell in the human body (14). The malady was termed *yuppie flu*. Although the acquired immunodeficiency syndrome (AIDS) epidemic soon swept CFS from the headlines, chronically fatigued patients were so numerous and perplexing that the Centers for Disease Control (CDC) increased its involvement. A working group was convened to establish a definition for this illness, which they recommended naming *chronic fatigue syndrome*. Their criteria for inclusion were published in 1988 (15) and revised in 1994 (16) (Tables 25.1, 25.2). The revised criteria show that investigators had turned away from their earlier emphasis on

postinfectious causes of CFS and had discarded any reliance on physical signs.

The CDC criteria have been examined and validated for research purposes in several studies (17–19). These criteria show that patients meeting these guidelines are clinically distinct from people with good health and from patients with multiple sclerosis, depression, and other chronic illnesses (17). This heterogeneity, however, challenges efforts to create homogeneous groups for study (20–22).

Although many physicians seem reluctant to make the diagnosis of CFS, it is beneficial to validate the patient's illness with a single coherent and appropriate diagnosis (23–26). Schooley notes an important caveat, stating that the CDC definition " . . . should not be used as a rigid checklist with which to rule the syndrome in or out in an individual patient. The diagnosis remains one of exclusion . . . " (27,28).

## EPIDEMIOLOGY OF CHRONIC FATIGUE SYNDROME

From the 19th century, it was thought that fatigue syndromes were an affliction or an affectation of women of the wealthy class (5). These patients may simply reflect those who could afford to seek care. Modern studies have shown that although CFS affects a preponderance of women, by a relative risk of 1.3 to 1.7 (29), CFS is not an illness of the affluent. Well executed telephone surveys in Chicago (30) and San Francisco (31) agree that the highest levels are found among women, some minorities, and persons of less education and lower income.

The prevalence of CFS has repeatedly been studied. Across broad population groups, the point prevalence in the United States may be 0.075% to 0.267% (32), 0.2% (31), or 0.42% (30). Rates in England were similar at 0.5% (33), but much lower in Japan at just 0.85 per 100,000 (34), correlating with an observation that in the United States the lowest prevalence is among Asians (31).

Certainly, patients who meet the CDC criteria for CFS are far outnumbered by patients who simply are fatigued.

**A. B. McDaniel and W. W. Gabhart:** Ohio Valley Integrated Medicine, New Albany, Indiana.

## TABLE 25.1. 1987 CENTERS FOR DISEASE CONTROL CRITERIA FOR DIAGNOSIS OF CHRONIC FATIGUE SYNDROME

**Major Criteria**
  Persistent or relapsing fatigue, not resolved with bed rest or reducing daily activity at least 50% for at least 6 months, and exclusion of other chronic medical and psychiatric illnesses.

**Minor Criteria**
  Symptoms
    Mild fever or chills
    New, generalized headache
    Sleep disturbance
    Myalgias
    Migratory arthralgias
    General muscle weakness
    Sore throat
    Painful nodes
    Prolonged fatigue after exercise
    Symptom onset acute or subacute
    Neuropsychiatric symptoms, including photophobia, scotomata, forgetfulness, irritability, confusion, difficulty thinking or concentrating, depression
  Physical signs:
    Low-grade fever (37.6°C to 38.6°C)
    Nonexudative pharyngitis
    Palpable or tender lymphadenopathy, cervical or axillary, <2 cm, physician documented at lease twice, at least 1 month apart
  *Cases of chronic fatigue syndrome should have at least two physical signs and (a) meet both major criteria or (b) meet six minor criteria.*

From Holmes GP, Kaplan JE, Gantz NM, et al. Chronic fatigue syndrome: a working case definition. *Ann Intern Med* 1988; 108:387–389.

## TABLE 25.2. 1994 REVISED CASE DEFINITION OF CHRONIC FATIGUE SYNDROME, AN ALGORITHM FOR EVALUATION

Severe fatigue that persists or relapses for at least 6 months

Exclude if patient found to have:
  1. Active medical condition that may explain the chronic fatigue, such as untreated hypothyroidism, sleep apnea, narcolepsy
  2. Previously diagnosed medical conditions that have not clearly fully resolved, such as previously treated malignancies or unresolved cases of hepatitis B or C virus infections
  3. Any past or current major depressive disorder with psychotic or melancholic features, bipolar affective disorders, schizophrenia, delusional disorders, dementias, anorexia nervosa, or bulimia nervosa
  4. Alcohol or other substance abuse within 2 years before the onset of chronic fatigue and at any time afterward
  5. Severe obesity, defined by a body mass index [weight in kg/ (height in meters)$^2$] of 45 or more.

Classify as **chronic fatigue syndrome** if:
  Sufficiently severe: of new or definite onset (not lifelong)
  Not substantially alleviated by rest, and results in
  Substantial reduction in previous levels of occupational, educational, social or personal activities;
*And*
  Four or more of the following symptoms are concurrently present for at least 6 months:
  1. Impaired memory or concentration
  2. Sore throat
  3. Tender cervical or axillary lymph nodes
  4. Muscle pain
  5. Multi-joint pain
  6. New headaches
  7. Unrefreshing sleep
  8. Post-exertional malaise

Classify as **idiopathic chronic fatigue** if fatigue severity or symptom criteria for chronic fatigue syndrome are not met.

From Fukuda K, Strauss SE, Hickie I, et al. The chronic fatigue syndrome: a comprehensive approach to its definition and study. *Ann Intern Med* 1994; 121:953–959.

Indeed, the complaint of chronic fatigue is one of the most common in many illnesses and may occur in as many as 20% of patients attending a general medical clinic (35). The ratio of patients with "true" CFS to those with idiopathic chronic fatigue (16) varies among reports, with a range of 1:3 to 1:24 (31–33,36), suggesting that application of the CDC criteria in an accurate and uniform manner may be difficult (32). This difficulty has been confirmed by Fukuda et al. (37).

Some epidemiologic studies have rejected the suggestion that CFS could be a postviral syndrome (38,39), although one notes an increased seasonal onset of illness, which the authors interpret as supporting an infectious etiology (40). There are, however, statistically significant associations between the onset of CFS and antecedent stress, either physical or psychological (38,41). This finding may have a significant bearing on later discussion of the roles, both adaptive and maladaptive, of the adrenal and thyroid glands.

## Association with Fibromyalgia

One disorder with significant overlap with CFS is fibromyalgia (FM). Goldenberg has described this syndrome in a thorough review (41). He notes that between 10% and 12% of the general population has chronic, widespread pain. The need to study these patients has led to the formulation of diagnostic criteria for FM.

The American College of Rheumatology classification of 1990 (42) was based on a blinded study comparing 293 patients with FM and persistent, generalized idiopathic pain with 265 "control" patients with regional chronic musculoskeletal pain or a systemic rheumatic disease. The symptom of chronic widespread pain and the finding of mild or greater tenderness to finger pressure in at least 11 of 18 specified locations gave a sensitivity of 88% and specificity of 81% in distinguishing between FM and the other causes of chronic pain.

Goldenberg illustrates a conceptual difference between FM and CFS: FM is accepted as coexisting with many illnesses, rather that being a "diagnosis of exclusion." It is, for example, found in 10% to 40% of patients with systemic lupus erythematosus and 10% to 30% of patients with rheumatoid arthritis.

Other investigators have examined the epidemiology of FM. Buchwald et al. recorded a significant sex difference in diagnosis of FM among 348 patients with CFS. Women with CFS had significantly more FM than men, 36% versus 12% (43). This sex bias was not apparent in a smaller Canadian study (44).

Reports have specifically studied the coincidence of CFS and FM. One group of 402 chronically fatigued clinic patients could be subdivided into CFS (37%), FM (7%), or both (15%). The remainder was considered to have idiopathic chronic fatigue (45). Recently, 74 patients with FM were found to meet 1988 CDC criteria for CFS in 58% of the women and 80% of the men. These percentages were considerably higher than those of two control groups (44).

Goldenberg addresses the debate over the exact relationship between FM and CFS (41). Citing various reports, he states that FM, CFS, and irritable bowel syndrome overlap so extensively that they ought to be considered different presentations of the same general condition. This statement is supported elsewhere in at least three other review articles (46–48). A multicenter study compared the frequency of 10 clinical conditions among patients with CFS, FM, and temporomandibular disorder. They found that the three syndromes share many key symptoms with irritable bowel syndrome (49). This finding was reaffirmed by a British study of 1,797 chronically fatigued patients, of whom 63% fulfilled criteria for irritable bowel syndrome (50).

Klein and Berg report a study of autoantibodies that shows close correlation between FM and CFS (51). Antibodies to serotonin (5-HT) were closely related with FM/CFS. Antibodies to gangliosides and phospholipids were common, but also could be detected in other disorders.

Levels of substance P (a cytokine associated with pain) in the cerebrospinal fluid of patients with FM usually are elevated, but not in patients with CFS (52). In addition, the level of somatomedin C [a breakdown product of growth hormone (GH) with much longer plasma life, also called *insulin-like growth factor-1* (IGF-1)] was found to be higher in 49 patients with CFS than in 30 healthy matched control subjects, whereas it was lower in patients with FM (53). The authors state that different abnormalities in the somatotropic neuroendocrine axis or sleep must exist for CFS and FM.

Again, Goldenberg provides a framework for resolution of these disparate facts (41). He states that patients with FM are found to have a generalized hypervigilance to both pain and auditory stimuli, with qualitatively altered nociception. This characteristic now is generally believed to be a manifestation of altered central nervous system (CNS) processing of nociceptive stimuli (41), which can explain the diversity of causal associations with the onset of this

syndrome. It also may explain the observed relationship between such seemingly disparate entities as FM and interstitial cystitis, which are found to overlap significantly (54).

In summary, then, it seems that FM syndrome is interwoven with CFS. There are some differences, primarily in pain perception, between patients with CFS with and without FM.

## DIAGNOSTIC CONSIDERATIONS

Chronic fatigue syndrome is a diagnosis of exclusion. No current single laboratory test can diagnose CFS or gauge its severity. A careful history must be taken from the patient, with consideration not only of medical disorders but psychiatric status and sleep history. A list of some conditions that can lead to chronic fatigue is offered by the National Institute of Allergy and Infectious Diseases NIAID (55). These are shown in Table 25.3.

Studies suggest that unsuspected illnesses can lead to chronic fatigue. These disorders may be grouped into rough categories for this review. Immunologic problems include familial dysfunction of natural killer (NK) cells (56), celiac disease (57), dermatomyositis (58), and "seronegative" Sjögren's syndrome (59). Various toxic conditions are cited as well, including fungal disease, which may either stimulate the immune system or poison through mycotoxins (60). Also noted are environmental toxins, including lead (61), for which our standard blood tests are arguably imperfect (62), and carbon monoxide (63). Other, more exotic toxins include chronic ciguatera poisoning in Australia (64) and

**TABLE 25.3. SOME CONDITIONS THAT CAN EXPLAIN CHRONIC FATIGUE**

Hypothyroidism
Sleep apnea
Narcolepsy
Unresolved hepatitis B or C
Alcohol or substance abuse
Severe obesity
Iatrogenic, medication side effects
Systemic lupus erythematosus
Multiple sclerosis
Cancer
Major depressive disorder
Anorexia nervosa
Bulimia nervosa
Schizophrenia
Bipolar disorder
Dementia
Lyme disease

From National Institute of Allergy and Infectious Diseases, National Institutes of Health. *Chronic fatigue syndrome: information for physicians.* NIH publication no. 97-484. Bethesda, MD: National Institutes of Health, 1997.

**TABLE 25.4. NATIONAL INSTITUTES OF HEALTH RECOMMENDED INITIAL LABORATORY WORKUP**

Urinalysis
Complete blood count with differential
Chemistry panel
Thyroid function test (thyroid-stimulating hormone may suffice)
Erythrocyte sedimentation rate
Alanine aminotransferase
Total protein
Albumin
Globulin
Alkaline phosphatase
Calcium
Phosphorus
Glucose

From National Institute of Allergy and Infectious Diseases, National Institutes of Health. *Chronic fatigue syndrome: information for physicians.* NIH publication no. 97-484. Bethesda, MD: National Institutes of Health, 1997.

the eosinophilia myalgia syndrome from contaminated l-tryptophan (65).

Various disorders may be grouped into "metabolic problems" of varied cause. These disorders include the syndrome of inappropriate antidiuretic hormone (66), phosphate diabetes from abnormal renal tubular reabsorption, causing changes in mitochondrial respiration (67), and primary chronic magnesium deficiency (68). Downey also speculates on the possible role of abnormal porphyrin metabolism (69).

The list of possible differential diagnoses for CFS is extensive. It is noteworthy that many authors cite failure of standard laboratory tests to make the correct diagnosis.

## Laboratory Evaluation

The National Institutes of Health (NIH) has suggested an initial laboratory workup for CFS (55) (Table 25.4). From the perspective of an infectious diseases specialist, Schooley also suggests a purified protein derivative, an enzyme-linked immunosorbent assay for human immunodeficiency virus, and serologic studies for EBV, cytomegalovirus, and hepatitis A, B, or C, as indicated by abnormal hepatic aminotransferases (27). The current review includes both standard and nonroutine tests in an attempt to explain the many facets of CFS.

## AN ETIOLOGIC APPROACH TO UNDERSTANDING CFS

### Psychiatric and Neurologic Studies

The description of what is now called CFS predated the birth of modern psychiatry. Although Beard refused to ac-

cept a psychogenic explanation for neurasthenia, the disorder was gradually incorporated into 20th century psychiatry. CFS was considered to be a functional somatic disorder, an illness that after appropriate medical assessment cannot be explained in terms of a conventionally defined medical disease (70). Psychiatrists therefore have traditionally been primary caregivers for patients with CFS.

In 1999, Barsky and Borus presented a review (71) in which they agree that the number of specific somatic syndromes is largely an artifact of medical specialization. They further present an analysis of psychosocial factors that amplify symptoms. Prospective studies of patients with herpes zoster, heart disease, postviral fatigue, and CFS are cited that suggest that patients' beliefs about their disease at the outset strongly influence the reporting of symptoms at follow-up. They also cite evidence that anxiety and depression amplify and perpetuate somatic symptoms.

Although patients with chronic fatigue are at greater risk for psychiatric disorder than those without chronic fatigue (72), one review states that in every study, between one third to one half of CFS cases do not fulfill primary criteria for psychiatric illness (73). Efforts also have been made to validate psychometric instruments for the study of CFS (74–77).

One significant issue involves the frequent coexistence of CFS and depression. Using questionnaires, three series report significant qualitative differences between CFS and depressed patients (78–80). Only one recent study failed to show a difference between these two groups (81). It therefore appears that although patients with CFS often are depressed, CFS is not caused by depression.

A variety of other psychiatric disorders have been examined in relation to CFS. Interest in posttraumatic stress disorder also has been expressed (73). A possible link with seasonal affective disorder is noted for a subgroup of patients (82), but is dismissed in an NIH study (83). Mention also is made of a possible association between CFS and obsessive–compulsive disorder (84).

## Central Nervous System: Cognitive and Neurologic

Patients with CFS frequently note that they have impaired cognition. Nine reports of cognitive testing from 1994 to 1999 have validated abnormalities in patients with CFS compared with various carefully chosen control groups. These patients with CFS demonstrated significant problems in performance of visuomotor search and logical memory (85), attentional capacity (86), auditory processing (87), and learning and memory (88), as well as psychomotor slowing, impaired attention, learning rate, and delayed recall (89), and problems with motor cognition and cognitive processing (90), information processing (91), memory, attention, and information processing (92), and information processing and attention (93). Standing virtually alone against this preponderance of positive results is a single negative report in which no differences could be found (94).

Physiologic measures of CNS function have been further evaluated. Two studies show significant gait abnormalities, which are thought to strengthen the hypothesis of a direct involvement of the CNS in the onset of CFS (95,96). Reports of other forms of testing that have been positive for CNS dysfunction include impaired acquisition of the classically conditioned eyeblink response, indicating an associative deficit (97). Vestibular testing has shown central-type abnormalities (98). Cortical motor potentials have shown slowed reaction times and reduced premovement-related potentials (99). To the contrary, a test of P300 auditory potentials showed no difference between patients with CFS and control subjects (100).

## Studies of Sleep

A common complaint among patients with CFS is lack of high-quality, refreshing sleep, primarily noted as difficulty in staying asleep (101). A Welsh study found that 80% of patients with CFS fulfilled both *Diagnostic and Statistical Manual of Mental Disorders,* 3rd edition (revised) and International Classification of Diseases-10 (ICD-10) criteria for sleep disorders (75). Polysomnography has been performed in a variety of well controlled studies and has consistently provided abnormal results. Findings in the CFS groups include disturbances in sleep initiation and sleep maintenance and a decrease in stage 4 sleep (102,103), with significantly more time in bed, less efficient sleep architecture, and longer time awake after sleep onset (104). Only 20% of patients with CFS reported sleep continuity complaints before the onset of CFS symptoms (103).

Researchers have also studied sleep electroencephalograms in groups of patients with CFS. Several studies have reported alpha-wave intrusions into non–rapid eye movement sleep (alpha-delta sleep) and K-alpha sleep to be significantly more common among patients with CFS (105,106). A negative study was reported and discussed the importance of the electrode placement array (107). Some disorders of excessive sleep, daytime fatigue, and disturbed night sleep are thought at least in part to involve immunopathologic mechanisms (108). A note of caution was raised (109). Four patients who had been diagnosed with CFS were found actually to have narcolepsy. Two were cured of symptoms and two improved significantly with methylphenidate treatment.

## Central Nervous System Imaging Studies

In a 1994 review article, Bell cites the technique of single-photon emission computed tomography (SPECT) scanning, which demonstrates cerebral perfusion (110). Of several studies, one demonstrated abnormal perfusion in several areas of the brain and brain stem in 80% of 60 patients with CFS who were compared with 14 healthy control subjects. Three studies have confirmed significant perfusion abnormalities in various regions of the brain and brain stem (111–113). One of these groups compared SPECT to magnetic resonance imaging (MRI) and found no significant association of MRI abnormalities in 16 patients with CFS compared with 15 control subjects (114). Although one of three other recent MRI studies showed a positive correlation (115), it is clear that MRI does not consistently show abnormalities in patients with CFS (116,117).

Brain positron emission tomography (PET) also has been used to study brain glucose metabolism. Tirelli and coworkers report a statistically significant hypometabolism in both mediofrontal cortex and brain stem in patients with CFS compared with both healthy and depressed control subjects (118). Although valuable, the PET scan was less sensitive than SPECT scanning, indicating that it is possible to have perfusion abnormalities of the brain without a corresponding measurable decrease in glucose uptake (119). These two modalities clearly offer the best imaging evidence for CNS abnormalities in patients with CFS.

## Neurotransmitter Abnormalities

Neurotransmitter abnormalities have been studied. Demitrack and colleagues compared 19 patients with CFS with 17 healthy control subjects, testing both cerebrospinal fluid and peripheral blood for metabolites of neurotransmitters (120). Although no significant differences were found in the cerebrospinal fluid, plasma levels of 5-hydroxyindole acetic acid (5-HIAA), a metabolite of serotonin, were significantly higher and those of MHPG [from norepinephrine (NE)] were significantly lower in patients. These findings are opposite from those noted in depressed people.

Cleare et al. presented evidence that depressed patients have "hypothalamic–pituitary–adrenal (HPA) overdrive" with raised cortisol levels exerting an inhibitory effect on central 5-HT neurotransmitter function (121). Referring to Demitrack and colleagues' 1991 report, they suggested that CFS may be clinically the opposite of depression, with reduced HPA function and increased 5-HT function. Using 30 mg d-fenfluramine orally, a 5-HT–releasing agent, and measuring both plasma cortisol and plasma prolactin levels (as a measure of 5-HT function) in a well controlled trial, they obtained data that supported their hypothesis. Increased prolactin response to another 5-HT agonist (buspirone) also is reported in a controlled study (122). Unfortunately, a study similar to that of Cleare et al. using twice as large a dose of d-fenfluramine (60 mg) failed to note any significant differences (123).

Several other investigations relevant to 5-HT are interesting. Patients with CFS were found to have significantly higher levels of plasma free tryptophan (the 5-HT precursor) at rest, which did not change during or after exercise (124). These levels were similar to those seen after major surgery. The authors believed that their findings supported Cleare and colleagues' study.

## Pharmacotherapy Based on a Neuropsychiatric Paradigm

Because interest in 5-HT metabolism is active, selective serotonin reuptake inhibitors are a mainstay of medical treatment for the symptomatic relief of patients with CFS. Unfortunately, there is considerable disappointment in the results. One review has demonstrated poor outcomes with the use of these agents (125). A large, double-blind, randomized, placebo-controlled study of a large number of patients also was negative (126).

Monoamine oxidase inhibitors and tricyclic antidepressants also have been carefully studied. There may be some improvement, mostly to concurrent depressive rather than to CFS symptoms. Some improvement with the tricyclics may be due to their analgesic effects. Amitriptyline benefits appear independent of mood effect. Side effects of some drugs may be considerable (125). Overall, it seems wise to reserve antidepressants for the treatment of coexisting depression in patients with CFS.

## Cognitive Behavioral Therapy

Whatever triggers CFS may not perpetuate it (73). The rationale for cognitive behavioral therapy (CBT) is based on the understanding of the importance of perpetuating factors in maintaining the disorder. As previously cited, there are strong associations between expectations about illness and the eventual outcome (71).

In two randomized, controlled trials each of 60 patients, CBT has demonstrated success (127,128). Combined with medical care, 73% of patients on CBT achieved a satisfactory outcome, compared with just 23% with medical care alone (127). CBT was more effective than relaxation therapy in both functional impairment and fatigue measures. The improvements were sustained over 6 months of follow-up (128).

## Summary

Evidence of neurologic impairments seems sufficient to show that patients with CFS do demonstrate physiologic illness. Expectations and fears add to the burden of the illness. Previous history of psychiatric disorders may be common in these patients and comorbid depression occurs frequently. It often is helpful to enlist a psychotherapist's assistance for the long-term management of patients with CFS.

## THE POSTINFECTIOUS HYPOTHESIS

### Viruses

Many patients with CFS point to an infectious illness that immediately predated the onset of their symptoms. Concern

that CFS might be an after-effect of infection is reflected in the original CDC criteria for defining CFS (15). Many reports have offered connections between CFS and a variety of agents.

Every college student in the 1960s knew that some people who got mononucleosis might remain ill for months. With the interest in CFS that followed the reports from Nevada in the 1980s, it was natural to suspect EBV. This human herpesvirus may be highly pathogenic, yet it "benignly" infects and persists for life in more than 90% of the adult human population, being found in memory B cells (14).

Epstein-Barr virus has been studied extensively. Impairments of performance and mood are very similar between acutely infected and convalescent patients compared with healthy control subjects (129). Several early reports suggested a significant role for EBV in chronic illness (130, 131). A variety of small, controlled studies showed conflicting results. In a well designed, controlled study of 548 patients with CFS tested for antibodies to 13 viruses (in addition to medical and psychiatric evaluation), Buchwald et al. (132) demonstrated no differences in seropositivity or geometric mean titer of antibodies compared with control subjects on any subset of patients, including those with acute-onset or documented fever.

Interest in postinfectious causes of CFS has continued (133–136). Human herpesvirus-6 has been reportedly activated more often in patients with CFS (136–138). Interest persists, yet results still conflict (139).

Enterovirus infections may cause symptoms similar to CFS (140–145). The Glasgow group has found enterovirus traces using polymerase chain reaction (PCR) assay, including distinctly novel enterovirus sequences (141). The Dutch and Swedish groups also used PCR and found negative results. Borna disease virus was suggested in Japan as a possible link to CFS (146). It is a neurotropic single-strand RNA virus, naturally infecting horses and sheep. There has been a great discrepancy between reports, with one showing positive PCR assays in 8 of 25 patients with CFS (147), but another in 1999, using a new assay technique, finding no positives among 75 patients with CFS (148).

A scattering of reports mention other viruses. Included are parvovirus B19 (149,150) and coxsackie B virus, none different from control subjects in two large studies (151, 152). Finally, the postpolio syndrome is mentioned briefly in this context (153).

### Other Infectious Agents

One infection that has been of concern, especially in the northeastern United States, is Lyme disease. Although controlled studies have been performed, limitations are apparent. One study that described "post-Lyme syndrome," characterized by persistent arthralgias, fatigue, and neurocognitive impairment, appears to have done no more than compare a group of post-Lyme syndrome sufferers with a group of patients fully recovered from Lyme disease (154). The findings basically confirm only that the sicker patients were more symptomatic.

A recent study examined 1,156 healthy men for Lyme *Borrelia* antibodies using a prospective, double-blind methodology. Seropositive subjects who had never manifested clinical Lyme disease showed significantly more frequent chronic fatigue and malaise than seronegative subjects (155). The authors reasonably suggest consideration of an antibiotic for patients with CFS with positive *Borrelia* serology. Counterbalancing this report is a controlled study of 39 patients with CFS from the northeastern United States that found no reactivity on a Bb immune complex test (156). These authors state that patients lacking antecedent signs of Lyme disease are not likely to have laboratory evidence of *Borrelia* infection.

Two studies from California have examined *Mycoplasma* species in large cohorts of patients with CFS. Both report a significant number of atypical *Mycoplasma* genomes in DNA purified from blood samples using a PCR assay. In the first, Vojdani and associates found genomes for *Mycoplasma* species significantly more frequently in patients with CFS than in healthy control subjects (157). People with high genome copy numbers (i.e., numerous *Mycoplasma* genomes per unit of DNA) had higher immunoglobulin G (IgG) and IgM antibodies against *Mycoplasma*-specific peptides. Nasralla et al. also noted 91 patients with CFS who had a positive test for any *Mycoplasma* (158). Forensic PCR assay for five different *Mycoplasma* species showed that 30.8% had double infections (multiple species) and 22% had triple infections.

A British report suggested the existence of a chronic fatigue state after an outbreak of Q fever in England using a controlled, questionnaire method (159). Swanink et al. found no correlation between *Yersinia enterocolitica* and CFS in a controlled study of 88 patients. An immunoblot technique was used to detect IgG and IgA antibodies to various *Yerisnia* outer membrane proteins (160).

## Retrovirus

The AIDS epidemic introduced clinicians to the retrovirus. Naturally, attention was given to the possibility that this class of virus could be associated with CFS. Early studies were conflicting (161,162). In a sequence of six reports, Martin and colleagues described what they termed a "stealth" virus, a pathogen related to simian cytomegalovirus (163). Martin and Glass inoculated this virus into cats and produced acute neurologic illness (164), and Martin showed that some of these strains may have arisen from live poliovirus vaccines (165–167).

A group of electron microscopists in New Zealand reported structures similar in shape, size, and character to a lentivirus in 10 of 17 patients with CFS and in no control

subjects (168). They were unable to identify a lymphoid phenotype containing these structures, and results of a reverse transcriptase assay were equivocal in this blinded and case-controlled study.

## Epidemiologic Analysis

With the many conflicting reports of infectious etiologies in patients with CFS, epidemiologic methods have been used. A British review of patients with Q fever seemed to support the postviral assertion (159). Buchwald et al. compared demographic, clinical, and laboratory features in 717 patients with chronic fatigue with and without a self-reported postinfectious onset (169). They concluded that a postinfectious onset was not significant and could not differentiate between fatigued patients and those with CFS.

A prospective study of 245 patients with "glandular fever" or an upper respiratory infection stated that the empirically defined fatigue syndrome probably represents a valid condition 6 months after glandular fever (170). A better executed, controlled study compared 83 patients postviral meningitis with 76 nonmeningitic postviral patients (non-CNS and nonenteroviral) over a 6- to 24-month follow-up (171). Two observations were noted. First, there was a relatively high prevalence of CFS overall, 12.6%, although no difference existed between the groups. Second, the onset of CFS is predicted by psychiatric morbidity and prolonged convalescence, not by severity of the viral illness itself. Two other works (172,173) support the role of psychiatric comorbidity.

The most thorough work on postinfectious fatigue was presented by Wessely et al., who noted that common infectious episodes in primary care are not causative of CFS (174). Their prospective study followed 1,199 people 18 to 45 years of age who presented to their general practitioners with symptomatic infections for 6 months, and was controlled by 1,167 people who attended for other reasons. At 6 months, 9.9% of cases and 11.7% of control subjects reported chronic fatigue. No effect of infection was noted. The strongest predictors of "postinfectious fatigue" were fatigue or psychological problems at the baseline evaluation, in agreement with others (171–173).

## Treatment Based on Postinfectious Paradigm

Several strategies for antiviral therapy have been studied. Application of interferon-α to patients with CFS was reported by See and Tilles in 1996 (175). Thirty patients were treated with interferon-alfa 2a or placebo in a double-blind crossover study. Immunologic parameters and quality of life were measured. There was no effect of treatment except on a subset of seven patients whose only abnormality was isolated NK cell dysfunction. Their NK cell function improved, as did their symptom questionnaire scores. Antiviral drugs have been applied with varying results. Interferon and acyclovir were combined to treat successfully one patient with a dramatic presentation of well documented, chronic active EBV infection (176). This report supported the hypothesis of endogenous reactivation of EBV.

Strayer and colleagues' 1994, multicenter, randomized, placebo-controlled successful treatment of 92 patients with CFS with an antiviral and immunomodulatory drug, poly(I)-poly(C12U) (Ampligen; HEM Pharmaceutical, Philadelphia, PA), yielded significantly superior results across many measures, including increased treadmill work tolerance, reduced cognitive deficit, and reduction of daily medicines (177). From subsequent work by the same authors (178,179), it seems that the success of the drug was due to its immunomodulatory effect, not its antiviral action.

Amantadine has been used in two groups of patients. In one trial the results seemed promising, but only four patients were studied, one of whom had already obtained a good result with prior treatment with amantadine (180). A larger series of 30 patients, in contrast, not only demonstrated no statistically significant improvement, but the side effects of the drug were so intolerable that half of the study group dropped out (181).

## Summary

The postinfectious hypothesis has not been supported. There are no convincing data to conclude that CFS occurs as an outgrowth of viral or bacterial illnesses.

## IMMUNOLOGIC ABNORMALITIES

It has been speculated that an overproduction of one or more cytokines triggered by an infectious agent might be a factor in the pathogenesis of CFS (27). Some authors suggest that these agents might establish a regulatory imbalance of cytokines, which may disrupt neurotransmitter function and result in the symptoms of CFS (135). Immunologic abnormalities have also been postulated by Bennett et al. (182).

## Studies of Cytokines

Sixteen controlled studies of cytokines in patients with CFS have been conducted (183–198). Neopterin, a marker of macrophage activation, is the only cytokine that has shown abnormal results in every study reviewed (183,186,187). Its consistent elevation indicates immunologic stimulation in CFS.

Tumor necrosis factor-$\alpha$ (TNF-$\alpha$, cachectin) may cause symptoms of pain, inflammation, fatigue, and somnolence in vivo (198). Serum TNF-$\alpha$ was shown to be significantly elevated in a large, retrospective, controlled study of 240 patients with CFS and 240 control subjects. Thirty-two

percent of the patients and only 7% of control subjects had elevated levels above 50 pg/mL (198). Support for the role of TNF-$\alpha$ comes from two positive studies (186,195) and a third that showed that TNF-$\alpha$ response to endotoxin stimulation is abnormally reduced in patients with CFS (191). The only negative study merely showed no significant increase in TNF-$\alpha$ among patients with CFS (190).

The third cytokine that seems consistently abnormal is interleukin-6 (IL-6). Six reports have shown a significant elevation of IL-6 in patients with CFS (185,193,195–198), whereas two could detect no significant elevation (186,190). Several other cytokines have sufficiently consistent elevated levels to impress that they may be significantly abnormal in patients with CFS. IL-1$\alpha$ and IL-1$\beta$ have been found to be elevated (185,186) and their response to both endotoxin and physiologic stimulation also has been found to be abnormal (191,194). IL-2 was elevated in two series, and in one was abnormal in 15.6% of cases (186,188). Another study found normal IL-2 levels (189). Transforming growth factor-$\beta$ was one of the first cytokines to be identified as abnormal in CFS (183,192). Other reports note elevated C-reactive protein and $\beta_2$-microglobulin (193), $\alpha_2$-macroglobulin (196), IL-2 soluble receptor (186), and IL-1 soluble receptor (194); IL-1 receptor antagonist was high in the follicular phase of the menstrual cycle in patients tested by Cannon et al. (194).

Although these data are strong evidence that the immune system is activated or upregulated in patients with CFS, no authors would state that these tests are in any way diagnostic for CFS. In two publications, the authors note correlation of abnormal test results to severity of symptoms (186,187). No other groups can make any correlation of cytokine levels with severity of illness. These reports encourage further study of the immune system.

### Animal Model of Chronic Fatigue Syndrome Testing the Cytokine Paradigm

Sheng and coworkers injected 2 mg of *Corynebacterium parvum* antigen into mice of two different strains and measured daily running distance (before and after injection) to determine fatigue (199). One strain, C57BL/6 mice, showed a significant reduction in running activity. Injection of antibodies specific to either IL-1$\beta$ or TNF-$\alpha$ did not alter the apparent fatigue. It was found, however, that in the brains of the fatigued mice the expression of both TNF-$\alpha$ and IL-1$\beta$ messenger RNA (mRNA) was increased. The elevated CNS cytokine mRNA expression corresponded to the development of fatigue.

### Studies of Cellular Markers and Function

Cytokine elevations suggest upregulation of the immune system. Work has been done to investigate immune function on a cellular level, and the results are again complicated and conflicting. Guided by reviews by Evengard et al. (135),

Bell (110), and Gordon (200), 18 works are considered here (201–218).

Reduced NK cell function is the only abnormality that has been consistently reported in patients with CFS (201, 203,207,217), with a fifth study showing abnormal failure to increase NK cell activity after l-arginine stimulation (216). Evengard et al. cite an additional six reports all in agreement that NK cell function is reduced in patients with CFS (135). Only Mawle et al. from the CDC reported no significant decrease (212). Evengard et al. note that four publications have documented abnormalities in T-cell responses to stimulation (135). Responses to mitogens and specific antigens also have been depressed.

There are abnormalities that may be significant across all of these studies. Naive T-cells (CD4$^+$, CD45RA-bearing cells) usually are decreased (203,206,208). Adhesion markers (CD39, CD54, CD58) are a sign of activation, and reportedly are increased (206,208) or "slightly increased" (212). Two early studies showed a decreased T-helper to T-suppressor (CD4$^+$/CD8$^+$) ratio (203,206).

Vedhara et al. have tested immunologic function in patients with CFS in a novel way. They randomly allocated live poliovirus vaccine or placebo to 14 patients with CFS and compared them with each other and with 9 healthy control subjects who received the vaccine (219). They found evidence of altered immune reactivity and virus clearance in patients with CFS. They also found increased poliovirus isolation, earlier peak proliferative responses, lower T-cell subsets on certain days, and a trend toward reduced interferon-γ. No symptoms of CFS were exacerbated.

Cell-mediated immunity also has been tested. Evengard and colleagues cite Lloyd et al., who in 1992 found reduced cell immune competence (135). Two later reports contradict this, showing intact delayed hypersensitivity to childhood vaccines (220) and no difference in delayed hypersensitivity in a controlled study at the CDC (212). Lloyd's group, who had found reduced delayed hypersensitivity in 1992, reported in 1995 that cell-mediated immune function, measured at trial entry and follow-up in 103 patients, was unchanged and had no effect on outcome (221). Cell-mediated immunity would appear not to be a significant factor in CFS.

## Evidence for Autoimmune Activation

In discussing autoimmunity in CFS, we are dealing with conflicts in classification. If a patient is positive for a defined autoimmune disease then, by definition, he or she is not a patient with CFS. For example, a strongly positive anti-nuclear antibody moves the diagnosis away from CFS to systemic lupus erythematosus, one of the NIH's diagnoses of exclusion (55). Nevertheless, with so much evidence for immune system activation, it is of considerable interest to investigate autoimmune reactivity.

Von Mikecz et al. (222) found that in 60 patients with CFS, 68% had a positive anti-nuclear antibody and 47% were positive to cytoplasmic antigens. Overall, 83% of patients with CFS had at least one of these two antigens positive, significantly more than the 17% recorded in their control group. These elevated levels, however, have been considered too low to warrant treatment.

Other investigators report positive anti-serotonin antibodies along with weaker reactions to anti-gangliosides (seen in Guillain-Barré syndrome) and anti-phospholipids. Plioplys found no anti-muscle or anti-CNS reactive autoantibodies in ten patients compared with ten control subjects (223). Finally, Berg et al. suggest that CFS and FM are variants of antiphospholipid syndrome (224). They suggest using a panel of five tests of coagulation activation, but offer no results.

Hashimoto's autoimmune thyroiditis is common in allergic patients. This diagnosis and its implications for CFS are discussed in depth later in this review. Insulin resistance and adrenal insufficiency also may be linked to autoimmune processes, and are discussed subsequently.

In another review, Vincent et al. examined autoantibodies to neural proteins with disorders such as myasthenia gravis (anti-acetylcholine receptor autoantibodies) and Lambert-Eaton myasthenic syndrome (LEMS) (autoantibodies to the P/Q voltage-gated calcium channels) (225). LEMS is associated with significant autonomic dysfunction (226), which may have some relevance to patients with CFS. Furthermore, LEMS IgG has been shown to reduce hormone release in rats from both anterior pituitary cells and insulinoma cells, although this was not found in a small human study (227). This also could have relevance to patients with CFS.

Vincent and colleagues discuss the fact that the CNS is protected from autoimmune diseases by the blood–brain barrier. They raise the possibility that cytokines or other circulating factors could cause these disturbances if the blood–brain barrier is breached (225). It seems that the activated immune system may effect the CNS in many ways.

## Apoptosis, RNase L, and Interferon-induced Proteins

Apoptosis is a form of programmed cell death initiated by extracellular or intracellular signals in which enzymes in the IL-1 family are activated to degrade nuclear DNA, causing the cell to shrink and finally break up. In the immune system, this process is used to delete autoreactive lymphocytes (228). Swanink et al. found no increased apoptosis in leukocyte cultures from 76 patients with CFS compared with 69 healthy control subjects in 1996 (211). Vojdani et al., in a smaller group of 29 patients, studied peripheral blood lymphocytes and found increased apoptotic cells compared with 15 control subjects (229).

Suhadolnik et al. presented a series of papers documenting significant dysregulation in several components of the

$2',5'$-oligoadenylate (2-5A) synthetase/RNase L and protein kinase (PKR) antiviral pathways in CFS (228). Various subsets of patients are described. Their study suggests that the RNase L enzyme dysfunction in CFS is more complex than previously reported. This work is supported by two studies from Vojdani's group (229,230).

## Allergy and Chronic Fatigue

The interconnection of allergy and chronic fatigue appears robust. Although the high rate of allergies in patients with CFS, 66% to 83%, has been repeatedly noted (190, 231–233), with increased nickel sensitivity (233) and elevated serum eosinophilic cationic protein (231), relatively little has been made of this association. Borish et al. have used PCR to demonstrate that cytokines (TNF-α) in peripheral blood mononuclear cells are similarly and significantly elevated in both CFS and allergic patients (232). They also note a significant decrease in IL-10 (232). They proposed that allergic inflammation could produce CFS symptoms in susceptible individuals.

A number of reports suggesting a link between allergy and fatigue appeared as early as 1928 (234–236). These papers usually cite food allergy as the causative agent. Persistent limitation of the concept of "allergy" to IgE-mediated type I Gel and Coombs reactions can hinder research in this area. Expanding the definition of "allergy" to include all Gel and Coombs immune pathways opens broad avenues of research and therapy (237).

## Treatment Based on an Immunologic Paradigm

In one study, terfenadine did not benefit a small group of 28 patients with CFS (238), confirming that this condition is not a simple IgE-mediated problem. An aggressive trial studied 99 patients with CFS in a double-blind, randomized, placebo-controlled trial of intravenous immunoglobulin (239). No significant improvement was noted, and adverse reactions were reported by 70% of patients.

Transfer factor has been used to treat patients with CFS. Transfer factor is an active component of dialysates of human leukocyte extracts. It can transfer antigen-specific delayed hypersensitivity and cell-mediated immunity as well as enhance T-cell responses to mitogens and increase the percentage and total numbers of circulating T cells and T helper cells (240). Three studies of transfer factor and a review article were published in a single issue of *Biotherapy* in 1996 (241–244). Of these, a Czech study of 222 patients was most ambitious. This open-treatment trial showed that older patients (54 to 77 years of age) fared less well with treatment than did two younger subsets (243). Rea and coworkers at the Environmental Health Center in Dallas, Texas have considerable experience with transfer factor, reporting mostly good results using it as a maintenance rather than a curative treatment (240).

## Summary

Many immunologic abnormalities have been well documented among patients with CFS. Of these, the single most commonly reported finding was allergy, uniformly seen in most patients. It is safe to state that patients with CFS have a significantly activated, or "overactive" immune system compared with healthy control subjects. These data support the role of immune dysfunction in CFS, but cannot be considered diagnostic for CFS.

## FUNGAL HYPERSENSITIVITY THEORY, OR *CANDIDA*-RELATED COMPLEX

The "yeast" hypothesis is related to the immunologic rather than to the infectious paradigm of CFS. Kroker has reviewed the role of *Candida* hypersensitivity in patients with CFS (245). The proposed mechanism involves an infestation of the gastrointestinal tract with an allergenic fungus. Symptoms are caused by an immune response to the fungus in the gut with consequent inflammation of the gut mucosa and systemic immune dysfunction. Types I, III, and IV immune responses are involved (245).

The recommended treatment based on this hypothesis is the elimination of the fungus from the gut. A well known protocol is recommended by Crook (246), and includes a low-carbohydrate diet, antifungal medications, probiotics (beneficial normal gastrointestinal flora like *Lactobacillus acidophilus*), and high-potency vitamins and nutritional supplements. Normal bacterial flora may play a significant role in gastrointestinal homeostasis (247–250). Kroker cites Bolivar and Bodey's work showing that broad-spectrum antibiotics alter the flora and permit overgrowth of fungus (245). The repeated use of broad-spectrum antibiotics is thought to be instrumental in the genesis of the yeast problem. Oral supplementation with normal gut flora is believed to combat the growth of the fungus. In replenishing the gut bacteria, the treatment also restores any benefits of a healthy gut ecology.

Antifungal medications are thought to be an important part of this complex regimen. Kroker discusses a variety of antifungal treatments, both pharmaceutical and "natural," systemic and nonabsorbable. With emerging fungal resistance against these agents, at least one reference laboratory offers stool fungus culture and sensitivity panels (251).

One blinded prospective study of the yeast hypothesis has been published (252). In this negative trial, the single intervention studied was oral nystatin versus placebo. All other aspects of the recommended treatment were omitted, presumably to limit the otherwise large number of variables. From these data, we can state that the use of nystatin alone is not an adequate treatment for these patients. At this time, only anecdotal evidence supports the continued use of this protocol for chronically fatigued patients (253).

## NEURALLY MEDIATED HYPOTENSION AND DYSAUTONOMIA

Hypotension rarely is considered a pathologic disease state by Western practitioners (254). Indeed, it may be difficult to identify patients with episodes of markedly low blood pressure. Bou-Holaigah and colleagues from Johns Hopkins have reviewed the many synonyms and the proposed mechanism of action for neurally mediated hypotension (NMH) expressed as syncope and near-syncope (255). Episodes of hypotension are thought to result from a paradoxical reflex initiated by venous pooling on prolonged standing, leading to reduced ventricular preload. Susceptible people then produce high levels of catecholamines, which augment inotropism and excessively stimulate mechanoreceptors in the left ventricle of the heart. Mechanoreceptor activation then causes withdrawal of sympathetic and increased vagal tone, causing vasodilatation, bradycardia, and syncope or near-syncope. After such an event, patients remain fatigued for a surprisingly long time.

Wilke et al. suggest a more complex set of possible outcomes in addition to the aforementioned condition, which they term a *vasovagal reaction*. These outcomes include vasodepressor reactions with suddenly decreased blood pressure but increased heart rate, progressive orthostatic hypotension with or without altered heart rate, orthostatic tachycardia alone, and chronotropic insufficiency, in which the BP changes normally but the heart rate remains unchanged (256). These authors agree that fatigue may be significantly associated with these events. This large number of possible responses makes comparisons between series of patients in the medical literature more difficult.

The first reports of tilt-table testing of patients with CFS came from Rowe, Bou-Holaigah, and colleagues at Johns Hopkins in 1995 (255,257). Reviewing relevant literature, they support the observations that the symptoms of CFS and NMH overlap to a great extent. They propose that some patients with CFS actually have NMH. The authors then validate the head-up tilt test as a measure of NMH in a literature review. Combining published data, they note that approximately 50% of patients believed to have NMH and only 8% of control subjects demonstrate an abnormal response to upright tilt testing. The reproducibility of tilt testing results ranges from 77% to 90%. Adjunctive use of isoproterenol to augment the subject's own catecholamine production increases the rate of positive tests to 65% of patients with NMH and 27% of control subjects. The authors advocate its use, even though this infusion disproportionately increases the rate of false-positive results from 8% to 27% (a change of 19%, or 2.37-fold increase) while im-

proving the true-positive rate only from 50% to 65% (a 15% change, or 0.3-fold increase) (255).

The Hopkins group's first report showed that in a group of seven adolescent patients, all had significant hypotension on tilt-table testing (257). In the same year, their most significant series was published. Twenty-three unselected patients with CFS were tested and compared with 14 healthy control subjects. All patients complained of orthostatic symptoms and increased fatigue on tilting, compared with none of the control subjects. Sixteen (70%) with CFS became hypotensive with upright tilt, compared with none of the control subjects. With isoproterenol intravenous infusion, 22 of 23 (96%) of patients with CFS but only 4 of 14 (29%) healthy subjects had abnormal responses (255). All of the patients' abnormal responses conform to Wilke and colleagues' vasovagal category (256). Similar patient series have subsequently been reported and note an overall rate of hypotensive abnormalities of 42% of patients (258–263).

It is doubtful that NMH could be the sole cause of CFS, although CFS certainly seems to be associated with hypotension. The physiologic changes in patients with CFS that have been associated with NMH may arise from different sources.

### Dysautonomia

Given the preceding findings, the possibility that CFS is caused by an idiopathic autonomic neuropathy must be considered. In two studies, blood pressure and heart rate while at rest and in performing various tasks were studied (267,268). Neither study demonstrated any significant autonomic abnormality. Electrocardiographic R-R interval variability has been tested in two roughly comparable studies with conflicting results, one showing more variability in CFS (268,269). Results of paced breathing also have given inconsistent results (267). A treadmill test of 11 patients with CFS showed significantly reduced vagal power compared with control subjects (270). Even the simplest measurement of heart rate at rest has been inconsistently reported, with three groups finding that patients with CFS have higher resting heart rates (263,264,268) and four stating that there was no difference between patients and control subjects (255,265,267,271).

With such variability in even the most basic vital signs, there is profound disagreement among authors in interpretation of their data. Two groups state that there is no significant abnormality in autonomic function among patients with CFS (267,268), three others write that vagal power is decreased (269–271), and two more believe that sympathetic activity is increased in CFS (266,269).

### Treatment Based on the Hypotensive Paradigm

The Hopkins group designed a treatment protocol to address their NMH hypothesis and used it with good preliminary results, although no follow-up data are published (255). Therapy was designed to increase blood volume through increased salt intake or use of fludrocortisone, a synthetic corticosteroid with strong mineralocorticoid (aldosterone) properties. If needed, a second tier of treatment may be used. The inotropic effects of adrenergic stimulation are decreased with β-adrenergic antagonists (atenolol) or disopyramide. The bradycardia and vasodilatation of the vasovagal response may be mitigated using anticholinergic antagonists (disopyramide). The specific indications, doses, sequence, and some contraindications are given by Wilke et al (256).

Using this protocol, 9 of 19 (47%) patients reported complete or nearly complete resolution of all symptoms within 1 month. Seven more felt at least somewhat better (255). Seven patients were intolerant of some or all of the medications. DeLorenzo and coworkers used a simpler treatment, giving sodium chloride 1,200 mg daily for 3 weeks. Of their 22 patients, repeat tilt-table testing demonstrated 11 (50%) were no longer hypotensive with reported improvement of their CFS symptoms (262). They also observed that those patients who failed treatment had significantly lower plasma renin activity compared with both the control and successfully treated groups. The authors state that an abnormal renin–angiotensin–aldosterone system could explain both their symptoms and treatment failure.

A novel treatment trial involved application of military antishock trousers (MAST) to patients with CFS who tested abnormally on the tilt test (259). Inflation of the MAST during tilting prevented all symptoms. In addition, the group reports finding that although patients have normal circulating plasma volume, their erythrocyte volume is low. Although not proving any particular etiology, this finding shows that excessive gravitational venous pooling and subnormal circulating erythrocyte volume are frequent in patients with CFS; they may play a role in its pathogenesis. Wilke et al. state that venous pooling is an important feature (256). Rowe et al. agree, identifying a subset of Ehlers-Danlos syndrome (abnormal connective tissue permitting excessive dilatation of veins) among adolescent patients with CFS with orthostatic intolerance (272).

## Summary

There is little doubt that approximately 40% of patients with CFS have orthostatic intolerance. Treatment designed to expand circulating blood volume appears to help. Despite a plausible hypothesis of NMH, little evidence consistently supports the presence of autonomic dysfunction.

In a study of 431 fatigued patients, each subsequently diagnosed with one of eight neurologic or endocrine disorders, Streeten and Anderson concluded that chronic fatigue is common in delayed orthostatic hypotension and all forms of hypocortisolism but is much less common in the other disorders (273).

Chronic fatigue syndrome shares at least 36 features with Addison's disease (274). Deficiency of aldosterone may occur with hypocortisolism or in isolation, and its symptoms and features also suggest a role in CFS. Hypoaldosteronism may be associated with high renin levels, possibly related to prolonged cortical stimulation (275). Elevated renin has been noted in tilt test–positive patients with CFS by DeLorenzo et al. (262). Investigators of NMH do not report results of adrenocortical workup in their patients, yet their treatment protocol is fundamentally the same as the medical treatment for hypoaldosteronism: adequate salt intake and fludrocortisone (275).

In summary, patients with CFS who are tested using the tilt-table show signs of orthostatic intolerance that might be of autonomic, adrenal or other origin. There are no clear data about these patients' adrenal status. They respond to treatment that is equally effective for autonomic and adrenal disorders. No consistent autonomic abnormalities have been found in multiple studies. It seems that evaluation of adrenal function may be important.

## ADRENAL GLAND AND HYPOTHALAMIC–PITUITARY–ADRENAL AXIS

In their current review article, Petzke and Clauw comment that the most consistent finding regarding autonomic dysfunction among patients with FM is an impaired ability to respond to stress (276). These comments again implicate the primary role of the adrenal glands in metabolic homeostasis and response to stress.

In the 1930s, Hans Selye described the association of stress and the activation of the HPA axis with the increased secretion of cortisone from the adrenal glands (6). It is relevant to the study of CFS that Selye suggested that through the chronic stress of a severe disease of any etiology, a patient could present with anorexia, loss of weight, depression, hypogonadism, peptic ulcers, and immunosuppression (276). A great volume of work has been produced studying the stress response and has been recently reviewed (276–278).

The adrenal gland is composite, having two distinct regions. The center, or medulla is essentially a sympathetic ganglion, producing epinephrine in times of acute stress (the "fight-or-flight" response). This hormone of immediate stress contrasts with the products of the outer part of the adrenal gland, the cortex, which are distinct biochemically and physiologically. The cortical hormones are based on the cholesterol molecule and therefore are called *steroids*. Of these, cortisol is the most important. It is the hormone of chronic stress and one of the few hormones necessary to sustain life. The synthesis of steroid hormones is displayed in Fig. 25.1.

The HPA regulates production of adrenal steroids. Corti-

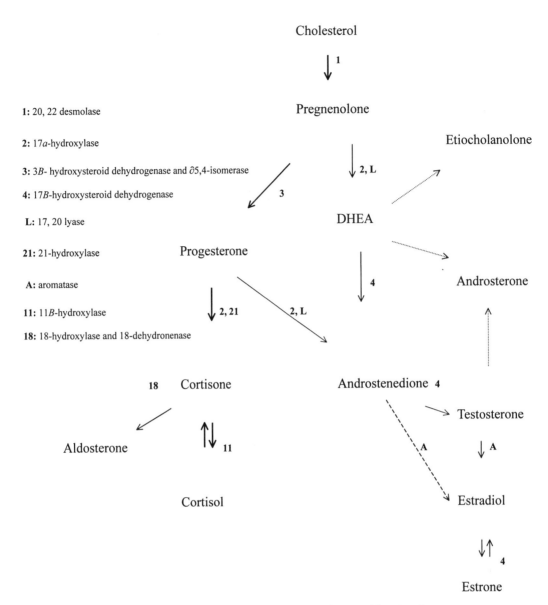

**FIG. 25.1.** Adrenal steroid synthetic pathways, abbreviated.

cotropin-releasing hormone (CRH) from the hypothalamus and other locations in the brain stimulates release of adreno-corticotropic hormone (ACTH) from the anterior pituitary. ACTH stimulates the adrenal conversion of cholesterol to pregnenolone, which is believed to be the rate-limiting step in the synthetic cascade. The fate of pregnenolone may then be directed by need. Increased demand for cortisol may result in diminished production of other steroids. It is well known that stressed women may temporarily stop menstruating. The British have termed the usurpation of sex hormones to produce cortisol *progesterone steal.* We see that by downregulating either 17α-hydroxylase or 17,20 lyase, all precursors move toward cortisol synthesis and the sex steroid paths are inhibited.

Heim et al. note some of the beneficial effects of cortisol as the organism is stressed (277). It induces gluconeogenesis, mobilizes free fatty acids, reduces amino acid use in protein synthesis, and increases cardiovascular tone, blood pressure, heart rate, and respiratory rate, thus increasing overall available energy. In large amounts, it reduces the immune response in many ways, including lymphocyte function, macrophage activity, antigen presentation, T-cell proliferation, NK cell function, and cytokine secretion. By inhibiting phospholipase, it also inhibits production of various proinflammatory prostaglandins and leukotrienes (276,277). It also restrains growth and reproduction (276). Rabin and Jefferies each emphasize the dose-related nature of immune system alterations by cortisol (278,279). At usual physiologic levels, cortisol enhances normal immune function.

Chronic activation of the adrenals by stress leads to adaptive responses. These adaptations involve various mechanisms. Blood levels of cortisol and tissue cortisol receptor numbers and sensitivity are complexly interrelated (277, 278). Cortisol effects brain CRH secretion and is involved with feedback loops influencing the locus ceruleus–NE autonomic system, reproduction, growth, several cytokines (IL-1, IL-6 and TNF-α), and the thyroid axis (276,278). Some individuals experience maladaptive responses to the detriment of their health.

With failure of adequate counterregulation, cortisol levels may stay high. What began as a temporary and protective response becomes maladaptive. Arousal transforms into anxiety, and vigilance becomes hypervigilance and insomnia. Assertiveness becomes excessive caution. The decreased emphasis on feeding and reproduction that is beneficial in acute stress is harmful when stress is sustained. This results in a syndrome of anorexia, hypothalamic hypogonadism, and decreased libido characteristic of melancholic depression (276). Studies have demonstrated that lifelong problems may be established early in life and even *in utero* (277,278).

The other significant form of maladaptive adrenal response is hypocortisolism (276,277). This has been well described in patients with posttraumatic stress disorder and also in patients with physical disorders, including CFS, FM, chronic pelvic pain, and asthma (277,280,281). Hypocortisolism may be a result of simple adrenal exhaustion, and a chronic decrease in CRH production in patients with CFS is clearly demonstrated (280,281). Responses of both ACTH and cortisol to CRH stimulation are blunted in another controlled series of patients with CFS (282). The neuroendocrine correlates of this response can be summarized as hypocortisolism and increased feedback inhibition of the pituitary–adrenal level of the HPA axis with apparent hyperactivation of the central CRH system (277). Various glucocorticoid receptor alterations (through adaptations, cytokines, or isoforms) may contribute to resistance to cortisol as well (277,279).

If simple hypocortisolism plays a major role in CFS, how can CFS seem a mysterious illness? The reasons are multiple. First, as observed by Jefferies, adrenal cortical insufficiency has come to be viewed exclusively by its most severe manifestation: Addison's disease. Nowhere in current texts is there a discussion of a borderline deficiency state or description of a syndrome of inadequate adrenal functional reserve (275, 283,284). Harrison's 7th edition in 1974 defined adrenocortical hypofunction as "all conditions in which the secretion of adrenal steroid hormones falls below the requirements of the body" (285). This definition was accurate in its lack of specificity, but it has been deleted in the 14th edition, which defines the condition strictly by an abnormal ACTH stimulation test result (275).

The second reason, then, is the difficulty in accurately testing the function of the adrenal gland. Unlike the thyroid gland, which stores a large amount of hormone and has relatively little diurnal variation in output, the adrenal stores no hormone but releases it promptly on synthesis. Further,

there is a strong diurnal variation and even hourly pulsatile fluctuation in ACTH release and cortisol synthesis (279, 283). Tests for ACTH and cortisol blood levels therefore must be done based on the patient's sleep pattern. A blood test shows only the blood level at the moment that the needle has pierced the vein. Also, published "normal" values may give an excessively broad range (286). Williams and Dluhy state that plasma cortisol values in patients with Addison's disease vary from zero into the lower range of normal; therefore, some patients have normal blood cortisol levels despite their disease state (275). Urine free cortisol is thought by some inaccurate because the detection limit of the assay lies in the normal range of cortisol excretion (283). Because of these difficulties, the standard diagnostic test for adrenal insufficiency is designed to measure adrenal response to ACTH stimulation.

As originally performed, the ACTH stimulation test required 8-hour continuous drips of ACTH daily for 4 or 5 days, during which time consecutive 24-hour urine specimens were collected for measurements of creatinine, 17-hydroxycorticoid, and 17-ketosteroid levels (285). The inconvenience and expense of this protocol are excessive, necessitated by insensitive laboratory tests of the early 1970s. It is very important to note that Harrison's 1974 text mentions "incomplete adrenal insufficiency" as a variant test response. These patients responded with small increments in steroid excretion on the first 3 days of the 5-day infusion test, and on the last 2 days there was an actual decline in the level of steroids. The authors state "these results suggest that the limited adrenal tissue has been maximally stimulated and has insufficient steroid reserve capacity." This statement is supported in clinical practice with patients with CFS.

With the development of superior assays, the ACTH stimulation test has been abbreviated to a single intravenous or intramuscular injection of ACTH with measurement of cortisol before injection and at 30 (or 45) and 60 minutes later. If the serum level of cortisol exceeds 20 μg/dL, the result is considered normal by some (283). Others require a stimulated cortisol level of at least 18 μg/dL and a minimal stimulated increment of more than 7 μg/dL (275). For the patient with CFS, this test is inadequate. Many patients with CFS relate that they felt well for a few hours after this test, then experienced a significant exacerbation of their CFS symptoms for many hours afterward.

Given that hypocortisolism in patients with CFS may be accompanied by an inhibited HPA axis, depressed ACTH release, glucocorticoid receptor resistance, and blunted response to ACTH stimulation, as described previously, it is understandable that a single test may not suffice. Salivary assays have been studied with mixed results, perhaps because of estradiol effects on cortisol-binding globulin (277, 287–289). A low-dose ACTH test using not 250 μg but 1 μg of ACTH designed to detect subtle abnormalities does not fully meet expectations (290,291).

A useful test has been a 24-hour urine assay using gas

chromatography–mass spectroscopy technique. This assay is available through the Mayo Clinic and through Meridian Valley Clinical Laboratories (Kent, WA). The latter laboratory provides more data that include free cortisol, cortisone [a less active prehormone, as thyroxine ($T_4$) is to triiodothyronine ($T_3$)], aldosterone, two precursors [pregnenolone and dehydroepiandrosterone (DHEA)], and two metabolites (etiocholanolone and androsterone), along with creatinine and total volume. When combined with routine blood tests for progesterone, testosterone, and estradiol as indicated, a very complete picture of steroid hormone synthesis is realized. Urine testing may be very sensitive if "renal sparing" exists for steroid products. Reuptake by the kidney maintains normal blood levels longer during times of shortages. This method may be used for a 24-hour urine ACTH stimulation test. Many patients with CFS actually demonstrate a decrease in cortisol production after stimulation. This seems to demonstrate decreased adrenal functional reserve and may correspond to the 1974 observations cited previously (285).

Another issue involving the treatment of adrenal dysfunction in patients with CFS is that of overtreatment or inappropriate treatment. Gordon cites a 1989 trial of aggressive glucocorticoid treatment that showed no positive and some deleterious results (200). Fludrocortisone is helpful when given to patients with CFS with postural hypotension. A small, blinded trial giving 0.1 to 0.2 mg fludrocortisone to unselected patients with CFS was disappointing, however (292). A report in 1998 claimed to use a low dose of hydrocortisone but actually gave suppressive doses. Patients showed significant improvement on treatment without significant adverse symptoms, but 12 of 30 taking hydrocortisone showed suppression of glucocorticoid responsiveness (293). Jefferies summarizes work reporting good symptom improvement in truly small, "subreplacement" (or subsuppressive, subphysiologic) doses of hydrocortisone (279). In a low-dose, controlled treatment trial giving 5 or 10 mg daily to 32 patients with CFS, there was significant improvement with treatment without suppression (294).

A final reason for the lack of recognition of adrenal involvement in CFS is the complexity of associated abnormalities. Patients with Addison's disease have increased incidence of autoimmune thyroiditis (AIT; both hypothyroidism and hyperthyroidism), premature ovarian failure, and type 1 diabetes mellitus (275,283). Increased association of hypocortisolism with vulnerability to asthma, allergies, and autoimmune disorders clearly is significant (277). These are compounded by ongoing stress, which alone decreases thyroid-stimulating hormone (TSH) production and inhibits conversion of low-potency $T_4$ to high-potency $T_3$ (276).

Future treatment for this problem may include the steroid precursors, DHEA and pregnenolone, which currently are under study (295–299). Early findings suggest that these agents may be useful tools in practice. It is most useful to use them in conjunction with a nutritional supplement designed to supply the cofactors for the cortical synthetic enzymes.

## Summary

The most consistent finding among patients with CFS is their inability to respond normally to stress. The HPA axis is of prime importance in the adaptive response to stress. Major stressful events or repeated smaller stresses may lead to maladaptive responses that can result in adrenal cortical insufficiency. This produces a plethora of symptoms, and indeed there is much overlap between symptoms of CFS and Addison's disease, the most severe adrenal disorder. The diagnosis of the role of adrenal cortical insufficiency is more difficult because of the complexity of neuroendocrine pathophysiology, the types of testing commonly used, and our current conceptualization of adrenal insufficiency as an all-or-none phenomenon. Successful treatment may be accomplished by judicious use of small doses of supplementary hormones and nutrients. Results will be best when associated disorders also are treated. Three of these, ovarian dysfunction, insulin resistance, and thyroid dysfunction are importantly, even inextricably interrelated with the adrenal disorder.

## OVARIAN DYSFUNCTION AND POLYCYSTIC OVARY SYNDROME

There are a variety of insults that impair normal ovarian function. Foremost of these is stress. It is well known that highly stressed women may temporarily stop menstruating. This result may occur with hypercortisolism. Hypocortisolism is a maladaptive response to chronic stress and also is associated with conditions known to interfere with the menstrual cycle, including adrenal insufficiency, hypothyroidism, and CFS (300).

It seems that rather than simply being a casualty of disease, the ovarian imbalances may play an active part in the production of symptoms in patients with CFS. An association between CFS and menstrual problems has been noted (301,302). Dalton's work with premenstrual syndrome in Britain in the 1950s called attention to the role of steroid sex hormones in both physical and mental health (303). A great amount of practical experience in hormone use and familiarity with side effects was gained with the advent of the oral contraceptive pill and postmenopausal hormone replacement therapy. In addition to the clear physical advantages, the psychotherapeutic benefits of estrogen treatment on both depression and cognitive functioning are now well accepted (304).

The controversy about postmenopausal hormone replacement therapy is elaborated by physician authors of popular books (303,305–307). Each advocates the advan-

## TABLE 25.5. ESTROGEN DOMINANCE SYMPTOMS

| | |
|---|---|
| Allergy symptoms | Headaches |
| Autoimmune disorders | Hypoglycemia |
| Breast cancer | Increased blood clotting |
| Breast tenderness (peripheral) | Infertility |
| Cervical dysplasia | Irregular menstrual cycling |
| Copper excess | Irritability |
| Diminished libido | Insomnia |
| Depression with anxiety or agitation | Magnesium deficiency |
| | Memory loss |
| Dry eyes | Mood swings |
| Early onset of menarche | Osteoporosis |
| Endometrial cancer | Premenstrual syndrome |
| Fat gain: abdomen, hips, and thighs | Polycystic ovaries |
| | Thyroid dysfunction |
| Fatigue | Uterine cancer |
| Fibrocystic breasts | Uterine fibroids |
| Foggy thinking | Water retention |
| Gallbladder disease | |
| Hair loss | |

tages of proper hormone replacement therapy, although their methods are diverse. It is apparent that imbalances between the steroid sex hormones may cause many symptoms, as in premenstrual syndrome. It also is clear that changing hormone ratios cause many symptoms in the perimenopausal woman. A substantial number of patients with CFS are perimenopausal women. Because these patients with CFS are affected by fluctuating hormone ratios, it may be useful to evaluate the steroid sex hormones.

Progesterone appears to play a central role. Its deficiency relative to estradiol produces symptoms usually described as *estrogen dominance* (305) (Table 25.5). Progesterone is both a hormone and a precursor of cortisol. As noted, it may be usurped by the adrenal under stress, creating a relative imbalance. As the patient enters her fifth decade, this may become more noticeable with diminished ovarian production and therefore increased demand on the adrenal gland. Progesterone supplementation, sometimes in prodigious doses, is recommended by some authors as a cure for many perimenopausal symptoms, including fatigue (303,305). This progesterone may supplement adrenal production of cortisol as well.

When indicated by history and symptoms, assays for three steroid sex hormones, progesterone, testosterone, and estradiol, give useful information about the female patient with CFS. When specimens are collected in the midluteal phase of menstruation, approximately the 20th day of the cycle, blood tests for these three hormones are strikingly consistent with the 24-hour urine adrenal steroid profile results.

One problem with synthetic steroid sex hormones is that they cannot be routinely measured. The estrogenic compounds in the oral contraceptive pill and some equine estrogens in conjugated estrogen (Premarin; Wyeth-Ayerst Labo-

ratories, Philadelphia, PA) are too different from human estrogens to be detected by standard blood tests for estradiol (307). The presence of many estrogenic chemicals in the environment has been repeatedly mentioned in the popular press, and these may add to our estrogenic exposure (305, 308). Progestins like medroxyprogesterone acetate (Provera, Pharmacia & Upjohn, Kalamazoo, MI) and agents in the oral contraceptive pill also are invisible to laboratory assays for human progesterone. Many patients with CFS come to the clinic taking synthetic hormones, and potentially significant imbalances may be difficult to detect.

## Polycystic Ovary Syndrome

Polycystic ovary syndrome (PCOS) is increasingly of interest to clinicians (309). The syndrome is common, with an incidence of up to 5% to 10% of all women. It has been popularized by the press as "syndrome X" (310). The most comprehensive review is by Dunaif (311). These patients often are chronically fatigued. Overlapping features in CFS and PCOS have been noted (301,312). Characteristically, serum insulin levels are elevated (313). This is the principal underlying disorder causing the syndrome (309).

Consequences of hyperinsulinemia include excessive production of androgens (not always testosterone) from increased ovarian stromal hyperthecosis, causing acne and hirsutism. An abnormality of particular interest is reduced sex hormone–binding globulin (309). This means that a test for "total testosterone" may fail to reveal the patient's elevated unbound testosterone, the biologically active form. The most accurate test is for "free testosterone." Standard laboratory tests for progesterone and estradiol also are tests of total hormone, so their results also may be inaccurate in patients with PCOS. Testing 24-hour urine samples or saliva samples may be valid alternatives to blood tests. Although these do reflect levels of free hormone, they also are excretory tests affected by total production of hormone as well as blood levels.

Although muscle and adipose cells are insulin resistant, the ovaries may have increased insulin sensitivity. Most patients have menstrual irregularities, usually starting with menarche. They have imbalances of luteinizing hormone and follicle-stimulating hormone (hyperprolactinemia), and often are infertile. Many patients are obese, at least partly because of the effects of insulin resistance. The frequent finding of elevated cholesterol also is related to high insulin (309). Insulin has an aldosterone-like effect on renal function and may contribute to hypertension (314). These effects act synergistically to create at least a sevenfold increased lifetime risk of myocardial infarction and an equally increased risk for diabetes mellitus (309). Because this syndrome responds well to treatment, it obviously is important to make an early diagnosis.

Dunaif notes that the inherent bias in studies of PCOS is the presence of polycystic ovaries as a diagnostic criterion (usually by ultrasound) (311). Not all patients with PCOS express all features of the disorder, including polycystic ovaries. Family studies show that beyond an increased incidence of PCOS in female relatives of patients, some brothers also are insulin resistant (310). The association of men and this disorder conceptually links PCOS and CFS with the syndrome of insulin resistance.

## Summary

Ovarian hormone imbalances and their consequent symptoms are common in women with CFS. These syndromes may be secondary to the same stress that seems to precipitate CFS or simply to the stress of being sick with CFS. The interrelation between ovarian and adrenal hormones is readily apparent. Insulin receptors in the ovaries may be overly activated to complicate clinical symptoms further. It is possible that ovarian disease with imbalance of the steroid sex hormones may be a primary contributor to the clinical picture of CFS.

## INSULIN RESISTANCE AND HYPERINSULINEMIA

Insulin resistance without diabetes mellitus may be of considerable importance in patients who are chronically fatigued. In controlled studies, Allain et al. found elevated insulin levels in patients with CFS and Hotamisligil showed in mice that TNF-α (elevated in a large group of patients with CFS cited previously) induces insulin resistance (315, 316). Luo et al. reported individual and interactive effects producing insulin resistance and hyperinsulinemia when the ventromedial hypothalamus of hamsters is infused with NE and 5-HT (317). Both NE and 5-HT play roles in CFS.

Serotonin is a potent stimulator of the CRH neurons in the lateral paraventricular nuclei as well as the locus ceruleus–NE autonomic system (276). Demitrack and Crofford stated that decreased 5-HT activation of the HPA in patients with CFS is an essential neuroendocrine feature of CFS (318), and this observation is supported by others (319). In work differentiating CFS from depressed patients, Cleare et al. suggest that CFS may be associated with increased 5-HT function and hypocortisolemia (320). These mediators, which are important in CFS, also contribute to insulin resistance.

A brief review of the physiologic roles of insulin is appropriate. Insulin permits glucose transport into cells. It activates anabolism through stimulating glucose utilization, by both forming glycogen and breaking glucose down to precursors for fat and protein synthesis. It moves fats from circulation into storage, causing hydrolysis of circulating triglycerides to provide fatty acids for adipose uptake, then stimulates synthesis of triglycerides in adipose tissue and liver. It increases ribosomal protein synthesis. In addition,

insulin inhibits catabolism. It blocks glycogenolysis and gluconeogenesis. It reduces lipolysis, the mobilization and oxidation of free fatty acids (321).

Other hormones contribute to the control of carbohydrate metabolism. In addition to insulin, the acute effect of GH decreases blood glucose. This is opposed by the chronic effect of GH, ACTH and glucocorticoids, epinephrine, glucagon, and $T_4$. The net direction and activity of catabolism or anabolism is governed primarily by the relative concentrations of insulin and glucagon. Hypoglycemia is a brisk stimulus for production of glucocorticoids and GH, useful for laboratory provocation testing (321).

Patients with CFS have been observed to have abnormalities in these relationships. Decreased GH release in response to insulin-induced hypoglycemia has been reported in controlled studies of patients with CFS by Allain et al. and Moorkins et al., although not observed in a smaller study by Cleare et al. (315,322,323). Conflicting data exist regarding the GH metabolite IGF-1, also called *somatomedin C* (52,324). The larger series showed that somatomedin C in patients with CFS was lower than in healthy control subjects (52).

Causes of insulin resistance are heterogeneous. Autoimmunity can play a role, directed against circulating insulin (common but usually insignificant) and insulin receptors (rare). Cross-reactivity of insulin and IGF-1 exists with low-affinity binding of little consequence (325). Decreased numbers of insulin receptors (downregulation) are seen in obesity, after glucocorticoid therapy, oral contraceptive therapy, and in acromegaly (326). Hypercortisolism from chronic or maladaptive stress predictably also might decrease numbers of insulin receptors. Hypothyroidism causes reduced binding of insulin to rat liver membranes (327). Receptor downregulation is caused by insulin-secreting tumors and is a feature of both a severe form of ovarian dysfunction with virilization and acanthosis nigricans in young women, and PCOS (320).

The insulin receptor in the cell membrane surface seems of less consequence than the glucose transporters. There are five isoforms of these glucose transporters located in different tissues and having different properties. The most important of these is Glut-4, highly expressed only in skeletal muscle, adipose tissue, and heart muscle. The isoforms Glut-1 (erythrocytes and other tissues) and Glut-3 (brain) have a high affinity for insulin and are thought less likely effected by insulin resistance. Glut-4, which accounts for most postprandial glucose uptake (skeletal muscle absorbs 80% to 90% of all insulin-stimulated glucose uptake) has a much lower affinity for insulin, and Glut-2 (liver and pancreatic β cells) has the lowest affinity for insulin (320, 326). The skeletal muscle, liver, and β cells therefore may be most affected by insulin resistance. This may explain some of the clinical features of insulin-resistant nondiabetic patients.

Unfortunately, there is no real discussion of clinical

symptoms in hyperinsulinemic insulin-resistant patients. Endocrinology texts seem to discuss the phenomenon solely as a prediabetic condition (326). From the foregoing discussion of PCOS, in which insulin resistance is the underlying cause of the disorder, and through the preceding paragraphs, it is evident that insulin resistance and hyperinsulinemia can cause symptoms.

Pullen in 1985 described hyperinsulinemia mimicking Ménière's disease and causing migraine headache (328). Clinical experience confirms that symptoms include and far exceed vertigo and headache. Prominent are CFS symptoms and hypoglycemic symptoms in which patients feel anxious, irritable, and lightheaded (brain = Glut-3), whereas peripheral blood is hyperinsulinemic but euglycemic (muscle, liver, and β cells = Glut-4 and Glut-2). Patients usually are physically obese, but they may be very slender indeed. As has often been observed about patients with CFS, these patients are the sickest ones. Pullen advocated the 4-hour oral glucose tolerance test (oGTT) with paired glucose and insulin assays to diagnose hyperinsulinemia (328). Normative data are provided by a 1987 study of 100 healthy volunteers, evaluated with both a euglycemic insulin clamp test and standard oGTT, then given a 75-g oGTT with blood aliquots divided for both glucose and insulin assay (329). These data are consistent with work cited by Olefsky (326). As a rule of thumb, serum insulin normally should not exceed 100 μU/mL after the 75-g oral challenge. Many patients demonstrate significant hypoglycemia when the high levels of insulin suddenly seem to break through the resistance. A large series of patients will show a spectrum of responses grading to type 2 diabetes mellitus.

Treatment of symptomatic insulin resistance involves nutritional supplementation, reduction of dietary carbohydrates (because they stimulate further hyperinsulinemia), and prescription drugs designed to increase insulin receptor sensitivity (metformin and rosiglitazone) (330). These steps are basically the same as the treatment for PCOS, which shares the same underlying pathologic process (309,311). Patients' results often are dramatic and improvement is sustainable.

## Summary

Insulin resistance and hyperinsulinemia are significantly associated with CFS. Studies have shown elevated insulin levels in patients with CFS. Insulin resistance may be induced by TNF-α, NE, and 5-HT, all abnormal in patients with CFS. Insulin is opposed by both glucocorticoids and epinephrine, both of which are elevated by the chronic stress important in the histories of many patients with CFS. Causes of insulin resistance are complex and multiple, with insulin receptor sites reduced in number after therapeutic doses of glucocorticoids and steroid sex hormones. The most vulnerable parts of the receptor apparatus are the glucose transporters with insulin affinity that varies by tissue-specific isoform. The high insulin affinity of brain receptors compared with the low affinity of pancreas and liver receptors may explain the hypoglycemic symptoms in insulin-resistant patients with normal values of blood glucose.

A conceptually simple and relatively inexpensive test seems to be diagnostic for the condition of symptomatic insulin resistance and hyperinsulinemia. Treatment also is conceptually simple and gives results that are most gratifying both to patient and physician.

## THYROID HORMONE DYSFUNCTION

The role of the thyroid gland in CFS involves more than a simple model of hypothyroidism. In addition, measurements of TSH and $T_4$ are inadequate to evaluate thyroid hormone function in the patient with CFS. Fortunately, newer concepts about thyroid hormone function are now being discussed. To preface, a brief review of thyroid physiology is useful.

The hypothalamus synthesizes thyrotropin-releasing hormone (TRH), which is conveyed through the hypophysial stalk to the anterior pituitary, where it stimulates production of thyrotropin (TSH). In turn, TSH is the major regulator of the morphology of the thyroid gland and stimulates production and release of thyroid hormones. These hormones are made using the thyroid peroxidase (TPO) enzyme to bind iodine onto tyrosyl residues, which are then coupled to form thyroid hormones and stored, bound on thyroglobulin (TG). The thyroid is the only endocrine gland that stores hormone—approximately 100 days' supply. Lysosomal proteases later cleave the bond to TG and release the thyroid hormone into circulation (331). At least three important forms of thyroid hormone exist, and it is crucial to understand their properties. $T_4$ (3,5,3',5' tetraiodothyronine) is the most plentiful product of the thyroid gland, followed distantly by 3,5,3' triiodothyronine ($T_3$) and then by a tiny amount of 3,3',5' triiodothyronine (reverse $T_3$, $RT_3$). Thyroid hormone feeds back to depress TSH production. This occurs at both the hypothalamus, where TRH synthesis is inhibited, and at the pituitary, where the release of TSH is blocked. It seems that low $T_4$ is the strongest stimulant of TSH production, whereas high $T_3$ is the strongest inhibitor (332).

The biologic effects of thyroid hormone are many, affecting virtually every organ system. The primary binding site is on the nuclear membrane. Mitochondrial activity is stimulated and cellular oxidation increases, along with many adenosine triphosphate–dependent activities and thermogenesis. Thyroid hormone acting on the nucleus controls expression of genetic information, and thereby all other activities of the cell may be influenced. It has generalized actions on RNA and protein synthesis, with specific actions on transcription of certain proteins. Thyroid hormone acts through generalized and concerted effects with other hormones, including cortisol, GH, and insulin (333).

Circulating thyroid hormone is bound to plasma proteins with such affinity that very little is metabolically available. Only 0.025% of $T_4$ and 0.3% of the less tightly bound $T_3$ are found as free and biologically active hormones. Hormones are primarily bound to thyroid-binding globulin, thyroid-binding prealbumin (transthyretin), and albumin. Only $T_4$ is bound to transthyretin, whereas albumin carries proportionally more $T_3$ than $T_4$, 25% versus 5% (334). The most abundant hormone, $T_4$, has little effect. In fact, it is often called a "prohormone" because it is so weak compared with $T_3$ (334,335). The fate of $T_4$, however, determines the rate of metabolism. To increase available energy, peripheral tissues (mainly the liver) can remove an iodine from the outer (prime) ring of $T_4$, creating $T_3$, which is five to seven times more powerful. The enzyme involved is a 5′-deiodinase. On the other hand, if a 5-deiodinase cuts an iodine from the inner ring, the result will be $RT_3$, which usually is considered biologically inactive (331) (Fig. 25.2). Thus, the metabolic rate may be controlled by altering the ratio of products of $T_4$.

The deiodinase enzymes exist in three tissue-specific isoforms that are clinically relevant (331). Specifically, the function of hepatic type I 5′-deiodinase depends on selenium, and deficiency can compromise the primary source of $T_3$ (335). The counterbalancing 5-deiodinase does not depend on selenium, which would further reduce $T_3$ availability in case of selenium deficiency (331). Pharmaceuticals, including corticosteroids and propylthiouracil, can inhibit the 5′-enzyme but not the 5-enzyme. The other enzyme isoforms, types II (5′-deiodination) and III (5-deiodination) are found in the CNS and pituitary. As yet, they have no identified rate-limiting cofactors. They vary in sensitivity to drugs and to other biologic agents, including the neurotransmitters NE and 5-HT (336). Marked changes of $T_3$ levels in brain tissue may not be reflected in the peripheral blood (336).

In addition to controlling thyroid hormone effects by differentially converting $T_4$ to either $T_3$ or $RT_3$, further metabolism of these hormones downregulates the system (331). Progressive deiodination of $T_3$ and $RT_3$ produces first $T_2$ isomers (which may have varying biologic effects) and, finally, $T_1$ isomers. Hepatic metabolism also alters potency and plasma half-life by decarboxylation, deamination, and conjugation, either glucuronidation or sulfation.

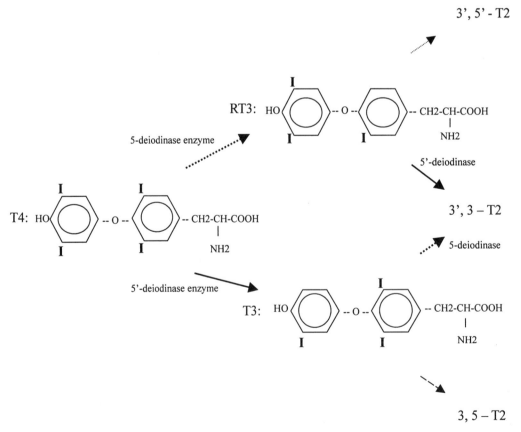

**FIG. 25.2.** Thyroid metabolic pathways, abbreviated.

## Thyroid Hormone Deficiency

Thyroid hormone deficiency causes a clinical syndrome consistent with CFS (337). Although it is stated that "tiredness and lethargy are common and lead to difficulty in performing a full day's work," chronic fatigue is not listed in a lengthy table of symptoms. Other common consequences of hypothyroidism include pallor, dry skin, thin hair, easy bruising, and brittle nails. Cardiac changes are multiple, featuring decreased inotropic and chronotropic effects. Weight gain is variable and appetite is reduced. Peristalsis is decreased and patients have symptoms of colitis, including constipation and gas. Gastric mucosa may atrophy and 12% of patients have overt pernicious anemia.

The nervous system is particularly vulnerable. Psychiatric disorders, in particular depression but also agitation, are common, with all intellectual functions slowing. Neurologic symptoms include headaches, reduced night vision, syncope, hearing loss, and numbness and tingling of the extremities. Carpal tunnel problems are increased. Muscles show stiffness and aching. Hyperirritability may be seen on electromyography and type 1 muscle fibers predominate in pale, swollen muscles with reduced striations. Renal blood flow is reduced. The red cell mass is decreased. Lipid metabolism is altered so that serum cholesterol rises, with increased low-density lipoprotein (LDL) cholesterol and decreased high-density lipoprotein (HDL) cholesterol.

Interaction with the neuroendocrine system is significant. Turnover of cortisol is reduced and 24-hour cortisol excretion is decreased, although normal plasma cortisol levels are maintained. Both pituitary and adrenal function may be secondarily decreased. Adrenal insufficiency can be precipitated by stress in long-standing cases of hypothyroidism, even by overly rapid replacement of thyroid hormone. A state of decreased adrenergic responsiveness is inferred. Plasma cyclic adenosine monophosphate response to glucagon and parathyroid hormones is decreased. NE functions are increased; 5-HT may be effected. Both secretion and function of GH are impaired, and IGF-1 may be reduced. Insulin effect is altered and the oGTT has a characteristically flat curve. Of course, the steroid sex hormones are affected. Menstrual abnormalities, including irregular and excessive bleeding and endometrial proliferation, infertility, and decreased libido are seen. Men experience impotence, oligospermia, and loss of libido.

## Laboratory Tests for Thyroid Function

It is apparent that hypothyroidism creates a clinical picture quite comparable with CFS. Laboratory testing of the thyroid must be wisely ordered and carefully interpreted. The tests discussed in this chapter serve as tools to validate a clinical impression rather than to dictate a particular outcome or approach to therapy (338).

The highly sensitive test for TSH is familiar to all physicians. The clinician must bear in mind, however, that it measures only pituitary production of TSH, not adequacy of thyroid hormone effects in the body. Also, it may not reflect hypothalamic or pituitary problems. Tests of $T_4$ and $T_3$ are available as free ($fT_4$, $fT_3$) or total, including both protein-bound and free hormone assays ($tT_4$ and $tT_3$). Because we are interested in testing metabolically available hormone, it is appropriate to order the free hormone assay (339).

The most often misunderstood test on a "thyroid panel" is the $T_3$ uptake. This generally obsolete test is not even a test for $T_3$, just for unoccupied binding sites on the carrier proteins (338), analogous to the "total iron-binding capacity" test. It is relevant only if there is a real question about carrier protein abnormalities.

Reverse $T_3$ may be assayed to great clinical advantage, but is reported in a way that may be misinterpreted. The tests for TSH, $T_4$, and $T_3$ discussed previously are all reported against a normal range, determined through a statistical analysis of samples from normal patients. The $RT_3$, however, is reported as an analysis of all samples received by the laboratory, both normal and abnormal. The problem is that no one knows which patients are normal and which are not. Therefore, a patient may show a value within the stated laboratory range and yet have a significant problem. The crucial parameter seems to be the relative amounts or ratio of $RT_3$ to $T_3$, as discussed later.

Underlying all of this is the concern that we are measuring only the blood levels of these hormones, not their biologic effect. Refetoff notes, "Thus, ideally, the adequacy of hormonal supply should be assessed by tissue responses rather than by parameters of thyroid gland activity or serum hormone concentration, which are several steps removed from the site of thyroid hormone action" (338). Unfortunately, without a well funded metabolic laboratory, the most convenient test is the basal temperature (340). The physician must remember that basal temperatures may be effected by ovarian, adrenal, metabolic, and immunologic parameters in addition to thyroid gland function.

Thyroid autoantibodies are a useful marker for a diseased thyroid. Unfortunately, approximately 10% of patients with AIT are negative for both anti-TPO antibody and anti-TG antibodies (341,342). Evidence argues for a much broader scope of autoimmune reactivity than tests for these two antibodies can define (343–345). Ultrasound studies are increasingly used and are useful (338).

There is a provocative test for pituitary, or secondary hypothyroidism, the TRH stimulation test. In this test, TRH is administered and the response in TSH and thyroid hormones is measured with serial blood tests. Protocols for the test are given by Thorner et al. and Refetoff (332,338). Popular enthusiasm for this test seems focused on a 1981 report of 250 depressed and fatigued psychiatric inpatients

(346). In this group, 20 patients were found to have an abnormal response to TRH, but only half had an elevated baseline TSH value. Two patients with a normal TSH but positive TRH stimulation received a trial of thyroid hormone treatment for their atypical depression, both successfully. This study has been cited as evidence that measurements of TSH and $T_4$ are not sensitive indicators of hypothyroidism (347).

## Thyroid-stimulating Hormone Levels May Not Be Reliable Indicators of Function

Chrousos and Gold state that stress decreases production of TSH (276). Kelly cites many studies that support this assertion (331). Evidence suggests that the HPA axis may be depressed in CFS. Can the hypothalamic–pituitary–thyroid axis also be depressed in CFS? Certainly, a variety of pharmaceuticals may decrease serum TSH concentration or its response to TRH, including glucocorticoids, dopaminergic agents (including dopamine, l-dopa, pyridoxine, and others), α-noradrenergic blockers (phentolamine), 5-HT agents, both agonists and antagonists, opiates, fenclofenac, and the hypolipidemic drug clofibrate (338).

The production of TSH may be reduced by central suppression in the euthyroid sick syndrome (ESS) or the "low $T_3$ syndrome" ($LT_3S$) (348,349). These two are essentially the same condition, seen in critically ill patients with nonthyroid diseases and well defined recently as low free $T_3$ with normal or subnormal TSH levels (350). Low thyroid hormone levels correlate strongly with poor prognosis. Many reports agree that $ESS/LT_3S$ is caused by the effects of IL-6 and TNF-α (350–355), two of the three cytokines consistently abnormal in patients with CFS.

Although most $LT_3S$ studies focus on the peripheral metabolism of $T_3$ and $RT_3$, evidence for central suppression of the hypothalamic–pituitary–thyroid axis exists. A study of patients perfused with recombinant TNF-α showed decreased TSH, believed to be a central effect (356). Two German studies, respectively of severely traumatized and of septic patients, found decreased TSH, and both suggest that this central suppression is caused by cytokines IL-6 or TNF-α (357,358).

Another possible mechanism of TSH suppression is suggested by two larger studies of patients with ESS involving 34 of 66 elderly people requiring emergency surgery and 36 of 199 patients with chronic heart failure (352,359). Significantly elevated serum NE levels were found in both studies, consistent with a stress response. Eravci et al. have shown that type II 5′-deiodinases in the CNS (and pituitary) are enhanced by NE. Tissue concentrations of $T_3$ in the pituitary rise by local conversion from $T_4$ to exceed blood levels (336). High levels of $T_3$ in the pituitary are the strongest inhibitor of TSH release (332). Relatively high levels of $T_3$ in the pituitary compared with the peripheral circulation may excessively inhibit TSH in ESS.

Strong evidence of central suppression of TSH is noted in a controlled study of ten patients with ESS given a TRH stimulation test both when acutely ill and after recovery (360). The response of TSH to the TRH bolus was significantly depressed when ill but returned to normal after recovery. In contrast, two reports show normal TSH levels in smaller groups of 16 patients with congestive heart failure and 11 with severe trauma and ESS (361,362). Other studies have excluded patients with low TSH in their study protocol.

A report of 1,434 healthy men with normal TSH and no history of thyroid disease emphasizes that such thyroid issues are not limited to critically ill patients with ESS (363). These men were divided according to the degree of atherosclerotic cardiovascular disease (ASCVD) in their carotid arteries. Free $T_4$ levels were significantly lower for patients with carotid ASCVD, and low $fT_4$ was identified as an independent risk factor for ASCVD in euthyroid (normal TSH) hyperlipidemic men.

In summary, patients with low thyroid hormone levels and insufficient function may have normal, even low TSH. This means that a patient with a "normal TSH" may still have insufficient thyroid hormone function.

## Thyroid Hormone Levels May Not Be Reliable Measures of Function

Patients with "normal" blood levels of thyroid hormones also may not have adequate thyroid hormone function. The best known clinical condition that supports this statement is subclinical hypothyroidism, most accurately defined as a combination of normal $fT_4$ and $fT_3$ with increased levels of TSH (364). The term *subclinical* is quite misleading. Patients do indeed have clinical symptoms of hypothyroidism that are significantly more frequent than in control subjects (364). The name seems inaccurately to imply that when $T_4$ and $T_3$ levels are in the normal laboratory range, there can be no clinical problem.

Three studies demonstrate improved cardiac function after treatment with levothyroxine (l-$T_4$), including significant improvements in systolic time intervals, systemic vascular resistance, diastolic function, and even symptoms (365–367). It is noted that although $fT_4$ and $fT_3$ were in the normal range, they were significantly lower compared with control subjects (367). Another study of 61 patients with idiopathic dilated cardiomyopathy evaluated the subjects with both blood tests and thyroid ultrasonography (368). Only 2 patients showed completely normal thyroid morphology and function, with 59 abnormal in one or both measures. There was no significant hypothyroidism or hyperthyroidism in the group, and 53 patients showed morphologic abnormalities on ultrasonography with significant correlation between duration of idiopathic dilated cardiomyopathy and thyroid volume.

Subclinical hypothyroidism was an independent risk factor and strong indicator of risk for atherosclerosis and myocardial infarction in a study of 1,149 elderly women (369), perhaps because of associated elevations of plasma cholesterol (370). A controlled study of 29 younger women noted significant increases in HDL cholesterol with l-$T_4$ treatment (371). Another study tested 40 subjects, 26 of whom had normal levels of TSH but an abnormal response to the TRH stimulation test (372). Twenty-two percent had hyperlipoproteinemia and, with l-$T_4$ treatment, their total and LDL cholesterol decreased significantly. All of these patients had thyroid hormone values in the normal range at entrance into the studies.

Subtle and overt psychiatric symptoms are significantly associated with subclinical hypothyroidism as well. A group of 14 "subclinical" patients who were originally thought free of symptoms were tested (373). On several standard scales they showed significant impairments in memory-related abilities and differences from control subjects in hysteria, anxiety, somatic complaints, and depressive features. This is a pattern suggestive of CFS. After l-$T_4$ treatment, patients showed improvements in memory skills, somatic complaints, and obsessionality compared with untreated patients. Another group of inpatients with "treatment-resistant depression" showed that subclinical hypothyroidism may play a role in the development of some treatment-resistant disorders (374).

Other reports suggest that neuromuscular symptoms are significantly more common in subclinical hypothyroidism, and calcium values, although still in the "normal" range, were significantly lower in patients than in control subjects (375). Another controlled study of 171 women with various thyroid disorders showed that the rate of associated oligomenorrhea and menorrhagia was not significantly different between patients with subclinical hypothyroidism and those with severe hypothyroidism (376).

In contrast, subclinical hyperthyroidism is shown to cause psychiatric morbidity. Forty-six manic patients were studied and all were clinically euthyroid, although baseline $T_4$ levels were at the upper end of the normal range (377). Baseline levels of f$T_4$ and f$T_3$ significantly correlated with past psychiatric morbidity and scores on two scales. Treatment with lithium, a thyroid inhibitor, produced progressively decreasing TSH, f$T_4$, and f$T_3$ levels that correlated significantly with a decrease in psychiatric symptoms. This suggests that either the range of "normal" values of thyroid hormone tests is too broad at the upper end as well as the lower, or that thyroid hormones may interact with other physiologic factors to create symptoms of either deficiency or excess at levels usually considered normal.

Subclinical hypothyroidism is a common problem. An Italian study found subclinical hypothyroidism the most common thyroid disorder (378). In groups of 1,001, 1,149, and 1,191 subjects, the prevalence among women was 6.1%, 10.8%, and 7.6%, respectively, and lower among men: 3.4%, data not given, and 1.9% (364,369,370,379).

All of these studies report significant correlation with pathologic states, as noted previously. Only one negative study seems to refute these findings.

## Importance of the Percentile Value of "Normal" Thyroxine

Pop et al. studied the effects of maternal f$T_4$ concentrations during early pregnancy on psychomotor development of the child (380). The fetal thyroid is unable to produce any $T_4$ before 12 to 14 weeks' gestation. Values for maternal TSH, f$T_4$, and TPO antibody status were measured at 12 and 32 weeks' gestation; neurodevelopment then was assessed at 10 months of age in 220 healthy infants. After correction for confounding variables, f$T_4$ concentrations below the 10th percentile at 12 weeks' gestation were a significant risk for impaired infant psychomotor development. This supports the previous suggestion that "normal" $T_4$ may not be adequate.

## Consequences of Imbalances of $T_4$, $T_3$, and Reverse $T_3$

The disposition of $T_4$ significantly affects the rate of metabolism. The conversion of $T_4$ to $T_3$ may be reduced and production of $RT_3$ increased by a variety of stressful situations, including starvation and fasting (331,381–383), ESS/L$T_3$S from trauma, surgery (331,362,384), and chronic illness (348,381), sleep deprivation (331), stressors, including cold exposure and medical school examinations (331), endotoxins (385), pharmacologic doses of corticosteroids (338,386), and toxic agents, including lead, cadmium, and carbon tetrachloride (331). The consensus is that the activity of type I 5'-deiodinase is inhibited. Because the 5-deiodinase is not inhibited, $T_4$ is converted more into $RT_3$, less into $T_3$. In addition, $RT_3$ levels remain higher because it cannot be degraded into 3,3'-$T_2$, which also is a function of the 5'-deiodinase enzyme (338), throwing into question the role of $RT_3$ as a possible competitive inhibitor of $T_3$.

Attention in the 1970s was focused on the question of receptor site individuality and affinities for $T_3$ and $RT_3$. Results have shown separate $RT_3$ receptors in rat liver plasma membranes (387) and in nuclei of pig liver (388), rat brain (389), rat liver (390), rat and pig liver (391), and human liver and placenta (392). An additional two studies, one of rat brain and liver and the other of human endometrium, showed the same binding affinity for thyroid hormones to nuclear $T_3$ receptors that Kobayashi et al. reported (389), $T_3 > T_4 > RT_3$ (390,393,394).

Receptor status is plastic. Kobayashi et al. found $RT_3$ receptor type differences between the cerebral cortex and the thalamus and hypothalamus and reported that the density of $RT_3$ binding sites significantly decreased from birth to age 9 weeks (389). Receptors can be upregulated in cases of starvation (anorexia nervosa), hypothyroidism, and L$T_3$S

(383,395). The drug dithiothreitol increased binding of $T_3$ and reduced binding of $RT_3$ to nuclear receptors (391). In response to various stimuli, the number and binding affinities of receptor sites can change, which may alter the effects of thyroid hormone.

In summary, specific $RT_3$ receptors seem to exist on the nuclear membrane, and $T_3$ receptors have some affinity for $RT_3$. Lavin writes, " . . . the presence of the nuclear thyroid hormone receptor may allow a response but does not ensure it . . . other factors must control function . . . " (333). It is possible that interplay of $T_3$ and $RT_3$ may contribute to this control of function. Work with TSH receptor-stimulating and -inhibiting antibodies seems to show that there are two receptors involved—one stimulatory, the other inhibitory. It is possible that $RT_3$ might act on an inhibitory receptor to block the effect of $T_3$.

Three studies have shown that reverse $T_3$ may be a competitive inhibitor of $T_3$. First, a study of β-adrenoreceptors in the rat heart compared the effects of in vivo $T_4$, $T_3$, or $RT_3$ with the effects of hypothyroidism (396). Pretreatment of rats with $RT_3$ produced changes similar to those seen in hypothyroid rats. Second, a 1991 study of a line of rat pituitary cells showed that although the stimulant effect of $RT_3$ is 1,000 times less potent than that of $T_3$ and unlikely to have significance, $RT_3$ may block $T_3$ (397). When a cell was superfused with $RT_3$ (10 nM), the subsequent effect of $T_3$ was prevented, even in a concentration of 10 nM. Finally, a 1998 study on human lymphocyte function and $RT_3$ was stimulated by findings of increased serum $RT_3$ in response to cold exposure (398). It demonstrated that $RT_3$ binding on nuclear receptors is competitive with $T_3$. $RT_3$ uptake on receptors increased as the $RT_3$ concentration increased. Importantly, there was an indication that lymphocyte function is depressed by increasing serum concentrations of $RT_3$.

In contrast, one report reaches a contrary conclusion. In 1980, Smith et al. tested the ability of various iodothyronines, including $RT_3$, to displace labeled $T_3$ from binding sites in isolated pig liver nuclei (399). They wrote that these were unlikely to modulate the interaction of $T_3$ with its receptor. This may be an overstatement; antihistamines, for example, cannot displace histamine from its receptor, but certainly are competitive inhibitors of histamine.

In his 1991 book, Wilson popularized the concept that elevated $RT_3$ levels can cause symptoms of hypothyroidism in a patient who seems euthyroid by all laboratory tests (400). Wilson claims excellent therapeutic results from treatment with synthetic $T_3$. Three reports may support this assertion. The first is a controlled study of cardiomyopathic left ventricle myocytes (401). Pretreatment with $T_3$ improved myocyte contractile performance after hypothermic cardioplegic arrest and rewarming. The second is a study of $LT_3S$ in a model of chronically calorie-deprived rats (402). Supplementation with $T_3$ significantly normalized both car-

diac function and phenotype of the calorie-restricted animals, suggesting a role for $LT_3S$ in the pathophysiologic response to starvation. Finally, a study of six children undergoing complex cardiac operations under cardiopulmonary bypass showed that normalizing serum $T_3$ levels were reflected in a marked decrease in requirement for inotropic support, conversion to normal sinus rhythm, and a progressively improving clinical course (403). A manuscript given to the French Fibromyalgia Association in May, 2000 reports a group of 77 euthyroid patients with FM treated with an open trial of $T_3$ to test the hypothesis of partial cellular resistance to thyroid hormone (404). Fifty-eight (75%) reported some degree of improvement. Differences between pretreatment and posttreatment pressure/pain thresholds at 18 sites showed significant improvement.

It appears from these studies that the ratio of $T_3$ to $RT_3$ is important. Correction of an unfavorable balance through judicious dosing of $T_3$ may give excellent results. Several reports mention the ratio of $T_3$ to $RT_3$. A report of $LT_3S$ in 100 bone marrow transplant recipients used the ratio of $RT_3$ to $T_3$ (405). Other reports seem hindered by their failure to compare $RT_3$ with $T_3$, relying instead on some determination of "normal" levels of $RT_3$ (406,407). Intuitively, in an either/or case such as the deiodination of $T_4$, it makes sense to review both products, $T_3$ and $RT_3$, in relative proportion. Low levels of $RT_3$ may be quite significant when offset by even lower levels of $T_3$.

Therapy with $T_3$ may be successful, although its short half-life must be considered. Wilson recommends every–12-hour dosing using a preparation compounded with a resin to delay absorption and prolong its functional half-life (400). Clinically, it seems that most patients do well with commercially available $T_3$ on a 12-hour dosing schedule. A few people prefer dosing every 8 hours. Concerns are voiced about risks of treatment. In a 1997 review of the literature, Chopra states that he found no evidence of harm by treatment of patients with ESS with up to replacement doses of $T_3$ (348).

From the foregoing discussion, the relative levels of $T_4$ to $T_3$ to $RT_3$ must be considered when evaluating a chronically fatigued patient who is being treated for hypothyroidism. It is easy to collect a series of patients who are taking synthetic $T_4$ preparations ($l$-$T_4$) but are still symptomatic (data in preparation). Some of these patients will simply be taking the wrong dose of $LT_4$. A British group analyzed 91 patients taking $T_4$ and found a high TSH in 26.8% and a low TSH in 20.6% (408). Similar results may be present in CFS, indicating that it is difficult to achieve optimal dosing of $l$-$T_4$. With further testing, some of these patients have considerably lower levels of $fT_3$ than $fT_4$, which suggests faulty 5′-deiodinase function. Most of these also have relatively more $RT_3$ than $fT_3$. The results of treatment directed to correct these imbalances often are very good.

## Peripheral Resistance to Thyroid Hormone

Like insulin resistance, cases of resistance to thyroid hormone (RTH) at the receptor level are well documented (409). Unlike insulin resistance, RTH is thought to be rare, with only approximately 600 cases reported. It is caused by point mutations in the thyroid hormone receptor gene (409, 410). Resistance can exist with normal baseline laboratory findings (410). In addition, mutations of the TSH receptor have been reviewed by DuPrez et al. (411). Different phenotypes exist, ranging from asymptomatic TSH resistance to overt congenital hypothyroidism. RTH merits consideration in the context of CFS. Cases of genetic mutations causing insulin receptor resistance are well documented and seem to be similar to RTH. Could there also exist a type of RTH that, like most cases of insulin resistance, is acquired instead of hereditary? In this circumstance, the lack of tests for thyroid hormone function seems a particularly significant issue. Because the mechanisms of insulin resistance are not well known, it may be possible that RTH can exist in an as-yet occult form. If so, autoimmunity may play some role.

## Autoimmune Disorders of the Thyroid

The thyroid system is subject to many sorts of autoimmune attack. Most common is AIT, a group of conditions characterized by the presence of circulating thyroid antibodies and immunologically competent cells capable of reacting with certain thyroid constituents (412). The incidence of AIT is increasing in frequency (412–415). The reasons for this increase probably are multiple, including dietary iodine excess from iodized commercial bread and exposure to radioactive fallout (416–418). AIT is the most common cause of spontaneous hypothyroidism in areas of iodine sufficiency. The incidence in women is approximately 3.5 cases per 1,000, and in men, 0.8 per 1,000 (413). The prevalence increases with age, although the peak incidence of new cases occurs in the fourth and fifth decades. There is a weak association with certain human leukocyte antigen markers, and AIT is strongly familial (413).

Autoimmune thyroiditis is significantly increased in a number of other disorders. Approximately 40% of patients with nontuberculous adrenocortical insufficiency have circulating thyroid autoantibodies (412). There usually is an increase in AIT among patients with autoimmune disorders, including type 1 insulin-dependent diabetes mellitus (412, 419,420), pernicious anemia, idiopathic hypoparathyroidism, vitiligo and alopecia areata, primary biliary cirrhosis, rheumatoid arthritis, lupus erythematosus, progressive systemic sclerosis, Sjögren's syndrome (412), multiple sclerosis (421), celiac disease (422), ankylosing spondylitis (423), and others. Hotze tested 697 consecutive allergic pa-

tients in Texas and found 24% of women positive for thyroid autoantibodies (424). Allergy, the most common form of immune dysregulation, is a marker for increased risk of AIT.

Cell-mediated AIT also exists (412). Attention has focused, however, on a wide variety of specific autoantibodies directed against the thyroid system. Most commonly tested are the anti-TG and anti-TPO (formerly anti-microsomal) antibodies that may cause cell damage and activate killer cells. Others include antibodies directed against "second colloid antigen," cell surface antigen, and both $T_4$ and $T_3$ (412). It seems that the anti-$T_4$ antibody may not cross-react with $T_3$ (425). Antibodies against the TSH receptor site cause Graves' disease when they stimulate the receptor, and atrophic Hashimoto's thyroiditis when they do not (412). It seems possible that other autoantibodies against other targets in the thyroid system might exist.

Kim et al. offer evidence that seemingly euthyroid AIT may be associated with unpredictably severe consequences. In their report, 28 euthyroid women who tested positive for AIT with anti-TPO or anti-TG antibodies but no other immunologic diseases underwent in vitro fertilization (426). Compared with 51 control subjects without antibodies, the patients with AIT had significantly fewer pregnancies and more miscarriages. Harris reviews the association of thyroid autoantibody status in postpartum depression (427). He notes effects of AIT on the infant, the family, and later development of the child, and emphasizes the importance of treatment (427). A Danish study of 207 centenarians found that the presence of thyroid autoantibodies correlated with poor physical functioning independent of TSH, $T_4$, or $T_3$ (428). McGregor and Hall state that a significant reduction in thyroid function cannot be excluded on the basis of normal thyroid function test results alone, which seems to be supported in these studies (412). Indeed, the report of Kim et al. demonstrating tissue responses to thyroid hormone may reflect Refetoff's ideal measurement of thyroid hormone adequacy, discussed previously (338).

There may be application of Kim and colleagues' work with AIT to CFS as well. One outcome study appears to demonstrate significant consequences of AIT in the absence of any other abnormal thyroid study result. There seems to be an increased frequency of AIT in chronically fatigued, multiply allergic patients (429). Another series showed that fine-needle aspiration cytology of indurated thyroid glands in 50 patients with idiopathic chronic fatigue showed a spectrum from AIT to nodular goiter (342). Although autoimmune blockade of insulin receptors is known to exist, reports of thyroid receptor blockade have not been found. In addition, thyroid cells effected by AIT can release both IL-1 and IL-6 (430,431), and IL-1 inhibits thyroid function (430). The interconnection of cytokines, thyroid disease, and CFS might be considered.

## Miscellaneous Inhibitors of Thyroid Hormone Function

A number of agents alter the extrathyroidal metabolism of thyroid hormone (338). Among the most potent and commonly encountered inhibitors of conversion of $T_4$ to $T_3$ are β-adrenergic blockers like propranolol. These drugs are commonly used for migraine headache, hypertension, and heart disease and have significantly effected thyroid function among some patients. Glucocorticoids, propylthiouracil, amiodarone, the tricyclic antidepressant clomipramine, and iodinated contrast agents have the same effect. Others stimulate hormone degradation or fecal excretion, including phenytoin, carbamazepine, phenobarbital, cholestyramine resins, and soybeans.

Organophosphate poisoning may result in ESS (432). In a series of 22 patients, 7 (31.8%) had ESS. The hormone levels returned to normal values after resolution of the poisoning. A British controlled study of sheep fed pesticides from birth to sacrifice at 67 weeks demonstrated that pentachlorophenol consistently disrupted thyroid function, probably through a direct effect on the thyroid gland (433). Reductions in serum values for $tT_4$ and $fT_4$ and in the magnitude and duration of response of $T_4$ to TSH were significant. The $T_3$ but not $RT_3$ response to TSH also was markedly reduced after pentachlorophenol. As discussed in Chapter 23, pesticides in our food chain may effect people with impaired or "saturated" hepatic detoxication pathways at quite low doses.

## Treatment Considerations

From the foregoing discussion, it can be seen that setting the treatment goal for either overt or subclinical hypothyroidism as solely the normalization of TSH is no longer valid (434). Williams' recent review enumerated the consequences of excessive L-$T_4$ dosing as defined by depressed TSH levels, without even mentioning blood levels of $T_4$ or $T_3$ (435). Such use of TSH alone is overly simplistic. In the preceding paragraphs, it can be clearly seen that TSH levels are not the most important indicators of an euthyroid state. A low TSH does not prove excessive levels of thyroid hormone.

The goal of thyroid hormone treatment is restoration of normal thyroid hormone function. This requires attention to patients' clinical symptoms and physical findings as well as to their laboratory studies (436). The physician must consider which preparation of thyroid hormone best fits the patient's clinical situation. Available options include $T_4$, $T_3$, or mixes, both natural and synthetic. A discussion of relative merits and disadvantages exceeds the scope of this chapter. Any preparation containing $T_3$ is most effective if used in divided doses at least every 12 hours because of its short half-life.

Before starting treatment, the patient must be evaluated for other problems, especially adrenal. If abnormalities of both thyroid and adrenal coexist, it is wise to stabilize the adrenal first. The dose of thyroid hormone in a chronically fatigued patient must be built up by small increments. Dosing is individualized, based on "lean" body mass (437). As the dose of thyroid hormone is increased, patients must taper off and stop other stimulants. Many untreated hypothyroid patients use caffeine, stimulants, or herbal preparations. These agents can interact with thyroid hormone and make it difficult to find the optimal thyroid dose.

From the discussion of hypothalamic and pituitary dysfunction, it is evident that in certain circumstances, the physician must give doses of thyroid hormone sufficient to suppress TSH to achieve good results. A small dose of hormone may quickly be offset by a reduction in the already inadequate amount of TSH. In such circumstances, the patient's circulating thyroid hormone levels remain unchanged until the escalating treatment dose fully suppresses TSH. This factor emphasizes the importance of measuring thyroid hormone levels—$T_4$, $T_3$, and sometimes $RT_3$—as these patients are followed through their treatment course. Lacking concise data regarding peak and trough levels in thyroid treatment, many clinicians draw blood levels midway between doses (438). This gives a useful average blood level to assess the safety of the patient's dose. Understanding that the normal levels of thyroid hormone may be imprecise at the high end as well as the low, several reports find no harm from doses of thyroid hormone that suppress TSH while giving normal levels of $T_4$ and $T_3$ (348,439).

## Summary

The model of primary hypothyroidism is oversimplified and inadequate for dealing with patients with CFS. Insufficient thyroid hormone effect creates a clinical condition that is consistent with CFS. After a careful history and physical examination, the laboratory evaluation is very important. There is no single definitive test for adequacy of thyroid hormone function. Thyroid tests must be inclusive and the results interpreted with an eye to the relative proportions of $T_4$, $T_3$, and $RT_3$. The presence of thyroid autoantibodies often is significant. The interaction of other illnesses with thyroid hormone function always must be considered.

Every patient treated with thyroid hormone ought to know that he or she is on a treatment trial—even those whose tests show frank hypothyroidism. Patients with CFS must be given the hormone preparation best suited to their needs as indicated by their laboratory results. In some cases, L-$T_4$ simply will not work. Blood levels must be tested to ensure safety.

## NUTRITION AND CFS

Nutritional interventions may help the symptoms of many patients. A multivitamin of quality and extra B-complex vitamins and antioxidants make good clinical sense. Adrenal nutritional supplements such as desiccated bovine adrenal gland (or its equivalent) and DHEA or pregnenolone show anecdotal success. From a cost–benefit evaluation, however, it is troubling to see disabled patients pay large amounts of money for so many bottles of substances recommended by various well intentioned parties. In suggesting any nutritional supplement, the clinician should have a specific goal and be able somehow to monitor improvement. If an intervention does not help, be willing to discontinue it as ineffective.

## PROGNOSIS FOR CFS PATIENTS

Most reports with 18 months or longer follow-up of patients with CFS are not encouraging. Reported rates of "cure" are low: 2% of 445 patients, 3% of 246 patients, 4% (1 of 23), 6% (6 of 103), and 12% (21 of 177) (440–444). In other papers, a larger number of patients state an improvement in their condition: 64%, 17%, 39% (9/23), and 63% (440–443). Only one report of a small group of patients with CFS afforded intensive multidisciplinary intervention gives better results: 88% (46/51) returned to employment or an equivalent level of activity, with only 12% disabled (445). Their management included medical, psychiatric, and cognitive–behavioral treatment.

These studies are hindered by the difficulties in defining these patients' status, first as patients with CFS and then functionally. There are no clear lines drawn between "disabled" and "impaired." Also, many patients have some difficulty with serial questionnaires. From these studies, however, it appears that patients with CFS do not respond well to conventional management (446,447).

## SUMMARY

Chronic fatigue syndrome remains a difficult illness to diagnose, characterize, and effectively treat. The evidence suggests that CFS reflects a multisystem dysfunction, involving the immunoneuroendocrine axis, and that it can be refractory to a variety of interventions. Concurrent illnesses such as FM, depression, and allergic diseases complicate the clinical picture of CFS and present challenges to even experienced clinicians. The pathophysiologic process of CFS is coming under better understanding, but the pathogenesis of the disorder remains a mystery.

Of all forms of intervention, the validation of the patient's perception that he or she is afflicted by a confirmed physiologic illness can offer the most relief. A multimodal approach using medical, behavioral, and psychosocial interventions can result in maximizing return to function by most patients with CFS. A complete allergy evaluation, including attention to inhalants, foods, and chemical triggers,

may assist in reducing the burden of the disease and improving symptoms.

Clinical trials of new and adapted interventions are necessary to obtain a consistent and valid approach to patients with this debilitating disease. Information presented in this chapter can assist clinicians and researchers in designing and carrying out these critical studies so that in the coming decades, a reliable and effective treatment protocol for patients with CFS can be established.

## REFERENCES

1. DaCosta JM. On irritable heart: a clinical study of a form of functional cardiac disorder and its consequence. *Am J Med Sci* 1871;121:17–52.
2. Beard G. Neurasthenia, or nervous exhaustion. *Boston Med Surg J* 1869;80:217–220.
3. Wessely S. Old wine in new bottles: neurasthenia and "ME." *Psychol Med* 1990;20:35–53.
4. Abbey SE, Garfinkel PE. Neurasthenia and the chronic fatigue syndrome: the role of culture in the making of a diagnosis. *Am J Psychiatry* 1991;148:1638–1646.
5. Kim E. A brief history of chronic fatigue syndrome. *JAMA* 1994;272:1070–1071.
6. Selye H. A syndrome produced by diverse noxious agents. *Nature* 1936;138:32–36.
7. Gilliam AG. Epidemiologic study of an epidemic, diagnosed as poliomyelitis, occurring among the personnel of the Los Angeles County General Hospital during the summer of 1934. *Public Health Bull* 1938;240:1–90.
8. Sigurdsson B, Sigurjonsson JHJ, Sigurdsson JT, et al. A disease epidemic in Iceland simulating poliomyelitis. *Am J Hyg* 1950; 52:222–238.
9. The Medical Staff of the Royal Free Hospital. An outbreak of encephalomyelitis in the Royal Free Hospital group, London. *BMJ* 1957;2:895–904.
10. Poskanzer DC, Henderson DA, Kunkle EC, et al. Epidemic neuromyasthenia: an outbreak in Punta Gorda, Florida. *N Engl J Med* 1957;257:356.
11. Hoad A. Coming to terms with ME. *Health Visit* 1994;67: 302–303.
12. Holmes GP, Kaplan JE, Stewart JA, et al. A cluster of patients with a chronic mononucleosis-like syndrome: is Epstein Barr virus the cause? *JAMA* 1987;257:2297–2302.
13. Daugherty SA, Henry BE, Peterson DL, et al. Chronic fatigue syndrome in northern Nevada. *Rev Infect Dis* 1991;13[Suppl]: S39–S44.
14. Thorley-Lawson DA, Babcock GJ. A model for persistent infection with Epstein-Barr virus: the stealth virus of human B cells. *Life Sci* 1999;65:1433–1453.
15. Holmes GP, Kaplan JE, Gantz NM, et al. Chronic fatigue syndrome: a working case definition. *Ann Intern Med* 1988;108: 387–389.
16. Fukuda K, Strauss SE, Hickie I, et al. The chronic fatigue syndrome: a comprehensive approach to its definition and study. *Ann Intern Med* 1994;121:953–959.
17. Komaroff AL, Fagioli LR, Geiger AM, et al. An examination of the working case definition of chronic fatigue syndrome. *Am J Med* 1996;100:56–64.
18. Anderson JS, Ferrans CE. The quality of life of persons with chronic fatigue syndrome. *J Nerv Ment Dis* 1997;185(6): 359–367.
19. Nisenbaum R, Reyes M, Mawle AC, et al. Factor analysis of

unexplained severe fatigue and interrelated symptoms: overlap with criteria for chronic fatigue syndrome. *Am J Epidemiol* 1998; 148:72–77.

20. Kakumanu S, Yeager M, Craig TJ. Chronic fatigue syndrome. *J Am Osteopath Assoc* 1999;99[10 Suppl Pt.1]:S1–S5.
21. Hickie I, Lloyd A, Hadzi-Pavlovic D, et al. *Psychol Med* 1995; 25:925–935.
22. Buchwald D, Wener MH, Pearlman T, et al. Markers of inflammation and immune activation in chronic fatigue and chronic fatigue syndrome. *J Rheumatol* 1997;24:372–376.
23. Finestone AJ. A doctor's dilemma: is a diagnosis disabling or enabling? *Arch Intern Med* 1997;157:491–492.
24. Woodward RV, Broom DH, Legge DG. Diagnosis in chronic illness: disabling or enabling: the case of chronic fatigue syndrome. *J R Soc Med* 1995;88:325–329.
25. Morriss RK, Wearden AJ, Mullis R. Exploring the validity of the Chalder Fatigue Scale in chronic fatigue syndrome. *J Psychosom Res* 1998;45:411–417.
26. Myers C, Wilks D. Comparison of Euroqol EQ-5D and SF-36 in patients with chronic fatigue syndrome. *Qual Life Res* 1999;8:9–16.
27. Schooley RT. Chronic fatigue syndrome. In: Mandell GL, Bennett JE, Dolin R, eds. *Principles and practice of infectious diseases*, 4th ed. New York: Churchill Livingstone, 1995.
28. Sharpe M, Archard LC, Banatvala JE. A report: chronic fatigue syndrome—guidelines for research. *J R Soc Med* 1991;84: 118–121.
29. Wessely S. The epidemiology of chronic fatigue syndrome. *Epidemiol Rev* 1995;17:1–13.
30. Jason LA, Richman JA, Rademaker AW, et al. A community-based study of chronic fatigue syndrome. *Arch Intern Med* 1999; 159:2129–2137.
31. Steele L, Dobbins JG, Fukuda K, et al. The epidemiology of chronic fatigue in San Francisco. *Am J Med* 1998;105(3A): 83S–90S.
32. Buchwald D, Umali P, Umali J, et al. Chronic fatigue and the chronic fatigue syndrome: prevalence in a Pacific Northwest health care system. *Ann Intern Med* 1995;123:81–88.
33. Wessely S, Chalder T, Hirsch S, et al. The prevalence and morbidity of chronic fatigue and chronic fatigue syndrome: a prospective primary care study. *Am J Public Health* 1997;87: 1449–1455.
34. Minowa M, Jaimo M. Descriptive epidemiology of chronic fatigue syndrome based on a nationwide survey in Japan. *J Epidemiol* 1996;6:75–80.
35. Straus SE. Chronic fatigue syndrome. In: Fauci AS, Braunwald E, Isselbacher KJ, et al., eds. *Harrison's principles of internal medicine*, 14th ed. New York: McGraw-Hill, 1998.
36. Conti F, Priori R, DePetrillo G, et al. Prevalence of chronic fatigue syndrome in Italian patients with persistent fatigue. *Ann Ital Med Int* 1994;9:219–222.
37. Fukuda K, Dobbins JG, Wilson LJ, et al. An epidemiologic study of fatigue with relevance for the chronic fatigue syndrome. *J Psychiatr Res* 1997;31:19–29.
38. Salit IE. Precipitating factors for the chronic fatigue syndrome. *J Psychiatr Res* 1997;31:59–65.
39. Hall GH, Hamilton WT, Round AP. Increased illness experience preceding chronic fatigue syndrome: a case control study. *J R Coll Physicians Lond* 1998;32:44–48.
40. Zhang QW, Natelson BH, Ottenweller JE, et al. Chronic fatigue syndrome beginning suddenly occurs seasonally over the year. *Chronobiol Int* 2000;17(1):95–99.
41. Goldenberg DL. Fibromyalgia syndrome a decade later: what have we learned? *Arch Intern Med* 1999;159:777–785.
42. Wolfe F, Smythe HA, Yunus MB, et al. The American College of Rheumatology 1990 criteria for the classification of fibromy-

algia: report of the Multicenter Criteria Committee. *Arthritis Rheum* 1990;33:160–172.
43. Buchwald D, Pearlman T, Kith P, et al. Gender differences in patients with chronic fatigue syndrome. *J Gen Intern Med* 1994; 9:397–401.
44. White JP, Speechley M, Harth M, et al. Co-existence of chronic fatigue syndrome with fibromyalgia syndrome in the general population: a controlled study. *Scand J Rheumatol* 2000;29: 44–51.
45. Bombardier CH, Buchwald D. Chronic fatigue, chronic fatigue syndrome, and fibromyalgia: disability and health-care use. *Med Care* 1996;34:924–930.
46. Dunne FJ, Dunne CA. Fibromyalgia syndrome and psychiatric disorder. *Br J Hosp Med* 1995;54:194–197.
47. Buchwald D. Fibromyalgia and chronic fatigue syndrome: similarities and differences. *Rheum Dis Clin North Am* 1996;22: 219–243.
48. Breau LM, McGrath PJ, Ju LH. Review of juvenile primary fibromyalgia and chronic fatigue syndrome. *J Dev Behav Pediatr* 1999;20:278–288.
49. Aaron LA, Burke MM, Buchwald D. Overlapping conditions among patients with chronic fatigue syndrome, fibromyalgia, and temporomandibular disorder. *Arch Intern Med* 2000;160: 221–227.
50. Gomborone JE, Gorard DA, Dewsnap PA, et al. Prevalence of irritable bowel syndrome in chronic fatigue. *J R Coll Physicians Lond* 1996;30:512–513.
51. Klein R, Berg PA. High incidence of antibodies to 5-hydroxytryptamine, gangliosides and phospholipids in patients with chronic fatigue and fibromyalgia syndrome and their relatives: evidence for a clinical entity of both disorders. *Eur J Med Res* 1995;1:21–26.
52. Evengard B, Nilsson CG, Lindh G, et al. Chronic fatigue syndrome differs from fibromyalgia: no evidence for elevated substance P levels in cerebrospinal fluid of patients with chronic fatigue syndrome. *Pain* 1998;78:153–155.
53. Bennett AL, Mayes DM, Fagioli LR, et al. Somatomedin C (insulin-like growth factor I) levels in patients with chronic fatigue syndrome. *J Psychiatr Res* 1997;31:91–96.
54. Clauw DJ, Schmidt M, Radulovic D, et al. The relationship between fibromyalgia and interstitial cystitis. *J Psychiatr Res* 1997;31:125–131.
55. National Institute of Allergy and Infectious Diseases, National Institutes of Health. *Chronic fatigue syndrome: information for physicians.* NIH publication no. 97-484. Bethesda, MD: National Institutes of Health, 1997.
56. Levine PH, Whiteside TL, Friberg D, et al. Dysfunction of natural killer activity in a family with chronic fatigue syndrome. *Clin Immunol Immunopathol* 1998;88:96–104.
57. Empson M. Celiac disease or chronic fatigue syndrome: can the current CDC working case definition discriminate? *Am J Med* 1998;105:79–80.
58. Fiore G, Giacovazzo F, Giacovazzo M. Three cases of dermatomyositis erroneously diagnosed as "chronic fatigue syndrome." *Eur Rev Med Pharmacol Sci* 1997;1:193–195.
59. Nishikai M, Akiya K, Tojo T, et al. "Seronegative" Sjögren's syndrome manifested as a subset of chronic fatigue syndrome. *Br J Rheumatol* 1996;35:471–474.
60. Sorenson WG. Fungal spores: hazardous to health? *Environ Health Perspect* 1999;107[Suppl]3:469–472.
61. Mesch U, Lowenthal RM, Coleman D. Lead poisoning masquerading as chronic fatigue syndrome. *Lancet* 1996;347:1193.
62. David Quig, Doctors' Data Laboratory, Chicago, IL. Personal communication.
63. Knobeloch L, Jackson R. Recognition of chronic carbon monoxide poisoning. *WMJ* 1999;998:26–29.

64. Pearn JH. Chronic fatigue syndrome: chronic ciguatera poisoning as a differential diagnosis. *Med J Aust* 1997;166:309–310.
65. Priori R, Conti F, Luan FL, et al. Chronic fatigue: a peculiar evolution of eosinophilia myalgia syndrome following treatment with L-tryptophan in four Italian adolescents. *Eur J Pediatr* 1994;153:344–346.
66. Peroutka SJ. Chronic fatigue disorders: an inappropriate response to arginine vasopressin? *Med Hypotheses* 1998;50:521–523.
67. DeLorenzo F, Hargreaves J, Kakkar VV. Phosphate diabetes in patients with chronic fatigue syndrome. *Postgrad Med J* 1998;74:229–232.
68. Durlach J, Bac P, Durlach V, et al. Neurotic, neuromuscular, and autonomic nervous form of magnesium imbalance. *Magnes Res* 1997;10:169–195.
69. Downey DC. Fatigue syndromes revisited: the possible role of porphyrins. *Med Hypotheses* 1994;42:285–290.
70. Wessely S, Nimnuan C, Sharpe M. Functional somatic syndromes: one or many? *Lancet* 1999;354:936–939.
71. Barsky AJ, Borus JF. Functional somatic syndromes. *Ann Intern Med* 1999;130:910–921.
72. Wessely S, Chalder T, Hirsch S, et al. Psychological symptoms, somatic symptoms, and psychiatric disorder in chronic fatigue and chronic fatigue syndrome: a prospective study in the primary care setting. *Am J Psychiatry* 1996;153:1050–1059.
73. Brunello N, Akiskal H, Boyer P, et al. Dysthymia: clinical picture, extent of overlap with chronic fatigue syndrome, neuropharmacological considerations, and new therapeutic vistas. *J Affect Disord* 1999;52:275–290.
74. Swanink CM, Versoulen JH, Bleujenberg G, et al. Chronic fatigue syndrome: a clinical and laboratory study with a well matched control group. *J Intern Med* 1995;237:499–506.
75. Farmer A, Jones I, Hillier J, et al. Neurasthenia revisited: ICD-10 and DSM-III-R psychiatric syndromes in chronic fatigue patients and comparison subjects. *Br J Psychiatry* 1995;167:503–506.
76. Buchwald D, Pearlman T, Kith P, et al. Screening for psychiatric disorders in chronic fatigue and chronic fatigue syndrome. *J Psychosom Res* 1997;42:87–94.
77. Morriss RK, Wearden AJ. Screening instruments for psychiatric morbidity in chronic fatigue syndrome. *J R Soc Med* 1998;91:365–368.
78. Johnson SK, DeLuca J, Natelson BH. Personality dimensions in the chronic fatigue syndrome: a comparison with multiple sclerosis and depression. *J Psychiatr Res* 1996;30:9–20.
79. Komaroff AL, Fagioli LR, Doolittle TH, et al. Health status in patients with chronic fatigue syndrome and in general population and disease comparison groups. *Am J Med* 1996;101:281–290.
80. Morriss RK, Ahmed M, Wearden AJ, et al. The role of depression in pain, psycho-physiological syndromes and medically unexplained symptoms associated with chronic fatigue syndrome. *J Affect Disord* 1999;55:143–148.
81. Schmaling KB, DiClementi JD, Cullum CM, et al. Cognitive functioning in chronic fatigue syndrome and depression: a preliminary comparison. *Psychosom Med* 1994;56:383–388.
82. Terman M, Levine SM, Terman JS, et al. Chronic fatigue syndrome and seasonal affective disorder: comorbidity, diagnostic overlap, and implications for treatment. *Am J Med* 1998;105(3A):115S–124S.
83. Garcia-Borreguero D, Dale JK, Rosenthal NE, et al. Lack of seasonal variation of symptoms in patients with chronic fatigue syndrome. *Psychiatry Res* 1998;77:71–77.
84. Magnusson AE, Nias DK, White PD. Is perfectionism associated with fatigue? *J Psychosom Res* 1996;41:377–383.
85. Krupp LB, Sliwinski M, Masur DM, et al. Cognitive functioning and depression in patients with chronic fatigue syndrome and multiple sclerosis. *Arch Neurol* 1994;51:705–710.
86. Joyce E, Blumenthal S, Wessely S. Memory, attention, and executive function in chronic fatigue syndrome. *J Neurol Neurosurg Psychiatry* 1996;60:495–503.
87. Johnson SK, DeLuca J, Diamond BJ, et al. Selective impairment of auditory processing in chronic fatigue syndrome: a comparison with multiple sclerosis and healthy controls. *Percept Mot Skills* 1996;83:51–62.
88. Marcel B, Komaroff AL, Fagioli LR, et al. Cognitive deficits in patients with chronic fatigue syndrome. *Biol Psychiatry* 1996;40:535–541.
89. Michiels V, Cluydts R, Fischler B, et al. Cognitive functioning in patients with chronic fatigue syndrome. *J Clin Exp Neuropsychol* 1996;18:666–677.
90. Marshall PS, Forstot M, Callies A, et al. Cognitive slowing and working memory difficulties in chronic fatigue syndrome. *Psychosom Med* 1997;59:58–66.
91. DeLuca J, Johnson SK, Ellis SP, et al. Sudden vs. gradual onset of chronic fatigue syndrome differentiates individuals on cognitive and psychiatric measures. *J Psychiatr Res* 1997;31:83–90.
92. Deluca J, Johnson SK, Ellis SP, et al. Cognitive functioning is impaired in patients with chronic fatigue syndrome devoid of psychiatric disease. *J Neurol Neurosurg Psychiatry* 1997;62:151–155.
93. Michiels V, deGucht V, Cluydts R, Fischler B. Attention and information processing efficiency in patients with chronic fatigue syndrome. *J Clin Exp Neuropsychol* 1999;21:709–729.
94. Wearden A, Appleby L. Cognitive performance and complaints of cognitive impairment in chronic fatigue syndrome (CFS). *Psychol Med* 1997;27:81–90.
95. Boda WL, Natelson BH, Sisto SA, et al. Gait abnormalities in chronic fatigue syndrome. *J Neurol Sci* 1995;131:156–161.
96. Saggini R, Pizzigallo E, Vecchiet J, et al. Alteration of spatial-temporal parameters of gait in chronic fatigue syndrome patients. *J Neurol Sci* 1998;154:18–25.
97. Servatius RJ, Tapp WN, Bergen MT, et al. Impaired associative learning in chronic fatigue syndrome. *Neuroreport* 1998;9:1153–1157.
98. Ash-Bernal R, Wall C III, Komaroff AL, et al. Vestibular function test anomalies in patients with chronic fatigue syndrome. *Acta Otolaryngol (Stockh)* 1995;115:9–17.
99. Gordon R, Michalewski HJ, Nguyen T, et al. Cortical motor potential alterations in chronic fatigue syndrome. *Int J Mol Med* 1999;4:493–499.
100. Polich J, Moore AP, Wiederhold MD. P300 assessment of chronic fatigue syndrome. *J Clin Neurophysiol* 1995;12:186–189.
101. Schafer KM. Sleep disturbances and fatigue in women with fibromyalgia and chronic fatigue syndrome. *J Obstet Gynecol Neonatal Nurs* 1995;24:229–233.
102. Fischler B, LeBon O, Hoffmann G, et al. Sleep anomalies in the chronic fatigue syndrome: a comorbidity study. *Neuropsychobiology* 1997;35:115–122.
103. Morriss RK, Wearden AJ, Battersby L. The relation of sleep difficulties to fatigue, mood, and disability in chronic fatigue syndrome. *J Psychosom Res* 1997;42:597–605.
104. Sharpley A, Clements A, Hawton K, et al. Do patients with "pure" chronic fatigue syndrome (neurasthenia) have abnormal sleep? *Psychosom Med* 1997;59:592–596.
105. Manu P, Lane TJ, Matthews DA, et al. Alpha-delta sleep in patients with a chief complaint of chronic fatigue. *South Med J* 1994;87:465–470.
106. MacFarlane JG, Shahal B, Mously C, et al. Periodic K-alpha sleep EEG activity and periodic limb movements during sleep:

comparisons of clinical features and sleep parameters. *Sleep* 1996;19:200–204.

107. Flanigan MJ, Morehouse RL, Shapiro CM. Determination of observer-rated alpha activity during sleep. *Sleep* 1995;18:702–706.

108. Pollmacher T, Mullington J, Korth C, et al. Influence of host defense activation on sleep in humans. *Adv Neuroimmunol* 1995;5:155–169.

109. Ambrogetti A, Olson LG. Consideration of narcolepsy in the differential diagnosis of chronic fatigue syndrome. *Med J Aust* 1994;160:426–429.

110. Bell DS. Chronic fatigue syndrome update: findings now point to CNS involvement. *Postgrad Med* 1994;96(6):73–81.

111. Schwartz RB, Komaroff AL, Garada BM, et al. SPECT imaging of the brain: comparison of findings in patients with chronic fatigue syndrome, AIDS dementia complex, and major unipolar depression. *AJR Am J Roentgenol* 1994;162:943–951.

112. Costa DC, Tannock C, Brostoff J. Brainstem perfusion is impaired in chronic fatigue. *QJM* 1995;88:767–773.

113. Fischler B, D'Haenen H, Cluydts R, et al. Comparison of 99m Tc HMPAO SPECT scan between chronic fatigue syndrome, major depression and healthy controls: an exploratory study of clinical correlates of regional blood flow. *Neuropsychobiology* 1996;34:175–183.

114. Schwartz RB, Garada BM, Komaroff AL, et al. Detection of intracranial abnormalities in patients with chronic fatigue syndrome: comparison of MR imaging and SPECT. *AJR Am J Roentgenol* 1994;162:935–941.

115. Lange G, DeLuca J, Maldjian JA, et al. Brain MRI abnormalities exist in a subset of patients with chronic fatigue syndrome. *J Neurol Sci* 1999;171:3–7.

116. Cope H, Pernet A, Kendall B, et al. Cognitive functioning and magnetic resonance imaging in chronic fatigue. *Br J Psychiatry* 1995;167:86–94.

117. Greco A, Tannock C, Brostoff J, et al. Brain MR in chronic fatigue syndrome. *AJNR Am J Neuroradiol* 1997;18:1265–1269.

118. Tirelli U, Chierichetti F, Tavio M, et al. Brain positron emission tomography (PET) in chronic fatigue syndrome: preliminary data. *Am J Med* 1998;105(3A):54S–58S.

119. Abu-Judeh HH, Levine S, Kumar M, et al. Comparison of SPET brain perfusion and 18F-FDG brain metabolism in patients with chronic fatigue syndrome. *Nucl Med Commun* 1998;19:1065–1071.

120. Demitrack M, Gold PW, Dale JK, et al. Plasma and cerebrospinal fluid monoamine metabolism in patients with chronic fatigue syndrome: preliminary findings. *Biol Psychiatry* 1992;32:1065–1077.

121. Cleare AJ, Bearn J, Allain T, et al. Contrasting neuroendocrine responses in depression and chronic fatigue syndrome. *J Affect Disord* 1995;35:283–289.

122. Sharpe M, Clements A, Hawton K, et al. Increased prolactin response to buspirone in chronic fatigue syndrome. *J Affect Disord* 1996;41:71–76.

123. Yatham LN, Morehouse RL, Chisholm BT, et al. Neuroendocrine assessment of serotonin (5-HT) function in chronic fatigue syndrome. *Can J Psychiatry* 1995;40:93–96.

124. Castell LM, Yamamoto T, Phoenix J, et al. The role of tryptophan in fatigue in different conditions of stress. *Adv Exp Med Biol* 1999;467:697–704.

125. Reid S, Wessely S. Chronic fatigue and fibromyalgia: approaches to management. *Curr Opin Psychiatry* 1999;12:727–732.

126. Vercoulen JH, Swanink CM, Zitman FG, et al. Randomized, double-blind, placebo-controlled study of fluoxetine in chronic fatigue syndrome. *Lancet* 1996;347:858–861.

127. Sharpe M, Hawton K, Simkin S, et al. Cognitive behaviour therapy for the chronic fatigue syndrome: a randomized controlled trial. *BMJ* 1996;312:22–26.

128. Deale A, Chalder T, Marks I, et al. Cognitive behavior therapy for chronic fatigue syndrome: a randomized controlled trial. *Am J Psychiatry* 1997;154:408–414.

129. Hall SR, Smith AP. Behavioral effects of infectious mononucleosis. *Neuropsychobiology* 1996;33:202–209.

130. Strauss SE, Tosato G, Armstrong G, et al. Persisting viral illness and fatigue in adults with evidence of Epstein-Barr virus infection. *Ann Intern Med* 1985;102:7–16.

131. Jones JF, Ray CG, Minnich LL, et al. Evidence for active Epstein-Barr virus infection in patients with persistent unexplained illnesses: elevated anti-early antigen antibodies. *Ann Intern Med* 1985;102:1–7.

132. Buchwald D, Ashley RL, Pearlman T, et al. Viral serologies in patients with chronic fatigue and chronic fatigue syndrome. *J Med Virol* 1996;50:25–30.

133. Westin J, Rodjer S, Turesson I, et al. Interferon alfa-2b versus no maintenance therapy during the plateau phase in multiple myeloma: a randomized study. Cooperative Study Group. *Br J Haematol* 1995;89:561–568.

134. Oberg K. Interferon-alpha versus somatostatin or the combination of both in gastro-enteropathic tumors. *Digestion* 1996;57[Suppl 1]:81–83.

135. Evengard B, Schacterle RS, Komaroff AL. Chronic fatigue syndrome: new insights and old ignorance. *J Intern Med* 1999;246:455–469.

136. DiLuca D, Zorzenon M, Mirandola P, et al. Human herpesvirus 6 and human herpesvirus 7 in chronic fatigue syndrome. *J Clin Microbiol* 1995;33:1660–1666.

137. Patnaik M, Komaroff AL, Conley E, et al. Prevalence of IgM antibodies to human herpesvirus 6 early antigen (p41/38) in patients with chronic fatigue syndrome. *J Infect Dis* 1995;172:1364–1367.

138. Abashi DV, Eastman HB, Owen CB, et al. Frequent HHV-6 reactivation in multiple sclerosis (MS) and chronic fatigue syndrome (CFS) patients. *J Clin Virol* 2000;16:179–191.

139. Wallace HL Jr, Natelson B, Gause W, et al. Human herpesvirus in chronic fatigue syndrome. *Clin Diagn Lab Immunol* 1999;6:216–223.

140. Clements GB, McGarry F, Nairn C, et al. Detection of enterovirus-specific RNA in serum: the relationship to chronic fatigue. *J Med Virol* 1995;45:156–161.

141. Galbraith DN, Nairn C, Clements GB. Phylogenetic analysis of short enteroviral sequences from patients with chronic fatigue syndrome. *J Gen Virol* 1995;76:1701–1707.

142. Galbraith DN, Nairn C, Clements GB. Evidence for enteroviral persistence in humans. *J Gen Virol* 1997;78:307–312.

143. Swanink CM, Melchers WJ, van der Meer JW, et al. Enteroviruses and the chronic fatigue syndrome. *Clin Infect Dis* 1994;19:860–864.

144. Lindh G, Samuelson A, Hedlund KO, et al. No findings of enterovirus in Swedish patients with chronic fatigue syndrome. *Scand J Infect Dis* 1996;28:305–307.

145. McArdle A, McArdle F, Jackson MJ, et al. Investigation by polymerase chain reaction of enteroviral infection in patients with chronic fatigue syndrome. *Clin Sci (Colch)* 1996;90:295–300.

146. Kitani T, Kuratsune H, Fuke I, et al. Possible correlation between Borna disease virus infection and Japanese patients with chronic fatigue syndrome. *Microbiol Immunol* 1996;40:459–462.

147. Nakaya T, Takahashi H, Nakamura Y, et al. Detection of Borna disease vires RNA in peripheral blood mononuclear cells derived

from Japanese patients with chronic fatigue syndrome. *FEBS Lett* 1996;378:145–149.

148. Yamaguchi K, Sawada T, Nakari T, et al. Detection of Borna virus-reactive antibodies from patients with psychiatric disorders and from horses by electrochemiluminescence immunoassay. *Clin Diagn Lab Immunol* 1999;6:696–700.

149. Jacobson SK, Daly JS, Thorne GM, et al. Chronic parvovirus B19 infection resulting in chronic fatigue syndrome: case history and review. *Clin Infect Dis* 1997;24:1048–1051.

150. Ilaria RL, Komaroff AL, Fagioli LR, et al. Absence of parvovirus B19 infection in chronic fatigue syndrome. *Arthritis Rheum* 1995;38:638–641.

151. Miller NA, Carmichael HA, Calder BD, et al. Antibody to coxsackie B virus in diagnosing postviral fatigue syndrome. *BMJ* 1991;302:140–143.

152. Nairn C, Galbraith DN, Clements GB. Comparison of coxsackie B neutralisation and enteroviral PCR in chronic fatigue patients. *J Med Virol* 1995;46:310–313.

153. Bruno RL, Creange SJ, Frick NM. Parallels between post-polio fatigue and chronic fatigue syndrome: a common pathophysiology? *Am J Med* 1998;105(3A):66S–73S.

154. Bujak DI, Weinstein A, Dornbush RL. Clinical and neurocognitive features of the post-Lyme syndrome. *J Rheumatol* 1996;23:1392–1397.

155. Treib J, Grauer MT, Haass A, et al. Chronic fatigue syndrome in patients with lyme borreliosis. *Eur Neurol* 2000;43:107–109.

156. Schutzer SE, Natelson BH. Absence of Borrelia burgdorferi-specific immune complexes in chronic fatigue syndrome. *Neurology* 1999;53:1340–1341.

157. Vojdani A, Choppa PC, Tagle C, et al. Detection of Mycoplasma genus and Mycoplasma fermentans by PCR in patients with chronic fatigue syndrome. *FEMS Immunol Med Microbiol* 1998;22:355–365.

158. Nasralla M, Haier J, Nicolson GL. Multiple mycoplasmal infections detected in blood of patients with chronic fatigue syndrome and/or fibromyalgia syndrome. *Eur J Clin Microbiol Infect Dis* 1999;18:859–865.

159. Ayres JG, Flint N, Smith EG, et al. Post-infection fatigue syndrome following Q fever. *QJM* 1998;91:105–123.

160. Swanink CM, Stolk-Engelaar VM, van der Meer JW, et al. *Yersinia enterocolitica* and the chronic fatigue syndrome. *J Infect* 1998;36:269–272.

161. DeFreitas E, Hilliard B, Cheney PR, et al. Retroviral sequences related to human T-lymphotropic virus type II in patients with chronic fatigue immune dysfunction syndrome. *Proc Natl Acad Sci USA* 1991;88:2922–2926.

162. Khan AS, Heneine WM, Chapman LE, et al. Assessment of a retrovirus sequence and other possible risk factors for the chronic fatigue syndrome. *Ann Intern Med* 1993;118:241–245.

163. Martin WJ, Zeng LC, Ahmed K, et al. Cytomegalovirus-related sequence in an atypical cytopathic virus repeatedly isolated from a patient with chronic fatigue syndrome. *Am J Pathol* 1994;145:440–451.

164. Martin WJ, Glass RT. Acute encephalopathy induced in cats with a stealth virus isolated from a patient with chronic fatigue syndrome. *Pathobiology* 1995;63:115–118.

165. Martin WJ. Simian cytomegalovirus-related stealth virus isolated from the cerebrospinal fluid of a patient with a bipolar psychosis and acute encephalopathy. *Pathobiology* 1996;64:64–66.

166. Martin WJ. Genetic instability and fragmentation of a stealth viral genome. *Pathobiology* 1996;64:9–17.

167. Martin WJ. Severe stealth virus encephalopathy following chronic fatigue syndrome–like illness: clinical and histopathological features. *Pathobiology* 1996;64:1–8.

168. Holmes MJ, Diack DS, Easingwood RA, et al. Electron microscopic immunocytological profiles in chronic fatigue syndrome. *J Psychiatr Res* 1997;31:115–122.

169. Buchwald D, Umali J, Pearlman T, et al. Postinfectious chronic fatigue: a distinct syndrome? *Clin Infect Dis* 1996;23:385–387.

170. White PD, Grover SA, Kangro HO, et al. The validity and reliability of the fatigue syndrome that follows glandular fever. *Psychol Med* 1995;25:917–924.

171. Hotopf M, Noah N, Wessely S. Chronic fatigue and minor psychiatric morbidity after viral meningitis: a controlled study. *J Neurol Neurosurg Psychiatry* 1996;60:504–509.

172. Cope H, David A, Pelosi A, et al. Predictors of chronic "postviral" fatigue. *Lancet* 1994;344:864–868.

173. Cope H, Mann A, Pelosi A, et al. Psychosocial risk factors for chronic fatigue and chronic fatigue syndrome following presumed viral illness: a case-controlled study. *Psychol Med* 1996;26:1197–1209.

174. Wessely S, Chalder T, Hirsch S, et al. Postinfectious fatigue: prospective cohort study in primary care. *Lancet* 1995;345:1333–1338.

175. See DM, Tilles JG. Alpha-Interferon treatment of patients with chronic fatigue syndrome. *Immunol Invest* 1996;25:153–164.

176. Drago F, Ranieri E, Pastorino A, et al. Epstein-Barr virus-related primary cutaneous amyloidosis: successful treatment with acyclovir and interferon-alpha. *Br J Dermatol* 1996;134:170–174.

177. Strayer DR, Carter WA, Brodsky I, et al. A controlled clinical trial with a specifically configured RNA drug, poly(I)-poly(C12U), in chronic fatigue syndrome. *Clin Infect Dis* 1994;18[Suppl 1]:S88–S95.

178. Suhadolnik RJ, Reichenbach NL, Hitzges P, et al. Changes in the 2-5A synthetase/RNase L antiviral pathway in a controlled clinical trial with poly(I)-poly(C12U) in chronic fatigue syndrome. *In Vivo* 1994;8:599–604.

179. Suhadolnik RJ, Peterson DL, O'Brien K, et al. Biochemical evidence for a novel low molecular weight 2-5A-dependent RNase L in chronic fatigue syndrome. *J Interferon Cytokine Res* 1997;17:377–385.

180. Bowman MA, Kirk JK, Michielutte R, et al. Use of amantadine for chronic fatigue syndrome (letter). *Arch Intern Med* 1997;157:1264–1265.

181. Plioplys AV, Plioplys S. Amantadine and L-carnitine treatment of chronic fatigue syndrome. *Neuropsychobiology* 1997;35:16–23.

182. Bennett AL, Fagioli LR, Schur PH, et al. Immunoglobulin subclass levels in chronic fatigue syndrome. *J Clin Immunol* 1996;16:315–320.

183. Chao CC, Gallagher M, Phair J, et al. Serum neopterin and interleukin-6 levels in chronic fatigue syndrome. *J Infect Dis* 1990;162:1412–1413.

184. Chao CC, Janoff EN, Hu SX, et al. Altered cytokine release in peripheral blood mononuclear cell cultures from patients with the chronic fatigue syndrome. *Cytokine* 1991;3:292–298.

185. Linde A, Andersson B, Svenson SB, et al. Serum levels of lymphokines and soluble cellular receptors in primary Epstein-Barr virus infection and in patients with chronic fatigue syndrome. *J Infect Dis* 1992;165:994–1000.

186. Patarca R, Fletcher MA, Klimas NG. Immunological correlates of chronic fatigue syndrome. In: Goodnick PJ, Klimas NG, eds. *Chronic fatigue and related immune deficiency syndromes.* Washington, DC: American Psychiatric Press, 1993:14–22.

187. Lutgendorf SK, Brickman A, Antoni MG, et al. Immune functioning predicts cognitive difficulties in chronic fatigue syndrome. *Psychosom Med* 1993;55:100(abstr).

188. Rasmussen AK, Nielsen H, Andersen V, et al. Chronic fatigue syndrome: a controlled cross-sectional study. *J Rheumatol* 1994;21:1527–1531.

189. Natelson BH, Ellis SP, Braonain PJ, et al. Frequency of deviant

immunological test values in chronic fatigue syndrome patients. *Clin Diagn Lab Immunol* 1995;2:238–240.

190. MacDonald KL, Osterholm MT, DeDell KH, et al. A case-controlled study to assess possible triggers and cofactors in chronic fatigue syndrome. *Am J Med* 1996;100:548–554.

191. Swanink CM, Vercoulen JH, Galama JM, et al. Lymphocyte subsets, apoptosis, and cytokines in patients with chronic fatigue syndrome. *J Infect Dis* 1996;173:460–463.

192. Bennett AL, Chao CC, Hu S, et al. Elevation of bioactive transforming growth factor-beta in serum from patients with chronic fatigue syndrome. *J Clin Immunol* 1997;17:160–166.

193. Buchwald D, Wener MH, Pearlman T, et al. Markers of inflammation and immune activation in chronic fatigue and chronic fatigue syndrome. *J Rheumatol* 1997;24:372–376.

194. Cannon JG, Angel JB, Abad LW, et al. Interleukin-1 beta, interleukin-1 receptor antagonist, and soluble interleukin-1 receptor type II secretion in chronic fatigue syndrome. *J Clin Immunol* 1997;17:253–261.

195. Gupta S, Aggarwal S, See D, et al. Cytokine production by adherent and non-adherent mononuclear cells in chronic fatigue syndrome. *J Psychiatr Res* 1997;31:149–156.

196. Cannon JG, Angel JB, Ball RW, et al. Acute phase responses and cytokine secretion in chronic fatigue syndrome. *J Clin Immunol* 1999;19:414–421.

197. Gupta S, Aggarwal S, Starr A. Increased production of interleukin-6 by adherent and non-adherent mononuclear cells during natural fatigue but not following experimental fatigue in patients with chronic fatigue syndrome. *Int J Mol Med* 1999;3:209–213.

198. Moss RB, Mercandetti A, Vojdani A. TNF-a and chronic fatigue syndrome. *J Clin Immunol* 1999;19:314–316.

199. Sheng WS, Hu S, Lamkin A, et al. Susceptibility to immunologically mediated fatigue in C57BL/6 versus Balb/c mice. *Clin Immunol Immunopathol* 1996;81:161–167.

200. Gordon BR. Chronic fatigue syndrome: an allergic entity? *Curr Opin Otolaryngol Head Neck Surg* 2000;8:253–259.

201. Straus SE, Dale JK, Wright R, et al. Allergy and the chronic fatigue syndrome. *J Allergy Clin Immunol* 1988;81:791–795.

202. Lloyd A, Wakefield D, Boughton CR, et al. Immunological abnormalities in chronic fatigue syndrome. *Med J Aust* 1989;151:122–124.

203. Klimas NG, Salvato FR, Morgan R, et al. Immunologic abnormalities in chronic fatigue syndrome. *J Clin Microbiol* 1990;28:1403–1410.

204. van Greune CHJ, Bouic PJD. Aberrant in-vitro HLA-DR expression in patients with chronic fatigue. *S Afr Med J* 1990;78:219–220.

205. Landay AL, Jessop C, Lennette ET, et al. Chronic fatigue syndrome: clinical condition associated with immune activation. *Lancet* 1991;338:707–712.

206. Straus SE, Fritz S, Dale JK, et al. Lymphocyte phenotype and function in the chronic fatigue syndrome. *J Clin Immunol* 1993;13:30–40.

207. Masuda A, Nozoe SI, Matsuyama T, et al. Psychobehavioral and immunological characteristics of adult people with chronic fatigue and patients with chronic fatigue syndrome. *Psychosom Med* 1994;56:512–518.

208. Tirelli U, Marotta G, Improta S, et al. Immunological abnormalities in patients with chronic fatigue syndrome. *Scand J Immunol* 1994;40:601–608.

209. Bates DW, Buchwald D, Lee J, et al. Clinical laboratory test findings in patients with chronic fatigue syndrome. *Arch Intern Med* 1995;155:97–103.

210. Bennett AL, Fagioli LR, Schur PH, et al. Immunoglobulin subclass levels in chronic fatigue syndrome. *J Clin Immunol* 1996;16:315–320.

211. Swanink CM, Vercoulen JH, Galama JM, et al. Lymphocyte subsets, apoptosis, and cytokines in patients with chronic fatigue syndrome. *J Infect Dis* 1996;173:460–463.

212. Mawle AC, Nisenbaum R, Dobbins JG, et al. Immune responses associated with chronic fatigue syndrome: a case-controlled study. *J Infect Dis* 1997;175:136–141.

213. Peakman M, Deale A, Field R, et al. Clinical improvement in chronic fatigue syndrome is not associated with lymphocyte subsets of function or activation. *Clin Immunol Immunopathol* 1997;82:83–91.

214. Hassan IS, Bannister BA, Akbar A, et al. A study of the immunology of the chronic fatigue syndrome: correlation of immunologic parameters to health dysfunction. *Clin Immunol Immunopathol* 1998;87:60–67.

215. Natelson BH, LaManca JJ, Denny TN, et al. Immunologic parameters in chronic fatigue syndrome, major depression, and multiple sclerosis. *Am J Med* 1998;105(3A):43S–49S.

216. Ogawa M, Nishiura T, Yoshimura M, et al. Decreased nitric oxide-mediated natural killer cell activation in chronic fatigue syndrome. *Eur J Clin Invest* 1998;28:937–943.

217. Whiteside TL, Friberg D. Natural killer cells and natural killer cell activity in chronic fatigue syndrome. *Am J Med* 1998;105(3A):27S–34S.

218. Natelson BH, Denny TN, Zhou XD, et al. Is depression associated with immune activation? *J Affect Disord* 1999;53:179–184.

219. Vedhara K, Llewelyn MB, Fox JD, et al. Consequences of live poliovirus vaccine administration in chronic fatigue syndrome. *J Neuroimmunol* 1997;75(1–2):183–195.

220. Steinberg P, Pheley A, Petersen PK. Influence of immediate hypersensitivity skin reactions on delayed reactions in patients with chronic fatigue syndrome. *J Allergy Clin Immunol* 1996;98:1126–1128.

221. Wilson A, Hickie I, Lloyd A, et al. Cell-mediated immune function and the outcome of chronic fatigue syndrome. *Int J Immunopharmacol* 1995;17:691–694.

222. von Mikecz A, Konstantinov K, Buchwald DS, et al. High frequency of autoantibodies to insoluble cellular antigens in patients with chronic fatigue syndrome. *Arthritis Rheum* 1997;40:295–305.

223. Plioplys AV. Antimuscle and anti-CNS circulating antibodies in chronic fatigue syndrome. *Neurology* 1997;48:1717–1719.

224. Berg D, Berg LH, Couvaras J, et al. Chronic fatigue syndrome and/or fibromyalgia as a variation of antiphospholipid antibody syndrome: an explanatory model and approach to laboratory diagnosis. *Blood Coagul Fibrinolysis* 1999;10:435–438.

225. Vincent A, Lily O, Palace J. Pathogenic autoantibodies to neuronal proteins in neurological disorders. *J Neuroimmunol* 1999;100:169–180.

226. O'Suilleabhain P, Low PA, Lennon VA. Autonomic dysfunction in the Lambert-Eaton myasthenic syndrome. *Neurology* 1998;50:88–93.

227. Maddison P, Pinto A, Newsom-Davis J. Endocrine function in Lambert-Eaton myasthenic syndrome. *Ann Neurol* 1999;45:414–415.

228. Suhadolnik RJ, Peterson DL, O'Brien K, et al. Biochemical evidence for a novel low molecular weight 2-5A-dependent RNase L in chronic fatigue syndrome. *J Interferon Cytokine Res* 1997;17:377–385.

229. Vojdani A, Ghoneum M, Choppa PC, et al. Elevated apoptotic cell population in patients with chronic fatigue syndrome: the pivotal role of protein kinase RNA. *J Intern Med* 1997;242:465–478.

230. Vojdani A, Choppa PC, Lapp CW. Downregulation of RNase L inhibitor correlates with upregulation of interferon-induced proteins (2-5A synthetase and RNase L) in patients with chronic

fatigue immune dysfunction syndrome. *J Clin Lab Immunol* 1998;50:1–16.

231. Conti F, Magrini L, Priori R, et al. Eosinophil cationic protein serum levels and allergy in chronic fatigue patients. *Allergy* 1996; 51:124–127.

232. Borish L, Schmaling K. DiClementi JD, et al. Chronic fatigue syndrome: identification of distinct subgroups on the basis of allergy and psychologic variables. *J Allergy Clin Immunol* 1998; 102:222–230.

233. Marcusson JA, Lindh G, Evengard B. Chronic fatigue syndrome and nickel allergy. *Contact Dermatitis* 1999;40:269–272.

234. Rowe AH. Allergic toxemia and migraine due to food allergy: report of cases. *Calif West Med* 1928;33:785–793.

235. Randolph TG. Allergy as a causative factor of fatigue, irritability and behavior problems of children. *J Pediatr* 1947;31:560–572.

236. Rowe A. Allergy toxemia and fatigue. *Ann Allergy* 1950;8: 72–79.

237. Randolph TG. *Environmental medicine: beginnings and bibliographies of clinical ecology.* Ft. Collins, CO: Clinical Ecology Publications, 1987.

238. Steinberg P, McNutt BE, Marshall P, et al. Double-blind placebo-controlled study of the efficacy of oral terfenadine in the treatment of chronic fatigue syndrome. *J Allergy Clin Immunol* 1996;97:119–126.

239. Vollmer-Conna U, Hickie I, Hadzi-Pavlovic D, et al. Intravenous immunoglobulin is ineffective in the treatment of patients with chronic fatigue syndrome. *Am J Med* 1997;103:38–43.

240. Rea WJ. Tolerance moderators. In: *Chemical sensitivity: tools of diagnosis and methods of treatment,* vol 4. Boca Raton, FL: CRC Lewis, 1997.

241. Ablashi DV, Levine PH, DeVinci C, et al. Use of anti-HHV-6 transfer factor for the treatment of two patients with chronic fatigue syndrome (CFS): two case reports. *Biotherapy* 1996;9: 81–86.

242. DeVinci C, Levine PH, Pizza G, et al. Lessons from a pilot study of transfer factor in chronic fatigue syndrome. *Biotherapy* 1996;9:87–90.

243. Hana I, Vrubel J, Pekarek J, et al. The influence of age on transfer factor treatment of cellular immunodeficiency, chronic fatigue syndrome and/or chronic viral infections. *Biotherapy* 1996;9:91–95.

244. Levine PH. The use of transfer factor in chronic fatigue syndrome: prospects and problems. *Biotherapy* 1996;9:77–79.

245. Kroker GF. Chronic candidiasis and allergy. In: Brostoff J, Challacombe SJ, eds. *Food allergy and intolerance.* London: Bailliere Tindall, 1987:850–872.

246. Crook WG. *The yeast connection,* 2nd ed. Jackson, TN: Professional Books, 1984.

247. Pauling L. *Eat right and live longer.* New York: Hurst Books, HarperCollins, 1986.

248. Mallinson CN. Basic functions of the gut. In: Brostoff J, Challacombe SJ, eds. *Food allergy and intolerance.* London: Bailliere Tindall, 1987:51.

249. Toskes PP, Donaldson RM Jr. Enteric bacterial flora and bacterial overgrowth syndrome. In: Sleisinger MH, Fordtran JS, eds. *Gastrointestinal disease,* 5th ed. Philadelphia: WB Saunders, 1993:1106–1118.

250. Gorbach SL. Function of the normal human microflora. *Scand J Infect Dis Suppl* 1986;49:17.

251. Great Smokies Diagnostic Laboratory. 63 Zillicoa Street, Asheville, NC 28801-1074.

252. Dismukes W, Wade S, Lee J, et al. A randomized, double-blinded trial of nystatin therapy for the candidiasis hypersensitivity syndrome. *N Engl J Med* 1990;323:1717–1723.

253. Carter RE II. Chronic intestinal candidiasis as a possible etio-

logic factor in the chronic fatigue syndrome. *Med Hypotheses* 1995;44:507–515.

254. Owens PR, O'Brien ET. Hypotension: a forgotten illness? *Blood Press Monit* 1997;2:3–14.

255. Bou-Holaigah I, Rowe PC, Kan JS, et al. The relationship between neurally mediated hypotension and the chronic fatigue syndrome. *JAMA* 1995;274:961–967.

256. Wilke WS, Fouad-Taraze FM, Cash JM, et al. The connection between chronic fatigue syndrome and neurally mediated hypotension. *Cleve Clin J Med* 1998;65:261–266.

257. Rowe PC, Bou-Holaigah I, Kan JS, et al. Is neurally mediated hypotension an unrecognized cause of chronic fatigue? *Lancet* 1995;345:623–624.

258. DeLorenzo F, Hargreaves J, Kakkar VV. Possible relationship between chronic fatigue and postural tachycardia syndromes. *Clin Auton Res* 1996;6:263–264.

259. Streeten DH, Thomas D, Bell DS. The roles of orthostatic hypotension, orthostatic tachycardia, and subnormal erythrocyte volume in the pathogenesis of the chronic fatigue syndrome. *Am J Med Sci* 2000;320:1–8.

260. Lapp CW, Glenn F, Davis P. Neurally mediated hypotension and systemic orthostatic tachycardia in chronic fatigue syndrome. In: *Proceedings of the American Association for Chronic Fatigue Syndrome Research Conference.* 1996;23(abstr).

261. Schondorf R, Benoit J, Wein T, et al. Orthostatic intolerance in the chronic fatigue syndrome. *J Auton Nerv Syst* 1999;75: 192–201.

262. DeLorenzo F, Hargreaves J, Kakkar VV. Pathogenesis and management of delayed orthostatic hypotension n patients with chronic fatigue syndrome. *Clin Auton Res* 1997;7:185–190.

263. Freeman R, Komaroff AL. Does the chronic fatigue syndrome involve the autonomic nervous system? *Am J Med* 1997;102: 357–364.

264. LaManca JJ, Peckerman A, Walker J, et al. Cardiovascular response during head-up tilt in chronic fatigue syndrome. *Clin Physiol* 1999;19:111–120.

265. Yataco A, Talo H, Rowe P, et al. Comparison of heart-rate variability in patients with chronic fatigue syndrome and controls. *Clin Auton Res* 1997;7:293–297.

266. DeBecker P, Dendale P, DeMeirleir K, et al. Autonomic testing in patients with chronic fatigue syndrome. *Am J Med* 1998; 105(3A):22S–26S.

267. Soetekouw PM, Lenders JW, Bleijenberg G, et al. Autonomic function in patients with chronic fatigue syndrome. *Clin Auton Res* 1999;9:334–340.

268. Duprez DA, Buyzere ML, Drieghe B, et al. Long- and short-term blood pressure and RR-interval variability and psychosomatic distress in chronic fatigue syndrome. *Clin Sci (Colch)* 1998;94:57–63.

269. Pagani M, Lucini D, Mela GS, et al. Sympathetic overactivity in subjects complaining of unexplained fatigue. *Clin Sci (Colch)* 1994;87:655–661.

270. Sisto SA, Tapp W, Drastal S, et al. Vagal tone is reduced during paced breathing in patients with the chronic fatigue syndrome. *Clin Auton Res* 1995;5:139–143.

271. Cordero DL, Sisto SA, Tapp WN, et al. Decreased vagal power during treadmill walking in patients with chronic fatigue syndrome. *Clin Auton Res* 1996;6:329–333.

272. Rowe PC, Barron DF, Calkins H, et al. Orthostatic intolerance and chronic fatigue syndrome associated with Ehlers-Danlos syndrome. *J Pediatr* 1999;135:494–499.

273. Streeten DH, Anderson GH Jr. The role of delayed orthostatic hypotension in the pathogenesis of chronic fatigue. *Clin Auton Res* 1998;8:119–124.

274. Baschetti R. Investigations of hydrocortisone and fludrocorti-

sone in the treatment of chronic fatigue syndrome. *J Clin Endocrinol Metab* 1999;84:2263–2264.

275. Williams GH, Dluhy RG. Diseases of the adrenal cortex. In: Fauci AS, Braunwald E, Isselbacher KJ, et al., eds. *Harrison's principles of internal medicine,* 14th ed. New York: McGraw-Hill, 1998:2040–2054.

276. Petzke F, Clauw DJ. Sympathetic nervous system function in fibromyalgia. *Curr Rheumatol Rep* 2000;2:116–123.

277. Heim C, Ehlert U, Hellhammer DH. The potential role of hypocortisolism in the pathophysiology of stress-related bodily disorders. *Psychoneuroendocrinology* 2000;25:1–35.

278. Rabin BS. *Stress, immune function, and health: the connection.* New York: Wiley-Liss, 1999.

279. Jefferies WM. Mild adrenocortical deficiency, chronic allergies, autoimmune disorders and the chronic fatigue syndrome: a continuation of the cortisone story. *Med Hypotheses* 1994;42:183–189.

280. Demitrack MA, Dale JK, Straus SE, et al. Evidence for impaired activation of the hypothalamic-pituitary-adrenal axis in patients with chronic fatigue syndrome. *J Clin Endocrinol Metab* 1991;73:1224–1234.

281. Scott LV, Dinan TG. Urinary free cortisol excretion in chronic fatigue syndrome, major depression and in healthy volunteers. *J Affect Disord* 1998;47:49–54.

282. Scott LV, Medbak S, Dinan TG. Blunted adrenocorticotropin and cortisol responses to corticotropin-releasing hormone stimulation in chronic fatigue syndrome. *Acta Psychiatr Scand* 1998;97:450–457.

283. Loriaux DL. Adrenal cortex. In: Bennett JC, Plum F, eds. *Cecil textbook of medicine,* 20th ed. Philadelphia: WB Saunders, 1996:1245–1257.

284. Nelson DH. Adrenal insufficiency. In: DeGroot LJ, ed. *Endocrinology,* 2nd ed. Philadelphia: WB Saunders, 1989:1731.

285. Williams GH, Dluhy RG, Thorn GW. Diseases of the adrenal cortex. In: Wintrobe MM, Thorn GW, et al., eds. *Harrison's principles of internal medicine,* 7th ed. New York: McGraw-Hill, 1974:514–521.

286. Sonka J, Sucharda P, Limanova Z, et al. Factors affecting normal levels of insulin, cortisol, STH, thyroxine and triiodothyronine [in Czech]. *Sb Lek* 1990;92(10):289–394(abstr).

287. Strickland P, Morriss R, Wearden A, et al. A comparison of salivary cortisol in chronic fatigue syndrome, community depression, and healthy controls. *J Affect Disord* 1998;47:191–194.

288. Wood B, Wessely S, Papadopoulos A, et al. Salivary cortisol profiles in chronic fatigue syndrome. *Neuropsychobiology* 1998;37:1–4.

289. Young AH, Sharpe M, Clements A, et al. Basal activity of the hypothalamic-pituitary-adrenal axis in patients with the chronic fatigue syndrome (neurasthenia). *Biol Psychiatry* 1998;43:236–237.

290. Scott LV, Medbak S, Dinan TG. The low dose ACTH test in chronic fatigue syndrome and in health. *Clin Endocrinol (Oxf)* 1998;48:733–737.

291. Hudson M, Cleare AJ. The 1 μg short Synacthen test in chronic fatigue syndrome. *Clin Endocrinol (Oxf)* 1999;51:625–630.

292. Peterson PK, Pheley A, Schroeppel J, et al. A preliminary placebo-controlled crossover trial of fludrocortisone for chronic fatigue syndrome. *Arch Intern Med* 1998;158:908–914.

293. McKenzie R, O'Fallon A, Dale J, et al. Low-dose hydrocortisone for treatment of chronic fatigue syndrome: a randomized controlled trial. *JAMA* 1998;280:1061–1066.

294. Cleare AJ, Heap E, Malhi GS, et al. Low-dose hydrocortisone in chronic fatigue syndrome: a randomised crossover trial. *Lancet* 1999;353:455–458.

295. Tagawa N, Tamanaka J, Fujinami A, et al. Serum dehydroepiandrosterone, dehydroepiandrosterone sulfate, and pregnenolone sulfate concentrations in patients with hyperthyroidism and hypothyroidism. *Clin Chem* 2000;46:523–528.

296. DeBecker P, DeMeirleir K, Joos E, et al. Dehydroepiandrosterone (DHEA) response to i.v. ACTH in patients with chronic fatigue syndrome. *Horm Metab Res* 1999;31:18–21.

297. Scott LV, Salahuddin F, Cooney J, et al. Differences in adrenal steroid profile in chronic fatigue syndrome, in depression and in health. *J Affect Disord* 1999;54:129–37.

298. Kuratsune H, Yamaguti K, Sawada M, et al. Dehydroepiandrosterone sulfate deficiency in chronic fatigue syndrome. *Int J Mol Med* 1998;1:143–146.

299. Kodama M, Kodama T, Murakami M. The value of the dehydroepiandrosterone-annexed vitamin C infusion treatment in the clinical control of chronic fatigue syndrome (CFS): I. A pilot study of the new vitamin C infusion treatment with a volunteer CFS patient. *In Vivo* 1996;10:575–584.

300. Chrousos GP. Seminars in medicine of the Beth Israel Hospital, Boston: the hypothalamic-pituitary-adrenal axis and immune-mediated inflammation. *N Engl J Med* 1995;332:1351–1362.

301. Harlow BL, Signorello LB, Hall JE, et al. Reproductive correlates of chronic fatigue syndrome. *Am J Med* 1998;105(3A):94S–99S.

302. Saifer PL, Becker N. Allergy and autoimmune endocrinopathy: APICH syndrome. In: Brostoff J, Challacombe SJ, eds. *Food allergy and intolerance.* London: Bailliere Tindall, 1987:781–793.

303. Dalton K. *Once a month: understanding and treating PMS.* Alameda, CA: Hunter House, 1999.

304. Panay N, Studd JW. The psychotherapeutic effects of estrogens. *Gynecol Endocrinol* 1998;12:353–365.

305. Lee JR, Hanley MD, Hopkins V. *What your doctor may not tell you about premenopause.* New York: Warner Books, 1999.

306. Whitaker J. *Dr. Whitaker's guide to natural hormone replacement.* Potomac, MD: Phillips Publishing, 1996.

307. Wright JV, Morgenthaler J. *Natural hormone replacement for women over 45.* Petaluma, CA: Smart Publications, 1997.

308. Lemonick MD. Teens before their time. *Time Magazine* 2000;Oct 30:156(18):66–70, 73–74.

309. Hopkinson ZEC, Sattar N, Fleming R, et al. Polycystic ovarian syndrome: the metabolic syndrome comes to gynaecology. *BMJ* 1998;317:329–332.

310. Challem J, Berkson B, Smith MD. *Syndrome X: the complete nutritional program to prevent and reverse insulin resistance.* New York: John Wiley & Sons, 2000.

311. Dunaif A. Insulin resistance and the polycystic ovary syndrome: mechanism and implications for pathogenesis. *Endocr Rev* 1997;18:774–800.

312. Chaudhuri A, Watson WS, Pearn J, et al. The symptoms of chronic fatigue syndrome are related to abnormal ion channel function. *Med Hypotheses* 2000;54:59–63.

313. Prelevic GM, Wurzburger MI, Balint-Peric L, et al. Twenty-four-hour serum growth hormone, insulin, C-peptide and blood glucose profiles and serum insulin-like growth factor-1 concentrations in women with polycystic ovaries. *Horm Res* 1992;37(4–5):125–131.

314. Haenni A, Lind L, Reneland R, et al. Blood pressure changes in relation to sodium and calcium status in induced hyperinsulinemia. *Blood Press* 2000;9:116–120.

315. Allain TJ, Bearn JA, Coskeran P, et al. Changes in growth hormone, insulin, insulin-like growth factors (IGFs), and IGF-binding protein-1 in chronic fatigue syndrome. *Biol Psychiatry* 1997;41:567–573.

316. Hotamisligil GS. Mechanisms of TNF-alpha-induced insulin resistance. *Exp Clin Endocrinol Diabetes* 1999;107:119–125.

317. Luo S, Luo J, Cincotta AH. Chronic ventromedial hypotha-

lamic infusion of norepinephrine and serotonin promotes insulin resistance and glucose intolerance. *Neuroendocrinology* 1999; 70:460–465.

318. Demitrack MA, Crofford LJ. Evidence for and pathophysiologic implications of hypothalamic-pituitary-adrenal axis dysregulation in fibromyalgia and chronic fatigue syndrome. *Ann NY Acad Sci* 1998;840:684–697.

319. Dinan TG, Majeed T, Lavelle E, et al. Blunted serotonin-mediated activation of the hypothalamic-pituitary-adrenal axis in chronic fatigue syndrome. *Psychoneuroendocrinology* 1997;22: 261–267.

320. Cleare AJ, Bearn J, Allain T, et al. Contrasting neuroendocrine responses in depression and chronic fatigue syndrome. *J Affect Disord* 1995;34:283–289.

321. Fitzgerald PA. Diabetes mellitus. In: *Handbook of clinical endocrinology,* 2nd ed. London: Prentice Hall International, 1992: 464–473.

322. Moorkens G, Berwaerts J, Wynants H, et al. Characterization of pituitary function with emphasis on GH secretion in the chronic fatigue syndrome. *Clin Endocrinol (Oxf)* 2000;53: 99–106.

323. Cleare AJ, Sookdeo SS, Jones J, et al. Integrity of the growth hormone/insulin-like growth factor system is maintained in patients with chronic fatigue syndrome. *J Clin Endocrinol Metab* 2000;85:1433–1439.

324. Buchwald D, Umali J, Stene M. Insulin-like growth factor-1 (somatomedin C) levels in chronic fatigue syndrome and fibromyalgia. *J Rheumatol* 1996;23:739–742.

325. Gammeltoft S, Kahn CR. Hormone signaling via membrane receptors. In: DeGroot LJ, ed. *Endocrinology,* 3rd ed. Philadelphia: WB Saunders, 1995:56–58.

326. Olefsky JM. Diabetes mellitus (type II): etiology and pathogenesis. In: DeGroot LJ, ed. *Endocrinology,* 3rd ed. Philadelphia: WB Saunders, 1995:436–463.

327. Mackowiak P, Ginalska E, Nowak-Strojec E, et al. The influence of hypo- and hyperthyreosis on insulin receptors and metabolism. *Arch Physiol Biochem* 1999;107:273–279.

328. Pullen FW. Hyperinsulinism associated with migraine and Meniere's disease. In: Myers E, ed. *New dimensions in otorhinolaryngology—head and neck surgery,* vol 2. Proceedings of the XIIIth World Congress. Amsterdam: Elsevier Science Publishers BV, Excerpta Medica, 1985.

329. Hollenbeck C, Reaven GM. Variations in insulin-stimulated glucose uptake in healthy individuals with normal glucose tolerance. *J Clin Endocrinol Metab* 1987;64:1169–1173.

330. Kelly GS. Insulin resistance: lifestyle and nutritional interventions. *Altern Med Rev* 2000;5:109–132.

331. Kelly GS. Peripheral metabolism of thyroid hormones: a review. *Altern Med Rev* 2000;5:306–333.

332. Thorner MO, Vance ML, Laws ER, et al. The anterior pituitary. In: Wilson JD, Foster DW, Kronenberg HM, et al., eds. *Williams textbook of endocrinology,* 9th ed. Philadelphia: WB Saunders, 1998:264–266.

333. Lavin TN. Mechanisms of action of thyroid hormone. In: DeGroot LJ, ed. *Endocrinology,* 2nd ed. Philadelphia: WB Saunders, 1989:562–573.

334. Safrit HF. Thyroid disorders. *Handbook of clinical endocrinology,* 2nd ed. London: Prentice Hall International, 1992:156–161.

335. Berry MJ, Banu L, Larsen PR. Type I iodothyronine deiodinase is a selenocysteine-containing enzyme [Letter]. *Nature* 1991; 349:438–440.

336. Eravci M, Pinna G, Meinhold H, et al. Effects of pharmacological and nonpharmacological treatments on thyroid hormone metabolism and concentrations in rat brain. *Endocrinology* 2000; 141:1027–1040.

337. Larsen PR, Davies TF, Hay ID. Thyroid hormone deficiency. In: Wilson JD, Foster DW, Kronenberg HM, et al., eds. *Williams textbook of endocrinology,* 9th ed. Philadelphia: WB Saunders, 1998:460–467.

338. Refetoff S. Thyroid function tests and effects of drugs on thyroid function. In: DeGroot LJ, ed. *Endocrinology,* 2nd ed. Philadelphia: WB Saunders, 1989:590–639.

339. Fantz CR, Dagogo-Jack S, Ladenson JH, et al. Thyroid function during pregnancy. *Clin Chem* 1999;45:2250–2258.

340. Barnes BO, Galton L. *Hypothyroidism: the unsuspected illness.* New York: Harper & Row, 1976.

341. Nagataki S. The concept of Hashimoto disease. In: Nagataki S, Mori T, Torizuka K, eds. *80 Years of Hashimoto disease.* Amsterdam: Elsevier Science Publishers BV, 1993:539–545.

342. McDaniel AB. Fine needle aspiration for cytological diagnosis of the indurated thyroid gland. Presented at the American Academy of Otorhinolaryngic Allergy Spring Meeting. Palm Beach, FL, May, 1995.

343. Cho BY, Chung JH, Lee HK, et al. Immunogenetic heterogeneity of atrophic autoimmune thyroiditis according to thyrotropin receptor blocking antibody. In: Nagataki S, Mori T, Torizuka K, eds. *80 Years of Hashimoto disease.* Amsterdam: Elsevier Science Publishers BV, 1993:45–50.

344. Zakarija M, Egeland JA, Lacy LG, et al. Autoimmune thyroid disease in Old Order Amish. In: Nagataki S, Mori T, Torizuka K, eds. *80 Years of Hashimoto disease.* Amsterdam: Elsevier Science Publishers BV, 1993:51–57.

345. Pinchera A, Mariotti S, Chiovato L. Current concepts of Hashimoto disease. In: Nagataki S, Mori T, Torizuka K, eds. *80 Years of Hashimoto disease.* Amsterdam: Elsevier Science Publishers BV, 1993:533–538.

346. Gold MS, Pottash ALC, Extein I. Hypothyroidism and depression: evidence from complete thyroid function evaluation. *JAMA* 1981;245:1919–1922.

347. Gaby AR. Treatment with thyroid hormone [Letter]. *JAMA* 1989;262:1774.

348. Chopra IJ. Clinical review 86: euthyroid sick syndrome—is it a misnomer? *J Clin Endocrinol Metab* 1997;82:329–334.

349. McIver B, Gorman CA. Euthyroid sick syndrome: an overview. *Thyroid* 1997;7:125–132.

350. Kimura T, Kanda T, Kotajuma N, et al. Involvement of circulating interleukin-6 and its receptor in the development of euthyroid sick syndrome in patients with acute myocardial infarction. *Eur J Endocrinol* 2000;43:179–184.

351. Nagaya T, Fujieda M, Otsuka G, et al. A potential role of activated NF-kappa B in the pathogenesis of euthyroid sick syndrome. *J Clin Invest* 2000;106:393–402.

352. Girvent M, Maestro S, Hernandez R, et al. Euthyroid sick syndrome, associated endocrine abnormalities, and outcome in elderly patients undergoing emergency operation. *Surgery* 1998; 123:560–567.

353. Davies PH, Black EG, Sheppard MC, et al. Relation between serum interleukin-6 and thyroid hormone concentrations in 270 hospital in-patients with non-thyroidal illness. *Clin Endocrinol (Oxf)* 1996;44:199–205.

354. Boelen A, Maas MA, Lowik CW, et al. Induced illness in interleukin-6 (IL-6) knock-out mice: a causal role of IL-6 in the development of the low 3,5,3′-triiodothyronine syndrome. *Endocrinology* 1996;137:5250–5254.

355. Boelen A, Platvoet-Ter Schiphorst MC, Wiersinga WM. Soluble cytokine receptors and the low 3,5,3′-triiodothyronine syndrome in patients with nonthyroidal disease. *J Clin Endocrinol Metab* 1995;80:971–976.

356. Feelders RA, Swaak AJ, Romijn JA, et al. Characteristics of recovery from the euthyroid sick syndrome induced by tumor necrosis factor alpha in cancer patients. *Metabolism* 1999;48: 324–329.

357. Schilling JU, Zimmermann T, Albrecht S, et al. Low T3 syndrome in multiple trauma patients: a phenomenon or important pathogenetic factor? [in German]. *Med Klin* 1999;94[Suppl 3]: 66–69(abstr).

358. Monig H, Arnedt T, Meyer M, et al. Activation of the hypothalamo-pituitary-adrenal axis in response to septic or non-septic diseases: implications for the euthyroid sick syndrome. *Intensive Care Med* 1999;25:1402–1406.

359. Opasich C, Pacini F, Ambrosino N, et al. Sick euthyroid syndrome in patients with moderate-to-severe chronic heart failure. *Eur Heart J* 1996;17:1860–1866.

360. Duntas LH, Nguyen TT, Keck FS, et al. Changes in metabolism of TRH in euthyroid sick syndrome. *Eur J Endocrinol* 1999; 141:337–341.

361. Savastano S, Cannavale R, Valentino R, et al. Alpha-ANP, AVP, and pituitary-thyroid axis in patients with congestive heart failure and acute respiratory failure. *J Endocrinol Invest* 1999;22: 766–771.

362. Berger MM, Lemarchand-Beraud T, Cavadini C, et al. Relations between the selenium status and the low T3 syndrome after major trauma. *Intensive Care Med* 1996;22:575–581.

363. Bruckert E, Giral P, Chadarevian R, et al. Low free-thyroxine levels are a risk factor for subclinical atherosclerosis in euthyroid hyperlipidemic patients. *J Cardiovasc Risk* 1999;6:327–331.

364. Rivolta G, Cerutti R, Colombo R, et al. Prevalence of subclinical hypothyroidism in a population living in the Milan metropolitan area. *J Endocrinol Invest* 1999;22:693–697.

365. Ridgway EC, Cooper DS, Walker H, et al. Peripheral responses to thyroid hormone before and after L-thyroxine therapy in patients with subclinical hypothyroidism. *J Clin Endocrinol Metab* 1981;53:1238–1242.

366. Cooper DS, Halpern R, Wood LC, et al. L-thyroxine therapy in subclinical hypothyroidism: a double-blind, placebo-controlled trial. *Ann Intern Med* 1984;101:18–24.

367. Biondi B, Fazio S, Palmieri EA, et al. Left ventricular diastolic dysfunction in patients with subclinical hypothyroidism. *J Clin Endocrinol Metab* 1999;84:2064–2067.

368. Fruhwald FM, Ramschak-Schwarzer S, Pichler B, et al. Subclinical thyroid disorders in patients with dilated cardiomyopathy. *Cardiology* 1997;88:156–159.

369. Hak AE, Pols HA, Visser TJ, et al. Subclinical hypothyroidism is an independent risk factor for atherosclerosis and myocardial infarction in elderly women: the Rotterdam study. *Ann Intern Med* 2000;132:270–278.

370. Bindels AJ, Westendorp RG, Frolich M, et al. The prevalence of subclinical hypothyroidism at different total plasma cholesterol levels in middle aged men and women: a need for case-finding? *Clin Endocrinol (Oxf)* 1999;50:217–220.

371. Caron P, Calazel C, Parra HJ, et al. Decreased HDL cholesterol in subclinical hypothyroidism: the effect of L-thyroxine therapy. *Clin Endocrinol (Oxf)* 1990;33:519–523.

372. Bogner U, Arntz HR, Peters H, et al. Subclinical hypothyroidism and hyperlipoproteinemia: indiscriminate L-thyroxine treatment not justified. *Acta Endocrinol (Copenh)* 1993;128: 202–206.

373. Monzani F, DelGuerra P, Caraccio N, et al. Subclinical hypothyroidism: neurobehavioral features and beneficial effect of L-thyroxine treatment. *Clin Investig* 1993;71:367–371.

374. Hickie I, Bennett B, Mitchell P, et al. Clinical and subclinical hypothyroidism in patients with chronic and treatment-resistant depression. *Aust N Z J Psychiatry* 1996;30:246–252.

375. Monzani F, Caraccio N, DelGuerra P, et al. Neuromuscular symptoms and dysfunction in subclinical hypothyroid patients: beneficial effect of L-T4 replacement therapy. *Clin Endocrinol (Oxf)* 1999;51:237–242.

376. Krassas GE, Pontikides N, Kaltsas T, et al. Disturbances of menstruation in hypothyroidism. *Clin Endocrinol (Oxf)* 1999; 50:655–659.

377. Lee S, Chow CC, Wing YK, et al. Thyroid function and psychiatric morbidity in patients with manic disorder receiving lithium therapy. *J Clin Psychopharmacol* 2000;20:204–209.

378. Nardi M, DiBari M, Grasso L, et al. The "low-T3 syndrome" in unselected elderly home-dwellers: an epidemiological study in Dicomano, Italy. *J Endocrinol Invest* 1999;22[Suppl to no. 10]:40–41.

379. Lindeman RD, Schade DS, LaRue A, et al. Subclinical hypothyroidism in a biethnic, urban community. *J Am Geriatr Soc* 1999; 47:703–709.

380. Pop VJ, Kuijpens JL, van Baar AL, et al. Low maternal free thyroxine concentrations during early pregnancy are associated with impaired psychomotor development in infancy. *Clin Endocrinol (Oxf)* 1999;50:149–155.

381. Chopra IJ, Chopra U, Smith SR, et al. Reciprocal changes in serum concentrations of 3,3′,5-triiodothyronine (T3) in systemic illnesses. *J Clin Endocrinol Metab* 1975;41:1043–1049.

382. Scriba PC, Bauer M, Emmert D, et al. Effects of obesity, total fasting and re-alimentation on L-thyroxine (T4), 3,5,3′-L-triiodothyronine (T3), 3,3′,5′-L-triiodothyronine (rT3), thyroxine binding globulin (TBG), cortisol, thyrotrophin, cortisol binding globulin (CBG), transferrin, alpha 2-haptoglobin, and complement C′3 in serum. *Acta Endocrinol (Copenh)* 1979;91: 629–643.

383. Kvetny J. Thyroxine binding and cellular metabolism of thyroxine in mononuclear blood cells from patients with anorexia nervosa. *J Endocrinol* 1983;98:343–350.

384. Kunst G, Pfeilschifter J, Kummermehr G, et al. Assessment of sex hormone-binding globulin and osteocalcin in patients undergoing coronary artery bypass graft surgery. *J Cardiothorac Vasc Anesth* 2000;14:546–552.

385. van der Poll T, Endert E, Coyle SM, et al. Neutralization of TNF does not influence endotoxin-induced changes in thyroid hormone metabolism in humans. *Am J Physiol* 1999;276: R357–R362.

386. Chopra IJ, Williams DE, Orgiazzi J, et al. Opposite effects of dexamethasone on serum concentrations of 3,3′,5′-triiodothyronine (reverse T3) and 3,3′,5-triiodothyronine (T3). *J Clin Endocrinol Metab* 1975;41:911–920.

387. Arnott RD, Eastman CJ. Specific 3,3′,5′-triiodothyronine (reverse T3) binding sites on rat liver plasma membranes: comparison with thyroxine (T4) binding sites. *J Recept Res* 1983;3: 393–407.

388. Smith HC, Robinson SE, Eastman CJ. Binding of reverse T3 to hepatic nuclear protein. *Aust J Exp Biol Med Sci* 1980;58: 207–212.

389. Kobayashi A, Shimazaki M, Hamada N, et al. Reverse triiodothyronine nuclear binding in rat brain. *Osaka City Med J* 1990; 36:29–35.

390. Venkatraman JT, Lefebvre Y. Multiple thyroid hormone binding sites on male rat liver nuclear matrices. *Biochem Biophys Res Commun* 1987;148:1496–1502.

391. Wiersinga WM, Chopra IJ, Solomon DH. Specific nuclear binding sites of triiodothyronine and reverse triiodothyronine in rat and pork liver: similarities and discrepancies. *Endocrinology* 1982;110:2052–2058.

392. Kobayashi A, Shimazaki M, Kuwahara H, et al. Nuclear binding sites for reverse triiodothyronine in human placenta. *Osaka City Med J* 1989;35:137–144.

393. Gullo D, Sinha AK, Woods R, et al. Triiodothyronine binding in adult rat brain: compartmentation of receptor populations in purified neuronal and glial nuclei. *Endocrinology* 1987;120: 325–331.

394. Kirkland JL, Mukku V, Hardy M, et al. Evidence for triiodothy-

ronine receptors in human endometrium and myometrium. *Am J Obstet Gynecol* 1983;146:380–383.

395. Li DQ, Kuang AK, Ding T, et al. Nuclear 3,5,3'-triiodothyronine receptors (T3R) of circulating human lymphocytes in hyper- and hypothyroidism and nonthyroidal diseases. *Chin Med J (Engl)* 1990;103:355–358.

396. Szymanski PT, Nauman J. Effects of thyroid hormones and reverse-triiodothyronine (rT3) pretreatment on beta-adrenoreceptors in the rat heart. *Acta Physiol Pol* 1986;37:131–138.

397. du Pont JS. Is reverse triiodothyronine a physiological nonactive competitor for the action of triiodothyronine upon the electrical properties of GH3 cells? *Neuroendocrinology* 1991;54:146–150.

398. McCormack PD, Thomas J, Malik M, et al. Cold stress, reverseT3 and lymphocyte function. *Alaska Med* 1998;40(3):55–62.

399. Smith HC, Robinson SE, Eastman CJ. Binding of endogenous iodothyronines to isolated liver cell nuclei. *Endocrinology* 1980;106:1133–1136.

400. Wilson ED. *Wilson's syndrome.* Orlando, FL: Cornerstone Publishing, 1991.

401. Walker JD, Crawford FA Jr, Spindale FG. 3,5,3'-Triiodo-L-thyronine pretreatment with cardioplegic arrest and chronic left ventricular dysfunction. *Ann Thorac Surg* 1995;60:292–299.

402. Katzeff HL, Powell SR, Ojamaa K. Alterations in cardiac contractility and gene expression during low-T3 syndrome: prevention with T3. *Am J Physiol* 1997;273:E951–E956.

403. Chowdhury D, Parnell VA, Ojamaa K, et al. Usefulness of triiodothyronine (T3) treatment after surgery for complex congenital heart disease in infants and children. *Am J Cardiol* 1999;84:1107–1109.

404. Lowe JC, Honeyman-Lowe G. Fibromyalgia and thyroid disease. *Myalgias (in press).*

405. Schulte C, Reinhardt W, Beelen D, et al. Low T3-syndrome and nutritional status as prognostic factors in patients undergoing bone marrow transplantation. *Bone Marrow Transplant* 1998;22:1171–1178.

406. Burmeister LA. Reverse T3 does not reliably differentiate hypothyroid sick syndrome from euthyroid sick syndrome. *Thyroid* 1995;5:435–441.

407. Chopra IJ. Simultaneous measurement of free thyroxine and free 3,5,3'-triiodothyronine in undiluted serum by direct equilibrium dialysis/radioimmunoassay: evidence that free triiodothyronine and free thyroxine are normal in many patients with the low triiodothyronine syndrome. *Thyroid* 1998;8:249–257.

408. Parle JV, Franklyn JA, Cross KW, et al. Thyroxine prescription in the community: serum thyroid stimulating hormone level assays as an indicator of undertreatment or overtreatment. *Br J Gen Pract* 1993;43:107–109.

409. Pohlenz J, Schonberger W, Koffler T, et al. Resistance to thyroid hormone caused by a new mutation (V336M) in the thyroid receptor beta gene. *Thyroid* 1999;9:100–104.

410. Pohlenz J, Manders L, Sadow PM, et al. A novel point mutation on cluster 3 of the thyroid hormone receptor beta gene (P247L) causing mild resistance to thyroid hormone. *Thyroid* 1999;9:1195–1203.

411. DuPrez L, Parma J, van Sande J, et al. Pathology of the TSH receptor. *J Pediatr Endocrinol Metab* 1999;12[Suppl 1]:295–302.

412. McGregor AM, Hall R. Thyroiditis. In: DeGroot LJ, ed. *Endocrinology,* 3rd ed. Philadelphia: WB Saunders, 1995:683–701.

413. Larsen PR, Davies TF, Hay ID. Autoimmune and infectious thyroiditis. In: Wilson JD, Foster DW, Kronenberg HM, et al., eds. *Williams textbook of endocrinology,* 9th ed. Philadelphia: WB Saunders, 1998:475–479.

414. Slatosky J, Shipton B, Wahba H. Thyroiditis: differential diagnosis and management. *Am Fam Physician* 2000;61:1047–1052.

415. Ingbar SH, Woeber KA. Diseases of the thyroid. In: Wintrobe MM, Thorn GW, et al., eds. *Harrison's principles of internal medicine,* 7th ed. New York: McGraw-Hill, 1974:465–484.

416. Martino E, Safran M, Aghini-Lombardi F, et al. Environmental iodine intake and thyroid dysfunction during chronic amiodarone therapy. *Ann Intern Med* 1984;101:28–34.

417. Pacini F, Vorontsova T, Molinaro E, et al. Thyroid consequences of the Chernobyl nuclear accident. *Acta Paediatr Suppl* 1999;88:23–27.

418. Nagataki S, Shibata Y, Inoue S, et al. Thyroid diseases among the atomic bomb survivors in Nagasaki. *JAMA* 1994;272:364–370.

419. Roldan MB, Alonso M, Barrio R. Thyroid autoimmunity in children and adolescents with type I diabetes mellitus. *Diabetes Nutr Metab* 1999;12:27–31.

420. Hansen D, Bennedbaek FN, Hansen LK, et al. Thyroid function, morphology, and autoimmunity in young patients with insulin-dependent diabetes mellitus. *Eur J Endocrinol* 1999;140:512–518.

421. Karni A, Abramsky O. Association of MS with thyroid disorders. *Neurology* 1999;53:883–885.

422. Valentino R, Savastano S, Tommaselli AP, et al. Prevalence of coeliac disease in patients with thyroid autoimmunity. *Horm Res* 1999;51:124–127.

423. Lange U, Boss B, Teichman J, et al. Thyroid disorders in female patients with ankylosing spondylitis. *Eur J Med Res* 1999;4:468–474.

424. Hotze SF. Autoimmune thyroiditis and its relation to allergic disorders: a prospective clinical study. Presented at the American Academy of Otolaryngic Allergy annual meeting, Washington, DC, September 27, 1996.

425. Ohmori M, Harada K, Tsuruoka S, et al. Levothyroxine-induced liver dysfunction in a primary hypothyroid patient. *Endocr J* 1999;46:579–583.

426. Kim CH, Chae HD, Kang BM, et al. Influence of antithyroid antibodies in euthyroid women on in vitro fertilization-embryo transfer outcome. *Am J Reprod Immunol* 1998;40:2–8.

427. Harris B. Postpartum depression and thyroid antibody status. *Thyroid* 1999;9:699–703.

428. Andersen-Ranberg K, Jeune B, Hoier-Madsen M, et al. Thyroid function, morphology, and prevalence of thyroid disease in a population-based study of Danish centenarians. *J Am Geriatr Soc* 1999;47:1238–1243.

429. McDaniel AB. Autoimmune thyroiditis in the chronically fatigued, multiply allergic patient. Presented at the American Academy of Otolaryngic Allergy annual meeting, New Orleans, September 22, 1994.

430. Feldt-Rasmussen U, Krogh Rasmussen A, Kayser L, et al. A role of interleukin-1 and interleukin-6 in thyroiditis? In: Nagataki S, Mori T, Torizuka K, eds. *80 Years of Hashimoto disease.* Amsterdam: Elsevier Science Publishers BV, 1993:313–318.

431. Feldmann M, Dayan C, Quaratino S, et al. Mechanisms involved in the pathogenesis of thyroiditis: usefulness of T cell cloning to define antigens, epitopes and the role of anergy in disease induction. In: Nagataki S, Mori T, Torizuka K, eds. *80 Years of Hashimoto disease.* Amsterdam: Elsevier Science Publishers BV, 1993:279–284.

432. Guven M, Bayram F, Unluhizarci K, et al. Endocrine changes in patients with acute organophosphate poisoning. *Hum Exp Toxicol* 1999;18:598–601.

433. Beard AP, Rawlings NC. Thyroid function and effects on reproduction in ewes exposed to the organochlorine pesticides lindane or pentachlorophenol (PCP) from conception. *J Toxicol Environ Health* 1999;58:509–530.

434. Smallridge RC. Disclosing subclinical thyroid disease: an approach to mild laboratory abnormalities and vague or absent symptoms. *Postgrad Med* 2000;107:143–146, 149–152.

435. Williams JB. Adverse effects of thyroid hormones. *Drugs Aging* 1997;11:460–469.

436. Franklyn JA, Black EG, Betteridge J, et al. Comparison of second and third generation methods for measurement of serum thyrotropin in patients with overt hyperthyroidism, patients receiving thyroxine therapy, and those with nonthyroidal illness. *J Clin Endocrinol Metab* 1994;78:1368–1371.

437. Rezzonico JN, Pusiol E, Saravi FD, et al. Management of overt and subclinical hypothyroidism: factors influencing L-thyroxine dosage. *Medicina (B Aires)* 1999;59:698–704.

438. Koutras DA. The medical management of non-toxic goiter: several questions remain. *Thyroidology* 1993;5:49–55.

439. Franklyn JA, Betteridge J, Daykin J, et al. Long-term thyroxine treatment and bone mineral density. *Lancet* 1992;340:9–13.

440. DeRosa G, et al. Effect of suppressive L-thyroxine therapy on bone in women with nontoxic goiter. *Horm Metab Res* 1995; 27:503–507.

441. Ali M. Hypothesis: chronic fatigue is a state of accelerated oxidative molecular injury. *J Advancement Med* 1993;6:83–96.

442. Bombardier CH, Buchwald D. Outcome and prognosis of patients with chronic fatigue vs. chronic fatigue syndrome. *Arch Intern Med* 1995;155:2105–2010.

443. Vercoulen JH, Swanink CM, Fennis JF, et al. Prognosis in chronic fatigue syndrome: a prospective study on the natural course. *J Neurol Neurosurg Psychiatry* 1996;60:489–494.

444. Hill NF, Tiersky LA, Scavalla VR, et al. Natural history of severe chronic fatigue syndrome. *Arch Phys Med Rehabil* 1999; 80:1090–1094.

445. Wilson A, Hickie I, Lloyd A, et al. Longitudinal study of outcome of chronic fatigue syndrome. *BMJ* 1994;308:756–759.

446. Pheley AM, Melby D, Schenck C, et al. Can we predict recovery in chronic fatigue syndrome? *Minn Med* 1999;82(11):52–56.

447. Marlin RG, Anchel H, Gibson JC, et al. An evaluation of multidisciplinary intervention for chronic fatigue syndrome with long-term follow-up, and a comparison with untreated controls. *Am J Med* 1998;105(3A):110S–114S.

# ADDITIONAL ISSUES IN OTOLARYNGIC ALLERGY

# QUALITY OF LIFE IN ALLERGIC PATIENTS

## HELENE J. KROUSE

The efficacy of treating many illnesses in the past century has been evaluated by physical or clinical outcomes related to relief of symptoms, morbidity, mortality, and recurrence of disease. Since the 1980s, consensus has grown in the health care community that evaluating therapeutic outcomes of medical treatments without regard to the impact of the disease on the patient's quality of living is insufficient. Although allergic rhinitis is not a life-threatening condition that warrants sophisticated medical interventions or hospitalization, it nonetheless is a condition that can seriously affect people's daily lives. Therefore, examination of the efficacy of therapeutic regimens cannot be based solely on improvement of clinical symptomatology experienced by the person, but requires further evaluation of the person's perceptions of the effectiveness of treatment on his or her overall quality of life. This chapter attempts to develop a working definition of quality of life for the patient with allergic rhinitis that has utility to clinical practice and empiric analyses. A critical review of the various instruments used to measure quality of life among patients with allergic rhinitis is provided, with suggestions for future directions. Last, the body of research in this area is presented, with implications of findings for patients and practitioners.

## DEFINING QUALITY OF LIFE

The concept of quality of life has been recognized as an important component in the care of patients with many chronic conditions, such as arthritis, heart disease, or multiple sclerosis. Although widely referred to in the health care literature, the development of a consensus on the definition of quality of life has been quite challenging. The move toward a clear, uniform, and focused conceptual framework will facilitate communication regarding outcomes of care for patients and health professionals.

Currently, the World Health Organization's definition of health status is used frequently in conceptualizing quality of life because it refers to health as multidimensional in nature. Thus, a definition of the concept of quality of life, or, more specifically, health-related quality of life, most often encompasses multiple facets related to the person's overall health status. Shipper (1) defines quality of life in terms of four dimensions: physical and occupational function, psychological function, social and role interactions, and somatic complaints. A working definition of quality of life, therefore, encompasses such elements as overall health status and sense of well-being, work/school productivity, psychological well-being, physical well-being, social functioning, and level of performance.

## ALLERGIC RHINITIS

Patients with chronic conditions such as allergic rhinitis often are living with illnesses that routinely affect their feelings of well-being, vitality, sociability, and performance—central components in overall quality of life. Although not a life-threatening illness, allergic rhinitis can cause significant morbidity, affect functional status, and contribute to the development of other medical problems such as rhinosinusitis, otitis media, and asthma. These people are most concerned with receiving treatments that offers them the best chance for improvement or resolution of symptoms, so that other aspects of their lives such as work, school, social activities, and family life are not significantly impeded by their condition.

The nature of allergic rhinitis often necessitates prolonged medical management that may involve a combination of treatments, including antihistamines, decongestants, nasal steroid sprays, bronchodilators, and immunotherapy injections. In addition, patients often are encouraged to make substantial changes in lifestyle. Many people benefit from modifications in their diet, which may include eliminating or rotating certain allergenic foods. Modifications in home, work, or school environment also might be recom-

H. J. Krouse: College of Nursing, Wayne State University, Detroit, Michigan.

mended, depending on specific sensitivities. The close interaction of the physiologic consequences of allergic rhinitis with the person's functional, emotional, and psychological status necessitates the incorporation of not only physiologic indicators of positive outcomes but clinical and behavioral measurements of the multifaceted dimensions comprising quality of life. Therefore, the goal of therapy for patients with allergic rhinitis is to alleviate the symptoms that are most debilitating to the person and hence improve overall quality of life.

Allergic rhinitis often is viewed by health care providers as a benign health problem. In actuality, the contribution of allergic rhinitis to more serious conditions such as sinusitis, otitis media, and asthma is quite significant. The prevalence of allergic rhinitis has been steadily increasing, with the condition currently affecting an estimated 30% of the U.S. population (2). Allergic rhinitis is a very costly health care problem, resulting in over $3.5 billion spent on medications and office visits, as well as affecting work and school productivity, absenteeism, and overall quality of life (3).

Patients with seasonal or perennial allergies often complain that the disease or its treatments have a profound impact on their overall health, lifestyle, and psychological well-being. Primary goals of treatment for patients with allergies include (a) control of symptoms without altering functional ability; (b) preventing development of other medical conditions, such as respiratory diseases; and (c) improving each person's quality of life. In addition, the education of health care providers on the overall effects of allergic disease and its treatments on the patient is of vital importance.

Allergic rhinitis is frequently perceived simply as nasal congestion, stuffiness, and rhinorrhea, but many people also experience systemic symptoms. Several of the most common complaints include fatigue, irritability, malaise, mood changes, and effects on performance at school or work. The literature has even reported poorer psychological adjustment and difficulty in handling environmental pressures among allergic patients.

Practitioners have traditionally evaluated the effectiveness of their treatments by assessing the patient's physical status, specifically the condition of the nose and nasal cavity. Clinical indices such as nasal hyperreactivity, severity of nasal symptoms, nasal cytology, computed tomography scan, and rhinomanometry have been used as important clinical tools to evaluate the patient's anatomic structures and physical status. Clinical and diagnostic findings are important evaluative measures to assess physiologic responses to medical and surgical interventions. However, these indicators strictly assess the status of the sinonasal anatomy and physiology, and can be poorly correlated with the person's general sense of well-being, functional ability, and overall subjective evaluation of his or her health status. Hence, the patient's perceptions of the efficacy of treatment may significantly differ from those perceptions of the practitioner if

based only on objective clinical measurements. It therefore has become incumbent on the provider to incorporate indices representative of the person's health-related quality of life in determining the effectiveness of any treatment. Comprehensive assessment of the outcomes of medical treatment consists of both evaluating improvements in clinical symptomatology as well as examining patient perceptions of the effectiveness of treatments in their overall health status and functioning.

## MEASURING QUALITY OF LIFE

Measures of health-related quality of life for clinical evaluation of patient status incorporate both general and specific foci. Because health-related quality of life is multifaceted, the tools designed to measure this concept often are composed of questions to examine three or four of the dimensions identified by Shipper (1). Assessment of a person's health-related quality of life requires evaluation in several of these domains. In the dimension of functional status, areas that might be included are physical functioning, social functioning, role limitations related to physical problems, and role limitations related to emotional problems. Aspects related to a person's sense of well-being might focus on mental health, energy and fatigue, and pain. An overall evaluation of health in relation to quality of life incorporates general perceptions about a person's overall health status and changes in health in response to disease and its treatments.

Many instruments developed to assess quality of life, whether general or disease specific, evaluate several of these domains. Because of the complex nature of this construct, a single dimension such as somatic problems or functional status is insufficient in capturing its robustness. This factor represents a serious limitation of instruments that use a single domain to assess health-related quality of life. On the other hand, instruments that score various dimensions together for a total quality-of-life score collapse and lose valuable information and may hide the person's true status. For example, a patient may score well in physical status and poorly on social interactions. This valuable information is lost if only one score is generated or if subscale scores are combined.

General or generic measures assess more broad attributes that characterize various dimensions related to quality of life and span across disease state and treatments. These generic instruments are important in comparisons of different groups of patients relative to the impact of their diseases or treatments on their health status, functioning, and perceptions of well-being. Many of these general instruments have been adapted or developed specifically to assess quality of life and functional status among patients with allergic disease. For example, these general measures of health-related quality of life allow clinicians and researchers to compare patients with different conditions such as hypertension, cancer, and asthma on the same indices. Specific disease and treatment differences are not evaluated using these general measures. When used with specific patient populations, generic surveys may contain items that are irrelevant or lack items that assess specific situations important to that particular group.

To evaluate some of these unique aspects of disease processes and treatment, specific health-related quality-of-life instruments have been developed. Many of these scales are adaptations of generic surveys with modifications, deletions, and additions of items that assess specific quality-of-life issues for a particular disease and/or its treatments.

A major weakness of all health-related quality-of-life tools is that respondents are asked to rate the occurrence of an item without weighing the relative importance of that item to their overall quality of life. Rating the importance of an item provides additional information on the significance of that area to the person. For example, the presence of fatigue may be rated, but its relative importance in the person's quality of life not measured. The inclusion of a weighted score would provide additional information regarding patients' perceptions of their condition and the effectiveness of specific treatments.

## INSTRUMENTS

Several quality-of-life instruments have been used to assess outcomes of treatment among patients with allergic rhinitis (Table 26.1). Most of these tools are designed to measure various aspects of quality of life in this specific patient population. However one general instrument, the Medical Outcomes Study Short Form-36 (SF-36), has been used in many studies in the United States and abroad and therefore merits inclusion in this section. Most of the scales that have been developed specifically to measure quality of life in patients with allergic rhinitis are designed for adults, whereas one instrument is specifically designed for use with adolescents. Several instruments have been written for easy administration in the clinical setting so that the practitioner can include this information as part of the routine patient assessment. In selecting a tool to measure specific outcomes, it

## TABLE 26.1. QUALITY-OF-LIFE MEASURES

Adolescent Rhinoconjunctivitis Quality of Life Questionnaire
Allergy Outcome Survey (AOS)
Chronic Sinusitis Survey
Medical Outcomes Study Short Form-36 (SF-36)
Rhinoconjunctivitis Quality of Life Questionnaire (RQLQ)
Rhinosinusitis Disability Index (RSDI)
Sinonasal Outcome Test-20 (SNOT-20)

is important to consider the utility of the measurement for the particular purpose intended. Some instruments have good utility for research in comparing different treatment modalities or monitoring treatment outcomes. Other tools have been designed for use by practitioners as part of a patient assessment guide and may be less suited for scientific studies. Understanding the differences in the various measurements of quality of life assists in the appropriate selection and application of these instruments.

## Adolescent Rhinoconjunctivitis Quality of Life Questionnaire

The Adolescent Rhinoconjunctivitis Quality of Life Questionnaire (4) was developed specifically to measure changes in quality of life experienced by young people with seasonal allergic rhinitis. Instrument development with adolescents between the ages of 12 and 17 years revealed six domains that are most important in the evaluation of quality-of-life impairment in this age group. The 25-item questionnaire assesses practical problems, patient-specific activities, emotional problems, and physical symptoms, including non–hay fever symptoms, eye symptoms, and nose symptoms. Scores in each of these six domains are obtained, as well as an overall quality-of-life score. This instrument has demonstrated good psychometric properties compared with other conventional measures of symptom severity and clinical utility for measuring changes in various dimensions characterizing quality of life over time. This disease-specific quality-of-life measure is one of the few instruments exclusively designed and tested for use in an adolescent patient population. Identification of the various domains in quality of life among different age groups and development of instruments to measure these important characteristics will aid in understanding variations in quality of life and in measuring outcomes of care.

## Allergy Outcome Survey

The Allergy Outcome Survey (AOS) (5) was developed specifically to evaluate patients with allergic rhinitis. This brief, seven-item tool was developed for routine use in the clinical setting as an ongoing method of assessing patients' clinical progress during treatment. The AOS was constructed specifically to be a brief, practical measurement tool to evaluate symptoms and medication use among patients with allergic rhinitis. It is not intended to be a comprehensive assessment tool, and the authors therefore recommend using the AOS in combination with other measures for thorough outcome evaluation. With regard to the multidimensional definition of quality of life, this measurement specifically focuses on patients' allergic symptoms and medication use over time. In measuring these specific concepts, the tool demonstrated good test–retest reliability and is therefore a useful measure of temporal changes in these areas. Total score on the AOS correlated well with the total score on the Rhinoconjunctivitis Quality of Life Questionnaire ($r = 0.43$), providing one general score for patient assessment.

## Chronic Sinusitis Survey

The Chronic Sinusitis Survey (6) consists of six items included to measure outcomes specific to chronic rhinosinusitis and its treatments. The instrument contains a symptom section and a medication section, with each section scored separately. The Chronic Sinusitis Survey has been correlated with scores obtained on the SF-36 and is most consistent with scores related to physical and work activities and bodily pain. It is not designed to measure any aspects of social or emotional functioning. Used in conjunction with another tool such as the SF-36, this instrument can provide a comprehensive assessment of the patient with chronic rhinosinusitis.

## Medical Outcomes Study Short Form-36

The SF-36 (7) is a generic quality-of-life instrument designed for general evaluation of a person's health status. This 36-item survey measures eight domains of functioning and well-being relevant to quality of life. Specific domains include physical functioning, vitality (energy/fatigue), bodily pain, social functioning, mental health, role limitations due to physical and emotional problems, general perceptions of health, and change of health. Researchers using this tool sometimes separate role limitation into two discrete domains, physical role limitations and emotional role limitations, and report on nine domains of quality of life. Each domain is scored on a scale ranging from 0 to 100, with perfect health receiving a score of 100 points.

Although not a disease-specific quality-of-life measure for allergic rhinitis, the SF-36 has been widely used to evaluate outcomes in many patient populations, including patients with allergic rhinitis. The instrument is an excellent tool for quantifying the various domains included in this complex concept and has been useful in detecting differences between groups. The SF-36 is available in a French version and has been successfully administered to both adults and children. Psychometric properties of this instrument include good reliability and validity in measuring the concept of quality of life over time. The main disadvantages of using this tool for outcome assessment in general practice is its length because it includes items not relevant to patients with allergic rhinitis and therefore is more time consuming to administer in the office setting.

## Rhinoconjunctivitis Quality of Life Questionnaire

The Rhinoconjunctivitis Quality of Life Questionnaire (RQLQ) (8) is a disease-specific quality-of-life measure for adults and children with allergic rhinitis. In developing this instrument, the researchers measured both the frequency and importance of specific problems, including symptoms and impaired function. Six domains are used to summarize the various aspects of quality of life: sleep problems, nonnasal symptoms, nasal symptoms, practical problems, activity limitations, and emotional problems. There are two major parts to this questionnaire. The patient is first asked to select three specific activities as most restricted by his or her illness. The second section consists of the various domains pertinent to quality of life in allergic rhinitis. Lower scores indicate better quality of life for the person. This instrument has good utility for clinical practice and scientific investigation because it measures several of the identified domains necessary in the assessment of quality of life. It is specifically designed for repeated measurement of outcomes among patients with rhinitis. Because administration of the instrument takes an average of 10 minutes or less, it can be easily incorporated into the routine assessment of the patient.

## Rhinosinusitis Disability Index

The Rhinosinusitis Disability Index (RSDI) (9) is a disease-specific measure designed to assess the impact of rhinosinusitis on the daily life of the patient. In developing the RSDI, the investigators were concerned with designing a tool that would be sensitive to the person's level of disease-related disability in order to treat the patient effectively and facilitate desired outcomes. It is a measure of disease-specific and general quality-of-life measures of physical, emotional, and functional disabilities associated with rhinosinusitis. The RSDI has undergone a systematic development that has resulted in a well constructed, reliable, and validated comprehensive measure of quality of life specific for patients with rhinosinusitis. Three scores are obtained for the three disability domains: functional, physical, and emotional. The patient identifies how limiting nasal and sinus symptoms are to specific daily activities. The relative importance of these areas to the patient, however, is weighted in the patient's assessment.

The instrument is broadly constructed in that it covers major facets comprising quality of life with specificity to nasal and sinus diseases. Although designed specifically as a measure for rhinitis and sinusitis, the authors believe that it also may be effective in evaluating patient outcomes for allergic and nonallergic rhinitis and nasal obstructive disorders. Further scientific use of this instrument among patients with rhinitis is warranted to determine its full utility.

## Sinonasal Outcome Test-20

The Sinonasal Outcome Test-20 (SNOT-20) is a revised, shortened version of the Rhinosinusitis Outcome Measure (RSOM-31) (10). The original RSOM-31 is a disease-specific health status and quality-of-life instrument for use among patients with rhinosinusitis. The original 31-item instrument consisted of 7 domains: eye, ear, nasal, sleep, practical, emotional, and general health. The patient rates each item by the severity of the problem and the importance of the item to his or her life. The RSOM-31 has undergone three modifications to make it easier to use and to simplify scoring. There are three main modifications from the RSOM-31 to the SNOT-20: (a) reduction in number of items on the questionnaire; (b) the severity rating has been reduced from five to three categories; and (c) the importance rating was eliminated. Instead of rating the importance of each item to quality of life, the SNOT-20 simply asks the person to identify the five most important problems. A total score is obtained by adding the magnitude of all individual items and a second score is computed by adding only the five most important items selected by the patient. Psychometric evaluation of this shortened version suggests it has good reliability and validity with pertinent clinical utility.

## EMPIRIC INVESTIGATIONS

The investigative studies on quality of life among patients with allergic rhinitis are divided into three main categories. The largest group of studies is conducted using self-administered reports on the various domains of quality of life. The other two areas are those studies that focus on psychomotor tasks and those examining the effect on psychological and cognitive function.

### General Quality-of-Life Studies

This group of studies was conducted to compare patients with allergic rhinosinusitis with other patient groups or to evaluate specific treatment outcomes. Study design often involved a comparative group model of outcomes measures using one or more of the general or disease-specific rhinosinusitis quality-of-life questionnaires.

In one study conducted by Bousquet et al. (11), 111 patients with perennial allergic rhinitis were compared with 116 healthy subjects on a general measure of quality of life (SF-36). Subjects included in the allergic rhinitis group were diagnosed through history of perennial allergy and had a minimum of two self-reported symptoms of rhinitis. The 116 control subjects were recruited by 6 occupational health physicians and were screened for symptoms of rhinitis, significant medical condition, and any major treatment or life event, such as recent death of a relative, that might affect their quality of life. Results of this two-group comparison on the nine dimensions of the SF-36 revealed significant differences between the groups on eight of these scales. The subjects with allergic rhinitis scored significantly lower in the areas of physical functioning, energy/fatigue, general health perceptions, social functioning, role limitations resulting from both physical and emotional responses, bodily pain, and mental health.

Findings from this study suggest that people who experience moderate to severe symptoms from their perennial allergies perceive significant impairments in various aspects of their lives measured by a general quality-of-life instrument. The results of this study provided a preliminary understanding of the overall quality-of-life impairment that patients with allergic rhinitis experience.

Bousquet et al. (12) also collected data on quality-of-life scores using the SF-36 on a sample of 252 asthmatic patients, with varying degrees of severity of illness. A comparison of quality-of-life scores from patients with allergic rhinitis and patients with asthma showed that quality-of-life scores were poorer for the allergic patients in six of the nine domains examined. The domains in which the patients with allergic rhinitis scored lower were social functioning, physical role limitations, emotional role limitations, energy/fatigue, change in health over 1 year, and mental health. The three areas of quality of life on which patients with asthma scored lower were physical functioning, pain, and general health perceptions. Results of this comparative study revealed very interesting findings regarding the perceptions of patients with allergic rhinitis and quality of life. Although allergy often is perceived as a less serious condition by health providers, patients with allergy actually experienced reductions in more of the parameters that measure quality of life than patients with asthma. The importance of alleviating symptoms and improving outcomes related to quality of life in both of these patient groups presents a unique challenge for health professionals.

In another study done by Bousquet and his research team (13), 274 patients with perennial allergic rhinitis were compared on the SF-36 before beginning treatment with cetirizine, a second-generation antihistamine. Approximately half of the patients received the medication and one half received a placebo for 6 weeks. The subjects were readministered the SF-36 at 1- and 6-week intervals. At the end of 6 weeks, the subjects in the medication group noted significantly less symptomatic days or milder symptoms than the group receiving the placebo. The group receiving the antihistamine also demonstrated significant improvements on all nine dimensions of the quality-of-life instrument compared with the placebo group. This study demonstrates that patients with allergic rhinitis do experience impairments in their quality of life and that treatment with certain medications can improve patients' reported symptoms and perceptions related to quality of life. Duration of treatment has been shown to positively affect quality of life, with both initial improvement and further enhancement with additional therapy (14).

Several other studies have investigated the impact of nonsedating antihistamines on self-reported quality-of-life measures specifically designed for patients with allergic rhinitis. Studies by Van Cauwenberge and Juniper (15) and by Meltzer et al. (16) compared groups of patients with allergic rhinitis randomly assigned to either a treatment group receiving a daily nonsedating antihistamine or to a control group receiving a daily placebo. The collective results of these studies indicate that patients receiving treatment with a nonsedating antihistamine showed significant improvement in self-reported quality-of-life outcomes measured by the RQLQ. Specific scale scores that were most improved were the RQLQ domains related to work and school and daily functioning (16).

In a study by Bagenstose and Bernstein (17), a convenience sample of 19 patients was evaluated on several quality-of-life measures before treatment for chronic rhinitis and reevaluated after receiving treatment for 3 to 5 months. The treatment for all subjects included counseling on avoidance measures and a new medication regimen specifically determined for each patient based on his or her complaints. Four of the nine dimensions of the SF-36 significantly improved from pretreatment to posttreatment measurements for the group, including social functioning, vitality, general health, and changing health status. On the disease-specific quality-of-life scale, RQLQ, significant improvement was noted only in the measures of emotional problems and overall quality of life. Lack of a control group, inclusion of patients with different types of rhinitis, and variations in medications regimens limit interpretation of the results of this study for clinical practice.

One of the few studies designed to assess quality-of-life changes in patients who had received primary treatment of their allergic rhinitis with immunotherapy was conducted by Fell et al. (18). All patients were tested for allergy either through intradermal skin testing or in vitro testing before beginning immunotherapy. A total of 60 patients who had received allergy immunotherapy for their diagnosis of allergic rhinitis for at least 1 year were included in the study. A combination of patient interviews and chart reviews was used to collect the data. Because this study was designed as a retrospective review, subjects were asked to rate their nasal symptoms before beginning immunotherapy through recall, and then to rate these same symptoms at the present.

An interview questionnaire developed by the researchers and based on the SF-36 survey was used to assess quality of life in these subjects. Each person judged whether there was any improvement in general health and was questioned about the effects of immunotherapy on tolerance for exercise and outdoor activity, participation in social activities, energy level related to everyday activities, and work productivity. In addition, subjects were questioned about changes since initiation of immunotherapy on the number of days absent from work, physician visits for allergic symptoms or infections, current use of medications, and whether they felt that the allergy injections were worthwhile with regard to time and money.

Results of this comprehensive study revealed that 92% of patients perceived significant improvement in two or more nasal symptoms with immunotherapy. Of the patients experiencing three or more sinus or respiratory infections per year, 91% reported a decrease of 50% or more in these infections since beginning immunotherapy. With regard to exercise tolerance, 38% noted an increase in tolerance with immunotherapy, with many experiencing greater ease in performing specific activities. More than half of the patients also expressed significant improvements in social activities and energy level with allergy injections. Of those patients who reported that allergy symptoms affected their work productivity, all noted increases in their productivity since initiating therapy. Patients also rated the positive outcomes of symptom management and quality of life as worthy of the time and money invested in treatment with immunotherapy.

This study provides a multifaceted evaluation of patients on immunotherapy for a significant time. The many dimensions comprising quality of life as identified in the literature were clearly incorporated into the outcome interview. In addition, the investigators sought to discover further reasons for any identified improvements that patients had experienced over the course of their immunotherapy. Although this study is limited by its retrospective design and lack of a control group, it is the first study attempting to quantify quality-of-life outcomes in patients who had received immunotherapy for at least 1 year. The research clearly articulates a beginning framework for understanding the contributions of immunotherapy to improving quality of life. Further investigations using prospective, controlled studies as well as studies designed to compare various treatments for allergic rhinitis and their impact on quality of life and cost are warranted.

## Effects on Performance

Performance on specific tasks and productivity in work are other measures related to quality of life. Over the years, a number of studies have been conducted to evaluate both performance and productivity of people with allergic rhinitis. Some of these studies have used specific performance or cognitive tasks, whereas others have focused on morbidity in the work place. Comparisons between different groups of patients have been used to investigate effects on performance as a function of medical condition or treatment approach.

The prevalence of workers in the United States with allergic rhinitis was estimated at 12.6 million in the mid-1990s. Allergic rhinitis was the third most prevalent of common health conditions identified in both men and women in the workforce. Chronic sinusitis and hypertension were the only two conditions that were more prevalent in this group. The most common positions occupied by men with allergic rhinitis were in professional specialty, executive-managerial, precision production, sales, administration support, and machine operator categories. Positions occupied by women with allergic rhinitis were similar to the men and included administration support, professional specialty, service, sales, and executive-managerial responsibilities (19).

Allergic rhinitis can produce generalized symptoms such as malaise, fatigue, sleepiness, and headache in addition to nasal symptoms. Employee productivity related to job efficiency, cognitive and motor function, work injury, and days absent from work may be effected by both symptoms of allergic rhinitis and its treatment. More than 50% of people with allergic rhinitis rely primarily on over-the-counter (OTC) antihistamines for control of their allergic symptoms. These OTC medications are known to have significant sedative effects that may seriously impair cognitive and motor abilities. Based on this estimated use of OTC antihistamines by people with allergic rhinitis, Ross (19) estimated that 50% of the workforce would be treating their allergic rhinitis with these medications. Because these medications are sedating, causing drowsiness and central nervous system depression, efficiency in work-related activities and functioning may be impaired both through the disease and its treatment. The estimated cost of lost productivity in the workplace due to allergic rhinitis is in the billions of dollars annually.

The computerized patient and pharmacy records of a large health maintenance organization were reviewed by Gilmore and his research team (20) to investigate the relationship between use of specific medications and occurrence of traumatic work injuries. Medication use of employees with work-related injuries was compared with a group of similar employees who did not have any reported injuries. Findings of this correlational study revealed that both men and women showed an increased risk of injuries, particularly open wounds, fractures, and burns, if they were taking sedating antihistamines.

In another retrospective study, medical claims utilization records and daily output records on approximately 6,000 people employed in a large insurance company were examined to note the effect of antihistamine use on work productivity. Review of these records revealed that people taking sedating antihistamines were 7.8% less productive than patients not on these medications, whereas those using nonsedating antihistamines were 5.2% more productive (21).

The treatment of people with sedating antihistamines for allergic rhinitis profoundly affects work safety and productivity. Work-related injuries have been estimated to be 1.5 times greater in people using sedating antihistamines. Continued investigation with prospective, well controlled studies is necessary to understand better the impact of allergic rhinitis and its treatment on workplace injuries, safety, and job productivity.

In addition to affecting productivity and safety at work, treatment of allergic rhinitis with OTC medications such as sedating antihistamines can significantly impair performance on motor and cognitive tasks. Several studies have indicated that allergic rhinitis and its treatments not only may impair work-related performance, but can exert a profound effect on coordination, driving performance, cognitive function, and school performance.

Several investigations have evaluated the driving skills of people taking sedating versus nonsedating antihistamines. Using a standardized measure of driving skills, drivers were evaluated on specific performance tasks such as staying in the lane and maintaining a constant speed on the highway. Ramaekers et al. (22) conducted a double-blind study on 16 subjects to compare the effects of various antihistamines, placebo, and alcohol on driving performance. Impairment in driving performance was noted for people who had taken sedating antihistamines, even after the person felt he or she no longer was experiencing these sedative effects. Significant variability in maintaining a set speed and lateral weaving was noted in those people who were using sedating antihistamines. This impairment in driving performance was similar to effects noted in people driving under the influence of alcohol.

A similar investigation conducted by Weiler et al. (23) using a randomized, double-blind study design compared the effects of nonsedating and sedating antihistamines and alcohol on the driving abilities, responsiveness, and drowsiness of 40 subjects. Results of this study demonstrated that people taking a sedating antihistamine exhibited impairment in several driving tasks, including crossing the center line more frequently than with a nonsedating antihistamine or placebo, as well as less cohesiveness in car-following tasks. Similar impairments in performance also were noted in people who drove after ingesting alcohol. Participants also reported significantly higher levels of drowsiness both before and after driving when given sedating antihistamines.

Critical analysis of these studies on driving performance and related abilities reveals that many medications used by people to relieve symptoms related to allergic rhinitis cause significant impairment in functional ability. These well controlled experimental studies demonstrated significant impairment in specific driving tasks measured under standardized, controlled methods. Reported driving fatalities in which the driver was at fault revealed a 1.5 times greater likelihood of the driver having taken an antihistamine than not. These results have great significance for the use pattern of specific medications among patients with allergic rhinitis. Improved education of health professionals and the public regarding the serious adverse effects of sedating antihistamines on work and driving performance is necessary to decrease the untoward effects that may result from their continued use.

## Psychological and Cognitive Impact

Allergic rhinitis is a disease comprising many systemic symptoms in addition to the primary nasal symptoms. Patients often complain of fatigue, malaise, irritability, mood changes, sleep disturbances, and impairment of function.

In addition to the effects of allergic rhinitis on various aspects of job-related performance and specific behavioral tasks such as driving, impairment in cognitive abilities and psychological affect or mood also may occur.

Ten subjects with seasonal allergies were compared with eight control subjects both during and out of allergy season. Outcome measures used to compare the two groups included evaluation of memory, mood changes, verbal learning, and decision making. The researchers found that during seasonal exacerbations, patients with seasonal allergic rhinitis exhibited a significant decline in their ability to learn verbal material, along with negative affect scores. Scores of subjects in the control group experienced no impairments in cognition or mood in response to seasonal changes. In addition, cognitive abilities and affect improved during the winter months when allergic symptoms abated (24).

Impairments in performance related to allergic rhinitis and its treatment also have been demonstrated to occur in the learning activities of school-age children. Vuurman et al. (25) devised a measure to assess factual knowledge, conceptual knowledge, and knowledge application ability in school children. Fifty-two school children diagnosed with allergic rhinitis were compared with 21 children without allergies on various tasks to assess acquisition and application of knowledge. The authors found that children with allergic rhinitis had significant reductions in their factual knowledge compared with normal children as a result of their allergic condition alone. Treatment of allergic symptoms with a nonsedating antihistamine improved learning scores toward those of the normal children, whereas cognitive functioning and learning further deteriorated in those atopic children treated with a sedating antihistamine. These study results provide some very useful information regarding the negative impact of allergic rhinitis and its treatment on the learning ability of children. These negative consequences can be counteracted in part by administration of a nonsedating antihistamine, but performance can be further impeded by giving children an OTC sedating medication. The common practice of using OTC antiallergy medications to treat allergic symptoms in children can have serious negative implications regarding school performance. Proper education for parents, guardians, and educators regarding the adverse effects of sedating antihistamines therefore is essential.

Allergic rhinitis also may affect psychological adjustment and outlook on life. In a study by Gaucci et al. (26), 22 women with allergic rhinitis and 188 nonallergic women were administered a personality inventory to compare differences in psychological function. Women with allergic rhinitis scored poorer on several subscales designed to assess ego strength, ability to handle environmental pressures, and psychological adjustment. Their allergic disease, with its accompanying impairment in psychological functioning and coping, negatively affected the quality of life of these allergic patients. The small sample of patients who had allergic rhinitis unfortunately limits the generalizability of the results of this study. Further investigations into the impact of allergic rhinitis on psychological functioning and coping are needed to follow up on these preliminary findings.

## CONCLUSION

Allergic rhinitis cannot simply be conceptualized as a disease affecting only the eyes, ears, nose, and pharynx. Nasal symptoms as well as systemic manifestations such as fatigue, irritability, malaise, and sleep disturbances can have a profound impact on the patient's overall quality of life. This chapter has presented the current research on various measures of quality of life among patients with allergic rhinitis. Although research in this area is relatively recent, it is clear from these investigations that patients with allergic rhinitis perceive significant impairment in their quality of life as a result of their illness. In addition to patient identification of negative effects of this disease on their lives, impairments in cognitive performance, functional ability, and psychological adjustment also have been reported. Allergic rhinitis and its treatment can negatively affect work productivity. Cost in terms of days missed from work and work-related injuries suggests that the consequences of this disease can be quite serious.

The impact of allergic rhinitis and its treatment also has been shown to impair both cognitive abilities and performance in adults and children. This decline in learning of verbal information was most noticeable during allergy season with the exacerbation of symptoms. Treatment with sedating antihistamines results in significant impairments in function and performance. Patients seeking care for their allergic rhinitis require treatments that not only relieve physical symptoms but facilitate positive changes in their overall health status and quality of life. Patients with allergic rhinitis do experience significant impairment in their quality of life. Only through the use of outcome measures designed to assess patient improvement in quality of life and clinical symptoms related to allergic rhinitis will health professionals be able truly to evaluate the effectiveness of therapeutic regimens.

## REFERENCES

1. Shipper H. Guidelines and caveats for quality of life measurements in clinical practice and research. *Oncology* 1990;4:51–57.
2. Nathan RA, Meltzer EO, Selner JC, et al. Prevalence of allergic rhinitis in the United States. *J Allergy Clin Immunol* 1997;99: S808–S814.
3. Storms W, Meltzer EO, Nathan RA, et al. The economic impact of allergic rhinitis. *J Allergy Clin Immunol* 1997;99:S820–S824.
4. Juniper EF, Guyatt GH, Dolovich J. Assessment of quality of life in adolescents with allergic rhinoconjunctivitis: development and testing of a questionnaire for clinical trials. *J Allergy Clin Immunol* 1994;93:413–423.

5. Kemker BJ, Corey JP, Branca J, et al. Development of the allergy outcome survey for allergic rhinitis. *Otolaryngol Head Neck Surg* 1999;121:603–605.

6. Gliklich RE, Metson R. Techniques for outcomes research in chronic sinusitis. *Laryngoscope* 1995;105:387–390.

7. Ware JE Jr., Sherbourne CD. The MOS 36 item short-form health survey (SF-36): I. conceptual framework and item selection. *Med Care* 1992;30:473–483.

8. Juniper EF, Guyatt GH. Development and testing of a new measure of health status for clinical trials in rhinoconjunctivitis. *Clin Exp Allergy* 1991;21:77–83.

9. Benninger MS, Senior BA. The development of the rhinosinusitis disability index. *Arch Otolaryngol Head Neck Surg* 1997;123:1175–1179.

10. Piccirillo JF, Edwards D, Haiduk A, et al. Psychometric and clinimetric validity of the 31-item rhinosinusitis outcome measure (RSOM-31). *Am J Rhinol* 1995;9:297–306.

11. Bousquet J, Bullinger M, Fayol C, et al. Assessment of quality of life in patients with perennial allergic rhinitis with the French version of the SF-36 Health Status Questionnaire. *J Allergy Clin Immunology* 1994;94:182–188.

12. Bousquet J, Knani J, Dhivert H, et al. Quality of life in asthma: I. internal consistency and validity of the SF-36 questionnaire. *Am J Respir Crit Care Med* 1994;149:361–375.

13. Bousquet J, Duchateau J, Pignat JC, et al. Improvement of quality of life by treatment with cetirizine in patients with perennial allergic rhinitis as determined by a French version of the SF-36 questionnaire. *J Allergy Clin Immunol* 1996;98:309–316.

14. Burtin B, Duchateau J, Pignat JC, et al. Further improvement of quality of life by cetirizine in perennial allergic rhinitis as a function of treatment duration. *J Investig Allergol Clin Immunol* 2000;10:66–70.

15. Van Cauwenberge P, Juniper EF. Comparison of the efficacy, safety, and quality of life provided by fexofenadine hydrochloride 120 mg, loratadine, 10 mg and placebo administered once daily for the treatment of seasonal allergic rhinitis. *Clin Exp Allergy* 2000;30;891–899.

16. Meltzer EO, Casale TB, Nathan RA, et al. Once-daily fexofenadine HCl improves quality of life and reduces work and activity impairment in patients with seasonal allergic rhinitis. *Ann Allergy Asthma Immunol* 1999;83:311–317.

17. Bagenstose S, Bernstein JA. Treatment of chronic rhinitis by an allergy specialist improves quality of life outcomes. *Ann Allergy Asthma Immunol* 1999;83:524–528.

18. Fell WR, Mabry RL, Mabry CS. Quality of life analysis of patients undergoing immunotherapy for allergic rhinitis. *Ear Nose Throat J* 1997;76:528–536.

19. Ross RN. The cost of allergic rhinitis. *Am J Managed Care* 1996;2:285–290.

20. Gilmore TM, Alexander BH, Mueller BA, et al. Occupational injuries and medication use. *Am J Ind Med* 1996;30:234–239.

21. Cockburn IM, Bailit HL, Berndti ER, et al. Loss of work productivity due to illness and medical treatment. *J Occup Environ Med* 1999;41:948–953.

22. Ramaekers JG, Uiterwijk MMC, O'Hanlon JF. Effects of loratadine and cetirizine on actual driving and psychometric test performance and EEG during driving. *Eur J Clin Pharmacol* 1992;42:363–369.

23. Weiler JM, Bloomfield JR, Woodworth GG, et al. Effects of fexofenadine, diphenhydramine, and alcohol on driving performance: a randomized, placebo-controlled trial in the Iowa driving simulator. *Ann Intern Med* 2000;132:354–363.

24. Marshall PS, Colon EA. Effects of allergy season on mood and cognitive function. *Ann Allergy* 1993;71:251–258.

25. Vuurman E., van Veggel L, Uiterwijk M, et al. Seasonal allergic rhinitis and antihistamine effects on children's learning. *Ann Allergy* 1993;71:121–126.

26. Gaucci M, King MG, Saxarra H, et al. A Minnesota Multiphasic Personality Inventory profile of women with allergic rhinitis. *Psychosom Med* 1993;55:533–540.

## ADDITIONAL BIBLIOGRAPHY

**Blaiss MS.** Quality of life in allergic rhinitis. *Ann Allergy Asthma Immunol* 1999;83:449–454.

**Fireman P.** Treatment of allergic rhinitis: effect on occupation productivity and work force costs. *Allergy Asthma Proc* 1997;18:63–67.

**Gill TM, Feinstein AR.** A critical appraisal of the quality of quality-of-life measurements. *JAMA* 1994;272:619–626.

**Juniper EF.** Measuring health-related quality of life in rhinitis. *J Allergy Clin Immunology* 1997;99:S742–S749.

**King CR, Haberman M, Berry DL, et al.** Quality of life and the cancer experience: the state-of-the-knowledge. *Oncol Nurs Forum* 1997;24:27–41.

**Leopold D, Ferguson BJ, Piccirillo JF.** Outcomes assessment. *Otolaryngol Head Neck Surg* 1997;117:S58–S68.

**O'Hanlon JF, Ramaekers JG.** Antihistamine effects on actual driving performance in a standard test: a summary of Dutch experience, 1989–94. *Allergy* 1995;50:234–242.

**Storms WW.** Treatment of allergic rhinitis: effects of allergic rhinitis and antihistamines on performance. *Allergy Asthma Proc* 1997;18:59–61.

**World Health Organization.** *WHO chronicle.* Geneva: World Health Organization, 1947.

## 27

# ROLE OF NUTRITION IN ALLERGY MANAGEMENT

### BRUCE R. GORDON

Nutrition is a subject that rarely is emphasized as a therapeutic medical technique, although it has a critical role in maintenance of optimal health. Despite this neglect, the nutritional management of allergies has significant potential for improving results beyond those obtained with the traditional treatment triad of environmental controls, pharmacotherapy, and specific allergen immunotherapy. This is true because the pathologic common pathway of inflammation and tissue injury in allergy involves excess oxidation, a problem for which there are available nutritional treatment strategies. In addition, chemical toxicity may be an issue in any allergic patient, and nutritional treatment also can be effectively applied to mitigate a chemical load. Many types of nutritional interventions have been proposed, but the area of greatest current interest concerns the role of oxidant chemicals in the pathogenesis of allergic diseases, and in the potential to augment antioxidant defenses by nutritional means. General reviews of nutritional factors known to influence the severity of allergic diseases have been published previously (1,2). This chapter reviews and discusses current knowledge of nutrition as applied to treatment of both allergic diseases and chemical toxicity.

Nutritional management also is important for another broad aspect of allergy care, the design of therapeutic diets. When elimination or substitution diets are used to treat food allergy, it is important to identify and replace key nutrients that are omitted. This is most likely to be a problem in growing children, but also can become a problem in zealous adults who very rigidly follow a diet. Nutrient depletion is more likely to occur as the number of omitted foods increases, or whenever a food comprising more than half of the source of a particular nutrient is restricted. For example, a strict yeast-avoidance diet excludes so many common foods that it may lead to total calorie deficiency, whereas milk avoidance may cause calcium and vitamin D deficien-

cies because milk often supplies most of those nutrients in a typical American diet. Therefore, the essential nutrients that must always be considered during diet manipulations also are reviewed and discussed in this chapter. Finally, nutritional management can complement other allergy treatments, usually is inexpensive, and, in most cases, has a large margin of safety, with few side effects.

## PATHOLOGIC ROLE OF OXIDANTS IN ALLERGY

Oxidants are reactive chemicals that function as electron acceptors, and thus are capable of causing the destruction of cellular molecules such as lipids, proteins, and nucleic acids. Significant amounts of oxidant molecular damage can lead to metabolic inefficiency, DNA mutations (3), cell death (4), and, ultimately, to carcinogenesis, organ failure, or chronic illness. Oxidants are produced by normal cellular metabolism during mitochondrial aerobic respiration or hepatic microsomal detoxification. Also, oxidants are generated by leukocytes during phagocytosis and degranulation (5), during the spontaneous autoxidation of polyunsaturated lipids in cell membranes and fat stores, and when iron stores exceed normal limits. Preformed oxidants also can enter the body by consumption of rancid foods, by inhalation of smog, tobacco smoke, or other combustion products, or by exposure to oxidant or toxic chemicals (see Chapter 23). Even exposure to increased oxygen concentrations leads to increased oxidative injury (6). Finally, during allergic reactions, activated leukocytes release significant amounts of oxidants (7).

### Total Oxidant Load

Healthy, nutritionally normal cells possess sufficient capability to control and neutralize normal amounts of oxidants without incurring significant damage. However, cellular defenses can be stressed, and finally overwhelmed, when exposed to sufficiently large amounts of oxidants over a long

**B. R. Gordon:** Department of Otology and Laryngology, Harvard University, Cambridge; Associate Surgeon, Massachusetts Eye and Ear Infirmary, Boston; Chief of Otolaryngology, Cape Cod Hospital, Hyannis, Massachusetts.

enough time. Because all of these different sources of oxidants are additive, any single source of oxidants may be small enough to be easily contained by cellular antioxidant defenses, yet the sum may be too great, and lead to a pathologic state. Thus, the total personal oxidant load of each person at any point in time is a function of four factors: (a) their genetically determined ability to neutralize oxidants; (b) their personal chemical exposure history; (c) the presence of medical conditions, like allergy, that generate excess oxidants; and (d) nutritional factors that affect their antioxidant defenses. This concept of total personal oxidant load is one possible explanation for the current worldwide increase in allergic diseases: the steadily increasing oxidant burden imposed by environmental pollutants may be enough to increase both the incidence of symptomatic allergies and their severity (8). In fact, even small concentrations of atmospheric ozone have been found to be an important exacerbating factor in asthma (9).

## PROTECTIVE ANTIOXIDANT MECHANISMS

Cells possess two basic protective antioxidant mechanisms: first, enzymes that can neutralize oxidants with specific reducing cofactors, and, second, direct reaction of oxidants with small reducing molecules such as vitamin C or vitamin E (10). Enzymatic reactions are especially important for protecting cell organelles from structural and functional injury, and to operate at maximum efficiency, these enzymes require adequate nutritional sources of protein, mineral cofactors such as iron, zinc, copper, and molybdenum, and sufficient B vitamin cofactors to act as reducing agents. Direct neutralization requires substantial concentrations of vitamin C in the aqueous cell compartments, and vitamin E in the lipid phases of cell membranes, to ensure that oxidants preferentially react with the vitamins instead of with cell components. Other plant-derived antioxidants, such as carotenoids, polyphenols, and flavonoids, also are protective (4). These two defense mechanisms are linked because the reducing cofactors required by antioxidant enzymes are regenerated by glutathione, which is then recycled through the action of glutathione peroxidase and related enzymes. Adequate antioxidant levels can be maintained by this mechanism, provided that enough sulfur-containing amino acids, selenium, B vitamins, vitamin C, and vitamin E (11) are available in the diet, and are absorbed. For example, vitamin E supplements are an effective means to raise serum glutathione levels in otherwise well nourished people (12). Some common toxins, such as lead, excess levels of normal cell components, such as iron, and most exogenous organic chemical pollutants, increase the effective oxidant load by specifically inhibiting certain antioxidant enzymes, by preventing glutathione recycling, or by consuming glutathione and other cofactors and making them unavailable for recycling (10).

## BENEFITS OF NUTRIENTS IN ALLERGY TREATMENT

Although the observed effects of antioxidants on general health (13) and on the immune system (14) appear positive, there are few large, controlled studies demonstrating that specific nutrients have benefits in the treatment of allergy or chemical toxicity. The major difficulty in assessing benefits of individual nutrients is the great difficulty in controlling human behavior and diet for sufficiently long periods to allow observable effects. A second difficulty is that natural foods are complex, containing inconstant amounts of huge numbers of component nutrients, so that intake of specific antioxidants may be highly variable, both among different people and in individuals, over time. A third difficulty is that in many diseases, nutritional effects may be observed only if the intervention lasts for years or decades. Despite these problems, epidemiologic studies have identified specific antioxidants as having possible benefits in several disease states. For example, high levels of vitamin C are associated with fewer cataracts (15), vitamin E with reduced coronary disease, carotenoids with less lipid peroxidation (4), and vitamin C, vitamin E, and carotenoids all are linked with lowered risk of vascular disease and cancer (13).

There also is good epidemiologic evidence for the effects of both low cellular antioxidant levels and increased oxidant exposures causing a worsening of allergies. For example, dietary surveys have shown that there is a strong statistical probability that asthmatic patients will have low levels of vitamin C, magnesium, and manganese, and that people with seasonal hay fever will have low zinc levels compared with matched, nonallergic peers (16). A review of nutritional influences in asthmatic versus normal patients compiled relevant references and rated them for both positive clinical effects of nutritional treatment and for the presence of a demonstrated nutritional deficiency (17). Magnesium was positive in 3 of 6 quoted references, vitamin C was positive in 10 of 13 articles, selenium was positive in all of 6 studies, and omega-3 essential fatty acids (EFAs) were positive in 6 of 7 reports, suggesting strongly that these specific nutrients do have a role in mitigating allergic disease.

Vitamin C has been studied more than most nutrients. Recently, it has been shown to play an essential role in normal neutrophil function (18), and thus is critical in preventing infection-induced asthma flares. Furthermore, vitamin C reduces the inflammatory effects of inhaled or internally generated oxidants, prevents the formation of the allergic mediator, platelet-activating factor (19), and enhances the release of cytokines by stimulated lymphocytes (20). Vitamin C also shifts the cyclooxygenase pathway of arachidonic acid metabolism toward antiinflammatory, bronchodilating prostaglandins, and has been found to prevent exercise-induced asthma attacks in some patients (21). Finally, vitamin C has antihistamine activity. At plasma vitamin C levels achievable by taking oral supplements, histamine levels are decreased by vitamin C–mediated histamine oxidation (22).

Other nutrients also have been shown to have beneficial immunologic, respiratory, or antiallergic actions. For example, use of vitamin E supplements improves both cell-mediated immunity and specific antibody responses to vaccination (23), whereas dietary vitamin E intake is strongly correlated with preservation of lung function during aging (24). In addition, high vitamin E levels, combined with adequate vitamin C and selenium, appear to protect against allergic exacerbations (8,10). Isolated selenium deficiency increases both susceptibility to, and severity of, viral infections (25). Increasing the ratio of dietary omega-6 EFAs to omega-3 EFAs causes asthma to worsen, whereas increasing the proportion of omega-3 EFAs substantially improves asthma in approximately 40% of patients (26). Beta-carotene supplementation eliminates aging-associated declines in natural killer cell function (27), improves cell-mediated immunity (28), and inhibits release of histamine from stimulated mast cells (29). Compared with nonallergic people, both asthmatic and rhinitic patients have lower levels of selenium and glutathione peroxidase activity (30). Finally,

*N*-acetylcysteine, which is converted by the body into glutathione, both decreases the symptoms of chronic bronchitis and slows the decline in lung function in chronic obstructive pulmonary disease (31). Nutrients that are known to have beneficial effects on the severity of allergies are listed in Table 27.1, with an assessment of how common each deficiency is in the U.S. population (32).

## GENERAL NUTRITIONAL CONCERNS DURING ALLERGY MANAGEMENT

Patients with allergy share similar general nutritional requirements: (a) adequate water for replenishment of losses and removal of liquid wastes; (b) enough fiber for normal intestinal function; (c) adequate dietary total calories for energy; (d) sufficient amounts of high-quality protein, containing the essential amino acids, to maintain anabolic metabolism; (e) correct ratios and amounts of EFAs and other lipids to maintain cell membranes and provide raw materials for hormone biosynthesis; (f) adequate intake of minerals needed for structural, enzymatic, and electrochemical purposes; and (g) sufficient amounts of vitamins required by cell metabolism. Although patients with allergy have these nutritional requirements in common with the general population, certain aspects of allergic illness and treatments may make it more difficult for any particular patient to obtain his or her requirements. For example, elimination diets may make it difficult to obtain enough of key nutrients. Second, atopic people may differ biochemically from the general population, thus requiring increased quantities of nutrients (33). Finally, patients with allergy may live in stressful environments, and require greater than usual amounts of nutrients to keep up with their metabolic and detoxification demands. This is most likely for urban patients, who require increased amounts of antioxidant vitamins simply to cope with the pulmonary toxicity of air pollution (34).

## TABLE 27.1. BENEFICIAL NUTRIENTS FOR ALLERGY TREATMENT

| Nutrient | U.S. Deficiency Risk |
|---|---|
| Vitamins | |
| A | Common |
| B complex | Common |
| Folate | Common |
| C | Common |
| E | Common |
| Minerals | |
| Copper | Common |
| Iron | Common |
| Magnesium | Common |
| Manganese | Rare |
| Molybdenum | Rare |
| Selenium | Common |
| Zinc | Common |
| Amino acids | |
| Total protein | Common |
| Cysteine | ? |
| Cystine | ? |
| Glutathione | ? |
| Methionine | Common |
| Taurine | ? |
| Fatty acids | |
| Omega-3 | Common |
| Omega-6 | Common |
| Others | |
| Carotenoids | Common |
| Polyphenols | ? |
| Flavonoids | ? |

## SPECIFIC NUTRITIONAL REQUIREMENTS

### Water

The purity of the water supply for patients with allergy must be checked as part of the environmental evaluation. Because of the large daily intake, even small amounts of contaminants may have large cumulative effects, particularly for chemicals that accumulate, such as heavy metals and organochlorine compounds. Water contaminated with chemicals or organisms also may be a source of significant allergen exposure. Bottled water can be subject to the same contamination problems as tap water. At a minimum, the local water company or municipality should be asked for the most recent biologic and chemical analysis of the local water supply, and the type of distribution pipes should be determined. With this information, decisions can be made about the need for charcoal, ion exchange resin, or reverse osmosis home water purification systems.

## Fiber

Fiber has been believed to be essential for intestinal function since the African observations of Denis Burkitt and Hugh Trowell (35). Fiber is the nondigestible fraction of plant-derived foods. Fiber increases stool water content and bulk, and consequently decreases transit time, which may be a protective factor for tumorigenesis (36). Ion exchange and adsorptive properties, and the selective binding of bile salts, metals, and bacteria, may be protective. Fiber also has anti-oxidant, free radical–scavenging effects. Some fiber components may help determine which organisms predominate in the intestinal flora, and provide a source of digestion-resistant carbohydrates that are fermented by the colonic flora, producing short-chain fatty acids that nourish colonocytes.

Fiber also may have adverse effects (36). Large amounts reduce the absorption of foods. In a marginal diet, this may cause malnutrition. The increased stool bulk after a fiber-rich meal may trigger sigmoid volvulus in susceptible people. Presence of phytates in fiber may cause mineral or trace element deficiencies, particularly of zinc. Antinutrients in fiber, such as lectins, tannins, saponins, and enzyme inhibitors, may interfere with digestion, or injure the intestinal mucosa, increasing permeability. Fortunately, cooking inactivates most of these antinutrients. Finally, silica particles entrapped in cereal fiber may be etiologic agents of esophageal cancer. Specific recommendations for consumption of fiber do not yet exist, but increases in daily fiber as small as 5 to 40 g/day have shown benefits in some human studies.

## Total Calories

Humans have the unconscious capacity to adjust their caloric intake to their behavior, within a wide range of possibilities (37). Total caloric need is thus different from needs for all other nutrients because there is no evidence that humans can sense and adjust the intake of any specific nutrient. Energy requirements for young adults are shown in Table 27.2 (38).

**TABLE 27.2. YOUNG ADULT ENERGY NEEDS**[a]

| Activity Level | Men | Women |
| --- | --- | --- |
| Resting | 25 | 24 |
| Light | 40 | 37 |
| Moderate | 46 | 40 |
| High | 54 | 46 |
| Exceptional | 61 | 54 |

Energy needs decrease with age: age (y) 40–49, 95%; 50–59, 90%; 60–69, 80%; >70, 70%.
[a]In kilocalories/kilogram/day.

Energy needs can be met by any food. Usually, carbohydrates supply the bulk, typically at least 55% of total dietary calories. Carbohydrates may be entirely omitted from the diet because they can be synthesized from protein or from glycerol found in food. However, regular dietary carbohydrate is important for maintenance of maximum liver and muscle glycogen levels (38). Also, the specific type of carbohydrate eaten influences how any excess energy consumed is stored. Excess simple sugars are converted mainly into fat, whereas excess starch, which is absorbed more slowly, is converted preferentially into glycogen. In humans, there is no evidence that the quantity of carbohydrate consumed influences hunger, and therefore subsequent eating behavior (39). However, low-carbohydrate diets have been used very successfully in weight reduction programs, and recent evidence shows that high-carbohydrate diets are more atherogenic than high-fat diets (40,41).

Most carbohydrates are poor antigens. Allergic problems with carbohydrate foods come primarily from the fact that carbohydrate foods are not pure: they are mixed with allergenic plant proteins. Even highly processed foods such as table sugar and cooking starches contain significant amounts of protein. Furthermore, because of the quantity of carbohydrate foods normally eaten, and the frequency with which these foods are eaten, allergic sensitization often occurs. Consequently, carbohydrate-rich foods like cereal grains, sugars, and potatoes frequently require omission. If several of these are omitted, total calorie deprivation could occur.

## Essential Amino Acids

Turnover of body proteins results in the obligatory loss, for an average adult, of approximately 25 to 30 g/day of protein (38). At least this amount of high-quality protein is required to maintain anabolic metabolism, and because absorption of protein is not perfect, approximately twice as much protein must actually be eaten. Thus, the recommended minimum daily protein intake is approximately 44 g for women and 56 g for men, corresponding to approximately 12% of total dietary calories. Because of decreased digestibility and absorption of plant proteins, vegetarians need to increase their protein intake further over the recommended amounts (42). During dietary manipulation, particularly for children, major protein sources such as milk and eggs may need to be restricted, leading to possible deficiency. Variations in protein needs with age are shown in Table 27.3 (42).

Humans are unable to synthesize nine of the amino acids, and one more cannot be made in sufficient quantity for growing infants. These are essential, and must be obtained from the diet. Adults require approximately 20% of their total protein intake be in the form of essential amino acids, whereas preteens and infants require over twice as much (42). During severe illness, adult essential amino acid needs to increase to resemble those of infants. Of these ten amino

**TABLE 27.3. ADEQUATE DAILY PROTEIN INTAKE** [a]

| Age | Men | Women |
|---|---|---|
| 0–6 mo | 2.2 | 2.2 |
| 6–12 mo | 1.6 | 1.6 |
| 1–3 y | 1.2 | 1.2 |
| 4–6 y | 1.1 | 1.1 |
| 7–10 y | 1.0 | 1.0 |
| 11–14 y | 1.0 | 1.0 |
| 15–18 y | 0.9 | 0.8 |
| Adult | 0.8 | 0.8 |
| Pregnant | — | 0.8, +10 g |
| Lactating (0–6 mo) | — | 0.8, +15 g |
| Lactating (6+ mo) | — | 0.8, +12 g |

[a] In grams/kilogram/day.

acid requirements, lysine and the sulfur-containing amino acids methionine and cystine are present in significantly lower quantities in plant proteins compared with animal proteins. Combining different plant foods to approximate more closely the essential amino acid content of animal proteins is commonly practiced, usually by combining cereals (low in lysine) and legumes (low in methionine and cystine).

## Essential Fatty Acids

Fats (lipids) function in at least five distinct roles, as an energy source, forming membrane structures, as surfactants, as hormones, and as antioxidants (43). Two of these roles, as hormones and in protection from oxidative damage, are of particular interest in allergic patients. Both classes of lipid hormones, steroids and eicosanoids, have potent regulatory effects on allergic inflammation, whereas uncontrolled oxidation of fats (autoxidation) generates free radical compounds, which are, among other actions, immunotoxic and proinflammatory.

### Lipid Autoxidation

All lipids that contain unsaturated bonds have the potential for spontaneous oxidation and the production of toxic metabolites such as hydroperoxides, epoxides, dialdehydes, and free radicals. The oxidation-sensitive site is at the methylene carbon atoms adjacent to each unsaturated bond. Hydrogen atoms at these sites can be abstracted, forming free radicals that then trigger self-propagating chain reactions in cell membranes, leading to production of further unstable oxidation products (43). Some of these molecules, especially aldehydes and peroxides, can diffuse long distances before causing damage. These compounds cause molecular cross-linking and enzyme inhibition, and produce insoluble lipofuscin deposits from proteins, thus destroying macromole-

cules and interfering with cell functioning. They also directly damage DNA, and so are mutagenic and carcinogenic. Cellular aging, arteriosclerosis, malignant transformation, immune dysfunction, or cell death may be the ultimate result of extensive autoxidation.

Inside the cell, normal fatty acid oxidation for energy production is accomplished in peroxisomes and mitochondria. Both are specialized organelles that are capable of controlling the reactive compounds normally generated by lipid oxidation. Oxidation also is carefully controlled in lysosomes, during generation of reactive oxygen compounds to destroy microbes. All of these organelles contain protective antioxidant enzymes, including catalases, peroxidases, and superoxide dismutases. They also contain molecular antioxidants, including vitamins C and E, carotenoids, reduced glutathione, the essential peroxidase cofactors heme iron and selenium, and the essential superoxide dismutase cofactors copper, zinc, and manganese. Of these protective substances, all must be ingested in adequate amounts to have maximal protection from uncontrolled oxidation. The only exceptions are the enzymes and reduced glutathione, all of which can be synthesized, provided adequate essential amino acids are consumed.

Under the stress of a high-fat diet or vitamin E deficiency, peroxisomes proliferate in an attempt to compensate for the increased oxidative load (44). However, when large amounts of highly unsaturated fatty acids, cholesterol, or vitamin A are absorbed, uncontrolled autoxidation may occur outside of these organelles. Lipid autoxidation is further increased by exposure to other agents capable of generating free radicals, such as radiation, oxidants in smog, and chemical pollutants that require oxidative detoxification.

### Essential Fatty Acids

Essential fatty acids are unsaturated fatty acids with multiple double bonds, one of which is close to the methyl end of the molecule. Human enzymes are unable to work closer than seven carbon atoms from the methyl (omega) end, so that we are completely dependent on plants to synthesize these necessary lipids. There are two EFA families, the omega-6, or linoleic acid family, synthesized by all plants, and the omega-3, or linolenic acid family, synthesized by marine phytoplankton. EFAs may be ingested as linoleic or linolenic acids, and then enzymatically elongated and desaturated to form all of the EFAs humans require. Alternately, preformed polyunsaturated EFAs such as arachidonic acid, eicosapentaenoic acid, docosapentaenoic acid, and docosahexaenoic acid may be absorbed and used directly. In prevention or treatment of EFA deficiency, except for rare people with converting enzyme deficiencies, it is sufficient to supply adequate amounts of one member from each of the omega-3 and omega-6 EFA families. People with eczema also may convert omega-6 EFAs poorly because γ-linolenic acid supplements cause clinical improvement (45).

Essential fatty acid supplementation has complex effects on the balance of prostaglandin- and leukotriene-regulated immune functions. Synthesis of eicosanoid hormones from EFAs amounts to only milligrams per day, compared with a daily dietary consumption of approximately 10 g of EFAs, but eicosanoid production falls as soon as the regular dietary supply of EFAs is interrupted. In addition, modifying the relative amounts of omega-3 and omega-6 EFAs consumed influences tissue levels of both proinflammatory and antiinflammatory hormones, with omega-3 EFAs shifting the balance toward antiinflammation. For these reasons, feeding different absolute amounts of dietary EFA, as well as changing the omega-3 to omega-6 ratio, can have a profound effect on all eicosanoid functions, and can affect the activity of diseases such as asthma that are affected by leukotrienes and prostaglandins (46).

How much EFAs should be included in a prudent diet? Most authorities recommend limiting total EFA consumption to no more than 10% of total calories, but absolute minimal needs still are unknown (43). Clinical deficiency of EFAs can occur in several situations, including premature and young infants, fat malabsorption, multiple sclerosis, and several other illnesses. Greater amounts of EFAs may be safe, but there are concerns over possible carcinogenesis, and because fats are the most calorie-dense foods, control of total calories is difficult when any fat is increased. Experimental studies on prevention of nervous system or retinal injury in growing animals show that omega-6 to omega-3 EFA ratios between 4 to 1 and 10 to 1 are optimal. This range of ratios agrees exactly with analyses of human milk from mothers on a wide variety of diets, where omega-3 EFAs are a constant 1.5% to 2.5 % of total fat, and 0.7% to 1.3% of total calories. Based on these data, recommended levels of omega-3 EFA, given current average omega-6 EFA consumption of approximately 7% of total calories, would be approximately 1% of total calories, or approximately 4 g/day in adults. Childhood needs are not precisely known, but are significant because of nervous system growth requirements. How the omega-3 EFAs are ingested is as important as is the correct amount of supplementation. If pure fish liver oils are used, it is possible to ingest toxic overdoses of vitamins A and D. On the other hand, eating a half pound a day of wild-caught fatty fish, such as salmon, tuna, sardines, or mackerel, provides approximately 4 to 6 g of omega-3 EFA, but only small amounts of vitamins A and D, and is better tolerated. Omega-6 EFAs are easily supplied by ordinary polyunsaturated vegetable oils. For infants, breast-feeding is strongly recommended because it is not possible adequately to feed required amounts of long-chain EFAs using traditional formulas or solid foods.

A final concern is that adequate vitamin E also is consumed, so that EFA autoxidation is prevented. Fortunately, most natural plant sources of EFAs contain vitamin E in adequate amounts (34,35), but fish oils do not (43). Because vitamin E also can be destroyed by processing, heating, and improper storage, EFA supplements or oils may contain preformed oxidative toxins (37). In addition, because average vitamin E consumption is below recommended levels, many people need vitamin E supplements, particularly if they are treated with EFA concentrates.

## Major Minerals

### Calcium

Because major minerals are widely distributed in common foods, mineral needs seldom are considered in dietary planning. However, calcium always needs to be considered when planning allergy diets because milk products are simultaneously the major dietary source of calcium, as well as a major food allergen. Calcium deficiency actually is common even without any dietary modification because over two thirds of women in the United States do not ingest the recommended amounts of calcium. After 35 years of age, approximately three fourths of women are calcium deficient (47). Calcium requirements are imperfectly known, mainly because of the ability of the body to regulate calcium levels closely despite wide variations in calcium intake. The previous U.S. recommended dietary allowance (RDA) of 800 mg for adults was too low, and was raised in 1996 to 1,600 mg to protect against osteoporosis. Current estimates by the World Health Organization of calcium needs are shown in Table 27.4 (47), as modified by the new RDA.

Besides inadequate calcium intake, three other common factors tend to worsen calcium deficiency. First, high phosphate levels that are present in a diet rich in meats or carbonated soft drinks promote increased calcium excretion. Second, inadequate vitamin D levels because of limited sunlight exposure, as well as reduced gut efficiency due to aging, also decrease calcium absorption. These are important factors in the United States and, consequently, average calcium consumption should be further increased. Complications

**TABLE 27.4. ESTIMATED CALCIUM REQUIREMENTS**[a]

| Age | Men | Women |
|---|---|---|
| Newborn | 200 | 200 |
| 1 mo | 235 | 235 |
| 3 mo | 300 | 300 |
| 8 mo | 350 | 350 |
| 1 y | 600 | 600 |
| 1–10 y | 800 | 800 |
| Prepubertal | 1,000 | 1,000 |
| Puberty | 2,000 | 2,000 |
| Adult[b] | 1,600 | 1,600 |
|   Pregnant or lactating | — | 2,000 |
|   Potentially toxic | >2,500 | |

[a] In mg/day.
[b] See text: rare individuals may not tolerate high doses.

from excessive calcium intake do not occur in normal people at amounts up to 2,500 mg/day (47). However, patients with sarcoidosis or with calcium-containing renal stones may experience complications from ingesting as little as 800 mg/day, particularly if also given vitamin D supplements. All growing children, and many adults, should receive calcium supplements if taken off of milk products. Even young children usually will chew flavored calcium carbonate antacid tablets, and adults can take any inexpensive calcium supplement. The third factor that lowers body calcium stores is magnesium deficiency (see later).

### Phosphorus

In contrast, phosphorus, which ordinarily is considered together with calcium because of the joint regulation of their metabolism, is present in so many foods and food additives that deficiency seldom is seen (47). For adults, 800 to 1,500 mg/day of phosphorus is required, only a fraction of the average U.S. daily consumption. Phosphate deficiency may be a problem when its absorption is prevented, such as by the regular ingestion of large amounts of antacids, iron salts, or unsaturated fatty acids. Hereditary hypophosphatemia also occurs, and low phosphate levels also are common in hospitalized persons. But the much larger problem is that excess dietary phosphate stimulates excessive parathyroid hormone production, causing calcium mobilization and osteoporosis. With the exception of infants, who require more calcium than phosphorus, phosphorus should be ingested at the same level as calcium.

### Magnesium

Although it is widely distributed in foods, magnesium deficiency is common. Because magnesium has multiple roles in energy production, it is important for muscle function, and therefore deficiency can worsen serous otitis and asthma. In addition to enabling parathyroid hormone secretion, magnesium has been found to control osteoclast activity, so that bone resorption occurs when magnesium levels are low. This probably is an important factor in osteoporosis pathogenesis. Confirmation of suspected magnesium deficiency is by a three-step process. First, a serum magnesium level is done. When a patient has a deficiency risk factor, a normal serum level should be checked by measuring 24-hour urinary excretion (normal is >24 mg). A low serum level should also be confirmed by measuring 24-hour urinary excretion. If the serum and 24-hour urine results conflict, then a magnesium load test is performed (48).

Low daily intakes in U.S. adults of from 234 to 323 mg/day have been reported, with the adult RDA being set at 320 to 420 mg/day (48). The most frequent medical causes of magnesium deficiency are diabetes mellitus, alcoholism, and intestinal malabsorption syndromes. Because inflammatory bowel disease due to food allergies may cause malab-

**TABLE 27.5. ESTIMATED MAGNESIUM REQUIREMENTS[a]**

| Age | Men | Women |
|---|---|---|
| 0–6 mo | 30 | 30 |
| 6–12 mo | 75 | 75 |
| 1–3 y | 80 | 80 |
| 4–8 y | 130 | 130 |
| 9–13 y | 240 | 240 |
| 14–18 y | 410 | 360 |
| 19–30 y | 400 | 310 |
| 31–50 y | 420 | 320 |
| 51–70 y | 420 | 320 |
| >70 y | 420 | 320 |
| Pregnant | — | 350–400 |
| Lactating | — | 310–360 |
| Potentially toxic in renal deficiency (see text) | | |

[a]In mg/day.

sorption, magnesium deficiency should be considered in every allergy evaluation. Magnesium toxicity is rare because of the large capacity of normal renal excretion; however, magnesium supplements should not be given in renal impairment. Magnesium oxide is poorly absorbed, but large excesses of any magnesium salt are cathartic. Recommended daily magnesium intakes are listed in Table 27.5 (48).

### Iron

Still the most common nutrient deficiency, both in the United States and in the world, anemia due to low iron is a problem particularly in menstruating women, children, adolescents, and the elderly (49). Average iron intakes in the United States are approximately 10 to 20 mg, with average absorption of approximately 10%. These levels should be adequate, except during pregnancy. Although iron is common in many foods, it is poorly absorbed, especially from plant sources. Iron deficiency occurs when cereals make up a major portion of the diet owing to both low iron content and interference with absorption due to the presence of phytates. In allergy diets, iron deficiency may arise from exclusion of meats and eggs. Recommended daily iron intake is shown in Table 27.6 (49).

#### Iron Toxicity

Toxic accumulation can occur with prolonged administration of iron supplements to normal, nonmenstruating adults. For this reason, iron supplements should not be prescribed without prior evaluation. Furthermore, approximately 1 in 250 people is homozygous for hereditary hemochromatosis, and is at particular risk of iron overload. Because symptoms of iron overload occur late in the illness, many of these persons have no knowledge of their disease

**TABLE 27.6. RECOMMENDED IRON INTAKES**[a]

| Age | Men | Women |
|-----|-----|-------|
| 3–6 mo | 6.6 | 6.6 |
| 6–12 mo | 8.8 | 8.8 |
| 1–10 y | 10 | 10 |
| 10–18 y | 12 | 15 |
| Adult[b] | 10 | 10 |
| Menstruating | — | 15 |
| Pregnant[c] | — | 45 |
| Potentially toxic in adults | See text | |

[a] In mg/day.
[b] Always check iron level before supplementing.
[c] Average U.S. diets cannot meet pregnancy iron needs.

**TABLE 27.7. RECOMMENDED IODINE INTAKES**[a]

| Age | Men | Women |
|-----|-----|-------|
| 0–12 mo | 50 | 50 |
| 1–6 y | 90 | 90 |
| 7–12 y | 120 | 120 |
| Adult | 150 | 150 |
| Pregnant | — | 200 |
| Lactating | — | 200 |
| Potentially toxic | >2,000 | |

[a] In µg/day.

and do not know that they should never take iron supplements. Before prescribing iron, hematocrit and serum iron should be checked. If iron-binding capacity, transferrin saturation, and serum ferritin have not been determined within the past 10 years, these also should be done (49). However, even if all test results are normal or low, follow-up still is required because no available test, except liver biopsy, is absolutely diagnostic and able to identify all cases of hereditary hemochromatosis in the early stages (50). High levels of ionized iron are strongly prooxidant, potentially causing toxic free radical production. However, because of the strong protein binding of iron, significant radical production may not be a common clinical problem (49).

## Iodine

Worldwide, iodine deficiency probably is nearly as common as iron deficiency, but for a different reason: iodine is a rare element, is not uniformly distributed in soils, and is not concentrated in any common foods (51). Large areas of the world are depleted in iodine because of loss of topsoil or leaching by water, and crops grown in such areas are poor iodine sources. The best sources of iodine are in foods not widely consumed (seaweeds, marine fish, and shellfish), so the major source for most people is staple foods to which iodine supplements have been added. Average U.S. diets are adequate, containing between 400 and 800 µg/day, compared with an estimated minimum daily requirement of 50 µg. Intake of from 100 to 200 µg/day is probably sufficient, even when goitrogens, plant components that interfere with iodine absorption, are present in the diet (51). Exclusion of seafood and iodized salt from the diet may lead to iodine deficiency. Iodine toxicity can occur from frequent consumption of water that has been disinfected with iodine. Iodine status can be easily determined by measurement in a random urine sample (normal, 100 to 200 µg/L), and abnormal results are confirmed by measuring blood thyroid-stimulating hormone levels. Recommended iodine intakes are shown in Table 27.7 (51).

## Zinc

Only 2 to 3 g of zinc is present in the adult, but this small amount has many crucial roles in the body as an enzyme cofactor and membrane stabilizer. Because zinc acts as a cofactor in DNA, RNA, and protein synthesis, as well as in detoxification enzymes and immune cell functioning, zinc deficiency may be both insidious and serious. Zinc deficiency is common in hospitalized patients, and in outpatients with cancer or chronic illnesses, especially those affecting the intestinal tract, skin, or immune system. The major limiting factor in zinc metabolism usually is poor absorption due to inhibitory substances that are widely distributed in the diet. In addition to cereal phytates, tea and coffee, cow's milk products, soy protein, iron, calcium, and alcohol all impair zinc absorption. Human breast milk, zinfandel wine, and some organic acids, including citric, enhance zinc absorption. Meats, especially beef, lamb, mollusks, and crustaceans, are good zinc sources that are essentially free of inhibitory substances. Estimated guidelines for zinc intake are shown in Table 27.8 (52). Zinc status is difficult to assess because serum levels and urinary excretion of zinc may not decrease until deficiency is severe, and hair zinc may be falsely high in severe deficiency.

**TABLE 27.8. RECOMMENDED ZINC INTAKES**[a]

| Age | Men | Women |
|-----|-----|-------|
| Infant | 5 | 5 |
| Child | 10 | 10 |
| Adult | 15 | 12 |
| Pregnant | — | 19 |
| Lactating | — | 16 |
| Potentially toxic | >150 mg | |

[a] In mg/day.

Zinc toxicity can be a significant problem, either accidental or through overzealous use of supplements (52). Acid foods stored in galvanized containers can leach enough zinc to produce acute toxicity, with cramps, vomiting, headache, and seizures. Chronic overdose results in impaired copper absorption and copper deficiency anemia, although this competition can be used clinically to assist in control of Wilson's disease. Gastric ulcers may occur from slowly dissolving tablets. Daily zinc doses of only 150 mg may cause toxicity, and maximum daily doses of 40 mg, or less, are prudent.

### Copper

A critical enzymatic cofactor in multiple oxidation reactions, copper is vital both for energy production and for detoxification. There is only approximately 70 to 100 mg of copper in the average adult, so deficiency can occur easily, most commonly causing iron-resistant microcytic anemia, neutropenia, and impaired glucose tolerance (53). Because superoxide dismutase is a copper–zinc enzyme, deficiency of either metal seriously disrupts leukocyte oxidative killing, and possibly triggers neutrophils to autolyse by oxidative damage. Similar oxidative damage also may occur in hepatocytes because copper deficiency also decreases the detoxifying selenium enzyme, glutathione peroxidase. Even in the absence of Wilson's disease, high copper levels are implicated in free radical production and neurodegenerative diseases (53). Copper deficiency, like zinc deficiency, also impairs lymphocyte function. Copper deficiency is most likely to occur in infants fed mainly cow's milk or rice because both foods are extremely low in copper content. It also may occur because of regular use of antiacids, excess zinc supplementation (see earlier), or high levels of dietary phosphate. Malabsorption syndromes and chronic intestinal diseases also may cause copper depletion.

Important dietary sources of copper are copper water pipes and copper cooking utensils, mollusks, crustaceans, and legumes. Unlike cow's milk, human breast milk enhances copper absorption. Estimated copper needs are shown in Table 27.9 (53). Copper supplementation must be carefully approached because excess copper is significantly toxic. Doses of as little as 5 to 10 mg may produce nausea,

250 mg produces vomiting, and as little as 3.5 g may be fatal. Chronic daily doses of 10 mg may be tolerated. The ratio of copper to zinc is important: approximately ten times more zinc than copper is required. Copper status is assessed by measuring serum copper and ceruloplasmin levels; however, neither is sensitive to marginal deficiency and, as acute-phase reactants, they may be artificially elevated in numerous illnesses. Erythrocyte superoxide dismutase activity is an alternative measure.

## Trace Elements

### Selenium

Those elements currently known to be required, in small amounts, for normal nutrition are selenium, chromium, and manganese. Like iodine, the selenium concentration in soils and in foods varies significantly. However, in the United States, even low-selenium areas such as the Midwest have adequate selenium to prevent obvious deficiency, so it is primarily seen in patients requiring total parenteral nutrition, in patients with high systemic chemical loads, and in some patients with allergy and asthma (16). In selenium-deficient areas, minimum intakes of approximately 13 to 19 μg daily prevent Keshan deficiency disease (54). The adult total-body selenium content is minute, only 3 to 15 mg. Selenium is important because it is the cofactor for glutathione peroxidase, part of the oxidant protection system. Because this biologic action of selenium is complementary with those of other antioxidants, selenium deficiency is more likely to be evident if there also is concomitant vitamin E deficiency. Selenium also plays a role in detoxification of ingested heavy metals, and is necessary in the hepatic p450 microsomal detoxification system (54). The estimated safe range of dietary selenium is shown in Table 27.10 (54). Normal U.S. selenium intakes have been estimated to be from 62 to 224 μg/day. Selenium toxicity, with loss of hair or nails and central nervous system dysfunction, may occur with excess supplementation, but the lower

**TABLE 27.9. RECOMMENDED COPPER INTAKES**[a]

| Age | Amount |
| --- | --- |
| Infant | 0.4–0.6 |
| Child | 1.5–2.5 |
| Adult | 1.5–3 |
| Potentially toxic | >5 mg |

[a]In mg/day.

**TABLE 27.10. ESTIMATED TRACE ELEMENT REQUIREMENTS**[a,b]

| Age | Selenium | Chromium | Manganese |
| --- | --- | --- | --- |
| Infant | 10–15 | 10–60 | 300–1,000 |
| Child | 20–30 | 20–200 | 1,000–3,000 |
| Adolescent | 40–50 | 50–200 | 2,000–5,000 |
| Adult | 55–70 | 50–200 | 2,000–5,000 |
|   Pregnancy | 65 | — | — |
|   Lactation | 75 | — | — |
|   Potentially toxic | >750 | Unknown | >10,000 |

[a]In μg/day.
[b]Toxic levels may be only several times usual intake.
Do not exceed upper doses without measuring levels.

dose limit for toxicity is not precisely known. Doses of up to 400 μg/day probably are safe.

## Chromium

Overt deficiency of chromium, needed for carbohydrate, lipid, and nucleic acid metabolism, has been seen only in patients who are severely malnourished or on prolonged total parenteral nutrition. However, improvements in glucose tolerance and cholesterol metabolism have been shown to occur in a significant fraction of people given chromium supplements. Because average U.S. dietary chromium intakes are near or below the lower end of the recommended range, many apparently normal people may be subclinically deficient. Foods with high chromium content include mushrooms, brewer's yeast, prunes, nuts, asparagus, wines, and beer. Significant chromium also leaches into acidic foods from stainless steel cookware. The recommended intake of dietary chromium is shown in Table 27.10 (55). Chromium toxicity occurs with industrial exposure to hexavalent chromates, which damage DNA and increase the risk of lung cancer. Oral use of trivalent chromium compounds has not yet been shown to cause toxicity; however, high doses of chromium picolinate, but not chromium chloride or nicotinate, cause chromosome damage in tissue culture, and chromium may accumulate during clinical supplementation (32,55). For these reasons, prolonged supplementation without laboratory monitoring probably is unwise. Both hexavalent and trivalent chromium may cause chronic dermatitis due to allergic sensitivity (56).

## Manganese

Manganese is required in small amounts for normal growth and reproduction, and symptomatic deficiency has not been shown in humans except for patients on long-term parenteral nutrition. In some patients, low manganese levels were correlated with asthma (16). Manganese is an essential cofactor for several enzymes, including manganese superoxide dismutase, the enzyme that protects mitochondria from oxidative damage. The average adult contains approximately 12 to 20 mg of manganese, and tissue levels remain very constant throughout life despite poor absorption. Normal diets are believed to contain manganese levels significantly exceeding requirements. Good manganese sources include most plants, including tea. Recommended dietary levels are shown in Table 27.10 (57,58). Manganese has low toxicity, with no known toxicity due to dietary intake. High levels of dietary manganese, however, impair iron absorption. Miners exposed to manganese dust or fumes do develop eccentricity, and a central nervous system dysfunction similar to parkinsonism (57).

## Cobalt

The only known role for cobalt in human nutrition is as the active cofactor of vitamin $B_{12}$. Consequently, it is discussed in the section on water-soluble vitamins. Cobalt is a significant allergic sensitizer (56).

## Ultratrace Elements

Some other elements are necessary for normal nutrition, at levels of less than 1 μg/g of food consumed. Although at least 18 minerals have been proposed as essential ultratrace elements, there is good experimental evidence in animals to support essentiality only for 6 of these, and only minimal evidence in humans for 1 (molybdenum). In addition, a seventh ultratrace element, fluorine, although probably not essential, reduces dental caries. Those ultratrace minerals currently believed to be essential are molybdenum, arsenic, boron, nickel, silicon, and vanadium (58). With the exception of molybdenum, none of these has been shown to cause any deficiency symptoms in humans.

*Molybdenum* is an enzyme cofactor for important detoxifying enzymes, including aldehyde oxidase, sulfate oxidase, and others. Because it may be required at levels close to average dietary intakes, people with extra needs, such as chemically exposed individuals, may need supplements. *Arsenic* is believed to be required for taurine and sulfate production from methionine, and may be involved in other methyl transfer reactions. *Boron* is known to be essential in both plants and animals, but its specific role is not yet clear, although it may be a regulator of membrane transport. *Nickel* has no known definite role in mammals, but may play a role in methionine synthesis. Nickel is a significant allergic sensitizer (56). *Silicon* is required for connective tissue and bone structure to form properly, probably by influencing calcium deposition. *Vanadium* has no known definite role in mammals, but may affect iodine transfer in the thyroid, and it has insulin-like properties. It also is very toxic. *Germanium* has been thought by some researchers also to be essential, but the evidence to date is not convincing, and germanium is a significant nephrotoxin. Deaths from germanium supplementation have been reported (58). Estimated U.S. average dietary intakes and possible requirements for the ultratrace elements are shown in Table 27.11 (58). All of the ultratrace elements, except molybdenum, are normally present in the diet at levels that exceed their estimated requirements.

## Vitamins

### Fat-soluble Vitamins

#### Vitamin A
The fat-soluble vitamins include vitamin A and related carotenoid compounds, vitamin D, vitamin E, and vitamin K. Hundreds of chemically similar, naturally occurring compounds have vitamin A activity, and many of these can be absorbed and used by humans. Carotenoids are cleaved in cells to form vitamin A, but the rate of conversion is

**TABLE 27.11. ULTRATRACE ELEMENTS: AVERAGE ADULT INTAKES, POSSIBLE REQUIREMENTS[a], AND ACUTE TOXICITY[b]**

| Element | Intake | Requirement | Acute Toxicity |
|---|---|---|---|
| Molybdenum | 180 | 75–250 | >100,000 |
| Arsenic | 75 | 12–25 | >70,000 |
| Boron | 4 | >0.4 | >100,000 |
| Fluoride | 1,000–3,000 | 1,500–4,000 | >10,000 |
| Nickel | 400 | 35 | >250,000 |
| Silicon | 20,000+ | 20,000+ | Unknown |
| Vanadium | 15–30 | 10 | >4,500 |

[a] Precise requirements for ultratrace elements are not known.
[b] In µg/day.

limited, so that vitamin A toxicity due to ingestion of carotenoids has not been a problem (32). Retinoids are readily interconverted to form active vitamin A. Retinoids can serve as antioxidants, but also can autoxidize to form reactive compounds. Chronic overdose of vitamin A, usually from chronic consumption of greater than ten times the RDA, is immunotoxic, retinotoxic, dermatotoxic, and teratogenic, whereas acute overdose is toxic to the central nervous system, with coma and death possible (59). There also is some evidence for mild liver injury with chronic use of vitamin A supplements at twice the RDA, so that vitamin A supplementation should be approached cautiously (59). To prevent fetal malformations, before and during pregnancy, vitamin A doses over 10,000 IU/day must be prevented; however, the exact teratogenic dose is unknown, and may be less. Recommended daily total vitamin A doses in pregnancy are 31 IU/kg + 330 IU (i.e., 2,250 IU for a 62-kg woman). Carotene is not teratogenic in normal doses, and may be substituted for vitamin A during pregnancy. Vitamin A deficiency may occur when most vegetables and fruits are excluded from the diet, as in very–low-carbohydrate diets. Vitamin A status cannot be determined only from the serum retinol concentration because this value does not change greatly with large changes in vitamin A stores. The absence of retinyl esters in fasting plasma is a good indicator of deficiency, and can be confirmed with several types of loading tests (59). Both retinol and retinyl esters are elevated in hypervitaminosis A.

**Vitamin D**

Provitamins $D_2$ and $D_3$ are related steroid compounds that cannot be synthesized by humans, but are absorbed from fatty fish or fish liver oil meals and transported to the skin, where ultraviolet light opens the ring structure to form vitamin D. Vitamin D is then hydroxylated in the liver to form active 1,25-dihydroxyvitamin D. Active vitamin D is essential for absorption of calcium and phosphorus and maintenance of stable levels of these minerals. Excessive vitamin D intake, of 1,000 IU/day or greater, can lead to irreversible

damage to heart, aorta, and kidneys from ectopic calcification (60). If high vitamin D doses are given, serum and urine calcium levels must be monitored. Vitamin D deficiency is thought to be common, and can occur with milk exclusion, in the elderly, and from sun avoidance and sunscreen use. Vitamin D doses of 400 IU/day, or 50,000 IU weekly for 8 weeks, are adequate for repletion in deficient adults. Vitamin D levels in serum vary rapidly with dietary and solar exposure and cannot be used as a guide to therapy. Instead, vitamin D status is determined by measuring the serum level of the previtamin, 25-hydroxyvitamin D (60).

**Vitamin E**

The group of eight chemically similar natural tocopherols and tocotrienols that are produced by plants is termed *vitamin E*. Vitamin E is a free radical chain reaction–breaking antioxidant. It also has immune-stimulatory properties that may be biologically important (61). α-Tocopherol is the most potent of the natural vitamin E components (62). Synthetic vitamin E contains eight stereoisomers of α-tocopherol, and the isomer mixture is less active than the natural isomer. There may be distinct roles for each different molecular type of natural vitamin E. For example, γ-tocopherol has been found to be the primary vitamin E component to neutralize reactive nitrogen oxides (63). Because vitamin E is the major antioxidant capable of stabilizing membranes, it is required in greater amounts when intake of unsaturated lipids such as vitamin A or EFAs increases (see earlier). Vitamin E deficiency can easily occur when consumption of any polyunsaturated oil is high, especially fish and fish oils, which do not contain significant amounts of vitamin E. Premature infants often require vitamin E supplements. Vitamin E is not readily mobilized, so that rapid depletion of membrane levels occurs when dietary supplies are low. Supplements of 400 IU/day have been shown to decrease oxidation of serum low-density lipoproteins (62).

Adult doses of vitamin E up to 3,200 IU/day appear to be free of side effects, but the actual dose at which side

**TABLE 27.12. FAT-SOLUBLE VITAMINS: AVERAGE ADULT INTAKES, REQUIREMENTS, AND ACUTE TOXICITY[a]**

| Vitamin | Intake | Requirement | Acute Toxicity |
|---------|--------|-------------|----------------|
| A | 3,300–5,400 IU | 2,666–4,000 IU | 33,000 IU[b] |
| A (pregnant) | Use caution | 31 IU/kg + 330 IU | 25,000 IU[c] |
| D | 1,000–2,000 IU | 200–400 IU | >50,000 IU |
| E | 13.5 IU | 12–18 IU | See text |
| K | 100 µg | 45–80 µg | See text |

[a]In µg/day or IU/day.
[b]Dose possibly toxic to adults.
[c]See text: dose possibly embryotoxic.

effects may occur is unknown (37,54). Vitamin E can act as a prooxidant during in vitro experiments, although it has never been observed in this role in life (62). Consequently, there is some doubt about the safety of very large supplemental doses. Large doses also may cause flatulence, malabsorption of vitamins A and K, and interference with the procoagulant activity of vitamin K (64). Vitamin E overdose is suspected of depressing lymphocyte functions, and daily doses over 10,000 IU may be teratogenic (32). Short-term vitamin E status can be determined by measuring plasma levels, whereas levels in adipose tissue reflect long-term, average levels (61).

**Vitamin K**

Like vitamin E, vitamin K is not a single chemical entity but, rather, a group of chemically similar naphthoquinones with an unsaturated side chain composed of repeating isoprene units. Produced by plants, bacteria, and by some animals, approximately half of the daily human requirement for vitamin K is supplied by bacterial synthesis from the normal small intestinal flora (65). Prolonged or repeated antibiotic therapy, as is often seen in allergic patients with otitis or sinusitis, may produce vitamin K deficiency. Breastfed infants also have low levels, and should receive vitamin K at birth. Vitamin K supplements have never been reported to have toxic effects; however, vitamin K precursors, such as menadione, can cause hemolytic anemia and hyperbilirubinemia in infants (65).

Recommended daily doses, average dietary intakes, and toxic doses for the fat-soluble vitamins are shown in Tables 27.12 and 27.13 (59,60,62,65).

*Water-soluble Vitamins*

Water-soluble vitamins include the B vitamins, $B_1$ (thiamine), $B_2$ (riboflavin), $B_3$ (niacin), $B_6$ (pyridoxine), and $B_{12}$ (cyanocobalamin), biotin, vitamin C (ascorbic acid), folic acid, and pantothenic acid. Because of their water solubility and rapid excretion, safety margins are high, but storage is limited compared with the fat-soluble vitamins. Water-

soluble vitamins therefore must be consumed in adequate amounts on a regular basis to avoid deficiency. Fortunately, water-soluble vitamins are widely distributed in foods and are required in relatively small amounts, except for vitamin C, so that obvious deficiency is unusual in the absence of chemical exposure, malabsorption, chronic illness, malnutrition, or severe allergic disease. However, subclinical deficiency is very common. For example, thiamine deficiency can be induced by alcoholism, or by frequent ingestion of raw fish, which contains a thiaminase that is able to function in the intestinal tract. Similarly, biotin deficiency can be induced by frequent ingestion of raw egg whites, which contain avidin, a biotin-complexing substance. Vitamin $B_{12}$ deficiency due to impaired absorption is surprisingly common, and increases with age. Finally, vitamin C intake frequently is too low in teenagers, women, the elderly, and the chronically ill.

**Vitamin C**

Vitamin C is the most effective water-soluble antioxidant because it readily donates electrons to quench many oxidants, and also can be easily recycled (66). Only 5 to 10 mg/day of ascorbic acid is needed to prevent scurvy, but larger doses may have significant benefits, particularly in allergy and asthma (see earlier), and should always be strongly considered for supplementation (66,67). In smokers, vitamin C is depleted at approximately twice the usual rate, and their RDA is set 40 mg higher, at 100 mg/day. It is likely that the vitamin C RDA will be raised to 120 mg (68). There is a large body of evidence that suggests even higher doses of vitamin C may reduce the risk for development of chronic diseases such as cancer, circulatory disorders, eye diseases of aging, and neurodegenerative diseases (66).

Pharmacokinetic studies show that steady-state saturation of ascorbate plasma levels can be achieved by daily doses of 200 mg, with renal losses preventing sustained higher levels. Based on metabolic turnover and absorption studies, intestinal absorption of vitamin C is saturated by single doses above 3 g (69). Single doses greater than this

**TABLE 27.13. FAT-SOLUBLE VITAMINS RECOMMENDED DIETARY ALLOWANCES**[a]

| Category | Age | Vitamin A (IU/day) | Vitamin D (IU/day) | Vitamin E (IU/day) | Vitamin K (μg/day) |
|---|---|---|---|---|---|
| Infants | 0–1 | 1,250 | 300–400 | 4.5–6 | 5–10 |
| Children | 1–10 | 1,333–2,333 | 400 | 9–10.5 | 15–30 |
| Men | 11+ | 3,333 | 200–400 | 15 | 45–80 |
| Women | 11+ | 2,666 | 200–400 | 12 | 45–65 |
| Pregnant | | See text | 400 | 15 | 65 |
| Lactating | | 4,000 | 400 | 16.5–18 | 65 |

are cathartic, and some people tolerate only lower doses without cramping. Primate comparative diet studies suggest normal human consumption should be approximately 2.3 to 10 g/day (67), consumed in frequent, small doses. Megadoses of vitamin C appear to be safe for most people (32), although hemolysis may develop in people with glucose-6-phosphate dehydrogenase deficiency, and interference with the anticoagulant effects of heparin and warfarin have been reported (66). Vitamin C does enhance iron absorption (66), but this has not been shown to cause iron accumulation, and prior suggestions that ascorbate causes oxalate kidney stones and uricosuria have been disproved (32). However, vitamin C does increase aluminum absorption, and so it should not be taken with aluminum, including some common antacids. Vitamin C status can be assessed by its measurement in plasma or leukocytes.

Other water-soluble vitamins are of critical importance in energy production and detoxification pathways and always should be supplemented in chemical toxicity. B vitamins also play a significant role in prevention of arteriosclerosis and of birth defects, and may slow aging changes in the central nervous system.

Because of individual biochemical variability, actual requirements for specific water-soluble vitamins may vary significantly from the average. Also, these vitamins can have

pharmacologic actions when used in megadose amounts. Therefore, functional assays, such as serum amino acid analysis or specific enzyme activity determinations, rather than simple measurement of vitamin levels, may be needed to assess whether a particular vitamin needs to be supplemented, in a specific person, at higher-than-usual levels. Recommended average daily doses of water-soluble vitamins are shown in Table 27.14 (66,70).

## CONCLUSION

In summary, epidemiologic and experimental studies have shown that oxidants are involved in both the pathogenesis and exacerbation of allergic diseases. Relevant oxidants can be produced in the body by allergic reactions, and also may enter the body as environmental pollutants. Oxidants can even trigger a proinflammatory positive feedback loop of gene activation that can produce a chronic allergic reaction (71). Other studies have shown that adequate antioxidant defenses are beneficial in allergic diseases, particularly in asthma, and that a number of naturally occurring antioxidants found in food contribute to our oxidant defenses. However, consensus has not yet been reached, and the optimum dietary levels are not yet known for any of these substances. Because controlled long-term human dietary studies are exceedingly difficult to perform, specific antioxidant dose recommendations that are greater than RDA values may not be available in the near future.

In lieu of specific knowledge, physicians should recommend that patients consume a varied diet that includes a wide variety of vegetables, fruits, nuts, and other foods known to contain natural antioxidants (4), vitamin C, B vitamins, minerals, and EFAs, as well as enough high-quality protein to enable optimal antioxidant enzyme synthesis. Despite a varied diet, some patients, especially growing children, and anyone with increased metabolic needs, may be nutrient deficient (72,73), particularly when their foods may have low vitamin and mineral content from poor farming practices, food processing, or prolonged storage. In the elderly, where both intestinal absorption and diet quality

**TABLE 27.14. WATER-SOLUBLE VITAMINS; ADULT AVERAGE REQUIREMENTS AND ACUTE TOXICITY**[a]

| Vitamin | Requirement | Acute Toxicity |
|---|---|---|
| $B_1$ (thiamine) | 1.2–1.6 | >350 mg/kg |
| $B_2$ (riboflavin) | 1.2–1.8 | None |
| $B_3$ (niacin) | 13–20 | >1 g |
| $B_6$ (pyridoxine) | 1.6–2.2 | >2 g |
| $B_{12}$ (cyanocobalamin) | 2.0–2.6 | >40 g |
| Biotin | 0.03–0.1 | None |
| Folic acid | 0.18–0.4 | >15 mg |
| Pantothenic acid | 4.0–7.0 | >10 g |
| Vitamin C (ascorbate) | 60–200 | None (see text) |

[a] In mg/day.

often are poor, deficiencies are very common and should be expected. Also, in patients with allergy who are either following strict avoidance diets or who have significant malabsorption as a consequence of food allergies, important deficiencies may develop. For these reasons, most patients should use vitamin and mineral supplements as insurance that at least minimal quantities of critical vitamin and mineral cofactors are ingested. Third, use of pharmacologic amounts of individual nutrients, especially vitamins C and E, should be recommended for more severely symptomatic patients with allergy (74) and in other situations where the oxidant load is known to be either high or sustained. This is particularly likely to be helpful when treating severe asthma, chronic eczema or urticaria, chronic fatigue syndrome, or, in conjunction with other therapies, for treatment of patients with chemical sensitivity (73). Pharmacologic supplements of major minerals, particularly calcium, copper, magnesium, zinc, and organic forms of sulfur (essential amino acids), also are useful in many patients. Trace mineral deficiencies may contribute to many different ailments, but because of nonspecific symptoms, rarely are identified without specific laboratory testing. Finally, iron supplements should not be used unless there is documented iron deficiency.

Because chronic use of pharmacologic doses of some vitamin and mineral supplements can be toxic (13), and because some people may absorb nutrients poorly or have significantly higher nutrient needs than average, periodic determinations of serum or cellular nutrient levels (32) are necessary to practice safe and effective nutritional therapy. Laboratory assessment of many nutrients is difficult because serum levels do not always reflect either adequate tissue levels or effective enzyme saturation (73), and many concentrations are at such low levels that they are technically challenging to quantitate. Furthermore, the presence of many interdependent metabolic pathways means that a single deficiency can have multiple manifestations, making clinical diagnosis of deficiencies also very difficult. For these reasons, although serum nutrient levels can be used as a guide to severe deficiency or toxic levels, analysis of blood cell nutrient levels, nutrient loading tests, amino acid determinations, and assay of specific enzyme activities (73) may be required to determine the true nutritional status of some patients.

Because nutrition is a rapidly changing specialty, recommendations in this chapter should be considered as tentative. Other sources should be consulted, and, where appropriate, nutritional consultation should be obtained. Each patient should be systematically evaluated for nutritional risk factors, specific nutritional deficiencies should be identified by laboratory testing, and appropriate prescriptions made for dietary modifications and supplemental nutrients. Careful follow-up also is required to avoid either inadequate treatment or toxicity due to nutritional supplement overdose or conflicts. In addition, the biochemical variability of humans should be kept in mind, because what is an adequate dose of a nutrient for one person may be toxic for

some, and insufficient for still others. If attention is paid to these precepts, nutritional therapy will become a valuable addition to each physician's armamentarium, with significant health benefits for patients with allergy.

## ACKNOWLEDGMENTS

The author thanks June L. Bianchi, Beverly J. Flynn, Nancy E. Frazier, Sally C. Schumann, and Jeanie M. Vander Pyl, Cape Cod Hospital Medical Library, for their expertise in medical literature research.

## REFERENCES

1. Gordon BR. The importance of nutrition in allergy management. *Curr Opin Otolaryngol Head Neck Surg* 1997;5:53–54.
2. Gordon BR. Update on the importance of nutrition in allergy management. *Curr Opin Otolaryngol Head Neck Surg* 1998;6:67–69.
3. Collins AR, Duthie SJ, Fillion L, et al. Oxidative DNA damage in human cells: the influence of antioxidants and DNA repair. *Biochem Soc Trans* 1997;25:326–331.
4. Jacob RA, Burri BJ. Oxidative damage and defense. *Am J Clin Nutr* 1996;63:985S–990S.
5. Conner EM, Grisham MB. Inflammation, free radicals, and antioxidants. *Nutrition* 1996;12:274–277.
6. Lubec G, Widness JA, Hayde M, et al. Hydroxyl radical generation in oxygen-treated infants. *Pediatrics* 1977;100:700–704.
7. Sanders SP, Zweir JL, Harrison SJ, et al. Spontaneous oxygen radical production at sites of antigen challenge in allergic subjects. *Am J Respir Crit Care Med* 1995;151:1725–1733.
8. Hatch GE. Asthma, inhaled oxidants, and dietary antioxidants. *Am J Clin Nutr* 1995;61:625S–630S.
9. Delfino RJ, Coate BD, Zeiger RS, et al. Daily asthma severity in relation to personal ozone exposure and outdoor fungal spores. *Am J Respir Crit Care Med* 1996;154:633–641.
10. Greene LS. Asthma and oxidant stress: nutritional, environmental, and genetic risk factors. *J Am Coll Nutr* 1995;14:317–324.
11. Kidd PM. Glutathione: systemic protectant against oxidative and free radical damage. *Altern Med Rev* 1997;2:155–176.
12. Hu JJ, Roush GC, Berwick M, et al. Effects of dietary supplementation of alpha-tocopherol on plasma glutathione and DNA repair activities. *Cancer Epidemiol Biomarkers Prev* 1996;5:263–270.
13. Hathcock JN. Vitamins and minerals: efficacy and safety. *Am J Clin Nutr* 1997;66:427–437.
14. Kubena KS, McMurray DN. Nutrition and the immune system: a review of nutrient-nutrient interactions. *J Am Diet Assoc* 1996;96:1156–1164.
15. Jaques PF, Taylor A, Hanksinson SE, et al. Long-term vitamin C supplement use and prevalence of early age-related lens opacities. *Am J Clin Nutr* 1997;66:911–916.
16. Soutar A, Seaton A, Brown K. Bronchial reactivity and dietary antioxidants. *Thorax* 1997;52:166–170.
17. Monteleone CA, Sherman AR. Nutrition and asthma. *Arch Intern Med* 1997;157:23–34.
18. Levy R, Shriker O, Porath A, et al. Vitamin C for the treatment of recurrent furunculosis in patients with impaired neutrophil functions. *J Infect Dis* 1966;173:1502–1505.
19. Lehr HA, Weyrich AS, Saetzler RK, et al. Vitamin C blocks

inflammatory platelet-activating factor mimetics created by cigarette smoking. *J Clin Invest* 1997;99:2358–2364.

20. Jeng KCG, Yang CS, Sui WY, et al. Supplementation with vitamins C and E enhances cytokine production by peripheral blood mononuclear cells in healthy adults. *Am J Clin Nutr* 1996;64:960–965.

21. Cohen HA, Neuman I, Nahum H. Blocking effect of vitamin C in exercise-induced asthma. *Arch Pediatr Adolesc Med* 1997;151:367–370.

22. Johnson CS. The antihistaminic action of ascorbic acid. *Subcell Biochem* 1996;25:189–213.

23. Meydani SN, Meydani M, Blumberg JB, et al. Vitamin E supplementation and in vitro immune response in healthy elderly subjects. *JAMA* 1997;277:1380–1386.

24. Dow L, Tracey M, Villar A, et al. Does dietary intake of vitamins C and E influence lung function in older people? *Am J Respir Crit Care Med* 1996;154:1401–1404.

25. Beck MA, Levander OA. Oxidative stress and viral infection. *Nutr MD* 1999;25:1–3.

26. Broughton KS, Johnson CS, Pace BK, et al. Reduced asthma symptoms with n-3 fatty acid ingestion are related to 5-series leukotriene production. *Am J Clin Nutr* 1997;65:1011–1017.

27. Santos MS, Meydani SN, Leka L, et al. Natural killer cell activity in elderly men is enhanced by beta-carotene supplementation. *Am J Clin Nutr* 1996;64:772–777.

28. Hughes DA, Wright AJA, Finglas PM, et al. The effect of beta-carotene supplementation on the immune function of blood monocytes from healthy male nonsmokers. *J Lab Clin Med* 1997;129:309–317.

29. Schmutzler W, Gladis-Villanueva MM, Bolsmann K, et al. Effect of beta-carotene on histamine release from human mast cells and monocytes. *Int Arch Allergy Immunol* 1997;113:335–336.

30. Misso NLA, Powers KA, Gillon RL, et al. Reduced platelet glutathione peroxidase activity and serum selenium concentration in atopic asthmatic patients. *Clin Exp Allergy* 1995;26:838–847.

31. Repine JE, Bast A, Lankhorst I. Oxidative stress in chronic obstructive pulmonary disease. *Am J Respir Crit Care Med* 1997;156:341–357.

32. Werbach MR. *Foundations of nutritional medicine.* Tarzana, CA: Third Line Press, 1997:45–78, 133–160, 267–293.

33. Horrobin DF. Post-viral fatigue syndrome, viral infections in atopic eczema, and essential fatty acids. *Med Hypotheses* 1990;32:211–217.

34. Van Asbeck BS, Van der Wal WAA. Role of oxygen radicals and antioxidants in adult respiratory distress syndrome. *Resuscitation* 1989;18:S63–S83.

35. Trowell HC, Burkitt DP. *Western diseases: their emergence and prevention.* London: Edward Arnold, 1981.

36. Jenkins DJA, Wolever TMS, Jenkins AL. Fiber and other dietary factors affecting nutrient absorption and metabolism. In: Shils ME, Olson JA, Shike M, et al., eds. *Modern nutrition in health and disease,* 9th ed. Philadelphia: Lippincott Williams & Wilkins, 1999:679–698.

37. Beaton GH. Criteria of an adequate diet. In: Shils ME, Young VR, eds. *Modern nutrition in health and disease,* 7th ed. Philadelphia: Lea & Febiger, 1988:649–665.

38. Hultman E, Thomson JA, Harris RC. Work and exercise. In: Shils ME, Young VR, eds. *Modern nutrition in health and disease,* 7th ed. Philadelphia: Lea & Febiger, 1988:1001–1022.

39. Stubbs RJ, PR Murgatroyd, GR Goldberg, et al. Carbohydrate balance and the regulation of day-to-day food intake in humans. *Am J Clin Nutr* 1993;57:897–903.

40. Byers T. Hardened fats, hardened arteries? *N Engl J Med* 1997;337:1544–1545.

41. Hu FB, Stampfer MJ, Manson JE, et al. Dietary fat intake and the risk of coronary heart disease in women. *N Engl J Med* 1997;337:1491–1499.

42. Matthews DE. The proteins and amino acids. In: Shils ME, Olson JA, Shike M, et al., eds. *Modern nutrition in health and disease,* 9th ed. Philadelphia: Lippincott Williams & Wilkins, 1999:12–48.

43. Jones PJH, Kubow S. Lipids, sterols, and their metabolites. In: Shils ME, Olson JA, Shike M, et al., eds. *Modern nutrition in health and disease,* 9th ed. Philadelphia: Lippincott Williams & Wilkins, 1999:67–94.

44. Stott WT. Chemically induced proliferation of peroxisomes: implications for risk assessment. *Regul Toxicol Pharmacol* 1988;8:125–159.

45. Horrobin DF. Essential fatty acid metabolism and its modification in atopic eczema. *Am J Clin Nutr* 2000;71:367S–372S.

46. Kankaanpaa P, Sutas Y, Salminen S, et al. Dietary fatty acids and allergy. *Ann Med* 1999;31:282–287.

47. Avioli LV. Calcium and phosphorus. In: Shils ME, Young VR, eds. *Modern nutrition in health and disease,* 7th ed. Philadelphia: Lea & Febiger, 1988:142–158.

48. Shils ME. Magnesium. In: Shils ME, Olson JA, Shike M, et al., eds. *Modern nutrition in health and disease,* 9th ed. Philadelphia: Lippincott Williams & Wilkins, 1999:169–192.

49. Fairbanks VF. Iron in medicine and nutrition. In: Shils ME, Olson JA, Shike M, et al., eds. *Modern nutrition in health and disease,* 9th ed. Philadelphia: Lippincott Williams & Wilkins, 1999:193–221.

50. Specialty Laboratories. *Hemochromatosis: an aid to definite diagnosis.* Bulletin TN52. Santa Monica, CA: Specialty Laboratories, 1991.

51. Hetzel BS, Clugston GA. Iodine. In: Shils ME, Olson JA, Shike M, et al., eds. *Modern nutrition in health and disease,* 9th ed. Philadelphia: Lippincott Williams & Wilkins, 1999:253–264.

52. King JC, Keen CL. Zinc. In: Shils ME, Olson JA, Shike M, et al., eds. *Modern nutrition in health and disease,* 9th ed. Philadelphia: Lippincott Williams & Wilkins, 1999:223–239.

53. Turnlund JR. Copper. In: Shils ME, Olson JA, Shike M, et al., eds. *Modern nutrition in health and disease,* 9th ed. Philadelphia: Lippincott Williams & Wilkins, 1999:241–252.

54. Burk RF, Levander OA. Selenium. In: Shils ME, Olson JA, Shike M, et al., eds. *Modern nutrition in health and disease,* 9th ed. Philadelphia: Lippincott Williams & Wilkins, 1999:265–276.

55. Stoecker BJ. Chromium. In: Shils ME, Olson JA, Shike M, et al., eds. *Modern nutrition in health and disease,* 9th ed. Philadelphia: Lippincott Williams & Wilkins, 1999:277–282.

56. Adachi A, Horikawa T, Takashima T, et al. Potential efficacy of low metal diets and dental metal elimination in the management of atopic dermatitis: an open clinical study. *J Dermatol* 1997;24:12–19.

57. Levander OA. Manganese. In: Shils ME, Young VR, eds. *Modern nutrition in health and disease,* 7th ed. Philadelphia: Lea & Febiger, 1988:274–277.

58. Nielsen FH. Ultratrace minerals. In: Shils ME, Olson JA, Shike M, et al., eds. *Modern nutrition in health and disease,* 9th ed. Philadelphia: Lippincott Williams & Wilkins, 1999:283–303.

59. Ross AC. Vitamin A and retinoids. In: Shils ME, Olson JA, Shike M, et al., eds. *Modern nutrition in health and disease,* 9th ed. Philadelphia: Lippincott Williams & Wilkins, 1999:305–327.

60. Holick MF. Vitamin D. In: Shils ME, Olson JA, Shike M, et al., eds. *Modern nutrition in health and disease,* 9th ed. Philadelphia: Lippincott Williams & Wilkins, 1999:329–362.

61. Meydani M. Vitamin E. *Lancet* 1995;345:170–175.

62. Traber MG. Vitamin E. In: Shils ME, Olson JA, Shike M, et al., eds. *Modern nutrition in health and disease,* 9th ed. Philadelphia: Lippincott Williams & Wilkins, 1999:347–362.

63. Ralof J. Health benefits of another vitamin E. *Sci News* 1997; 151:207.
64. Bieri JG, Corash L, Hubbard VS. Medical uses of vitamin E. *N Engl J Med* 1983;308:1063–1071.
65. Olson RE. Vitamin K. In: Shils ME, Olson JA, Shike M, et al., eds. *Modern nutrition in health and disease,* 9th ed. Philadelphia: Lippincott Williams & Wilkins, 1999:363–380.
66. Jacob RA. Vitamin C. In: Shils ME, Olson JA, Shike M, et al., eds. *Modern nutrition in health and disease,* 9th ed. Philadelphia: Lippincott Williams & Wilkins, 1999:467–483.
67. Pauling L. *How to live longer and feel better.* New York: Avon Books, 1986.
68. Levine M, Rumsey SC, Daruwala R, et al. Criteria and recommendations for vitamin C intake. *JAMA* 1999;281:1415–1423.
69. Levine M, Dhariwal KR, Welch RW, et al. Determination of optimal vitamin C requirements in humans. *Am J Clin Nutr* 1995;62:1347S–1356S.
70. Bloch AS, Shils ME. Appendix. In: Shils ME, Olson JA, Shike M, et al., eds. *Modern nutrition in health and disease,* 9th ed. Philadelphia: Lippincott Williams & Wilkins, 1999:A3–A210.
71. Barnes PJ, Katin M. Nuclear factor kappa-B: a pivotal transcription factor in chronic inflammatory diseases. *N Engl J Med* 1997; 336:1066–1071.
72. Werbach, MR. *Nutritional influences on illness.* Tarzana, CA: Third Line Press, 1993:623–631.
73. Rea WJ. *Chemical sensitivity.* Boca Raton, FL: CRC Press, 1997; 1:221–479, 2541–2684, 2091–2185.
74. Hendler SS. *The doctor's vitamin and mineral encyclopedia.* New York: Simon and Shuster, 1990:416–419.

# COMPLEMENTARY AND ALTERNATIVE MEDICINE IN OTOLARYNGIC ALLERGY

## KAREN RHEW

The purpose of this chapter is to give a brief overview of alternative medical practices in the United States and present those that at this time are useful to the otolaryngic allergist. Some treatments that the reader already may be successfully using, or that will become accepted as standard treatment in the near future, may not be included if they are controversial or if there is not yet enough substantial data on their use. It is hoped that most physicians are following the literature on alternative medicine and are ready to incorporate measures into patient care as it becomes reasonable to do so.

*Alternative medicine* is a term that includes a variety of therapies, most of which predate the development of *modern medicine* that has evolved over only the past 200 years. Most of these old, even ancient, practices were discarded or suppressed in this country as science and technology directed the advances of medicine in the Western world. Other names used to describe alternative medicine are *traditional, natural, holistic, mind–body, unconventional,* or *unorthodox* medicine. The term *complementary* medicine has been added to emphasize that many of these methods can be used in conjunction with conventional or allopathic medicine to maximize health and healing benefits for patients.

The growing importance of alternative medicine, as well as its changing nomenclature, is reflected in the establishment of the National Institutes of Health (NIH) Office of Alternative Medicine (OAM) by Congressional mandate in 1992. In 1998, the OAM was elevated to the National Center for Complementary and Alternative Medicine (NCCAM), with the mission of conducting and supporting basic and applied research and training (see Appendix B). The Center also has a clearinghouse that disseminates information on complementary and alternative medicine (CAM) to practitioners and the public.

A recent term to be used widely in conjunction with

CAM is *integrative* medicine, which refers to the process and practice of interweaving the best methods of CAM into mainstream medicine. The potential of this process is demonstrated by the University of Arizona College of Medicine Program in Integrative Medicine, which was established in 1996 with objectives of "establishing integrative medicine as a new direction within academic medicine, not as a new specialty" (1). To support this goal, the Arizona program has established a model of medical education that trains physicians, nurses, pharmacists, and other health care providers in the theory and practice of integrative medicine. The fact that more and more medical schools are developing similar programs to incorporate CAM into their curriculum ensures that there will be a substantial working relationship between alternative and conventional medicine in the future. Future physicians will understand how to evaluate and integrate CAM practices that are effective in treating their patients. This should end the dichotomy in the care of the almost 50% of health care consumers who have used some form of CAM, often without the awareness, let alone the advice, of their physician (2). This also will lay the groundwork for more basic research into alternative medicines and treatments as well as clinical outcomes studies on their efficacy.

## FORMS OF ALTERNATIVE MEDICINE

### Complete Therapeutic Systems

To understand alternative medicine as it exists today, it is helpful to take a brief look at its origins in the ancient complete therapeutic systems. These traditional systems are considered complete because they (a) encompass a working theory of health/disease, (b) have methods to diagnose and treat illness, (c) have methods to prevent disease and maintain/improve wellness, and (d) use herbal medicines, body works, and diet/nutrition as therapy. What also links them to modern CAM is the understanding that the body has a natural ability to heal itself and any treatment must facili-

**K. Rhew:** Department of Otolaryngology–Head and Neck Surgery, University of Colorado School of Medicine, Denver, Colorado.

tate, and not interfere with, this process. Also central to the various treatment approaches is the holistic belief that health and healing require a balance of mind, body, and spirit (emotions or soul). Factoring in the influence that environment and social interactions have on the person's health is part of this philosophy as well.

*Shamanism* is the earliest form of medicine, as documented by prehistoric cave paintings in Europe. Shamanistic practices continued through time in tribal and village cultures, such as witches in Europe, witch doctors in Africa, yogis in India, and Native American medicine men. Shamanism usually is a melding of religion and medicine with methods that usually include rituals for eliciting altered states of consciousness through hypnotic techniques or hallucinogenic plants. This trance state is believed to facilitate supernatural connections that aid in physical, psychological, or spiritual healing. The use of herbal medicines and physical manipulations has roots in shamanism.

Elements of shamanism can be seen in our modern society. Evangelical religious healers of today seem to have certain shamanic characteristics. The emphasis on spirituality and the supernatural aspects of the earth and universe holds great appeal for some New Age practitioners, who aspire to heal through spirituality and mystical energy techniques using crystals or energy/aura fields. Physicians in certain areas of the country where there are concentrations of Native Americans or first-generation immigrants from Indonesia, Mexico, South America, or Africa, often find that familiarity with the shamanic practices and herbal remedies used by their patients in these groups is necessary to facilitate conventional approaches.

*Ayurveda* is perhaps the oldest medical system, with documentation back to circa 3000 b.c. It evolved in the context of ancient Indian civilization and Hindu philosophy. Of all the ancient healing systems, Ayurveda most emphasizes maintaining health through a deep mind–body connection, using the formalized practice of *yoga* with its posturing, breath control, and meditation to facilitate this. Ayurvedic medicine was banned in India in 1835 under British rule. However, it was reinstated in the first part of the 20th century and is practiced alongside Western medicine in India today.

Partly because of the common influence of Buddhism, Ayurveda and Chinese medicine share many philosophical and therapeutic similarities. Central to both is a concept of life force or energy, called *prana* in Ayurveda and *chi* or *qi* in Chinese medicine. In addition to highly developed pharmacopoeias of herbal remedies, both systems intertwine medicine and food by using dietary modifications as an important treatment modality.

In India, Ayurvedic physicians undergo 5 years of training. Most Ayurvedic medicine practiced in the United States is Maharishi Vedic Medicine, founded by Maharishi Mahesh Yogi, who is perhaps best known for also bringing Transcendental Meditation to this country in the 1960s.

This modernized version of Ayurveda is taught in a worldwide network of universities and at five Maharishi Vedic Medical Centers in the United States (see Appendix B).

*Oriental medicine* originated over 2,500 years ago in China and strongly influenced Japanese, Korean, Vietnamese, Tibetan, and Indonesian medicine.

Chinese medicine is based on the understanding that life-giving energy, qi or chi, flows throughout the body. When qi is blocked, pain or illness results. In turn, qi is regulated by a balance of the *yin* and *yang,* the opposing forces that govern the universe and all living things. Yang qualities are positive, such as heat, strength, and light; yin qualities are negative such as coldness, weakness, and dark. For example, a person who complains of fatigue and is observed to be pale and have cold hands is diagnosed as having an excess of yin. Conversely, a person complaining of severe pain and noted to be feverish with flushed face would be said to have an excess of yang. Treatment is designed to restore yin–yang balance and the natural flow of qi. Perhaps the yin and yang concept can be loosely correlated with the balance of sympathetic and parasympathetic domains in the autonomic nervous system.

The traditional Oriental medicine practitioner considers diet, herbal medicines, and physical therapies (i.e., acupuncture, acupressure massage, or therapeutic exercise such as tai chi), whether prescribing for the maintenance and enhancement of wellness or the treatment of illness. However, practice in the United States often is limited to acupuncture or acupressure. The meditative physical exercises such as tai chi often are taught by instructors in martial arts who may or may not practice other aspects of Oriental medicine.

*Traditional Arabic* or *Islamic medicine* dates back to the 7th century, when Islam expanded into areas of Europe that had formerly been part of the Greco-Roman Empires. The Greek fathers of Western medicine such as Hippocrates (c. 460–360 b.c.) and Galen (a.d. 130–200) had been influenced by Oriental medicine but are believed to have had a knowledge of human internal anatomy that had been forbidden to the Chinese. Greek and Arabic herbal medicines naturally were derived from the native plants in the Mediterranean and Middle East, which, in turn are similar to those found in Europe. The four humors of ancient Greek medicine—blood, phlegm, yellow bile, and black bile—also are found in the conceptual basis of Arabic medicine, as well as Western medicine as late as the 1700s. Islamic medicine was later influenced by Ayurveda when the Muslims invaded India in the 11th century. This form of Arabic medicine, known as Unani-Tibb, is still practiced by Muslims in India and Asia.

## Naturopathy

Modern naturopathy can be traced from the complete traditional medical system learned by the Greeks from the Orient, and adopted by Arabs who passed it on to Western

Europe during the Dark Ages (A.D. 500 to 900). Unfortunately, despite the rebirth of learning that came with the Renaissance, beginning in the 14th century, harsh treatments such as bloodletting, leeches, cathartics, and the use of toxic chemicals eventually seemed to take a more prominent role over more gentle healing methods. In the 1800s, several Germans pioneered systems of medical practice based the healing power of nature. Vincent Preissnitz founded the *Nature Cure,* based on the innate healing processes of the body and using natural therapies of clean air and water, foods, herbals, and bodywork. His work was brought to America by Benedict Lust, who emigrated from Germany in the early 1900s. Naturopathy managed to remain intact as a complete system of natural healing despite pressure from the scientific approach that came with the Industrial Revolution in the 18th and 19th centuries, and formed modern Western medicine (3). Today, three schools of naturopathy have 4-year postgraduate degree programs: the National College of Naturopathic Medicine in Portland, Oregon, the John Bastyr College of Naturopathic Medicine in Seattle, Washington, and the Southwest College of Naturopathic Medicine in Tempe, Arizona. These colleges produce well educated graduates who have backgrounds in basic sciences and a clinical curriculum that is similar to the standard in medical schools. In addition, they are trained in holistic methods, including clinical nutrition, botanical medicine, homeopathy, acupuncture, and psychological counseling, with strong emphasis on optimizing wellness and disease prevention. Graduates of these programs hold Doctor of Naturopathic Medicine (N.D. or N.M.D.) degrees and are eligible to apply for the naturopathic licensing examinations administered by the North American Board of Naturopathic Examiners, and any of the state licensing boards. Graduates also are eligible to join the American Association of Naturopathic Physicians (AANP), which ensures that the N.D. degrees of their members meet the educational criteria for licensure. State licensure allows a naturopathic physician to practice as a primary care physician.

The AANP is actively seeking to standardize the practice and licensure of naturopaths in all states by 2008. To date, only 12 states and Puerto Rico have such licensing laws. In the meantime, a great many of those who currently practice naturopathy have degrees obtained through correspondence schools, seminars, or short courses without the rigorous standards of the 4-year degree. Close attention to proper credentialing and licensing of naturopathic physicians is warranted because it allows them to practice as primary care physicians (see Appendix B). In addition, a qualified naturopathic physician may be considered a general practice CAM physician who is uniquely qualified to facilitate integration of alternative and allopathic medicine. Such a professional will be a valuable resource for the physician seeking appropriate CAM treatments for his or her patients (see Appendix B).

## Homeopathy

Although Hippocrates used remedies based on homeopathic methods, modern homeopathy was founded by Samuel Hahnemann, a German physician and chemist. In the late 1700s, Western medical practices were characterized by traumatic and ineffective treatments such as bloodletting. Dr. Hahnemann became disenchanted by the lack of scientific and clinical rationale for the medical practices of his day. This dissatisfaction, as well as his training in chemistry, eventually led him to develop the system of homeopathic medicine, at the heart of which is to effect a cure by matching a precise homeopathic remedy to the patient's history and symptom pattern. This requires a detailed history on each patient and thorough knowledge of the more than 3,000 homeopathic remedies that are compiled in standard pharmacopoeias such as the *Homeopathic Pharmacopoeia of the United States.* These remedies are based on the principal that substances that produce certain symptoms of illness in a well person can also cure the same symptoms if they are caused by illness. The first example of this phenomenon that Hahnemann investigated was quinine, which causes symptoms of malaria in a well person but relieves these same symptoms in a person with malaria. Hence the name *homeopathy,* which means "treating like with like."

The homeopathic remedies must be so specifically and meticulously prepared that most practitioners obtain them from pharmacies specializing in these preparations. Substances used in remedies come from plants, minerals, drugs (penicillin, cortisone), and nosodes (products of disease such as gonorrheal discharge, tuberculous granuloma, and influenza virus). Remedies are extremely dilute, with the premise that the greater the dilution, the more potent the remedy. For example, many remedies are diluted further than 1 millionth ($10^{-6}$ or $6\times$ potency). Some substances exceed the dilution of Avogadro's number ($10^{24}$ or $24\times$), which means that not even one molecule of the substance remains in the dilution. Conventional medicine is critical of unsubstantiated homeopathic theory, which maintains that "the energy which is contained in a limited form in the original substance is somehow released and transmitted to the molecules of the solvent. Once the original substance is no longer present, the remaining energy in the solvent can be continually enhanced *ad infinitum*" (4). At least it can be said that this extreme dilution makes homeopathic dilutions safe, nontoxic, and relatively inexpensive. Despite the criticisms of conventional medicine, homeopathy has been proven to work for many people. Certainly, this concept of serially dilute substances being efficacious when properly administered to a closely evaluated patient bears certain similarities to hyposensitization injections. In fact, there are a number of homeopathic remedies specifically for allergic conditions. Many homeopathic remedies can be purchased over the counter without the guidance of a homeopathic practitioner. The directions on the package should be followed exactly.

Homeopathy is considered by some to be a specialty in the medical system of naturopathy. Most practitioners come from backgrounds such as naturopathy or chiropractic, and some even are lay persons without formal degrees. There are only approximately 200 medical doctors practicing homeopathy in the United States. The fact remains that the modern science and art of homeopathy is exquisitely complicated when practiced in its purest form, requiring full commitment on the part of the practitioner. A true homeopath adheres strictly to the laws and standards of homeopathy because taking shortcuts will produce inconsistent results in patient benefit. Formal training usually involves a type of apprenticeship to an experienced practitioner, in addition to intensive, ongoing study (see Appendix B).

## Nutritional Therapy

In traditional Chinese medicine, diet is the first therapeutic intervention considered, followed by herbals, then physical therapy or acupuncture. In Ayurvedic medicine, impaired digestion is believed to be the primary cause of allergies. The practice of *fasting,* long a part of the Ayurvedic tradition, probably stems from the instinctive loss of appetite as a coping response to illness, experienced by people and animals alike. Other forms of dietary therapy considered to be on the "fringe" of alternative are *macrobiotic, vegetarian,* and *vegan* diets. Elimination and rotation diets are used by many CAM practitioners. Charged with managing patients with food allergies, otolaryngic allergists have always used dietary and nutritional methods that were not used in mainstream medicine. This practice was established as a mainstay of patient treatment largely because of the work of the two pioneers in the field of otolaryngic allergy, Herbert J. Rinkel and Theron Randolph, who developed the concept that food allergy could cause a multitude of systemic symptoms that could be controlled mainly with diet.

In the strictest definition, *nutritional therapy* involves the prescription of micronutrients (i.e., vitamins, minerals, and trace elements). The official view of the medical profession has recently become supportive of a daily multivitamin intake for adults (5). This is especially important for the allergic patient because food allergies and the constant stress of the hyperimmune state, often in the face of frequent antibiotics and steroids, can disrupt the digestive absorption process and deplete vitamin and mineral reserves. Without a diet that provides basic nutritional requirements needed for healing and optimum health, few of the other treatment measures, including hyposensitization injections, are likely to be maximally effective. Establishing a hypoallergenic, whole-foods diet for patients should include recommendations for basic nutritional supplements such as:

*Multivitamin–multimineral capsule*—This should be a hypoallergenic product that has adequate amounts of B-complex vitamins, antioxidants, and minerals in bioavailable forms. Supplements containing B vitamins should be taken early in the day because they stimulate metabolism and energy, which is desirable during the day but not at bedtime. An example of a reasonably priced, hypoallergenic multivitamin–multimineral capsule is TwinLab Daily Two (Twin Laboratories Inc., Ronkonkama, NY).

*Vitamin C*—Humans cannot store vitamin C, so it should be taken several times a day to be available when the body needs it. Most multivitamins provide at least 200 mg/day, which is the maximum amount the cells can absorb. However, during viral illnesses or certain disease states, the body may have an increased need for vitamin C. A superior form is Ester C (Inter-Cal, Prescott, AZ), which is buffered in such a way as to have over twice the absorption, with less chance of irritating the stomach, than unbuffered forms of vitamin C.

*Flax seed oil* 1,000 mg/day—This is a vegetarian source of the beneficial *omega-3 fatty acids* found in fish oil. These essential fatty acids are antiinflammatory and support the joints and cardiovascular system. The average American diet is deficient in these important nutrients.

NOTE: Rancid oils of any kind are unhealthy and even can be toxic. Supplements with an oil component should be kept in the refrigerator and discarded unless they have a fresh, nutty smell or are odorless. Oils in capsule form have a much longer shelf life than bottled oils.

As with all plant oils, the purity and healthful qualities are preserved if they are extracted by *cold pressing*, and not with the use of heat or chemicals.

*Evening primrose oil* (or black currant oil or borage oil) 90 mg GLA/day—These are sources of the *omega-6 fatty acids (γ-linolenic acid or GLA),* which support the production of antiinflammatory prostaglandins and are a nutrient for hair, skin, and nails.

*Chelated calcium* (500 to 1,000 mg) + *magnesium* (250 to 500 mg)—Calcium supplements are widely recommended and it is important to take magnesium along with calcium. Combination tablets with a ratio of half as much magnesium as calcium are commonly available. If constipation is a problem, additional chelated magnesium may be taken. The neuromuscular connections in the body depend on a balance of calcium and magnesium to function properly. Taking a calcium/magnesium supplement at dinner or bedtime promotes muscle relaxation and a more restful sleep. Also, the bones tend to take up calcium better when at rest. Chelated or citrated forms of calcium/magnesium are better absorbed than mineral salts such as calcium carbonate.

## Herbal Medicine

Also called *botanicals, herbals, phytotherapy,* and *phytomedicine,* herbal medicine refers to plants or parts of plants that are used as medicine. Herbs used as spices for flavoring food and for their aromatic oils in fragrances and soaps also are considered botanicals.

Herbalism is probably the oldest form of healing therapy, having evolved with humankind's reliance on plants as a food source. Ancient cultures throughout the world are known to have used botanicals as a main form of medical treatment. Indigenous herbs may have been originally chosen for medicinal purposes based on attraction to aroma, taste, or appearance, or perhaps by observing which plants were ingested by animals when they were sick or injured. The herbs that proved to be efficacious over the years were most likely to become part of a culture's traditional medicine.

## Ayurvedic Herbalism

The complex systems of use of the hundreds of herbs in Ayurvedic and Oriental medicine have resulted from thousands of years of study and refinement. Although the Ayurvedic tradition has a vast array of medicinal plants, the regulation of diet is equally important in therapeutic intervention. Ayurvedic herbs usually are prescribed in synergistic combinations, often with minerals. Most of the Ayurvedic herbals sold in health food stores in this country consist of single-herb ingredients such as ginger, gotu kola, licorice, *Boswellia,* ashwaganda, or turmeric (curcumin).

*Caution:* Heavy metals such as lead are used as part of the formula in some imported Ayurvedic preparations. Although advocates claim the metals are processed so as to be nontoxic, these preparations still should be avoided.

## Oriental Medicine Herbalism

Traditional Oriental medicine therapists are much more plentiful in this country than Ayurvedic practitioners. Oriental medicine practitioners usually prescribe mixtures of herbs that are tailored to the individual patient's needs. In addition to herbs, the concoction may contain minerals and ingredients from animals. When Oriental medicines are purchased in health food stores in the United States, single-herb preparations are more likely to be used, such as ginseng, astragalus, ginkgo, dong quai, and schizandra. As in Ayurveda, Oriental medicine values many of its herbs such as garlic, ginger, mushrooms (*Cordyceps,* zhu ling) for their culinary as well as medicinal attributes.

*Caution:* Currently, there are several problems with using herbals imported from China, most of which can be avoided by purchasing from a reputable source only those products that list their ingredients. For example:

■ A report by the California Department of Health Services in 1998 found 47% of imported traditional Chinese patent medicines sold in California contained contaminants such as heavy metals (lead, arsenic, mercury), unwanted pharmaceutical drugs (diazepam, phenylbutazone, ephedrine), and poisons (strychnine, belladonna) (6).

■ Substandard manufacturers often counterfeit labels to make their products appear to be from reputable manufacturers who follow Good Manufacturing Practice (GMP) standards (6).

■ Tibetan medicine balls may contain lead and mercury and there is no assurance that they have been prepared in a sanitary manner (7).

■ Certain species of herbs, particularly those that are weed-like and adaptable, may be grown in toxin-contaminated soil in some Eastern countries. Although the Chinese government is taking steps to establish regulation of herbs grown for export, it is not likely to be a rapid process (8).

■ Inclusion of animal parts in some preparations have endangered species such as tigers, the Siberian musk deer, rhinoceroses, and several species of bears (9).

■ Mushrooms and fungi, which are a frequent component in Oriental medicine remedies for their potent immune-enhancing properties, may cause problems for patients with mold allergies.

## Western Herbalism

When European settlers migrated in the 1700 and 1800s, they carried with them seeds of their most valued crop plants and medicinal herbs. In the North America, the climate was similar enough to that of Europe that the seeds often were viable. If not, similar indigenous plants could be found with the help of Native Americans who had considerable knowledge of their medicinal uses. This type of frontier setting encouraged the development of a simple blending of Native American and Western medicine such as that popularized by an unorthodox herbal practitioner named Samuel Thomson (1769–1843). Two more sophisticated naturopathic herbal systems were developed by groups known as *Eclectic Physicians* and *Physiomedicalism* practitioners who trained at medical schools teaching herbalism. This was a golden age of herbalism in the United States, which spread to Canada and Britain. However, the practice of herbal medicine went into decline after 1907, when the U.S. government began providing financial support only to conventional medical schools. Fortunately, research and government support of botanicals continued in other countries such as Germany, France, Japan, and China. It was not until the 1980s that public demand in this country started the revival of natural medicine alternatives. Congressional passage of the Dietary Supplement Health and Education Act in 1994 did not recognize herbals as medicines in their own right but did allow for their regulation as dietary supplements with limited but helpful information on use for the consumer. Moreover, the NIH Office of Dietary Supplements in collaboration the NCCAM has established four Centers for Dietary Supplement Research. These centers, located at Purdue University, University of Arizona, University of California at Los Angeles, and the University of Illinois, are funded $1.5 million per year for 5 years to promote scientific study of botanicals and to explore more fully the potential role of botanical dietary supplements. This type of government support constitutes a solid foundation for research, leading to clinical application of herbal medicines that should have far-reaching, cost-effective benefits in national health care.

It appears likely that by the year 2010, American medical schools will be preparing physicians to understand and integrate herbal and nutritional supplements into their conventional medical practices; but for now most physicians must seek such information in the form of self-conducted continuing education. Although dietary supplements can be considered part of the daily food intake, herbal medicines should be viewed as natural over-the-counter drugs. As such, taking botanicals should be reserved for when a therapeutic effect for a specific health problem is needed.

That being said, there are some *tonic* herbals in Oriental medicine that are prescribed on a routine basis to invigorate the healthy person and impart resilience in the debilitated:

Ginseng *(Panax ginseng)* is perhaps the best known of these, possibly for its reputation for increasing male sexual vigor.

Astragalus *(Astragalus membranaceus)* is a less expensive tonic herb used for general immune system support. It has been shown to stimulate nearly every phase of immune system activity, including increasing the number of stem cells in the marrow and lymphoid tissues, increasing the activity of macrophages, and increasing the production of interferon (10). It is used extensively for cancer treatment in China, and is being researched for that purpose in this country as well. Astragalus also can be used to decrease the severity and duration of colds and upper respiratory infections.

Other tonic herbs that are more familiar to Americans and can be simply included in the daily diet are *green tea, ginger,* and *garlic.*

Green tea has beneficial compounds (epigallocatechins) which have anticancer effects and lower cholesterol. It also has a natural form of the bronchodilator, theophylline. There is 40 to 70 mg of caffeine in a cup of tea, and decaffeinated green tea with the same benefits also is available. Black tea loses much of the beneficial catechin components when it is fermented; more important, however, *Aspergillus* fungus is used in the fermentation process, which can affect patients with mold allergies.

Ginger *(Zingiber officinale)* has many beneficial properties, but is used most frequently as an antiinflammatory for the gastrointestinal tract and the musculoskeletal system. It has been shown to decrease nausea in seasickness.

Garlic *(Allium sativum)* has substantial antimicrobial action, being effective against bacteria, viruses, and fungi (see later).

## NATURAL REMEDIES FOR SPECIFIC PROBLEMS

See Appendix A for sources of specific herbal supplements.

### Allergic Rhinitis and Hay Fever

Three natural substances that have antihistaminic properties without the undesirable side effects of dryness and drowsiness:

*Quercetin* 400 mg + *vitamin C* 1,400 mg—Take one capsule 20 minutes before each meal. Quercetin, a bioflavonoid, and high-dose vitamin C both have an antihistaminic effect. Quercetin stabilizes mast cells and inhibits immunoglobulin G–mediated histamine release.

*Fresh freeze-dried nettles* (*Urtica dioica* leaf)—The antihistaminic properties of the stinging nettles leaf are effectively preserved only with fresh freeze-drying (11) (see Appendix B).

*Zicam Allergy Relief*—Spray this gel inside each nostril every 4 hours while awake until hay fever symptoms subside. This is a homeopathic remedy that reduces severity and duration of symptoms of allergic rhinitis, and has no side effects (12).

### Upper Respiratory Infections

Start these measures at the first sign of symptoms:

*Vitamin C*—1,000 mg three times a day; use buffered vitamin C to avoid gastrointestinal upset.

*Garlic*—Two forms can be taken:

- Two garlic cloves finely chopped. Avoid "garlic breath" by washing down garlic particles with a glass of water without chewing them. Chewing parsley afterward also helps.
- One tablet two times a day of *Garlinase 4000* (Enzymatic Therapy) (Seacoast Natural Foods, Imperial Beach, CA)—a fresh-preparation garlic tablet standardized to 5,000 μg of allicin (the most beneficial component of garlic).

Garlic is antiviral, antibacterial, and stimulates the immune response in general.

*Echinacea (Echinacea purpurea)*—One capsule three times a day of 50 mg echinacea standardized for 2.4% fructofuranosides. Echinacea is the most frequently purchased botanical in the United States. There is a good deal of literature supporting its efficacy (13). It has been shown to increase the number and activity of the natural killer T cells, and increase production of interferon.

*Astragalus (A. membranaceus)*—One capsule three times a day of 250 mg astragalus root extract 10:1 standardized to contain 0.5% of the isoflavone 4' hydroxy 3' methoxy isoflavone 7. Astragalus stimulates the general immune response.

*Zicam Cold Remedy*—Spray this nasal gel to the inside of each nostril every 2 to 4 hours until symptoms subside. Reports show that this reduces severity and duration of symptoms of upper respiratory infections (14).

*Zinc lozenges*—Dissolve one lozenge in mouth every 2 to 4 hours. To obtain maximum ionization of zinc for best effect, choose a brand that has *glycine* and no citric acid, mannitol, or sorbitol (15). *Slippery elm* is beneficial in lozenges because of mucilages that cause secretion of mucus soothing to the mucous membranes of the throat and digestive tract.

### Green Tea, Herbal Teas

Drink four to six cups per day. Sipping warm, steamy liquids hydrates the respiratory tract and stimulates mucociliary action for clearing secretions.

- *Green tea* contains beneficial compounds (epigallocatechins) that have anticancer effects and lower cholesterol (see earlier). It also has a natural form of the bronchodilator, theophylline, which may be helpful during an upper respiratory tract infection.
- *Slippery elm* works by causing reflex stimulation of nerve endings in mucous membranes, resulting in secretion of a protective mucus coating. The inner bark of the elm is used and is not known to have cross-reactivity in people who are allergic to elm pollen.
- *Chamomile* has soothing, antiinflammatory properties. *Caution:* As a member of Compositae family, it has the potential to cross-react in people who are allergic to ragweed or related species.

*Caution: Comfrey (Symphytum officinale)* has been popular in folklore for making tea and still is sold, but it contains *pyrrolizidine alkaloids,* which are toxic to the liver and should never be taken internally in any form. However, comfrey can be used safely and effectively when applied externally in compresses for nonhealing wounds.

### Additional Natural Measures

Drink at least 2 quarts of noncaffeinated fluids a day.

*For nasal congestion*—Irrigate the nose with saline solution. The solution can be "snuffled" from a cupped hand rather than using bulb syringe, which cannot be thoroughly dried out between uses and usually is made of potentially allergenic latex or vinyl.

*For sinusitis*—Place a warm or cold pack (whichever feels better) over forehead and sinus areas. Sleep with head and upper body elevated.

*For congestion and cough:*

Breathe steam. Boil water in a small pot, remove from burner. Drape a towel over head to form a "tent" to catch the steam, and breathe it in.

Use a vaporizer or humidifier, especially at night. Direc-

tions should be followed for cleaning the machine to avoid mold and bacterial contamination.

*Rest!*—This allows the body to make more energy and resources available to the immune system to fight the infection.

## Latent Viral Infections (Herpes Simplex Virus), Shingles, Hepatitis

*L-lysine* 500 mg two times a day—Antagonizes arginine uptake necessary for viral replication.

*Garlic*—Two fresh minced cloves or one or two tablets of *Garlinase 4000* (Enzymatic Therapy) (see earlier). Garlic is antiviral and stimulates the immune response in general.

*Herpilyn* (Enzymatic Therapy, Green Bay, WI)—Apply topically to herpetic lesions two to four times a day, or more if needed. The active ingredient is allantoin 1% from comfrey. There is also a base of *Melissa* extract 70:1 that has antiviral properties of its own (16).

*Milk thistle (Silybum marianum)* standardized to contain 70% silymarin—This botanical has impressive ability to stimulate regeneration of liver cells and then protect them from toxic injury. It is nontoxic, well tolerated, and can be taken indefinitely for chronic viral infections such as hepatitis. It is recommended to be taken with any pharmaceuticals that tax the liver's detoxification capacity, such as systemic antifungals (see Appendix A).

## Oropharyngeal Lesions, Thrush, Geographic Tongue

*Grapefruit seed extract*—Five to ten drops in 5 oz water, swish and swallow three times a day after meals. This is a citricidal synthesized from the polyphenolic compounds found in grapefruit seed and pulp. This botanical inhibits growth of bacteria, fungi, and viruses and also has antiparasitic properties. It was originally developed as an alternative to chemical pesticides and antifungals for fruit and vegetable crops (see Appendix A).

*Paddock Nystatin Powder*—¼ Teaspoon in 8 oz water, swish and swallow three times a day after meals.

*Deglycyrrhizinated licorice root extract* (DLG)—Chew two tablets 20 minutes before each meal. This is a mucigogue, stimulating production of healthy mucin in the aerodigestive tract, which promotes healing of ulcerations. The glycyrrhetinic acid, which can raise blood pressure and cause loss of $K^+$, has been processed out of the licorice extract, making DLG safe to take.

## Musculoskeletal Pain

Pharmaceutical agents, such as nonsteroidal antiinflammatory drugs (NSAIDs) and steroids, that are taken for various chronic inflammatory conditions have many undesirable side effects, often adding to the underlying allergic state and interfering with hyposensitization therapy. It is useful to have natural medicine alternatives to help patients avoid these drugs when possible.

*Glucosamine sulfate* 500 mg and *chondroitin sulfate* 400 mg—One tablet three times a day. These natural compounds relieve arthritic joint pain, stiffness, and inflammation by stimulating joint repair and then serving as the substrate for the process. By contrast, NSAIDs do nothing to stop the destructive process in the joints, and even add to it by inhibiting the synthesis of the gel-like cartilage (proteoglycan). Glucosamine, the most important of the two substances, is produced synthetically and also is derived from marine exoskeletons. Chondroitin is also synthesized and from natural sources which are shark and bovine cartilage. As yet there have been no reports of people with shellfish allergy reacting to glucosamine, or people who are allergic to beef reacting to chondroitin. There is no cross-allergenicity to sulfa drugs with these two products. Not all glucosamine–chondroitin products are of good quality, and there still is controversy over whether glucosamine sulfate or glucosamine hydrochloride is superior. Even so, there are convincing data to show that these compounds reduce joint pain and rebuild cartilage (17,18). Even the American Academy of Orthopedic Surgeons has acknowledged glucosamine sulfate as an alternative to NSAIDs and as a first approach to joint support, especially for patients with osteoarthritis (19).

*Antiinflammatory herbal mixtures*—Combinations of herbs traditionally used by Ayurvedic practitioners for the relief of pain and inflammation can be found in health food stores. Usually included are *Boswellia (boswellin), turmeric (curcumin),* and *ginger.* Quercetin and bromelain also are used in such antiinflammatory mixtures (see Appendix A).

## Gastrointestinal Problems

More often than not, patients who seek out otolaryngic allergists have significant symptoms involving the gastrointestinal tract. One of the main causes is an imbalance of bowel flora from ingesting allergenic foods and taking antibiotics, steroids, NSAIDs, and gastric acid secretion inhibitors.

### Gastroesophageal Reflux Disease

Fortunately, mild to moderate reflux symptoms usually resolve within a week or two after the allergy patient begins in earnest on a hypoallergenic diet with probiotic supplements of beneficial bacteria. Unfortunately, drugs prescribed for gastroesophageal reflux disease (GERD; histamine type 2 receptor antagonists or proton pump inhibitors) work by suppressing gastric acid secretions. This tends to disrupt the digestive process that starts with hydrochloric acid lowering the stomach pH, activating digestive

enzymes and stimulating the pancreatic output. This disrupted process allows for undigested food to reach the gut, which already may be having problems with hyperpermeability, leading to more food allergies and intolerances.

To break this cycle, *digestive enzymes* with meals may be recommended. If *papaya* and *pineapple (bromelain)* are not acceptable or effective, a plant-based enzyme (that is not derived from fungi) is recommended.

*Caution:* Animal-derived enzymes are *not* recommended because of the increased threat of *prions* infecting animals raised for meat. These very small, nonliving proteins are responsible for "mad cow disease" (bovine spongiform encephalopathy), which is contracted from eating meat of infected animals. Besides the brain, prions are found in organ tissues, which is why enzymes and endocrine hormones from animals should be avoided. The main problem is in England, but cases are increasing in Europe, and infected animals have been found in the United States. At present, prions are difficult to detect and they are not easily killed by the usual disinfectants.

For gastritis and esophagitis caused by GERD, DLG is used. Chew two tablets 20 minutes before each meal and between meals as needed. This is a mucigogue, stimulating production of healthy mucin in the aerodigestive tract, which promotes healing of ulcerations. DLG protects the lining of the stomach and duodenum. With persistent gastric symptoms, *Helicobacter pylori* infection must be ruled out.

### Constipation

Staying adequately hydrated requires at least 2 quarts of fluid a day. Soluble and insoluble *dietary fiber* in the form of fruits, vegetables, bran, and so forth, is necessary. *Fiber supplements,* particularly those containing soluble fiber, may be helpful. Hypoallergenic soluble fiber is made from rice or buckwheat.

Taking an *extra supplement of magnesium* can help with constipation; start with 200 mg and increase the dose to "bowel tolerance" (loose stools), then reduce dose to level of comfort.

Consider any medications that might be contributing to constipation.

### Diarrhea

With acute, self-limited forms of infectious and "traveler's" diarrhea, it is important to stay well hydrated until the conditions begins to improve after a day or so. Then, *Pepto-Bismol* (Procter & Gamble, Cincinnati, OH) usually is safe to take.

A good preventative against becoming infected with bacteria and parasites that cause diarrhea is to maintain a healthy bowel flora by taking *probiotic supplements* containing beneficial bacteria such as *Lactobacillus, Acidophilus,* and

*Bifidobacterium.* Unfortunately, most brands of probiotic supplements do not have adequate amounts of live bacteria, no matter what the label says. Look for specific brands of these supplements made by companies known to have a guaranteed product. Probiotic supplements always should be stored in the refrigerator, both in the place of purchase or in the home.

Regular consumption of *fresh garlic* preparations helps suppress pathologic overgrowths of bowel organisms. However, large daily amounts of garlic over a long period can inhibit the normal flora.

*Ciprofloxacin* usually is the antibiotic of choice for diarrheal illness while traveling.

### Gas and Bloating

These symptoms are seen frequently in patients who have had frequent antibiotic or steroid ingestion. It is assumed that they indicate a fermentation excess caused by overgrowth of normal bowel yeast. Antifungals *(nystatin* or *fluconazole)* or natural remedies *(garlic, berberine, uva ursi, oregano)* may be needed to balance microorganisms. Excessive flatus also may indicate a deficiency of digestive enzymes or hydrochloric acid.

## Recurrent Fungal Skin Infections

Preparations effective against recurrent fungal skin infections include *grapefruit seed extract* (see Appendix A) and *100% tea tree oil (Melaleuca alternifolia);* the latter can be purchased at health food stores.

When jock itch, athlete's foot, tinea versicolor, and the like continue to recur after adequate treatment with oral and topical antifungal prescription medications, the routine daily use of antifungal soap and shampoo may be helpful in eradicating or keeping these organisms at bay. Shampoos and gel body soaps containing grapefruit seed extract or tea tree oil may be purchased, or five to ten drops of the grapefruit extract or tea tree oil can be added to the shampoo or soap gel normally used.

For *fungal nails,* tea tree oil can be rubbed into the cuticle and any thickened calluses daily while an oral antifungal is taken to speed up the eradication of the nail fungus. It is hoped that when other sources of fungal infection or overgrowth, such as in the bowel, are controlled, the patient's immune response will be improved so there will be less tolerance for the dermatologic fungal overgrowths.

*Note: Milk thistle* should be taken orally when oral antifungal medications are being taken.

## Chronic Disturbed Sleeping Patterns

Patients with debilitating allergic conditions frequently complain of disturbed sleep patterns. Reestablishing the diurnal rhythm is essential because hormone production,

the immune system, body temperature, and many other functions are adversely affected by irregular sleep patterns.

Sleep disorders known to be aggravated by allergy are *sleep-onset* and *sleep-maintenance disorders, insomnia, sleep apnea,* and *restless legs.*

Factors to be considered when evaluating sleep disorders include:

- The use of *pharmacologics,* particularly psychotropics, hormone therapy, nicotine patches, antihistamines, decongestants, and various bronchodilators are known to interfere with a normal sleep cycle.
- *Food intolerance* is a primary cause of daytime fatigue and insomnia. The use of caffeine and alcohol, known food allergens, excessive consumption of sugar, and overeating are all implicated.
- *Stress* should be evaluated as a causative factor. High nighttime levels of cortisol can be caused by chronic, long-term stress resulting from constant exposure to food or environmental allergens, as well as by mental or emotional factors. The 2:00 A.M. "wakeup call" is frequently a spike of cortisol secreted in response to the absorption of an undigested food protein into the bloodstream approximately 8 hours after the ingestion of the evening meal. Chronic stress may result in a maladapted adrenal response to stress. The normal cyclic cortisol rhythm becomes inverted, resulting in sleep-onset insomnia and a pattern of morning exhaustion. The adrenal reserve becomes depleted as a result of chronic high cortisol levels, and allergic responses become more frequent and severe.

Specific nutrients for supporting healthy rest are:

- *Calcium* and *magnesium* (500 to 1,000 mg at dinner or bedtime.)
- *Omega-3* and *omega-6 fatty acid supplements*
- *Phosphatidylserine* (Seriphos) (Interplexus, Kent, WA)—Two to four tablets every morning for approximately 4 months.
- *Potassium* supplementation may be helpful for leg cramps or restless legs.

### Temporary Problems Sleeping

*Melatonin* is an effective remedy for jet lag, especially for west-to-east travel. It is also useful for *occasional* insomnia—especially for people adjusting to working late shifts or who are in a temporary stressful situation. The dose is a 1-mg tablet dissolved under the tongue at bedtime. This dose can be repeated once more if awakening occurs during the night.

## Miscellaneous

### Stevia (Stevia rebaudiana)

This is a *natural sugar substitute* that is made from the leaves of a plant in the Asteraceae family. Stevia has been used in diet soft drinks in Japan for years and is very safe. It can be purchased in health food stores in liquid or crystalline form. Because it is important for allergic patients to avoid sugar and NutraSweet, it is helpful to have a safe substitute.

### Ginkgo (Ginkgo biloba)

The preparation should be standardized for 24% ginkgoflavonglycosides. Ginkgo increases blood flow in the microcirculation, which is why it has a positive effect in memory and brain function, especially in the elderly who are at risk for problems in this area. The heart also benefits from the increased capillary blood flow. Some patients insist that ginkgo decreases tinnitus; it may well have an effect if the tinnitus is secondary to decreased blood flow to the inner ear.

### Saw Palmetto (Serenoa repens)

The preparation should be standardized to contain 85% to 95% fatty acids and sterols. Although this herbal remedy is outside the area for which an otolaryngic allergist normally would be prescribing, it is so effective in reducing enlarged prostates and is so extremely well tolerated, it seems reasonable to assure a patient on this herbal to continue taking it if it helps. Saw palmetto is not known to cause allergic reactions or cross-react with other medications.

## Aromatherapy

Aromatherapy is the use of pure essential oils from fragrant plants to improve health. Although used in ancient Egypt, India, and China, modern aromatherapy was originated in the 1930s by a French chemist and perfumer named René-Maurice Gattefosse. In France, there continues to be a system of aromatherapeutic medicine where physicians prescribe aromatherapy and pharmacies routinely stock essential oils. In the United States, aromatherapy is mostly associated with the spa and beauty industries and is used as airborne fragrance or in massage oils.

It is reasonable that aromatherapy might be effective in stress reduction through the rapid psychological and physiologic effects that are possible through the olfactory pathways. The chemical reaction of the oil molecules with the smell receptors in the nose is instantly transmitted from the olfactory bulb to the limbic system, which provides interconnections with autonomic brain stem functions, emotional response, and memory. In this regard, oils with a tranquilizing effect (lavender, chamomile, lemon balm) or a stimulatory effect (peppermint, rosemary, eucalyptus) are used by aromatherapists to effect a desired change in mood or energy.

Although very little research has been done on aromatherapy at this point, there is considerable evidence of the effectiveness of some of the essential oils when used as anti-

microbials topically and for the gastrointestinal tract. *Tea tree oil (M. alternifolia)* has antibacterial, antiviral, and antifungal properties. Oregano oil has been used as an antibacterial, antifungal, and anthelmintic agent. Oils of peppermint, rosemary, thyme, and lemon balm *(Melissa officinalis)* are antibacterial, antifungal, and antispasmodic.

*Caution:* All of the essential oils are concentrated. To avoid overdose and gastrointestinal irritation, they should be ingested only in preparations made specifically for that purpose.

Preparations of oils of oregano and savory are used to treat intestinal conditions and should not be taken for longer than 10 days.

Essential oils that are toxic when taken internally and must be avoided include *thuja, wormwood, mugwort, tansy, hyssop,* and *sage.*

*Clove* and *cinnamon* may cause a rash when applied to the skin.

Many of the essential oils are in the mint or Lamiaceae family and may produce cross-allergenicity: *basil, bergamot, horehound, hyssop, lavender, lemon balm, marjoram, oregano, peppermint, rosemary, spearmint, savory, sage, thyme.*

## PHYSICAL THERAPIES

Many allergic patients have concomitant diagnoses of chronic fatigue syndrome, fibromyalgia, arthritis, headaches, chronic pain, and stress. There are a variety of CAM physical therapies that can help relieve many of the symptoms associated with these problems.

## Acupuncture

Acupuncture originated in China over 2,000 years ago and is an integral part of traditional and modern Chinese medicine today. Since the early 1980s, acupuncture has become increasingly popular in the United States, with the expectation that the 10,000 nationally certified acupuncturists practicing in this country in 1995 would double within 5 years. Approximately one third of certified acupuncturists are medical doctors (20) (see Appendix B).

Traditional Chinese medicine holds that the qi, or life force, in an individual circulates throughout the body along 12 main and 8 secondary defined pathways called *meridians.* These invisible meridians conduct qi between the body surface and the internal organs, enabling the latter to function properly. To correct health problems caused by blockage in the flow of qi, the meridians are accessed by inserting fine, solid metal needles into the more than 2,000 acupuncture points on the skin. The points are selected by history and examination with emphasis on tongue and pulse diagnosis. The needles simply may be left in place during treatment, or they may be gently stimulated by lifting, rotating, or flicking.

Clinical studies have shown that acupuncture is effective, by itself or in combination with conventional therapy, for certain conditions such as postoperative dental pain and nausea secondary to surgical anesthesia and cancer chemotherapy. Acupuncture also can be useful in treating addiction headaches, menstrual cramps, tennis elbow, fibromyalgia, myofascial pain, osteoarthritis, low back pain, carpal tunnel syndrome, and asthma (20).

The physiologic basis for acupuncture is unclear because the meridians do not directly correlate with nerve and blood circulation pathways. However, it has been shown that endogenous opioids may be released into the central nervous system during acupuncture, reducing pain (21). Acupuncture also can trigger the release of beneficial neurotransmitters and neurohormones that influence immune function and involuntary functions such as regulation of blood pressure, circulation, and body temperature (20).

There are other forms of treatment that are based on acupuncture points:

In *electroacupuncture,* weak electrical stimulation is applied at acupuncture sites, with or without needle insertion.

*Acupressure* uses fingertip pressure to acupuncture points. It is especially useful in patients fearful of needles and can be easily taught as a self-help technique.

*Moxibustion* involves stimulation of acupuncture sites with warmed ashes of dried moxa (*Artemesia vulgaris* or mugwort leaves).

In *cupping,* small cups or jars made of glass, bamboo, or metal are heated with a match, creating a vacuum. The cups are quickly applied to acupuncture points for 10 to 15 minutes while suction draws blood to the skin, leaving typical erythematous marks for up to 24 hours.

### Nambudripad's Allergy Elimination Techniques

*Nambudripad's Allergy Elimination Techniques* (NAET), a treatment for allergies that uses acupuncture points, was developed by a California chiropractor, Dr. Devi Nambudripad (22). A patient's sensitivity to various foods and substances is diagnosed by a kinesiology method in which the NAET practitioner tests muscle strength in the patient's arm while he or she is holding a closed vial containing a potential allergenic substance. Then, one at a time and in a specific order, each allergen is held near the body and "cleared" using acupressure or acupuncture, the treatment points being determined by the level of the sensitivity to the particular substance. After therapy, the patient abstains from the offending allergen for 25 hours. Advocates of this technique claim that 80% to 90% of patients experience complete and permanent relief from their allergenic symptoms caused by the items for which they have been treated. Critics of this technique point out that the claimed cure rates have not been substantiated by valid clinical outcomes studies. Furthermore, the muscle strength testing used to identify allergens and quantitate the patient's sensitivity to them is based on the subjective judgment of the examiner. Although the exact mechanism by which acupuncture treatment benefits other illnesses is not known, at least outcomes studies have documented its effectiveness. It is possible that acupressure and acupuncture could reduce hypersensitivity by affecting immune function or gastrointestinal function in general. However, proper studies must be carried out if NAET is to gain credibility as a treatment method.

### BioSet

Another chiropractor, Dr. Ellen Cutler, has developed a therapy call *BioSet* that elaborates on NAET (23). Instead of muscle testing, a computerized *BioMeridian Meridian Stress Assessment Machine* is used to identify allergens by measuring the electrical activity generated along the acupuncture meridians when a vial of antigen is held close to the body. This U.S. Food and Drug Administration–registered machine is used to test over 11,000 allergens. The patient then goes through a detoxification process using plant enzymes (many from fungal sources) to aid digestion and metabolic clearing. When detoxification is satisfactory, the acupressure clearing of allergens can be done. As with NAET, the BioSet method must be validated with properly conducted clinical studies before it is accepted by conventional medicine.

## Bodywork

Bodywork includes a number of "hands-on" systems of therapy in which the practitioner uses physical manipulation of a patient's body to effect beneficial changes. Most ancient cultures had some form of body work therapy, some of which have evolved into modern versions of physical therapies. The traditional basis of bodywork in the West comes from the *bone-setters,* who practiced healing techniques of massage and manipulation in Europe during the Middle Ages (3). Although this tradition virtually died out in Europe with the onset of modern medicine, new systems of bodywork were developed in the United States beginning in the late 1800s.

### Osteopathic Manipulative Therapy

Andrew Taylor Still was an Army surgeon when he founded osteopathic medicine in 1874. Like the founders of the naturopathic movement, he sought to replace some of the more brutal aspects of modern medicine with methods that used the natural healing powers of the body. From his premedical background as an engineer, Still was guided by the concept of "structure governs function" in devising a system of manipulations of the muscles and their bone and joint attachments designed to correct imbalances and maladjustments. His rationale for osteopathic manipulative therapy

(OMT) was that misalignment of the musculoskeletal system caused by injury, illness, or psychological strain could in turn produce other forms of illness. Doctors of Osteopathy (D.O.) are now indistinguishable from Medical Doctors (M.D.) in their education and practice of medicine. Only a few osteopaths use OMT as a significant part of their practice today (see Appendix B).

## Cranial Osteopathy

*Cranial osteopathy* was developed in the 1930s by an American osteopath, William Garner Sutherland. Cranial osteopathy involves fine, light touching of the skull and sacrum, manipulating any of the bones and sutures that still have mobility. Skilled practitioners can detect pulsations of the cerebrospinal fluid that fluctuate with breathing. Altering the flow of this fluid by gentle manipulation theoretically can relieve dysfunction in the central nervous system and other parts of the body. Much of pediatric OMT consists of these cranial manipulations. It is particularly aimed at treating headaches, sinus and facial pain, temporomandibular symptoms, and ear problems, including infection and tinnitus.

## Craniosacral Therapy

Craniosacral therapy is a recent extension of cranial osteopathic technique developed by John E. Upledger. The treatment goals of craniosacral therapy are the same as for cranial osteopathy, but the manipulations tend to follow a sequence of movements not dictated by symptoms.

## Chiropractic

Daniel David Palmer founded the first school of chiropractic in Davenport, Iowa, in 1895, although it is his son, Bartlet Joshua Palmer, who is known for establishing this form of therapy in the United States. The core concept of diagnosis and treatment in chiropractic is that pain and illness are caused by abnormal stress on the nervous system from mechanical, chemical, or psychological sources. Because of the close integration of nerves, bones, joints, and muscles, treatment is focused on manipulation and adjustment of the musculoskeletal system, especially the spine. The chiropractic profession is criticized by conventional medicine for inconsistent standards of education because not all Doctor of Chiropractic (D.C.) degrees require 4 years of postgraduate training. This becomes particularly relevant because many chiropractors also practice other forms of CAM, such as homeopathy, herbals, nutrition, and colonic cleansing. Nevertheless, chiropractic is the largest alternative medical profession and is licensed in all 50 states (24) (see Appendix B).

## Massage Therapy

Massage was practiced as a structured therapy over 5,000 years ago in China and Mesopotamia and was written about by Hippocrates in 500 b.c. Most modern methods of massage stem from Swedish massage, which was developed by a Swede, Per Henrik Ling, who observed Oriental techniques when he visited China in the 1800s (3). Therapeutic massage focuses on normalization of soft tissues affected by stress, injury, and illness through the use of manual techniques that improve circulation and enhance muscular relaxation. The beneficial effects of massage are likely related to stimulation and relaxing of the nervous system through musculocutaneous reflexes. The benefits of this type of integrative response to touch and stroking appear to be quite basic to the human physiology, as studies on development of premature infants have shown (25).

Depending on the therapeutic purpose of the massage, attention is directed to different parts of the body and various types and intensities of touch are used, including rubbing, stroking, kneading, and knuckling percussion. The American Massage Therapy Association is the professional organization that represents this field (see Appendix B).

There are other specialized forms of massage that require separate training and certification.

### Shiatsu Massage
*Shiatsu massage* is an ancient Japanese method based on acupuncture points and meridians.

### Reflexology
*Reflexology* refers to a method based on massage of the feet to correct health imbalances in other parts of the body. Although therapeutic manipulation of the feet was known to have been practiced in ancient Egypt and Greece, modern reflexology is based on the work of two Americans, Dr. William Fitzgerald and his follower, Eunice Ingham. The theoretic basis of this modern *reflex zone therapy* is that the entire body is divided into zones that have corresponding zones on the soles and sides of the feet. Stimulation of specific zones on both feet simultaneously is done by massage techniques, but carryover may be attempted by using special shoe inserts or having the patient use specially designed rollers.

### Rolfing
*Rolfing* is a form of deep, slow manual pressure to the muscles and connective tissue with the purpose of improving health through realigning and balancing body structure and posture. The full treatment course entails ten 1-hour sessions, each focusing on a different part of the body without regard to a set of symptoms, but with the goal of progressively reintegrating the body as a whole. Founded in 1971 by Dr. Ida P. Rolf, the Rolf Institute of Structural Integration trains and certifies qualified practitioners of Rolfing (see Appendix B.)

### Myotherapy (Trigger Point Therapy)

Tender spots in muscles with spasm or abnormal tautness were described in ancient Chinese medicine. However, it was not until the 1940s that Dr. Janet Travell described a specific therapy for relieving muscular pain caused by these trigger points called *trigger point injection therapy*. This concept was later modified by physical fitness expert, Bonnie Prudden, into myotherapy, which uses sustained firm pressure to the trigger point to release the muscle spasm (3).

### Therapeutic Touch

This *energy field* technique developed by Doris Krieger, Ph.D., R.N., is used by nurses and other health care practitioners. Therapeutic Touch does not involve direct physical contact between practitioner and patient. Instead, the practitioner's hands are held 2 to 6 inches away from the patient and moved in a slow, rhythmic fashion to feel the patient's energy flow and blockages. The practitioner then uses the electromagnetic energy present in his or her hands to "balance" the perceived energy fields in the patient. Research has shown that Therapeutic Touch can increase hemoglobin, reduce pain, and help correct dysfunction of the autonomic nervous system (26).

### Reiki

*Reiki* is an ancient Japanese healing modality based on channeling healing energy through a practitioner's hands, with or without contact with the patient's body.

## Movement and Balance Therapies

The human body evolved in the context of vigorous daily exercise, and the need for regular aerobic activity remains essential for health. Movement therapies teach proper use and posture during activity so that strength and flexibility of the body are maintained without undue wear and tear. They also aim to balance activity with mental and physical relaxation, a necessity for managing stress, which is a growing factor in health and aging in the modern world.

Ancient Eastern cultures developed various forms of "moving meditation"—that is, active systems of movement, balance, and mental focus based on the theory of life energy flow. Similar movement therapies were not developed in the West until the early 1900s. Although the various movement and balance systems may require initial training from a qualified instructor, their ultimate value is in the continuing independent practice by the person. By contrast, bodywork achieves musculoskeletal and nervous system relaxation passively through a skilled therapist and is more often used on a limited basis for acute problems.

### Yoga

There is evidence that yoga postures and meditation were practiced in India 5,000 years ago. The physical aspects of yoga include a number of postures *(asanas)* and breath control techniques *(pranayama)*. The mental concentration necessary to achieve these physical elements serves as a mind–body link, which can ultimately lead to a meditative state.

Although all of the movement therapies focus on breathing to some extent, breathing is the essence of yoga. Breath is viewed as one with the life energy force and the spirit. Control of breathing allows access to its brain stem source and from there to the unconscious central and autonomic nervous system processes that are not ordinarily under conscious control. Andrew Weil advocates using breathing exercises on a daily basis, stating that "breath is the master key to health and wellness, a function we can learn to regulate and develop in order to improve our physical, mental, and spiritual well-being" (27). In fact, many studies have examined the health benefits of yoga, such as reducing blood lipids, lowering blood pressure, decreasing anxiety, and facilitating musculoskeletal rehabilitation (28–31).

The most traditional practice of yoga is intertwined with a philosophical–religious system that includes Ayurvedic medicine, diet, and meditation, and views the life energy flow as being organized through seven *chakras* or centers corresponding to nerve plexuses along the spine. In the United States, yoga is mostly used as a healthful form of mind–body exercise that keeps the body toned and flexible and teaches relaxation. There are three forms of yoga that are most commonly practiced in this country. *Hatha yoga* emphasizes stretching positions and breathing, which lead to relaxation of the nervous system. *Raja yoga* primarily focuses on meditation. *Ashtanga yoga,* popularized as "power yoga," consists of a flowing sequence of more strenuous yoga positions with breath control. Heightened concentration is necessary to get through the continuous moves, which end in a period of deep relaxation, but not meditation.

### Tai Chi Chuan

Tai chi is one form of qi gong, the daily exercise routine done by millions of people of all ages in China. This exercise system consists of a series of gentle, flowing movements performed while standing upright. Reflecting origins in Oriental martial arts, the slow, graceful motions of tai chi can build strength while simultaneously promoting balance and relaxation. The underlying principle is that mental focus on the energy flow directs the precision movements and synchronized breathing:

MIND *leads* > ENERGY *leads* > BODY

The basic formalized positions and sequence of tai chi movements may be performed in full, requiring 30 to 45 minutes, or in a short form taking as little as 5 minutes.

Senior citizens have been especially receptive to taking up tai chi because of its positive effects on maintaining mental concentration, physical flexibility, and balance. A number of clinical studies have demonstrated these benefits in the elderly (32–34).

### Alexander Technique

The first well known Western movement therapy was developed by Frederick Matthias Alexander (1869–1955) in an effort to restore his voice, which had begun to fail during his performances of Shakespeare's works. Doctors diagnosed laryngitis but had no therapeutic recommendations other than voice rest. By observing himself in a mirror while reciting, Alexander was able to correct his posture and head position in such a way that optimal breathing, reduction of muscular tension, and speaking ability occurred naturally. He spent 10 years perfecting his methods, which he extended into a hands-on therapy for performers and others seeking the health benefits of good posture. He trained other *Alexander teachers,* and use of his techniques spread throughout his native Australia to the United Kingdom and other Western countries in the early 1900s. The Society of Teachers of the Alexander Technique was established in Britain in 1958 to supervise standards for teacher training and certification. This function is carried out in the United States by the American Society for the Alexander Technique, which was founded in 1987 (see Appendix B).

The Alexander teachers use gentle touch and verbal guidance to make the client aware of deeply ingrained and unconscious postural habits. The same nonmanipulative touch and instruction are then used to help the client use conscious control to reeducate the muscle sense of movement and position so that the proper function feels normal and is automatically used. Alexander Technique is beneficial for anyone who desires better posture and body alignment for health purposes, but it is especially sought out by performers whose careers depend on optimal bodily function and control.

### Trager Work

The Trager method was originated by Dr. Milton Trager, a California physician, to release tension and promote flexibility in patients with neuromuscular disorders. Trager sessions are tailored to the individual needs of the client, who lies on table while the therapist uses gentle, rhythmic rocking manipulations of the limbs.

Trager work is classified as a movement therapy because the recipient is encouraged to enter a completely relaxed, even dreamlike state and allow the freer body movements being facilitated by the therapist to imprint on the unconscious mind. At the end of the session, the client is instructed in *Trager Mentastics,* which are gentle, mind-directed movements designed to maintain the flexibility achieved during therapeutic manipulation. The Trager Institute establishes standards of practice and a certification program for Trager practitioners (see Appendix B).

### Feldenkrais Work

This is a form of combined bodywork and movement therapy created by Moshe Feldenkrais (1904–1984), a Russian-born engineer, physicist, and martial arts expert. There is emphasis on a mind–body connection during movements, with the idea that moving the body in the desired way will reprogram the brain, which will in turn direct proper whole-body movement. There are two forms, one of which is passive and the other active. The passive form is called *functional integration* and consists of a trained practitioner gently manipulating the recipient's body into an improved pattern of motion. This method is especially useful for patients with spasticity, stroke, and developmental mental retardation. The more active form of Feldenkrais is *awareness through movement,* which is taught in group classes. Students are instructed in movements during which they consciously attend to what the body is doing. This technique is useful for physical rehabilitation but also is used by performers such as athletes, dancers, and musicians. The Feldenkrais Guild of North America was established in 1977 and certifies Feldenkrais practitioners (see Appendix B).

### Pilates Method

German-born Joseph Pilates originally designed this system of exercise to help rehabilitate bedridden soldiers when he served as a nurse in England during World War I. The underlying principle of Pilates is to strengthen the body by focusing on the "core strength" of the torso, particularly the abdomen and pelvis. Pilates later started an exercise studio in New York, where he expanded his method into a general fitness program that uses a series of slow, stretching movements coordinated with focused awareness of breathing, spinal alignment, and balance. Special equipment with a moving platform and springs is used for part of the process. Pilates' program still is used today for rehabilitation, but perhaps is more popular as a workout regimen in health clubs. Pilates is particularly attractive for dancers and athletes who seek strength and flexibility to support movement rather than build muscle bulk (see Appendix B).

## PSYCHOLOGICAL THERAPIES

Stress often is the mediating factor that activates the immune system in an inappropriate "fight-or-flight" pattern, which can result in an allergic flare state. When stress seems to be a major contributing factor in a patient's allergic diathesis, it is important to offer direction as to how that patient might deal with the pressures.

The young science of psychoneuroimmunology has done

much to elucidate a physiologic basis for the mind–body connection by studying biochemical interactions of the mind and nervous system with the immune and endocrine systems.

In the 1970s, research at the NIH revealed that endorphins, the neuropeptide messenger molecules found in the brain, also were present in the immune and endocrine systems and throughout the body. A positive emotional state was found to correlate with a higher concentration of endorphins in all parts of the body. It was discovered that the ability of a virus to enter a cell was inversely related to the amount of neuropeptides present in the immediate environment. This finding confirmed the conventional wisdom that emotional state directly influences a person's immune response to viral infections such as influenza, colds, and herpes (35).

Research by Dr. Robert Adler showed that conditioning could alter immune response. His work suggests that the human body often cannot distinguish actual threatening events from those events that are present only in the thoughts. This implies that a wide variety of internal and external stimuli can alter a previously established immune response, resulting in such phenomena as exacerbation of allergies, asthma, or hives, and other disturbances of the autonomic system (36).

## Meditation

Hans Selye's pioneering research on stress emphasized that there are two kinds of stress—positive stress and negative stress. The difference between the two lies in the person's perception of *control* of the stress (37).

The practice of *meditation* is one technique a person can use to obtain an increased sense of internal control. Meditation involves entering a level of altered consciousness that quiets the mind and relaxes the body. There is emphasis on attention to breathing, which calms and focuses the mind. Studies have shown that during Transcendental Meditation, the body develops a deeper state of relaxation than during ordinary rest, with reduction of heart rate, blood pressure, and cortisol level (the main physiologic response to stress) (38). At the same time, electroencephalogram monitoring shows heightened awareness. There are many health benefits to meditation, not the least of which is the proper oxygenation of body tissues from the breathing exercises and the deep relaxation response that is elicited. Even without meditation, the average person is able to achieve significant benefit by learning some simple breathing techniques that elicit this type of relaxation response.

## Hypnosis, Self-hypnosis, and Relaxation Techniques

*Hypnosis, self-hypnosis,* and *relaxation techniques* are some of the modalities associated with the use of conditioning techniques to neutralize stress. These techniques all emphasize the role of the patient as an active participant in healing, rather than a passive recipient of medical intervention.

## Biofeedback

*Biofeedback* training is a process of learning consciously to regulate normally unconscious bodily functions (heart rate, blood pressure) to correct malfunction. It involves anything that offers the patient feedback (immediate information) from the body system, enabling the patient to alter that function consciously (35).

Effects can be measured by a variety of sources, including skin temperature (reflects capillary blood flow), galvanic skin response (measures electroconductivity of skin), electromyography (monitors muscle tension), electroencephalography (monitors brain waves), and electrocardiography (monitors cardiac function). Electrodes are placed at appropriate points on the patient's body. The patient is then taught various relaxation responses that can be observed to affect the electrical activity being monitored. Once learned, the response may be used indefinitely in "real-life" situations to control anxiety and responses to stress. Biofeedback has been shown to be effective in controlling a variety of disorders, including insomnia, migraine, temporomandibular joint syndrome, asthma, and hypertension.

## MEDICOLEGAL ASPECTS

As physicians become more informed about CAM practices and the benefits they offer patients, professional communication and referral patterns will increase. Clarification of the evolving malpractice liability issues regarding CAM will facilitate this process. In 1998, Studdert et al. published a review of relevant legal principles and case law, and made suggestions for physicians to use as guidelines when referring to CAM practitioners (39).

On the positive side, CAM practitioners are sued less often and for injuries less severe than those incurred in suits against physicians. As alternative medicine specialties are licensed by states, they are judged by the standards of their own particular school of medicine, making it less likely that a referring physician will be involved in the case. In addition, as states establish licensure status for CAM specialties, they also are more likely to mandate health care insurance coverage for their services. This factor further reduces the likelihood of a referring physician being sued. The trend for expanding licensure status is demonstrated by five of the largest groups of CAM practitioners (39).

- Chiropractors are licensed in all 50 states and District of Columbia; 42 states mandate coverage of chiropractic services in health insurance policies.
- Acupuncturists are licensed in 35 states; 7 states mandate health insurance coverage.

- Massage therapists are licensed in 27 states.
- Naturopaths are licensed in 12 states and Puerto Rico.
- Homeopaths are licensed in four states.

The following are causes for physicians being sued for referring to alternative medicine practitioners:

- If the physician's decision to refer the patient is *negligent* and the patient suffers *injury* related to the *substandard referral*. Besides physical harm, injury can include the referral delaying, decreasing, or eliminating the opportunity for the patient to receive other important care. A substandard referral includes referral made to a CAM practitioner who is known to be incompetent or the subject of disciplinary action by a professional board.
- The referring physician can be held liable for the treating CAM practitioner's negligence if the care given is a *joint undertaking* or the physician maintains a supervisory role over the patient's treatment.

Knowing these litigation risk circumstances, a physician referring to a CAM practitioner should make sure of certain conditions beforehand (39):

- Is there evidence to suggest that the therapy to be received by the patient as a result of the referral will offer no benefit or will subject the patient to unreasonable risks?
- Know the CAM practitioner to whom you are referring:

Does he or she have state licensure? Is he or she covered by malpractice insurance? Do you have any knowledge that the practitioner is incompetent or substandard?

- It should be made clear to the patient and the CAM practitioner that the referring physician's role in no way will involve supervision of the CAM treatment.

## CONCLUSION

Discussing the modern medicolegal aspects of using old or ancient medical practices inspires a certain perspective. For all the technological and biomedical advances that humankind has achieved, the human mind and body have not evolved beyond the fundamental needs that are met with a holistic and natural approach to health. Integrative medicine is an opportunity for physicians to take a most interesting and exciting trip "back to the future"—all aboard?

## APPENDIX A. SOURCES OF NATURAL REMEDIES

*Note:* Most of the supplement manufacturers listed here have Web sites that can be reached by using their name as a keyword or search phrase.

| Supplement/Dose | Source | Allergy Considerations |
|---|---|---|
| *Quercetin + C*<br>One to two capsules two times/day | TwinLab<br>Can be easily found in health food stores, or ordered from vitamin discount companies | Bioflavonoid derived from blue-green algae; vitamin C derived from sago palm (i.e., avoids citrus and corn) |
| *Fresh freeze-dried nettle leaf*<br>One to two capsules q2–4h as needed | Eclectic Institute, Inc. (888) 799-4372<br>Usually found in health food stores | Some patients complain of itching and increased nasal congestion, requiring stopping use |
| *Fresh Preparation Garlic*<br>    Garlinase 4000 | Enzymatic Therapy—health food stores, mail order companies | Garlic has anticoagulant effect, can potentiate pharmaceutical anticoagulant agents |
|     Garlitrin 4000<br>    One to two tablets/day | PhytoPharmica, sold to pharmacies and health care professionals (800) 553-2370 | |
| *Herpilyn* | Enzymatic Therapy—health food stores, mail order companies | Active ingredient is 1% allantoin from comfrey plant |
| *Herpalieve*<br>Apply to lesions two to four times a day, or as often as needed | PhytoPharmica—sold to pharmacies and health care professionals (800) 553-2370 | Contains *Melissa* extract (lemon balm), which also has antiviral properties |
| *Deglycyrrhizinated licorice*<br>    DLG (chocolate mint flavor) | Enzymatic Therapy—health food stores, mail order companies | Rhizinate comes in a sugar-free tablet as well as chocolate mint flavor |
|     Rhizinate<br>    Apply to lesions two to four times a day or as often as needed | PhytoPharmica—sold to pharmacies and health care professionals (800) 553-2370 | Licorice is a legume but is not known to cross-react with soy, peanuts, or other legumes |
| *Citricidal grapefruit seed extract*<br>    NutriBiotic Liquid Concentrate<br>    Five to ten drops mixed in 5 oz water. Swish and swallow two or three times a day | NutriTeam, Inc. (800) 785-9791<br>Usually found in health food stores | Derived from citrus |
| *Milk thistle (silymarin)*<br>    Milk Thistle X | Enzymatic Therapy—health food stores, mail order companies | Member of Asteraceae or Compositae family—may cross-react with ragweed |
|     Silybin Phytosome<br>    One or two tablets/day | PhytoPharmica—sold to pharmacies and health care professionals (800) 553-2370 | |
| *Herbal antiinflammatory mixture*<br>    Inflavonoid Intensive Care<br>    One or two tablets two times a day | Metagenics (800) 321-6382 Sold to health care professionals | Contains bioflavonoids derived from citrus<br>Cayenne pepper—*Solanaceae*, also contains *Boswellia*, ginger, turmeric, quercetin |

## APPENDIX B. DATABASES

There are numerous World Wide Web sites for complementary and alternative medicine, most of which can be accessed with keywords or search phrases. The following are several CAM Web sites with hyperlinks to other CAM-related Web sites with comprehensive databases.

**NCCAM, NIH**

http://nccam.nih.gov

The National Center for Complementary and Alternative Medicine, National Institutes of Health

**IBIDS**

http://odp.od.nih.gov/ods/databases/ibids.html

International Bibliographic Information on Dietary Supplements (IBIDS) is a database of published, international, scientific literature on dietary supplements, including vitamins, minerals, and botanicals.

Produced by the Office of Dietary Supplements at the National Institutes of Health

**PubMed**

http://www.ncbi.nlm.nih.gov/PubMed

National Library of Medicine's search service to access the 9 million citations in MEDLINE, and Pre-MEDLINE, and other related databases.

**Rosenthal Center for Complementary and Alternative Medicine**

http://cpmcnet.columbia.edu/dept/rosenthal/Botanicals.html

Rosenthal Center for Complementary and Alternative Medicine Columbia University, College of Physicians and Surgeons

**HerbMed**

http://www.herbmed.org

Evidence-based resource for herbal information, with

hyperlinks to clinical and scientific publications. Designed for the needs of physicians and pharmacists.

## Information Sources

### Acupuncture

The American Association of Acupuncture and Oriental Medicine (AAOM) is the umbrella organization representing the acupuncture profession in the United States. It is closely associated with the National Commission for the Certification of Acupuncturists and Oriental Medicine (NCCAOM). AAOM members are regarded as the highest qualified practitioners of Oriental medicine in the United States.

The American Academy of Medical Acupuncture (AAMA) is a physician-only professional acupuncture society in North America. Full-practice members of AAMA must have an active license to practice medicine under U.S. or Canadian jurisdiction as an M.D., D.O., or equivalent, as well as credentials showing adequate training in acupuncture.

AAOM
433 Front Street 5820
Catasauqua, PA 18032
(888) 500-7999
http://www.aaom.org
AAMA
Wilshire Boulevard, Suite 500
Los Angeles, CA 90036
(800) 521-2262 or (323) 937-5514
http://www.medicalacupuncture.org

### Alexander Technique

The American Society for the Alexander Technique (AmSAT) is the largest professional organization for teachers of the Alexander Technique in the United States. AmSAT also establishes and maintains standards for teacher training and certification. Membership requirements include 1,600 hours of training over a 3-year period in an AmSAT-approved teacher training program. For information or to obtain a list of Certified Alexander Teachers, contact:

American Center for the Alexander Technique
39 W. 14th Street, Room 507
New York, NY 10011
(212) 633-2229
American Society for the Alexander Technique
P.O. Box 60008
Florence, MA 01062
(800) 473-0620 or (413) 584-2359
http://www.alexandertech.org

### Ayurvedic Medicine

Although traditionally trained Ayurvedic physicians can be found, most Ayurvedic medicine practiced in the United States is Maharishi Vedic Medicine. This modernized version of Ayurveda is taught in a worldwide network of universities. The College of Maharishi Vedic Medicine in Fairfield, Iowa offers a bachelor's degree in Maharishi Vedic Medicine and a Ph.D. degree in Physiology with Specialization in Maharishi Vedic Medicine. The Center for Natural Medicine and Prevention, currently supported by an $8 million grant from the NIH, conducts the research program associated with the College of Maharishi Vedic Medicine.

College of Maharishi Vedic Medicine
1603 N. 4th Street
Fairfield, IA 52556
(641) 472-4600
http://mum.edu/CMVM

### Chiropractic

Chiropractors are easily found in most parts of the country. For more information on chiropractic or a list of chiropractors practicing in your locality, contact:

American Chiropractic Association
1701 Clarendon Blvd.
Arlington, VA 22209
(703) 276-8800
http://www.amerchiro.org

### Feldenkrais Method

The Feldenkrais Professional Training Program is a 3- to 4-year program leading to professional certification as a Feldenkrais Practitioner.

Feldenkrais Guild of North America
3611 SW Hood Avenue, Suite 100
Portland, OR 97201
(800) 775-2118 or (503) 221-6612
http://www.feldenkrais.com

### Homeopathy

There are many training programs in homeopathy and there are different certifying boards for the practice of homeopathy, depending on whether the applicant is an M.D., D.O., naturopath, chiropractor, or a lay person. Even so, no state recognizes any diploma or certificate from these schools as a license to practice homeopathy. For information on homeopathy and to locate practitioners, contact:

The National Center for Homeopathy (NCH)
801 North Fairfax Street, Suite 306
Alexandria, VA 22314
(877) 624-0613 or (703) 548-7790
http://www.homeopathic.org

## Massage Therapy

The American Massage Therapy Association (AMTA) is the professional organization that represents this field. Members of the AMTA have graduated from a program accredited by the Commission on Massage Therapy Accreditation (COMTA), which requires a minimum training of 500 hours of classroom instruction. Certification by the National Certification Board for Therapeutic Massage and Bodywork is an indication that the therapist has the required hours of education, has passed a comprehensive written examination, and is qualified to enter the field. So far, 29 states and the District of Columbia regulate and license massage therapists.

> American Massage Therapy Association
> 820 Davis Street, Suite 100
> Evanston, IL 60201
> (847) 864-0123
> http://www.amtamassage.org

## Naturopathic Medicine

Membership in the American Association of Naturopathic Physicians (AANP) ensures that the N.D. degrees of their members meet the educational criteria for licensure.

> American Association of Naturopathic Physicians (AANP)
> 8201 Greensboro Drive, Suite 300
> McLean, VA 22102
> (703) 610-9037
> http://www.naturopathic.org

## Osteopathy

The American Academy of Osteopathy is the professional organization of osteopaths who practice manipulation as a major method of treatment.

> American Academy of Osteopathy
> 3900 DePauw Boulevard, Suite 1080
> Indianapolis, IN 46268
> (317) 879-1881
> http://www.academyofosteopathy.org

## Pilates Method

Pilates, Inc., in New York City can provide information about Pilates, including a list of Pilates-certified studios.

> The Pilates, Inc.
> 2121 Broadway, Suite 201
> New York, NY 10023
> (800) 474-5283, or (212) 875-0189 in New York City
> http://www.pilates-studio.com

## Rolfing

The Rolf Institute is the only certifying body for Rolfers. Certification enables graduates of the training program to become members of The Rolf Institute and qualified to practice under the title of Certified Rolfer or Rolf Movement Practitioner.

> The Rolf Institute
> 205 Canyon Boulevard
> Boulder, CO 80302
> (800) 530-8875 or (303) 449-5903
> http://www.rolf.org

## Trager Work

The Trager Institute establishes standards of practice and certification program for practitioners.

> The Trager Institute
> 33 Millwood
> Mill Valley, CA 94941
> (415) 388-2688
> http://www.trager.com

## REFERENCES

1. Weil A. Testimony before Congressional Subcommittee on Labor, Health and Human Services and Education. Washington, DC, March 28, 2000.
2. Eisenberg DM, Davis RB, Ettner SL, et al. Trends in alternative medicine use in the United States, 1990–1997. *JAMA* 1998;280:1569–1575.
3. Shealy CN, ed. *The complete family guide to alternative medicine.* Rockport, MA: Element Books, 1996.
4. Vithoulkas G. *The science of homeopathy.* New York: Grove Press, 1980:104.
5. Oakley GP Jr. Eat right and take a multivitamin. *N Engl J Med* 1998;338:1060–1061.
6. Kaltsas HJ. Patent poisons: buyers beware. On-line: http://www.alternativemedicine.com./digest/issue32/chimed.shtml.
7. Weil A. Learning the mysteries of Tibetan medicine? On-line: http://www.pathfinder.com/drweil.com.
8. Halpern G. Do Western science and traditional Chinese medicine mix? Year 2000 Florence Strauss Lecture. Presented at the University of Colorado Health Science Center, Denver, CO, May 5, 2000.
9. World Wildlife Fund. On-line: http://www.wwf.org.
10. McCaleb R. Boosting immunity with herbs. The Herb Research Foundation. On-line: http://www.ibiblio.org/herbs/immune.html.
11. Mittman P. Randomized double-blind study of freeze-dried *Urtica dioica* in the treatment of allergic rhinitis. *Planta Med* 1990;56:44–47.
12. Nobel S. Daily application of the homeopathic remedy Zicam Allergy Relief significantly improves the quality of life and impairment in patients with seasonal allergic rhinitis. *Internet J Fam Pract* 2000;1(1). On-line: http://www.ispub.com/journals/IJFP.
13. Melchart D, et al. Immunomodulation with echinacea: a systematic review of controlled clinical trials. *Phytomedicine* 1994;1:245–254.

14. Hirt M, Nobel S, Barron E. Zinc nasal gel for the treatment of common cold symptoms: a double-blind placebo-controlled trial. *Ear Nose Throat J* 2000;79:778–780.

15. Zarembo JE, et al. Zinc(11) in saliva: determination of concentrations produced by different formulations of zinc gluconate lozenges containing common excipients. *J Pharm Sci* 1992;81(22): 128–130.

16. Wolbling RH, Leonhardt K. Local therapy of herpes simplex with dried extract from *Melissa officinalis. Phytomedicine* 1994; 1:25–31.

17. Muller-Fassbender H, et al. Glucosamine sulfate compared to ibuprofen in osteoarthritis of the knee. *Osteoarthritis Cartilage* 1994;2:61–69.

18. Forster KK, et al. Longer term treatment of mild to moderate osteoarthritis of the knee with glucosamine sulfate: a randomized, controlled, double-blind clinical study. *Eur J Clin Pharmacol* 1996;50:542.

19. Press release, 66th Annual Meeting of the American Academy of Orthopedic Surgeons, Anaheim, CA, February 5, 1999.

20. National Institutes of Health Consensus Panel. *Acupuncture: National Institutes of Health Consensus Development Statement.* Bethesda, MD: National Institutes of Health, November 3–5, 1997.

21. Han JS, Wang Q. Mobilization of specific neuropeptides by peripheral stimulation of identified frequencies. *News Physiol Sci* 1992:176–80.

22. Nambudripad DS. Nambudripad's allergy elimination techniques. On line: www.naet.com, 2001.

23. Cutler E. Bioset: the ultimate allergy cure. On line: www.drellencutler.com, 2001.

24. Kaptchuk TJ, Eisenberg DM. Chiropractic: origins, controversies, and contributions. *Arch Intern Med* 1998;158:1.

25. Scafidi FA, Field T, Schanberg SM. Factors that predict which preterm infants benefit most from massage therapy. *J Dev Behav Pediatr* 1993;14:176–180.

26. Glick MS. Caring touch and anxiety in myocardial infarction patients in intermediate cardiac care unit. *Intensive Care Nurs* 1986;(2):61–66.

27. Weil A. *Natural health, natural medicine,* rev. ed. New York: Houghton Mifflin, 1995.

28. Schmidt T, et al. Changes in cardiovascular risk factors and hormones during a comprehensive residential three month kriya yoga training and vegetarian nutrition. *Acta Physiol Scand Suppl* 1997; 640:158–162.

29. Vedanthan PK, et al. Clinical study of yoga techniques in university students with asthma: a controlled study. *Allergy Asthma Proc* 1998;19:3–9.

30. Garfinkel MS, et al. Yoga-based intervention for carpal tunnel syndrome: a randomized trial. *JAMA* 1998;280:1601–1603.

31. Garfinkel M, Schumacher HR. Yoga. *Rheum Dis Clin North Am* 2000;26:125–132.

32. Kessenich CR. Tai chi as a method of fall prevention in the elderly. *Orthop Nurs* 1998;17(4):27–29.

33. Lin YC, Wong AM, Chou SW, et. al. The effects of tai chi chuan on postural stability in the elderly: preliminary report [English abstract]. *Chang Keng I Hsueh Tsa Chih* 2000;23:197–204.

34. Lan C, Lai JS, Chen SY, et. al. Tai chi chuan to improve muscular strength and endurance in elderly individuals: a pilot study. *Arch Phys Med Rehabil* 2000;81:604–607.

35. Goldberg B. *Alternative medicine: the definitive guide.* Puyallup, WA: Future Medicine Publishing, 1998.

36. Adler R, Cohen N. Behaviorally conditioned immunosuppression. *Psychosom Med* 1997;37:333–340.

37. Selye H. *Stress without distress.* New York: Penguin, 1975.

38. Shapiro DH, Walsh RN. *Meditation: classic and contemporary perspectives.* New York: Aldine, 1984.

39. Studdert DM, Eisenberg DM, et al. Medical malpractice implications of alternative medicine. *JAMA* 1998;280:1610–1615.

## BIBLIOGRAPHY

**Jellin JM, Batz F, Hitchens K.** *Pharmacists's letter/prescriber's letter natural medicines comprehensive database.* Stockton, CA: Therapeutic Research Faculty, 1999.

*PDR for herbal medicines.* Montvale, NJ: Medical Economics Company, 1998.

**Tyler VE.** *Herbs of choice: the therapeutic use of phytomedicinals.* Binghamton, NY: The Haworth Press, 1994.

# A RESEARCH AGENDA FOR OTOLARYNGIC ALLERGY

## JOHN H. KROUSE
## BERRYLIN J. FERGUSON

Although the diagnosis and treatment of allergic diseases has been conducted for over a century, there are still many questions that remain unanswered. We have developed a number of effective treatment protocols based on observation and clinical experience, and have begun to characterize the immunologic mechanisms involved in these interventions. In this textbook, we have presented a number of these strategies, as well as the basic and clinical science supporting them.

The purpose of this final chapter is to examine some of the areas for future investigation in the field of otolaryngic allergy. There are many questions in both the science and the practice of our discipline that remain unanswered. These issues form the framework for many research inquiries over the next decade. This chapter reviews a number of these potentially fruitful areas.

## BASIC SCIENCE

### Mechanisms of Immunotherapy

In the past several years, there has been an increase in our knowledge of many of the underlying mechanisms involved in the allergic response. Much of this research has focused on a group of polypeptide proinflammatory agents known as *cytokines*. These agents have been shown to be important mediators in both seasonal and perennial allergic rhinitis (1, 2), and variations in the levels of specific cytokines known as *interleukins* have been shown in the onset and clearance of its symptoms. For example, Hayashi et al. (3) demonstrated a significant increase in interleukin-5 (IL-5) during pollen season compared with preseasonal levels in patients with allergic rhinitis. Similar elevations have been noted in both IL-4 and IL-5 by a number of researchers (4,5).

The specific mechanism involved in the therapeutic improvement in patients treated with inhalant desensitization immunotherapy has been an area of interest for many years. In the traditional view of immunotherapy, injections are thought to stimulate the production of an immunoglobulin G4 (IgG4)–blocking antibody that is involved in modulating specific IgE and therefore reducing sensitivity to antigens. Although such a mechanism may well contribute to the therapeutic effects seen in immunotherapy, it does not fully explain the events that do occur.

Several researchers have begun to examine the effects of immunotherapy on various cytokines. Ohashi and colleagues, for example, examined levels of specific IgE and IL-4 in patients with seasonal allergic rhinitis treated with immunotherapy (5). Their patients were divided into immunotherapy and pharmacotherapy groups, and assessed both before and during allergy season for Japanese cedar pollen. The researchers found that among patients treated with pharmacotherapy, there was a seasonal rise in specific IgE and IL-4 and a decrease in interferon-γ that corresponded with the pollen season. In the immunotherapy group, however, there was no change in any of these three factors during the allergy season. In addition, levels of specific IgE and IL-4 differed significantly between good responders and poor responders to immunotherapy.

In another study, Lu and colleagues examined the effects of immunotherapy on children with atopic asthma (6). In their study, patients sensitive to dust mite antigen, a perennial allergen, were treated over an 8-month period. The authors demonstrated that both IL-4 and IL-10 levels decreased after immunotherapy. In addition, IgG4 antibody to dust mite increased at 8 months after the initiation of immunotherapy. The authors also noted that serum levels of IL-13 increased with immunotherapy. They noted that IL-13 has an effect on inducing IgG4 production by B cells, and concluded that IL-13 may play a role in the generation of IgG4-blocking antibodies during immunotherapy.

In another study of the efficacy of immunotherapy, Durham and colleagues examined the effects of grass pollen

**J. H. Krouse:** Department of Otolaryngology, Wayne State University, Detroit, Michigan.

**B. J. Ferguson:** Department of Otolaryngology, University of Pittsburgh School of Medicine, Pittsburgh, Pennsylvania.

desensitization on the differential responses of type 1 (Th1) and type 2 (Th2) T helper lymphocytes (7). The authors noted that immunotherapy inhibited the expression of IL-4 and IL-5 by Th2 lymphocytes, while enhancing the local concentration of protective Th1 cells in the tissues. These findings suggest that immunotherapy may exert effects directly on T-cell function in a highly selective manner. Additional researchers have also examined the immunologic basis of immunotherapy, focusing on both cytokines and T-cell function and modulation (8–12).

In addition, although studies have shown the efficacy of immunotherapy for allergic rhinitis in the short term (13, 14), less is known about the maintenance of treatment effects after the cessation of therapy. A recent study has shown that after the administration of grass pollen immunotherapy over a 3- to 4-year period, clinical remission of symptoms can be maintained for at least 3 years (15). Long-term follow-up of patients treated with immunotherapy for allergic rhinitis clearly is necessary to assess the maintenance of clinical effects over time.

There is a great deal more information that would be relevant to understanding the mechanisms involved in inhalant desensitization immunotherapy. For example, it often has been observed that the onset of symptomatic improvement is more rapid in patients treated with immunotherapy based on skin endpoint titration than with other types of skin testing. A precise appreciation of the mechanisms involved in the efficacy of immunotherapy and their temporal behavior would allow a more objective determination of the validity of this frequent observation. In addition, the development of a temporal sequence of the kinetics involved in this process also would allow better prediction of the outcomes of immunotherapy, and assist in determining whether a patient is being adequately treated.

In addition, a comparison of various therapeutic modalities would be possible with a better appreciation of the mechanisms involved in immunotherapy. Objective appraisals of the efficacy of such diverse methods as oral immunotherapy, sublingual immunotherapy, and enzyme-potentiated desensitization (EPD) would also be possible. Further, an examination of immunotherapy based on differing in vivo and in vitro testing methods could be conducted. Objective serum markers for the evaluation of immunotherapy would be of great use in both clinical and research applications.

## Allergic Disease and Sleep

Research also has demonstrated the physiologic role of various cytokines in the regulation of sleep. The nocturnal rise and fall of various cytokines during sleep has been demonstrated in both normal and sleep-deprived subjects, yet the significance of these effects has not yet been determined. It is well known that sleep patterns frequently are disturbed in patients with increased upper airway resistance due to

allergic rhinitis and obstructive sleep apnea, yet the role of cytokine regulation in these patients has not been studied. It is unclear how sleep varies in patients with seasonal allergic rhinitis during pollen season compared with their preseasonal sleep patterns. Variations in sleep architecture and continuity may be profoundly altered during pollen season and significantly contribute to symptoms of malaise, fatigue, and decreased concentration exhibited by the allergic patient.

It further appears that the restorative functions of sleep may affect immunologic functioning (16). IL-1β also has been shown to be involved in physiologic regulation of sleep (17). The administration of exogenous IL-1β induces increased non–rapid eye movement sleep, whereas inhibition of IL-1β reduces spontaneous sleep. Uthgenannt and colleagues investigated the effects of sleep on IL-1β and IL-2 (16). They noted that as sleep proceeds through the night, levels of IL-1β diminish over time. In addition, production of IL-2 was enhanced during sleep, with this effect limited to the late nocturnal sleep phase, after 3:00 A.M.

It is frequently observed that among patients with allergic rhinitis, nasal complaints are more commonly noted on awakening than they are for the remainder of the day. Smolensky and colleagues confirmed this circadian variation of nasal congestion, sneezing, blocked nose, and rhinorrhea (18), and noted that an understanding of the mechanisms involved in this variability could maximize therapy among patients with allergic rhinitis. This morning symptomatology has been attributed to dust mite exposure in the bedroom overnight. In addition, patients with allergic rhinitis often are bothered by daytime somnolence, with significant effects on mood and daytime functioning. Although these daytime symptoms have been attributed to medication effects, it appears that the nighttime effects on sleep commonly seen in patients with nasal congestion and rhinitis may worsen these symptoms of fatigue (19).

The relationship between allergic rhinitis and sleep is a fruitful area for research over the next decade. Not only is the relationship important to understand in normal sleep, but in patients with sleep-disordered breathing and sleep apnea as well. In addition, the effects of various medications such as sedating and nonsedating antihistamines on sleep have not been fully examined. A better understanding of sleep in allergic patients may provide additional insight into the observed quality-of-life impairment common in patients with allergic rhinitis.

## CLINICAL SCIENCE

### Relationships with Concurrent Disease Processes

It has been clinically observed that patients with allergic diseases have a higher prevalence of certain other chronic diseases. This relationship has been well documented for several of these processes, but less well so for others. For example, it is well appreciated that patients with allergic rhinitis and other upper respiratory symptoms have a higher incidence of lower respiratory allergies and asthma (20). This finding has been well documented in both children and adults.

Several other diseases are seen more commonly in allergic patients than in nonallergic individuals. Several researchers have noted an increased prevalence of thyroid disease among patients with inhalant allergy, postulating a higher degree of autoimmunity among these people (21,22). Allergic symptoms often can be exacerbated in hypothyroid patients, and can be more difficult to treat. Screening for thyroid disease therefore is indicated in patients undergoing treatment for allergic rhinitis. In addition, many patients with inhalant allergy also complain of abdominal pain, reflux, diarrhea, and other gastrointestinal symptoms. There may be additional physical illnesses that are seen more frequently in patients with allergic rhinitis.

In addition, there has been a reported association between psychiatric disease and inhalant allergies. Although direct pathophysiologic relationships have been noted between chronic allergic disease and illnesses such as anxiety and depression (23,24), it is far more common for physicians to dismiss the physical, allergic basis of many disease processes as "functional somatic syndromes," and to attempt to treat them with behavioral or psychotropic interventions (25).

Krouse and Krouse (26) presented some preliminary work investigating the prevalence of various concurrent illnesses among patients with allergic rhinitis. In this study, the authors examined a group of patients who were skin-test positive for inhalant allergy with a contrast group of patients with cerumen impaction. They noted a higher frequency of several medical illnesses among allergic patients, as well as the more common use of various medications. Allergic patients had a higher incidence of sinusitis, hypothyroidism, and pulmonary diseases than nonallergic patients. In addition, allergic patients were treated more commonly not only with antihistamines and nasal steroids, as expected, but with thyroid replacement therapy and psychoactive medications. In fact, patients with inhalant allergy were treated three times as frequently with psychoactive medications. These findings suggest not only a higher prevalence of anxiety and depression among allergic patients, but that physicians may use these medications to treat the psychiatric manifestations of their disease, rather than recognizing the allergic and immunologic basis of their symptoms.

This preliminary study suggests that additional research is necessary to clarify the associations between allergic disease and other medical and psychiatric conditions. Initially, descriptive research would be indicated to assess these various interrelationships, and to explore other areas that may be yet unrecognized. Once these areas have been better char-

acterized, the effect of allergy management on these related chronic illnesses can be investigated.

## Oral/Sublingual Immunotherapy

An area of controversy in the treatment of both inhalant and food allergy has been the use of orally or sublingually administered sera for desensitization and neutralization. These approaches have found more common use in Europe than they have in the United States, and have been demonstrated in many studies to be both safe and efficacious (27, 28). Sublingual and oral therapies, however, are in general not well accepted by physicians in the United States.

This therapeutic option has potential benefit, but is not widely understood. Research is necessary both to describe the mechanisms involved in oral/sublingual immunotherapy, as well as to document the clinical safety and efficacy of the approach. This research provides an important area for additional study over the next decade.

## Enzyme-potentiated Desensitization

Another modality that has been introduced in recent years has been EPD. In this type of immunotherapy, β-glucuronidase is used as an immune response modulator to potentiate the effect of the antigenic treatment (29,30). Very small amounts of antigens to be treated are added to the β-glucuronidase, and a single injection is given before the onset of pollen season. Early studies in Europe have suggested that EPD can be effective in the treatment of seasonal allergy when used in a preseasonal manner. Several studies have shown changes in various cytokine levels in response to therapy.

Proponents of EPD believe that its utility is far broader than in the treatment of seasonal inhalant allergy. In fact, they believe that EPD may be of benefit in the treatment of diseases ranging from food sensitivities to rheumatoid arthritis. Although these claims are offered by proponents of the techniques, there is an absence of supporting research in the literature. This area of treatment must therefore be viewed currently as unsubstantiated. Controlled, double-blind studies are necessary to further examine the role of EPD not only in seasonal and perennial allergy, but in food sensitivities and related disorders.

## Immunostimulatory Conjugation

Recognizing the risks associated with immunotherapy, researchers have attempted chemically to modify antigens to decrease the likelihood of adverse reactions and anaphylaxis. In general, these attempts have been unsuccessful because of the decreased immunomodulatory effects of these modified antigens and their failure to provide symptomatic relief. One study has used immunostimulatory DNA fragments as adjuvants in stimulating the immune response (31). In this study, a short DNA fragment was coupled with ragweed antigen to enhance its immunogenicity. In this study performed with mice, this modified antigen was able to stimulate Th1 activity with secretion of interferon gamma, without stimulation of Th2 activity (IL-5 secretion). In addition, this modified antigen did not stimulate histamine release. There is a great potential for clinical use of this strategy in immunotherapy, with the maintenance of therapeutic activity without the accompanying risk of anaphylaxis. Additional work in both animals and humans is necessary to investigate further and develop this novel mechanism.

## Allergic Fungal Sinusitis

The recognition of allergic fungal sinusitis (AFS) as an important disease process continues to increase among otolaryngologists. A study by Ferguson and colleagues (32) shows that the incidence of AFS among patients treated with surgical therapy for chronic rhinosinusitis can be as high as 23%. This incidence is much higher in the southern United States than it is elsewhere in the country. The disease is recurrent despite aggressive medical and surgical treatment, often requiring numerous procedures to keep patients free of symptoms (33).

Recent work by Mabry and colleagues has strongly suggested that immunotherapy for fungal antigens can be an important adjunct in the treatment of patients with AFS (34,35). In their small clinical series, the authors noted no recurrence of symptoms of AFS with standard surgical debridement followed by immunotherapy. This area of research provides promise for providing long-term control among patients with this chronic disease. Prospective, controlled research studies are underway to examine this area scientifically. Additional work is necessary to characterize further the role of immunotherapy and other treatment methods in the management of patients with AFS.

## Id (Dermatophytid) Reaction

One of the clinical entities described by otolaryngic allergists is that of the id or dermatophytid reaction. In this entity, the presence of a cutaneous fungal process in one body site provokes an eczematoid eruption at another site distant from that involved by the primary infection. Although no fungus can be recovered from the distant symptomatic site, fungal organisms can be recovered at the primary site. Treatment for id reactions is offered through desensitization therapy for cutaneous fungal antigens through the use of TOE (*Trichophyton,* Oidiomycetes, and *Epidermophyton*) (36,37).

Despite the frequent observation of this phenomenon by otolaryngic allergists, its precise mechanism has never been described. In fact, there have been very few studies that have investigated this area scientifically. The id reaction may be a real pathologic entity, or it may be an artifactual observation. The specific pathophysiologic process of this phenom-

enon has not been determined. Research is necessary to confirm this observed process and describe its pathologic mechanism.

## Therapeutic Uses of Histamine

Otolaryngic allergists have used histamine both sublingually and subcutaneously for the treatment of both inhalant and food allergies. A number of physicians have thought that it has excellent utility with a very good safety profile. In fact, the use of low-dose histamine has been recommended for the treatment of disorders such as Bell's palsy, vertigo, headaches, and urticaria (38).

Unfortunately, there has never been a randomized, double-blind study that has investigated the efficacy of histamine therapy for the treatment of allergic symptoms. King reviewed 100 patients retrospectively, and described the use of low-dose histamine as a safe and effective treatment for a variety of disorders, but again this review suffers from being retrospective and lacking scientific controls (38). In addition, the mechanism by which such a treatment protocol would work has not been adequately described.

Although there appears to be clinical experience that suggests the efficacy of low-dose histamine therapy, a prospective, randomized, controlled, double-blind trial is necessary to demonstrate objectively that more than a placebo effect is functional in this treatment. Although it will admittedly be difficult to blind the histamine administration, an appropriate methodology must be implemented to answer this clinical question in a scientific manner.

## Novel Therapeutic Approaches

With the advance of our understanding of the molecular and cellular mechanisms involved in the immunology of allergic disease, it is clear that creative new therapeutic mechanisms may be developed to advance the treatment of these disorders. These interventions can be targeted to various points in the pathophysiologic mechanisms of allergy, and may show broad effectiveness with excellent safety.

With the increasing awareness of the importance of antigen-presenting cells (or antigen-processing cells), pharmacotherapeutic interventions could be directed toward these cells, disabling the presentation of antigens to T cells for processing. In addition, antiinterleukin medications also could be effective in preventing the cascade of immunologic events that lead to the development of symptoms. Alternately, the administration of exogenous interleukins such as IL-12 could downregulate the immune response through inhibiting the production of IgE antibodies, as demonstrated by Lee and colleagues (39). In addition, monoclonal antibodies directed toward IgE would present another approach to the control of allergic disease on the molecular level (40).

These are but a few of the areas that would be important

for future research. By controlling the development of the allergic response at the earliest cellular levels rather than blocking the symptoms with antihistamines and antiinflammatory medications, physicians would have the opportunity to provide a real cure of the hypersensitivity reactions associated with allergy. This area clearly will be important for research in the next decade and beyond.

## COST EFFECTIVENESS

In this era of rising concerns over the costs of health care, it is becoming increasingly important to document not only the clinical efficacy of various treatment modalities, but the relative costs of these treatment options. With decisions regarding health care being made frequently not by physicians or patients, but by the insurers themselves, certain medications or interventions will be approved with consideration of their economic impact as a key element of that decision.

### Costs of Pharmacotherapy

Not all medications offer the same therapeutic benefits and safety profiles. This statement is clearly true of antihistamines. Although sedating antihistamines are available for purchase over the counter (OTC) at costs less than those for nonsedating prescription antihistamines, there are more side effects to the OTC preparations than with the currently available nonsedating and minimally sedating medications. Managed care organizations have noted this price differential, and have advised the use of short-acting nonsedating antihistamines during the day and sedating medications at night. The flaw in this philosophy has been noted in a significant "hangover" effect of residual somnolence in the morning on awakening.

Another important issue is the optimal method for the prescription of pharmacotherapy for allergic rhinitis and related diseases. Not all patients need to be treated with several medications; a single agent may control the symptoms adequately and do so in a more cost-effective manner. The proper use of antihistamines and nasal steroid sprays reflects one such situation. It has been shown that although nonsedating antihistamines are both the most commonly used and the most expensive medications for treating nasal allergies, nasal steroid sprays have better efficacy at less cost (41). The concurrent use of the oral and nasal medications is of minimal addictive benefit, and adds significantly to the cost of therapy. Additional research is indicated to examine the proper use of pharmacotherapeutic agents and their impact on the costs of health care.

### Costs of Immunotherapy

An additional area for research involves the costs of immunotherapy. There has been little work done to investigate the direct costs of immunotherapy relative to other methods of treating allergic disease. For example, is immunotherapy a cost-effective management strategy compared with pharmacotherapy? The demonstration of the safety and efficacy of immunotherapy in combination with its cost effectiveness would be an important addition to otolaryngic allergy practice. One such study was recently published on the German experience, which showed significant savings in both direct and indirect costs with immunotherapy over a 10-year period (42). Additional studies of this focus are important in further clarifying the costs of immunotherapy.

Another related area concerns the cost effectiveness of various testing strategies for inhalant allergy. The use of screening panels for both skin testing and in vitro assays has been recommended as one method of decreasing the cost of allergy testing. Obviously, issues related to sensitivity of these screens become important in this discussion. A cost–benefit analysis of various screening panels in the detection of significant inhalant allergy would be very useful.

Along the same line of thought, the ideal number of antigens for testing and treatment has not been determined. Patients may be tested and treated for as few as 15 to 20 allergens, or as many as 50 or more allergens, depending on the allergist treating them. There are no good data investigating whether there is significant clinical advantage to panels with large numbers of antigens versus those with smaller numbers of allergens. One study demonstrated that patients with multiple inhalant allergies responded similarly to immunotherapy whether all positive antigens were included, or only a subset of those antigens (14). Do we see significant incremental improvement in patients with a panel of two to three times larger than that used in other patients? The efficacy of various panels and their related costs would also be an important clinical issue for assessment over the next decade.

## CONCLUSION

The issues discussed in this chapter are but a few areas that would be relevant for research over the coming years. They are meant to be only a broad canvas for topics in both clinical and basic science, and in the economics of treatment. As otolaryngic allergists, we must remain at the forefront of research, and strive to confirm our clinical observations with thoughtful, well designed research methodologies.

## REFERENCES

1. Fireman P. Cytokines and allergic rhinitis. *Allergy Asthma Proc* 1996;17:175.
2. Bachert C, van Kempen M, Van Cauwenberge P. Regulation of proinflammatory cytokines in seasonal allergic rhinitis. *Int Arch Allergy Immunol* 1999;118:375–379.

3. Hayashi M, Ohashi Y, Tanaka A, et al. Suppression of seasonal increase in serum interleukin-5 is linked to the clinical efficacy of immunotherapy for seasonal allergic rhinitis. *Acta Otolaryngol Suppl (Stockh)* 1998;538:133–142.

4. Moverare R, Rak S, Elfman L. Allergen-specific increase in interleukin (IL)-4 and IL-5 secretion from peripheral blood mononuclear cells during birch-pollen immunotherapy. *Allergy* 1998; 53:275–281.

5. Ohashi Y, Nakai Y, Okamoto H, et al. Serum level of interleukin-4 in patients with perennial allergic rhinitis during allergen-specific immunotherapy. *Scand J Immunol* 1996;43:680–686.

6. Lu FM, Chou CC, Chiang BL, et al. Immunologic changes during immunotherapy in asthmatic children: increased IL-13 and allergen-specific IgG4 antibody levels. *Ann Allergy Asthma Immunol* 1998;80:419–423.

7. Durham SR, Ying S, Varney VA, et al. Grass pollen immunotherapy inhibits allergen-induced infiltration of CD4+ T lymphocytes and eosinophils in the nasal mucosa and increases the number of cells expressing messenger RNA for interferon-gamma. *J Allergy Clin Immunol* 1996;97:1356–1365.

8. Benjaponpitak S, Oro A, Maguire P, et al. The kinetics of change in cytokine production by CD4 T cells during conventional allergen immunotherapy. *J Allergy Clin Immunol* 1999;103:468–475.

9. Ishii K, Asakura K, Kataura A. Effects of immunotherapy on cytokine production from peripheral blood mononuclear cells in patients with house dust mite allergic rhinitis. *Arerugi* 1999;48: 480–485.

10. Ohashi Y, Nakai Y, Okamoto H, et al. Serum level of interleukin-4 in patients with perennial allergic rhinitis during allergen-specific immunotherapy. *Scand J Immunol* 1996;43:680–686.

11. Tanaka A, Ohashi Y, Kakinoki Y, et al. Immunotherapy suppresses both Th1 and Th2 responses by allergen stimulation, but suppression of the Th2 response is a more important mechanism related to the clinical efficacy of immunotherapy for perennial allergic rhinitis. *Scand J Immunol* 1998;48:201–211.

12. Ohashi Y, Nakai Y, Tanaka A, et al. Allergen-specific immunotherapy for allergic rhinitis: a new insight into its clinical efficacy and mechanism. *Acta Otolaryngol Suppl (Stock)* 1998;538: 178–190.

13. Varney VA, Gaga M, Frew AJ, et al. Usefulness of immunotherapy in patients with severe summer hay fever uncontrolled by antiallergic drugs. *BMJ* 1991;302:265–269.

14. Krouse JH, Krouse HJ. Efficacy of immunotherapy based on skin end-point titration. *Otolaryngol Head Neck Surg* 2000;123: 183–187.

15. Durham SR, Walker SM, Varga EM, et al. Long-term clinical efficacy of grass-pollen immunotherapy. *N Engl J Med* 1999;341: 468–475.

16. Uthgenannt D, Schoolmann D, Pietrowsky R, et al. Effects of sleep on the production of cytokines in humans. *Psychosom Med* 1995;57:97–104.

17. Kreuger JM, Fang J, Taishi P, et al. Sleep: a physiologic role for IL-1 beta and TNF-alpha. *Ann NY Acad Sci* 1998;856:148–159.

18. Smolensky MH, Reinberg A, Labrecque G. Twenty-four hour pattern in symptom intensity of viral and allergic rhinitis: treatment implications. *J Allergy Clin Immunol* 1995;95:1084–1096.

19. Craig TJ, Teets S, Lehman EB. Nasal congestion secondary to allergic rhinitis as a cause of sleep disturbance and daytime fatigue and the response to topical nasal corticosteroids. *J Allergy Clin Immunol* 1998;101:633–637.

20. Borish L. Genetics of allergy and asthma. *Ann Allergy Asthma Immunol* 1999;82:413–424.

21. Heymann WR. Chronic urticaria and angioedema associated with thyroid autoimmunity: review and therapeutic implications. *J Am Acad Dermatol* 1999; 40:229–232.

22. Lindberg B, Ericsson UB, Fredriksson B, et al. The coexistence of thyroid autoimmunity in children and adolescents with various allergic disease. *Acta Paediatr* 1998;87:371–374.

23. Anderson JL. The immune system and major depression. *Adv Neuroimmunol* 1996;6:119–129.

24. Addolorato G, Marsigli L, Capristo E, et al. Anxiety and depression: a common feature of health care seeking patients with irritable bowel syndrome and food allergy. *Hepatogastroenterology* 1998;45:1559–1564.

25. Barsky AJ, Borus JF. Functional somatic syndromes. *Ann Intern Med* 1999;130:910–921.

26. Krouse JH, Krouse HJ. Concurrent medical illnesses in patients skin-test positive for allergy. Presented at the Annual Meeting of the American Academy of Otolaryngic Allergy, New Orleans, Louisiana, September 23–25, 2000.

27. Andre C, Vatrinet C, Galvain S, et al. Safety of sublingual-swallow immunotherapy in children and adults. *Int Arch Allergy Immunol* 2000;121:229–234.

28. Clavel R, Bousquet J, Andre C. Clinical efficacy of sublingual-swallow immunotherapy: a double-blind, placebo-controlled trial of a standardized five-grass-pollen extract in rhinitis. *Allergy* 1998; 53:493–498.

29. Ippoliti F, Ragno V, Del Nero A, et al. Effect of preseasonal enzyme potentiated desensitisation (EPD) on plasma-IL-6 and IL-10 of grass pollen-sensitive asthmatic children. *Allerg Immunol (Paris)* 1997;120:123–125.

30. Di Stanislao C, Di Berardino L, Bianchi I, et al. A double-blind, placebo-controlled study of preventive immunotherapy with E.P.D., in the treatment of seasonal allergic disease. *Allerg Immunol (Paris)* 1997;29:39–42.

31. Tighe H, Takabayashi K, Schwartz D, et al. Conjugation of immunostimulatory DNA to the short ragweed allergen amb a 1 enhances its immunogenicity and reduces its allergenicity. *J Allergy Clin Immunol* 2000;106:124–134.

32. Ferguson BJ, Barnes L, Bernstein JM, et al. Geographic variation in allergic fungal rhinosinusitis. *Otolaryngol Clin North Am* 2000; 33:441–449.

33. Kuhn FA, Javer AR. Allergic fungal sinusitis: a four-year follow-up. *Am J Rhinol* 2000;14:149–156.

34. Mabry RL, Mabry CS. Allergic fungal sinusitis: the role of immunotherapy. *Otolaryngol Clin North Am* 2000;33:433–440.

35. Mabry RL, Marple BF, Mabry CS. Outcomes after discontinuing immunotherapy for allergic fungal sinusitis. *Otolaryngol Head Neck Surg* 2000;122:104–106.

36. Derebery J, Berliner KI. Foot and ear disease—the dermatophytid reaction in otology. *Laryngoscope* 1996;106:181–186.

37. Iglesias ME, Espana A, Idoate MA, et al. Generalized skin reaction following tinea pedis (dermatophytids). *J Dermatol* 1994; 21:31–34.

38. King WP. The use of low-dose histamine therapy in otolaryngology. *Ear Nose Throat J* 1999;78:366–370.

39. Lee YL, Fu CL, Ye YL, et al. Administration of interleukin-12 prevents mite Der p 1 allergen-IgE antibody production and airway eosinophil infiltration in an animal model of airway inflammation. *Scand J Immunol* 1999;49:229–236.

40. Adelroth E, Rak S, Haahtela T, et al. Recombinant humanized mAb-E25, an anti-IgE mAb, in birch pollen-induced seasonal allergic rhinitis. *J Allergy Clin Immunol* 2000;106:253–259.

41. Stempel DA, Thomas M. Treatment of allergic rhinitis: an evidence-based evaluation of nasal corticosteroids versus nonsedating antihistamines. *Am J Manag Care* 1998;4:89–96.

42. Schadlich PK, Brecht JG. Economic evaluation of specific immunotherapy versus symptomatic treatment of allergic rhinitis in Germany. *Pharmacoeconomics* 2000;17:37–52.

# SUBJECT INDEX

*Note:* Page numbers followed by *f* indicate figures; page numbers followed by *t* indicate tables.

**437**